ACUTE MYELOGENOUS LEUKEMIA

CONTEMPORARY HEMATOLOGY

Judith E. Karp, MD, Series Editor

ACUTE MYELOGENOUS LEUKEMIA

Edited by

JUDITH E. KARP, MD

*The Sidney Kimmel Comprehensive Cancer Center
at Johns Hopkins, Baltimore, MD*

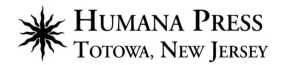

HUMANA PRESS
TOTOWA, NEW JERSEY

© 2007 Humana Press Inc.
999 Riverview Drive, Suite 208
Totowa, New Jersey 07512

humanapress.com

For additional copies, pricing for bulk purchases, and/or information about other Humana titles, contact Humana at the above address or at any of the following numbers: Tel: 973-256-1699; Fax: 973-256-8341; E-mail: orders@humanapr.com; website at humanapress.com

Due diligence has been taken by the publishers, editors, and authors of this book to ensure the accuracy of the information published and to describe generally accepted practices. The contributors herein have carefully checked to ensure that the drug selections and dosages set forth in this text are accurate in accord with the standards accepted at the time of publication. Notwithstanding, as new research, changes in government regulations, and knowledge from clinical experience relating to drug therapy and drug reactions constantly occurs, the reader is advised to check the product information provided by the manufacturer of each drug for any change in dosages or for additional warnings and contraindications. This is of utmost importance when the recommended drug herein is a new or infrequently used drug. It is the responsibility of the health care provider to ascertain the Food and Drug Administration status of each drug or device used in their clinical practice. The publisher, editors, and authors are not responsible for errors or omissions or for any consequences from the application of the information presented in this book and make no warranty, express or implied, with respect to the contents in this publication.

This publication is printed on acid-free paper. ∞
ANSI Z39.48-1984 (American National Standards Institute)
Permanence of Paper for Printed Library Materials.

Production Editor: Rhukea J. Hussain

Cover Illustration: Inset: Fig. 1, panels A and B from Chapter 14

Cover design by: Donna Niethe

Library of Congress Cataloging-in-Publication Data

Acute myelogenous leukemia / edited by Judith Karp.

    p. ; cm. -- (Contemporary hematology)

  Includes bibliographical references and index.

  ISBN-13: 978-1-58829-621-4 (alk. paper)

  ISBN-10: 1-58829-621-0 (alk. paper)

1. Acute myeloid leukemia. I. Karp, Judith. II. Series.

  [DNLM: 1. Leukemia, Myelocytic, Acute. WH 250 A1896 2007]

  RC643.A325 2007

  616.99'419071--dc22

                  2006039397

To my beloved husband, Stanley H. Freedman,
for unwavering support, understanding, and humor.

To my mentors: Stanley Schrier, MD, Philip J. Burke, MD, and Samuel Broder, MD.

To our patients, who give us the humility and inspiration to do better.

PREFACE

Acute myelogenous leukemia (AML) is a complex family of malignancies for which we need new treatment concepts and agents in order to increase the cure rates for all who suffer with these diseases. On the clinical level, AML is an important and devastating malignancy that affects all ages. On a biological level, AML is an outstanding model for understanding cancer biology and the challenges of cancer therapy in general.

This is an exciting time in leukemia research. The elegant basic science discoveries that have emerged over the preceding two decades are now leading to a heightened understanding of leukemia at its basic genetic and biochemical roots. This understanding in turn provides a springboard for developing new therapies that can modulate important factors in leukemia cell development and survival. There is a burgeoning application of new molecular concepts to the development of drugs that target critical leukemia-sustaining factors. In turn, there is rapid movement of these newly developed agents into the clinical testing arena and eventually into the effective armamentarium against AML.

The aim of *Acute Myelogenous Leukemia* is to bring new concepts and findings in the basic and clinical science of AML together "under one cover." This juxtaposition should serve basic and clinical investigators who are interested in AML with information that reaches from new concepts regarding leukemia pathogenesis to current and prospective advances in molecular therapeutics. This is the theme of Ravandi and Giles' overview chapter—the bidirectional flow of knowledge between the clinic and the laboratory, with the overarching goal of increasing AML cure rates.

Part II, Molecular Foundations of AML Pathogenesis and Pathophysiology, focuses on specific genetic lesions that disrupt the normal growth and survival in hematopoietic stem cells and subvert the cellular machinery to prevent differentiation and death. Toward that end, Friedman (Chapter 2) examines the disruption of orderly transcriptional regulation as a key mechanism of leukemogenesis, leading to loss of the normal obligatory link between proliferation, terminal differentiation and cell death. The next two chapters provide additional powerful insights into the complex process of leukemogenesis by discussing the multistep cellular changes that occur when AML evolves from myelodysplasia (Parker and Mufti, Chapter 3) or when it arises in the setting of previous cytotoxic therapies (Godley and LeBeau, Chapter 4). In Chapter 5, Steensma addresses the formative role that diminished repair of DNA damage (as exemplified by familial syndromes with heightened leukemia risk) can play in both the initiation and perpetuation of genomic instability, whereas in Chapter 6, Mesa and Kaufmann discuss the critical contributions of altered apoptotic responses to cellular stress to AML cell survival and inherent drug resistance. In the final chapter in this section, Ross expands on the issue of drug resistance as related to diverse transporter proteins that protect cells, perhaps most importantly stem cells, from cytotoxic drugs.

Part III emphasizes translation of AML biology into clinical application. In this context, Grimwade (Chapter 8) addresses the formative impact of specific cytogenetic aberrations (and, by extrapolation, the molecular results of those aberrations) on understanding clinical biology and individual prognosis. In no disease is this so well exemplified as in acute progranulocytic leukemia (APL), and Frankfurt et al., in Chapter 9, provide a detailed discussion of this remarkably sensitive disease and the "bench-to-bedside" (and back again) investigations that exemplify "molecular medicine" at its finest.

The theme of molecular medicine is carried forth in Part IV, beginning with Sausville's (Chapter 10) overview of mechanistically novel agents, both cytotoxic and "biological," that target selected key molecules or pathways and are now in clinical development for AML. This informative overview is followed by discussions of new agents that interrupt specific signal transduction effectors such as FLT-3 (Levis, Chapter 11) and farnesyltransferase (Lancet, Chapter 12), modulate the expression of inappropriately silenced genes by inhibiting DNA methyltransferases and/or histone deacetylases (Fandy et al., Chapter 13), and overcome the blockade to differentiation that characterizes the leukemic cell (Lin and Matsui, Chapter 14). The final two chapters of this section focus on immunomodulatory approaches including stem cell transplantation (Bolaños-Meade and Jones, Chapter 15) and vaccine development (Borrello, Chapter 16).

AML is a heterogenous disease and, as such, there are issues that demand special thera-peutic considerations. In this regard, Arceci (Chapter 17) addresses the unique biology of pediatric AML including distinctive drug development issues such as age-specific pharmaco-logical metabolism, the implications of long-term sequelae that may not arise in adults, and the importance of risk-stratification in clinical trial design. At the other end of the spectrum, Stone (Chapter 18) presents the unique challenges of treating AML in the elderly, where both host and disease factors contribute to an especially poor prognosis and where new strategies are desperately needed. In Chapter 19, Gotlib discusses the recently discovered *JAK2* mutation that serves as a unifying thread among the disparate family members of the so-called myelo-proliferative disorders, a group of myeloid malignancies that has been considered to be hetero-geneous but with a high propensity to evolve into AML.

Finally, as we continue to uncover new molecular pathways, we in turn develop new drugs to exploit and modulate those pathways. In the last chapter, Estey addresses the conun-drum that conventional clinical trials designs and classical clinical endpoints may not be applicable to effective and efficient drug development, and that new paradigms are needed to address the complexities underlying clinical outcome and response to new agents.

In summary, progress in curing AML will come ultimately from both an enhanced un-derstanding of the molecular foundations of these diseases and from rigorous clinical and correlative laboratory testing of new agents that alter those molecular foundations. I hope that *Acute Myelogenous Leukemia* will stimulate the reader to think about the diverse molecular components of AML pathogenesis and pathophysiology as a basis for new treatment strategies and multimodality approaches. It is through fluent translation between the laboratory and the clinic that we will be able to change the face of AML from a devastating disease to a highly curable one.

Judith E. Karp, MD

CONTENTS

CONTRIBUTORS

Robert J. Arceci • Director and King Fahd Professor of Pediatric Oncology,
  Kimmel Comprehensive Cancer Center at Johns Hopkins, Baltimore, Maryland
Javier Bolaños-Meade • Assistant Professor of Oncology, Sidney Kimmel Comprehensive
  Cancer Center at Johns Hopkins, Baltimore, Maryland
Ivan Borrello • Sidney Kimmel Comprehensive Cancer Center at Johns Hopkins, Balti-
  more, Maryland
Hetty Carraway • Division of Hematologic Malignancies, Sidney Kimmel Comprehensive
  Cancer Center at Johns Hopkins, Baltimore, Maryland
Elihu Estey • Leukemia Department, University of Texas M.D. Anderson Cancer Center,
  Houston, Texas
Tamer Fandy • Division of Hematologic Malignancies, Sidney Kimmel Comprehensive
  Cancer Center at Johns Hopkins, Baltimore, Maryland
Olga Frankfurt • Division of Hematology and Oncology, Northwestern University
  Feinberg School of Medicine, Robert H. Lurie Comprehensive Care Center
  of Northwestern University, Chicago, Illinois
Alan D. Friedman • Division of Pediatric Oncology, Johns Hopkins University,
  Baltimore, Maryland
Robert Gallagher • Montefiore Medical Center, Albert Einstein School of Medicine,
  Bronx, New York
Francis Giles • Department of Leukemia, University of Texas M.D. Anderson Cancer
  Center, Houston, Texas
Lucy A. Godley • Section of Hematology/Oncology and the University of Chicago Cancer
  Research Center, University of Chicago, Chicago, Illinois
Steven D. Gore • Associate Professor of Oncology, Division of Hematologic Malignancies,
  Sidney Kimmel Comprehensive Cancer Center at Johns Hopkins, Baltimore, Maryland
Jason Gotlib • Assistant Professor of Medicine (Hematology), Stanford Cancer Center,
  Stanford, California
David Grimwade • Department of Medical and Molecular Genetics, King's College
  London, and Department of Haematology, University College London Hospitals,
  London, United Kingdom
Richard J. Jones • Professor of Oncology, Sidney Kimmel Comprehensive Cancer Center
  at Johns Hopkins, Baltimore, Maryland
Scott H. Kaufmann • Division of Oncology Research, Mayo Clinic, Rochester, Minnesota
Jeffrey E. Lancet • Hematologic Malignancies Program, Department of Interdisciplinary
  Oncology, H. Lee Moffitt Cancer Center and Research Institute, University of South
  Florida, Tampa, Florida
Michelle M. Le Beau • Section of Hematology/Oncology and the University of Chicago
  Cancer Research Center, University of Chicago, Chicago, Illinois
Mark Levis • Sidney Kimmel Comprehensive Cancer Center at Johns Hopkins, Baltimore,
  Maryland
Tara L. Lin • Division of Hematologic Malignancies, Sidney Kimmel Comprehensive
  Cancer Center at Johns Hopkins, Baltimore, Maryland

William Matsui • Division of Hematologic Malignancies, Sidney Kimmel Comprehensive
    Cancer Center at Johns Hopkins, Baltimore, Maryland
Ruben A. Mesa • Division of Hematology, Mayo Clinic, Rochester, Minnesota
Jane E. Parker • Department of Haematological Medicine, Norfolk & Norwich University
    Hospital, Norwich; Guy's, King's Thomas' School of Medicine, London,
    United Kingdom; King's College Hospital, King's College London, United Kingdom
LoAnn C. Peterson • Division of Pathology, Northwestern University Feinberg School
    of Medicine, Robert H. Lurie Comprehensive Care Center of Northwestern University,
    Chicago, Illinois
Farhad Ravandi • Department of Leukemia, University of Texas M.D. Anderson Cancer
    Center, Houston, Texas
Douglas D. Ross • Program in Experimental Therapeutics, University of Maryland
    Marlene and Stewart Greenebaum Cancer Center, the Division of Hematology
    and Oncology, Department of Medicine, University of Maryland School of Medicine,
    Baltimore, Maryland, and the Baltimore Veterans Affairs Medical Center, Baltimore,
    Maryland
Edward A. Sausville • University of Maryland Marlene and Stewart Greenebaum Cancer
    Center, Baltimore, Maryland
David P. Steensma • Division of Hematology, Mayo Clinic, Rochester, Minnesota
Richard M. Stone • Clinical Director, Adult Leukemia Program, Dana Farber Cancer
    Institute, Associate Professor of Medicine, Harvard Medical School, Boston,
    Massachusetts
Martin S. Tallman • Division of Hematology and Oncology, Northwestern University
    Feinberg School of Medicine, Robert H. Lurie Comprehensive Care Center
    of Northwestern University, Chicago, Illinois

COLOR PLATES

Color plates follow p. 174

I OVERVIEW OF AML

1

Approaching the Treatment of AML from a Biological Perspective

An Overview

Farhad Ravandi and Francis Giles

CONTENTS

Summary

Current acute myeloid leukemia (AML) therapy is inadequate for the great majority of patients. Major challenges are peculiar to the elderly and the infirm. There is no prospect of further advances using current standard agents. At our current state of knowledge, all potential classes of agents merit clinical investigation. However, the empirical approach can certainly be refined by the application of recent data on the pathophysiology of AML, its molecular biology, the aberrations that drive the proliferative and antiapoptotic leukemia advantages, and the study of resistance to standard and novel agents. In this chapter we review some of the more promising novel agents in AML.

Key Words: Refractory; cloretazine; troxacitabine; clofarabine; mTOR; farnesylation; monoclonal antibodies; alkylating agents; nucleosides.

1. INTRODUCTION

Acute myelogenous leukemia (AML) is a highly heterogeneous group of diseases, and this diversity is reflected in the range of agents and approaches required for curative therapy *(1)*. The complexity and diversity of these diseases in terms of etiology and pathogenesis underlies the inadequate clinical results, namely the significant proportion of patients who are not cured by conventional cytotoxic regimens. Novel design of clinical studies may allow better allocation of different agents to different AML subgroups *(2)*. In this overview, we will review some of the more promising agents that we believe may advance AML therapy. These agents have been developed to a large degree from our enhanced understanding of leukemia biology on the molecular as well as clinical levels. Many agents will have multiple

From: *Contemporary Hematology: Acute Myelogenous Leukemia*
Edited by: J. E. Karp © Humana Press Inc., Totowa, NJ

cellular targets. For the sake of organization, we have arbitrarily divided our discussion into three areas: agents with more traditional cytotoxic activity, agents with putative biological modes of action, and agents that target cellular signaling pathways involved in cell proliferation, survival, and/or apoptosis. Many of these agents will be discussed in greater detail in subsequent chapters.

2. NUCLEOSIDE ANALOGS

Nucleoside analogs have been widely used in treatment of hematological malignancies. Generally, they gain entry into cells by a carrier and are then converted to their active metabolites by enzymes such as deoxycytotidine kinase (dCK). After they are incorporated, they inhibit DNA polymerase, which leads to decreased DNA synthesis and repair. Cytotoxicity correlates linearly with incorporation into DNA. Termination of the activity of nucleoside analogs is through their inactivation by enzymes such as deoxycytidine deaminase (dCD) or cytoplasmic 5-nucleotidase. Resistance to the antileukemic action of nucleoside analogs occurs either because of overexpression of the inactivating enzymes or because of suppression of the metabolizing enzymes. Modification of nucleoside analogs has led to new compounds that are similar in structure but that induce different antileukemic activity.

2.1. Clofarabine

Clofarabine (2-chloro-2-fluoro-deoxy-9–β-D-arabinofuranosyladenine) is a hybrid drug that retains the 2-halogenated aglycone of fludarabine and cladribine, which renders those analogs resistant to deamination by adenosine deaminase. A fluorine molecule at the $2'$-position of the carbohydrate inhibits the effect of purine nucleoside phosphorylase Clofarabine is metabolized to clofarabine $5'$-triphosphate. Clofarabine $5'$-triphosphate decreases cell replication and repair and causes cell death. To decrease cell replication and repair, clofarabine $5'$-triphosphate competes with deoxyadenosine triphosphate for the enzymes ribonucleotide reductase and DNA polymerase. Cell replication is decreased when clofarabine $5'$-triphosphate inhibits the reaction of ribonucleotide reductase with deoxyadenosine triphosphate to produce deoxynucleotide triphosphate, which is needed for DNA synthesis *(3)*.

In phase I studies, AML patients were administered an intravenous dose of 55 mg/m^2 of clofarabine over 1 hour each day for 5 days: every 3–6 weeks was the dose-limiting toxicity. The recommended dose for acute leukemia studies in adults was 40 mg/m^2 daily for 5 days *(4)*. In 32 patients with refractory or relapsed acute leukemia, the response rate was 16%, including 2 complete remissions (CRs) and 3 with marrow remission without a platelet recovery *(4)*. In a phase II study 62 patients with relapsed or refractory acute leukemia, high-risk myelodysplastic syndrome (MDS), or chronic myelogenous leukemia (CML) in blast phase (CML-BP) were treated with clofarabine 40 mg/m^2 daily for 5 days *(5)*. Seventeen of 31 (55%) patients with AML, 4 of 8 (50%) patients with MDS, and 7 of 11 (64%) patients with CML-BP achieved CR. Another 9 patients (15%) achieved CR without full platelet recovery.

Grade 3 and 4 toxicities included skin rashes, transient liver dysfunction, and nausea and vomiting *(5)*. More recently, the combination of clofarabine and ara-C was investigated in a phase I and II study *(6)* in 32 patients with relapsed acute leukemia, as follows: 25 patients with AML, 2 with acute lymphocytic leukemia (ALL), 4 with high-risk MDS, and 1 with CML-BP were treated with clofarabine 40 mg/m^2 given as a 1-hour intravenous infusion for 5 days (days 2–6) followed 4 hours later by ara-C at 1 g/m^2 per day as a 2-hour intravenous infusion for 5 days (days 1–5). Among all patients, 7 (22%) achieved CR, and 5 (16%) achieved

CR with incomplete platelet recovery, for an overall response rate of 38%. No responses occurred in 3 patients with ALL and CML. One patient (3%) died during induction. Adverse events were mainly grade 1 and 2, including transient liver test abnormalities, nausea and vomiting, diarrhea, and skin rashes. The authors concluded that the combination of clofarabine with ara-C is safe and active *(6)*.

In a phase I study in pediatric patients with refractory and relapsed leukemia, clofarabine was infused intravenously over 1 hour each day for 5 days. Six dosages between 11.25 and 70 mg/m^2 per day were evaluated in 25 patients. Five patients achieved CR, and 3 achieved partial response PR, for an overall response rate of 32%. The authors concluded that clofarabine is well tolerated and shows significant antileukemic activity in heavily pretreated children *(7)*. Clofarabine has been approved by the U.S. Food and Drug Administration (FDA) for pediatric patients with relapsed ALL.

2.2. Troxacitabine

All nucleoside analogs currently approved as anticancer agents exist in the D configuration *(8)*. Until recently the L-enantiomer nucleosides were thought not to have antineoplastic activity. The discovery of lamivudine as a potent inhibitor of human immunodeficiency virus led to the realization that unnaturally configured nucleoside analogs could be metabolized by humans, leading to the development of L-enantiomers as anticancer agents *(9,10)*. Exchange of the sulfur endocyclic atom with an oxygen in the structure of lamivudine resulted in the formation of troxacitabine. Troxacitabine was the first nucleoside L-enantiomer to show significant activity in myeloid leukemia *(11–13)*. Troxacitabine is activated by the enzyme dCK but is resistant to inactivation by dCD *(14,15)*.

In a phase I trial, Giles et al. reported that 42 patients with refractory or advanced hematological malignancies, 31 patients with AML, 6 patients with MDS, and 1 patient with CML-BP received escalating doses of troxacitabine. The maximum tolerated dose was 8 mg/m^2/day for 5 days. Three CR and one PR were observed in 30 evaluable patients with AML. Dose-limiting toxicities were stomatitis and hand–foot syndrome *(16)*.

In a phase II trial, troxacitabine 8 mg/m^2/day iv was tested in 42 patients with refractory or relapsed hematological malignancies *(12)*. Among the 16 evaluable patients, 2 patients had CR and 1 had PR *(12)*; the response rate was 37% in 16 patients with CML-BP. Combinations of troxacitabine with other cytotoxic agents (ara-C, idarubicin, or topotecan) were evaluated in patients with refractory AML, advanced MDS, or CML-BP *(13)*. Among 74 evaluable patients with AML or MDS, 10 (13%) achieved CR *(13)*. That group included 7 CR in 66 patients with AML: 4 with troxacitabine and ara-C, 2 with troxacitabine and idarubicin, and 1 with troxacitabine and topotecan. Four additional patients with AML achieved hematological improvement; all had received troxacitabine and ara-C *(13)*.

A randomized prospective study of troxacitabine plus ara-C (TA), troxacitabine plus idarubicin (TI), and ara-C plus idarubicin (IA) was conducted in newly diagnosed AML patients (≥50 years) with unfavorable karyotypes *(17)*. The CR rates were 10/18 (55%) for IA, 5/11 (45%) for TA, and 1/5 (20%) for TI. The IA group had a better cytogenetic profile, lower incidence of antecedent hematological disorder, and worse performance status than did patients who received TA and TI. No definite conclusions regarding the possibility of imbalances in the distribution of important prognostic covariates could be made because of the small number of patients randomized. Overall, troxacitabine-based regimens were not superior to standard induction chemotherapy *(17)*. New studies exploring the role of troxacitabine in treating patients with leukemia are in progress.

2.3. Epigenetic Therapy

Considerable data suggest that, in addition to genetic alteration, aberrant epigenetic regulation, such as silencing of tumor suppressors, is used by cancer cells to escape growth and death control mechanisms *(18–21)*. Hypermethylation of the promoters of genes such as p15 has been associated with disease progression and with worse outcome in myeloid malignancies *(22,23)*. Several agents—DNA methyl transferase inhibitors (DNMT) (e.g., decitabine and 5-azacytidine) and histone deacetylase inhibitors (phenylbutyrate, trichostatin A, SAHA, valproic acid, and depsipeptide)—are under investigation as single agents or for use in combination *(24–26)*. Decitabine (5-aza-2-deoxycitidine, DAC) is a pyrimidine analog that is activated by dCK and incorporated into DNA strands by a DNA polymerase. Once incorporated into DNA, decitabine irreversibly inhibits DNAMT enzymes that methylate newly synthesized DNA. In leukemia cells, this leads to the hypomethylation of the promoters of tumor suppressor genes, their activation, and cell differentiation *(27–30)*.

Decitabine is effective for treating patients with relapsed or refractory myeloid leukemias *(30–33)*. In a phase I study, 130 patients with CML, 64 patients in CML-BP, 51 with accelerated phase, and 8 with chronic phase received decitabine at a dose of 50–100 mg/m^2 every 12 hours for 5 days *(34,35)*. Eighteen of the 64 CML-BP patients (28%) achieved objective responses, including 6 CR, 2 partial recovery (PR), 7 hematological improvements, and 2 with return to chronic phase. Among the 51 patients with accelerated phase CML and the 8 patients with chronic phase CML, 28 (55%) and 5 (63%), respectively, achieved objective responses. The estimated 3-year survival rate was <5% in the blast phase and 27% in the accelerated phase *(35)*. The only significant toxicity was myelosuppression, which was delayed, dose dependent, and prolonged. Prolonged myelosuppression has been the dose-limiting toxicity of decitabine in other studies *(36–38)*. Decitabine has been used with amsacrine and idarubicin, and significant responses have been reported *(39,40)*.

Issa et al. investigated the "optimal biological dose" to achieve hypomethylation with minimal toxicity in patients with relapsed or refractory myeloid malignancies *(41)*. Fifty patients were treated with 5 mg/m^2 daily for 10 days, and the dose was increased to 10, 15, and 20 mg/m^2 daily for 10 days. Other cohorts received 15 mg/m^2 daily for 15 and 20 days. The drug was well tolerated, although there were 2 deaths from neutropenic sepsis and 8 asymptomatic elevations of liver indices. The overall response rate was 32%; 9 patients had CR and 7 had PR *(42)*. Eight of 35 (23%) patients with AML, 4 of 7 (57%) with MDS, and 4 of 5 (80%) with CML-BP achieved a response. The recommended dose for phase II and combination studies was 15 mg/m^2 for 10 days because dose and regimen were associated with the greatest responses.

Decitabine and the related drug 5-azacytidine (AZA) have significant activity in MDS. Silverman et al. conducted a randomized controlled trial of 191 MDS patients who either received AZA 75 mg/m^2 per day subcutaneously for 7 days every 28 days or were given supportive care *(43)*. Patients were allowed to cross over from the supportive care group to AZA upon disease progression. Responses were seen in 60% of patients treated with AZA (7% CR, 16% PR, 37% hematological improvement) compared to 5% in the supportive care ($p < 0.001$). The median time to transformation to AML or death was 21 months with AZA and 13 months with supportive care ($p = 0.007$). Landmark analysis after 6 months (to adjust for the confounding effect of early crossover to AZA) showed a significant improvement in survival for patients who received AZA (median 18 months vs 11 months: $p = 0.03$ *[43]*). Quality of life improved significantly with AZA *(44)*.

The use of decitabine has been investigated in elderly patients with MDS *(45,46)*. Sixty-six patients were administered a dose of 45 mg/m^2 per day for 3 days every 6 weeks for a maximum of six cycles *(46)*. The overall response rate was 49%. Patients with a high risk score for MDS on the international prognostic scoring system (IPSS) had a response rate of 64%. The median response was 31 weeks, and median survival times from diagnosis and from the start of therapy were 22 and 15 months, respectively *(46)*. Disappearance of chromosomal abnormalities present before start of therapy and reversal of hypermethylation were seen in the responding patients *(47–49)*.

Wijermans et al. have reported similar responses in 169 patients (median age 70) with intermediate or high-risk MDS *(50)*. The researchers reported a response rate of 49%, a median response duration of 40 weeks (95% CI 34.9–45.1 weeks), and a median survival of 15 months (95% CI 12.3–17.7 months). In a phase III trial, 170 patients with MDS (31% intermediate-1, 44% intermediate-2, 26% high risk disease by IPSS) were randomized either to receive decitabine in a 3-hour infusion (89 patients) at a dose of 15 mg/m^2 per hour every 8 hours for 3 days every 6 weeks or to receive supportive care (81 patients) *(51)*. The response rate was 17% for DAC (9% CR; 8% PR) compared with 0 for supportive care ($p < 0.001$). Durable responses occurred in all IPSS groups, lasting for a median of 9 months. Quality of life, including global health status, fatigue, and dyspnea, improved in the DAC group *(51)*.

The enzyme histone deacetylase (HDAC) acts by removing the acetyl group from DNA promoters to allow tighter binding of the histones to the DNA and prevent gene transcription. Several translocations in AML involve abnormal recruitment HDAC to promoters, leading to transcriptional repression *(52–55)*. Marcucci et al. conducted a phase I study in 9 AML patients who were treated with depsipeptide 13 mg/m^2 infused on days 1, 8, and 15 every 28 days *(56)*. One patient showed a transient decline in blast counts and tumor lysis syndrome. Histone acetylation was measured in 6 patients 4 hours after the infusion of depsipeptide. There was a median increase in acetylation for H3 histone of 40% (range 10–160%) and for H4 histone of 100% (range 0–240%). Byrd et al. reported no response in 10 patients with AML who received the same dose and schedule of depsipeptide *(57)*. Most patients had progressive fatigue and nausea, which prevented repeated treatment. HDAC inhibition and histone acetylation increases of at least 100% were noted *(57)*. Because of a cumulative increase in gastrointestinal and constitutional side effects associated with the weekly schedule, an alternative dosing schedule was recommended *(56,57)*.

2.4. Alkylating Agents

Alkylating agents can damage DNA, impair its replication, or both. Within that class there is a spectrum of antitumor activity and toxicity *(58)*. In view of the diversity of mechanisms that influence their efficacy and safety, new alkylating agents with distinct biological profiles and potential advantages over currently available drugs merit consideration for clinical evaluation in patients with hematological malignancies.

In preclinical studies a new sulfonylhydrazine alkylating agent, VNP40101M (101M, 1,2-bis methylsulfonyl-1-2-chloroethyl-2-methylamino carbonylhydrazine), has demonstrated potential advantages over existing alkylating agents *(59–66)*. VNP40101M first is activated to yield 90CE and methylisocyanate. The 90CE rapidly produces an alkylating, chloroethylating species, which is similar to the chloroethylating species generated by carmustine or BCNU. Unlike BCNU, VNP40101M does not generate a hydroxyethylating, vinylating, or aminoethylating species, and alkylation is relatively specific to the O6 position of guanine *(65,67,68)*. In vitro studies show that as a result of the different alkylating and isocyanate species generated by the agent, VNP40101M produces more crosslinks and fewer DNA single-strand nicks than does BCNU *(65)*. Giles et al. conducted a phase I study of 38 patients: 28 refractory or relapsed AML, with poor risk MDS, ALL, and 1 each with CLL and CML-BP. The patients were treated with VNP40101M as a single intravenous infusion over 15–70 minutes on day 1 *(69)*, and courses were repeated every 4 weeks according to antileukemic activity. The starting dose of 220 mg/m^2 was escalated by 33% in cohorts of 3–6 patients until a maximum tolerated dose was established. One additional cohort was treated with the maximum tolerated dose divided over days 1 and 8. Reversible infusion-related toxicities were the most frequent adverse event, occurring in 24 (63%) patients on the first course. Dose escalation was terminated at 708 mg/m^2 for prolonged myelosuppression in 1 of 7 patients, and 600 mg/m^2 was selected as the recommended phase II dose, with no significant extramedullary toxicity at that dose. Two patients—1 with MDS treated with 300 mg/m^2 and 1 with AML treated with 600 mg/m^2— achieved complete remission.

3. BIOLOGICAL AGENTS

3.1. CD33 Monoclonal Antibodies

Because CD33 is highly expressed on the surface of more than 90% of leukemic cells of patients with AML *(70,71)*, targeting CD33 using monoclonal antibodies has been the subject of intense research in myeloid malignancies *(72,73)*. To overcome the human antimouse antibody (HAMA)-neutralizing response, a human–mouse chimeric antibody with the human constant region and a mouse hypervariable region has been produced *(74)*. Such engineered antibodies can be given repeatedly without a loss in effectiveness, and they have longer circulation times. The expression of CD33 in tissues other than the hematopoietic system and in the normal pluripotent hematopoietic stem cells is not prominent *(75,76)*. CD33 expression is universal in acute promyelocytic leukemia (APL) with a high surface density of the antigen.

HuM195 (monoclonal antibodies to CD33) have demonstrated minimal toxicity, infusion reactions, and minimal HAMA response *(77,78)*. Jurcic et al. reported a higher polymerase chain reaction (PCR)-negative rate in APL patients treated with HuM195 (compared with all-*trans* retinoic acid [ATRA] alone) when the antibody was given to PCR-positive patients in hematological CR after an induction course of ATRA, with or without chemotherapy. Eleven of 22 (50%) became PCR negative, with HuM195 compared with 7 of 34 (21%) historical controls *(79)*. Feldman et al. reported using HuM195 as a single agent in patients with relapsed or refractory AML with minimal, but observable, antileukemic activity (2 CR and 1 PR with HuM195 in 50 patients) *(80)*. The same investigator reported a phase III study of 191 patients with primary refractory or first relapse AML randomized to receive MEC (mitoxantrone, etoposide, and cytarabine) plus HuM195 or MEC alone *(81)*. An overall response rate of 36% (27 CR and 13 CRp) was reported in patients receiving the combination vs 28% (20 CR and 5 complete remission with platelet recovery [CRp]) in patients given MEC alone. No increase in chemotherapy-related toxicity was reported for the combination, and no significant statistical differences in rates of CR, overall response, or survival were seen between the groups. HuM195 has been used as a vehicle for introducing toxins and radioisotopes to AML cells *(82)*. Gemtuzumab ozogamicin (GO), a conjugate of a CD33 antibody to calicheamicin, has received FDA approval for treatment of elderly patients (>60 years) with AML in first relapse and first CR duration greater than 3–6 months.

Sievers et al. reported a study of 142 patients with AML in first relapse treated with GO 9 mg/m^2 iv on days 1 and 15. Patients exhibited a CR rate of 16% and an overall response rate of 30%, and 23% of patients had grade 3 or 4 hyperbilirubinemia *(83)*. In another study, veno-occlusive disease (VOD) was seen in 12% patients treated with GO alone or in combination with other drugs *(84)*. The incidence of VOD with GO in the setting of a transplant could be higher, as seen by high incidence of liver toxicity (48%) in patients who received GO for relapsed AML after a stem cell transplant *(85)*. That outcome was associated with VOD-like findings (weight gain, ascites, jaundice) in 30% of patients *(85)*.

Nabhan et al. reported on 12 untreated AML patients over the age of 65 who were treated with OG. The response rate was 27%. Five (41%) developed cardiac toxicity, and 3 of those patients exhibited grade 3 or 4 toxicity. The response occurred irrespective of karyotype, and it lasted for a median of 7.6 months *(86)*. Piccaluga et al. reported on the use of GO in 24 AML patients. The overall complete response rate was 21%, for a median duration of 6 months. Four of the 5 patients with myeloid sarcoma showed a regression of the masses, in 2 cases also obtaining a clearance of marrow blasts *(87)*.

In another study in elderly patients (≥65 years) with newly diagnosed AML, CR rates were 45% in 20 patients with normal karyotypes and 6% in 31 patients with unfavorable karyotypes. Those results were inferior to those of historical controls treated with idarubicin and ara-C (IA) (corresponding CR rates of 54% and 44%, respectively) *(88)*. Furthermore, survival was better for IA than for GO with or without interleukin (IL)-11 to enhance platelet recovery ($p = 0.03$) *(88)*. The combination of GO and chemotherapy also has been investigated. Phase I–II studies of cytarabine and daunorubicin with GO in patients <60 years old with untreated AML have been reported *(89)*. The maximum tolerated dose in the phase I was ara-C 100 mg/m^2 per day on days 1–7, daunorubicin 45 mg/m^2 per day on days 1–3, and GO 6 mg/m^2 on day 4. The CR rate was 83% in 18 evaluable patients. The regimen was well tolerated; no VOD was reported *(89)*. Kell et al. investigated treatment with a lower dose of GO: 3 mg/m^2 was administered on day 1 of induction chemotherapy (1 of 3 regimens: DAT, DA, or FALG-IDA) *(90)*. In that study, 41 of 55 patients treated (85%) achieved CR with the first course. A higher incidence of liver toxicity was reported in patients who received thioguanine (TG): 22 of 39 with 6TG developed grade 3 or 4 liver toxicity, 1 of 16 patients without 6TG developed liver toxicity. GO was also administered with consolidation courses. A VOD-like syndrome was noted in 2 of 15 with GO in courses 1 and 2 but in none of the 17 patients receiving GO with course 3 *(90)*. GO in combination with cytarabine administered as continuous infusion was evaluated in nine elderly AML patients, untreated or with relapsed or refractory disease. Five patients achieved CR. The most common adverse event was myelosuppression. No VOD was recorded *(91)*.

3.2. Immunoconjugates and Other Monoclonal Antibodies

Monoclonal antibodies conjugated to α-emitting radioisotopes such as ^{213}(Bi) and ^{211}(At) have demonstrated preclinical promise *(92)*. Jurcic et al. conducted a phase I study of HuM195–^{213}(Bi) in 18 patients with relapsed or refractory AML or with chronic myelomonocytic leukemia. Reductions of circulating and bone marrow blasts were reported in 14 of 15 (93%) and in 14 of 18 (78%) evaluable patients, respectively *(93)*. Other radioimmunoconjugates, including β-particle-emitting agents (using ^{131}I and ^{90}Y) and radiolabeled antibodies against CD45 are being investigated with transplant therapy *(94,95)*.

Targeting leukemic cells by the catalytic and translocation subunits of diphtheria toxin (DT388) using granulocyte-macrophage–colony-stimulating factor (GM-CSF) receptor, which is strongly expressed in the leukemic cell, has been reported *(96)*. Leukemic progenitors isolated from patients with AML were sensitive to DT388–GMCSF irrespective of the clinical responsiveness of the patients to standard chemotherapeutic agents *(97)*. The fusion toxin DT388–GMCSF was investigated in a phase I study by Frankel et al. in 31 patients with resistant AML *(98)*. Those researchers reported 1 patient with CR and 2 with PR *(98)*. DT(388)IL3, another fusion toxin composed of DT388 and IL-3, is in preclinical development *(98,99)*.

3.3. Antiangiogenic Agents

Abnormalities in angiogenesis and angiogenic factors are now well documented in acute and chronic leukemias *(100)*. Vascular endothelial growth factor (VEGF) and basic fibroblast growth factor are positive regulators of angiogenesis that could be pathogenic in AML and MDS *(101–103)*. Agents such as bevacizumab, an anti-VEGF monoclonal antibody, are under evaluation in AML, MDS, and CML *(104)*. In a phase II clinical trial of 48 patients with relapsed or refractory AML, bevacizumab 10 mg/kg was administered in a timed sequential fashion on day 8 after ara-C 2 g/m^2/72 hours beginning on day 1 and mitoxantrone 40 mg/m^2 beginning on day 4. The overall response was 48%, with a CR of 33% *(104)*. Small molecule receptor tyrosine kinase inhibitors directed at the VEGF signaling pathway, such as SU5416, SU6668, ZD6474, ZK1222584, and CGP41251, also are in development *(105)*. Giles et al. reported on a mutlicenter phase II study of SU5416 as a single agent in 55 patients (33 AML, 22 MDS); 3 achieved PR and 1 exhibited hematological improvement *(106)*. Grade 3 or 4 toxicities included headaches (14%), infusion-related reactions (11%), dyspnea (14%), fatigue (7%), thrombotic episodes (7%), bone pain (5%), and gastrointestinal disturbance *(107)*. In another multicenter phase II trial of SU5416, 43 patients were treated. Some had refractory AML, and some were elderly patients not medically fit for intensive induction chemotherapy. One patient had a complete response without normalization of blood neutrophil and platelet counts, and 7 patients achieved a partial response *(107)*. Antiangiogenic agents may be more beneficial in combination with cytotoxic agents or in the setting of minimal residual disease.

4. CELL SIGNALING PATHWAYS AS A TARGET

Regulation of the cellular processes—proliferation, differentiation, and death—is tightly controlled by interactions among cells and through cell surface antigens, cytokines, and growth factors *(108)*. Cell surface receptors are important in communicating the extracellular stimulatory and inhibitory effects to cells, a process that ultimately affects gene transcription *(108)*. Defects in the intracellular pathways that control normal cellular processes can result in abnormal proliferation, increased survival, maturation arrest, and malignant transformation. Signal transduction cascades involve three major classes of proteins: kinases, adaptor or docking proteins, and transcription factors. Constitutive activation of kinases and dysfunction of adaptor proteins and transcription factors (such as Ras and Myc) have been linked to leukemic transformation *(109)*.

4.1. Constitutively Active Kinases as Targets of Therapy

Constitutive activation of diverse kinases involved in the regulation of downstream signaling cascades, such as the Jak–Stat pathway, the Ras/Raf/MAPK pathway, and the PI3K pathway leads to inappropriate cell proliferation and survival. As such, these kinases – c-ABL, c-FMS, FLT3, c-KIT, PDGFRα and PDGFRβ, as examples – are attractive therapeutic targets *(110)*, with the intent of such targeting leading to interference with malignant cell growth without causing significant clinical toxicity *(111)*. Subgroups of AML patients with specific cytogenic abnormalities leading to constitutive activation of tyrosine kinases have been described. The following tyrosine kinase inhibitors are under investigation.

c-Kit, a tyrosine kinase receptor, is expressed in 90% of AML patients. Cortes et al. investigated the efficacy of imatinib mesylate in 48 patients with myeloid disorders, including 10 patients with AML and 8 with MDS who were treated with imatinib 400 mg daily *(112)*. None of the patients with AML or MDS responded *(112)*. In a phase II pilot study, 21 patients with refractory AML and positive c-Kit received 600 mg imatinib mesylate orally once daily. Five responses were seen: Two patients had a complete hematological remission, 1 had no evidence of leukemia, and 2 achieved a minor response *(113)*.

FMS-like tyrosine kinase 3(FLT3) is a membrane bound receptor tyrosine kinases with a highly conserved intracellular domain. Constitutive activation of FLT3R stimulates signaling pathways to result in malignant transformation *(114,115)*. Two well-described molecular events that lead to such activation have been reported in more than 30% of patients with AML. The most common mutation involves internal tandem duplication of amino acids within the juxtamembrane domain of the receptor. Expression of a mutant FLT3 receptor in murine marrow cells results in a lethal myeloproliferative disorder *(116–119)*. Similarly, point mutations of codon 835 of the FLT3R gene, located in the activation loop of its tyrosine kinase domain, have been reported in 7% of patients with AML *(116–120)*. Those activating mutations of FLT3R confer a worse outcome.

SU11248 is an oral kinase inhibitor of FLT3, Kit, VEGF, and platelet-derived growth factor (PDGF) receptors. Fiedler et al. conducted a phase I study in which 15 patients with refractory AML received SU11248 for 4-week cycles followed by either a 2- or a 1-week rest period *(121)*. Thirteen patients received doses of 50 mg, and no dose-limiting toxicities were observed. The most frequent grade 2 toxicities were edema, fatigue, and oral ulcerations. Grade 4 fatigue, hypertension, and cardiac failure were observed in 2 patients who received a dose of 75 mg, and that dose was abandoned. All 4 patients with FLT3 mutations had morphological or partial responses, and the responses lasted longer than other responses. Only 2 of the 10 evaluable patients with wild-type FLT3 showed a response to SU11248 *(121)*. Inhibition of FLT3 phosphorylation was apparent in 50% of FLT3-wild-type patients and in 100% of FLT3-mutant patients *(122)*.

Stone et al. reported on 20 patients with mutant FLT3 and relapsed or refractory AML or high-risk MDS who received PKC412 (*N*-benzoylstaurosporine) at a dose of 75 mg three times a day orally *(123)*. The drug was generally well tolerated. The peripheral blast count decreased by 50% in 14 patients (70%); 7 (35%) experienced a greater than 2-log reduction in peripheral blast count for at least 4 weeks (median response, 13 weeks; range, 9–47 weeks). Bone marrow blast count was reduced by 50% in 6 patients (2 of them to ≥5%). FLT3 autophosphorylation was inhibited in most of the patients *(123)*.

CEP-701 is a selective FLT3 inhibitor tested in a phase I–II trial *(124)*. Fourteen patients with refractory, relapsed, or poor-risk AML expressing FLT3-activating mutations were treated with CEP-701 at an initial dose of 60 mg orally twice daily. CEP-701-related toxicities were minimal. Five patients had clinical evidence of biological activity and measurable clinical response, including significant reductions in bone marrow and peripheral blood blasts. Laboratory data confirmed that clinical responses correlated with sustained FLT3 inhibition by CEP-701 *(124)*.

SU5416 was assessed in a phase II trial *(125)*. Partial responses were observed in 2 of 33 patients. SU5416 concentration of 15 µM was associated with FLT3 inhibition *(125)*.

4.2. Ras Farnesylation as Target for Therapy

Because of its importance in carcinogenesis, the Ras signal transduction pathway has attracted considerable attention as a therapeutic target for AML and MDS. Prenylation of Ras by the enzyme farnesyltransferase (Ftase) is required for its association with the cell membrane and its transforming activity. Several pharmacological inhibitors of Ftase have been developed *(126–131)* that also have Ras-independent effects on other cellular signaling components that could contribute to their antileukemic action *(132)*. Karp et al. conducted a phase I study of Zarnestra in 35 adults with poor-risk acute leukemia *(130)*. Patients received oral Zarnestra at doses ranging from 100 to 1200 mg twice daily (bid) for 21 days every 4 weeks, for up to four full cycles *(130)*. A response rate of 29% (2 CR, 8 PR) was reported independent of Ras mutational status. Inhibition of Ftase activity was noted at or above the 300 mg bid dosing level, with a dose-limiting reversible neurotoxicity observed at the 1200 mg bid dosing. Responses were associated with all doses (100–900 mg bid) *(130)*. In a phase II study of 41 patients with untreated, poor-risk AML (defined as age ≥65 years, age ≥18 years with adverse cytogenetics, secondary AML) and MDS with IPSS score ≥1.5, Zarnestra 600 mg was given twice daily for 21 days *(133)*. A response rate of 33%, including 8 CR and 2 PR, was reported. Most of the responses occurred after one cycle of therapy. An additional 12 patients had stable disease after one cycle of therapy. Grade 4 toxicity occurring in 6 of 36 patients (17%) consisted mainly of infections associated with neutropenia *(133)*. Zimmerman et al. conducted a pharmacodynamic study in 42 patients with refractory hematological malignancies and bone marrow involvement *(134)*. Patients were randomly assigned to receive 1 of 4 doses: 100, 200, 300, or 600 mg bid orally for 12 days of a 28-day cycle. During cycle 1, peripheral blood and bone marrow mononuclear cells were analyzed at baseline and on day 21 for inhibition of HDJ2 prenylation. The greatest inhibition was noted for the 300-mg bid dose. After 1 cycle, 3 of 26 assessable patients exhibited significant decreases in total blast counts. The inhibition of farnesylation was greater in the 3 responders than in the nonresponders ($p = 0.03$) *(134)*.

In another trial in 21 MDS patients, Zarnestra was administered twice daily (3 weeks on, 1 week off) for 8 weeks *(135)*. Maintenance therapy at the dose and schedule tolerated during induction could be continued. The dose-limiting toxicity was fatigue, occurring at 900 mg total daily dose. A response rate of 30%, including 1 CR, was reported. Responses were independent of baseline Ras mutational status. Other Ftase inhibitors are also in clinical trials are SCH66336, L778123, and BMS214662 *(136–139)*.

4.3. Apoptosis Induction

Apoptosis (cell death) is an important physiological mechanism for normal tissue homeostasis, and suppression of apoptosis has been demonstrated in myeloid malignancies *(140,141)*. Resistance to the apoptotic machinery leads to prolonged leukemic cell survival, creating a permissive environment for genetic instability and accumulation of gene mutations. Resistance to apoptosis also confers resistance to cytotoxic agents in AML, and it is an important factor in determining the likelihood of response *(140–142)*. Thus, use of agents that induce apoptosis through downregulation of antiapoptotic proteins such as Bcl-2 can improve the response to chemotherapy and restore chemosensitivity to leukemia cells *(143–145)*. Marcucci et al. conducted a study in which 20 patients with refractory AML or ALL received G3139 (18-mer phosphorothioate oligodeoxynucleotide antisense, designed to bind the first six codons of human Bcl-2 mRNA) in combination with fludarabine and cytarabine and G-CSF (FLAG) *(146)*. The CR rate was 35%; G3139 was safe with no major side affects. Bcl-2 mRNA concentration were downregulated in 75% of patients evaluated *(146)*. The same investigators conducted a study with 26 previously untreated patients with high-risk AML *(147)*. The patients received G3139 at 7 mg/m^2/day by continuous infusion on days 1–10, 100 mg/m^2 cytarabine on days 4–10, one of two doses of daunorubicin (54 and 60 mg/m^2 per) on days 4–6. Ten patients achieved a CR (45.4%); 2 showed no evidence of disease but failed to maintain normal platelet and white blood cell counts *(147)*.

4.4. Proteasome Inhibition

Degradation of intracellular proteins is involved in regulation of a broad array of cellular processes, such as cell cycle and division, and regulation of transcription factors. The ubiquitin–proteasome pathway is central for degradation of intracellular proteins *(148,149)*. Important substrates for proteasome degradation include cyclins and CDKIs; transcription factors such as p53, NFκB, c-Myc, c-fos, and c-Jun; several of the apoptosis family of proteins; IAPs; and some caspases *(149–155)*. Bortezomib (PS341) is a specific and potent inhibitor of proteasome *(156)* with documented antitumor activity in MML malignancies. It induces apoptosis and overcomes resistance in several cell lines and in primary cells from patients with CLL *(157–161)*. Sustained clinical activity was not demonstrated in a phase I trial in 15 patients with acute leukemia and MDS, but transient decreases in blood or bone marrow blasts were reported *(162)*.

In a phase I study to determine the maximum tolerated dose of bortezomib in 15 patients with refractory or relapsing acute leukemia, patients were treated with 0.75, 1.25, or 1.5 mg/m^2 bortezomib administered twice weekly for 4 weeks every 6 weeks. Dose-limiting toxicity included orthostatic hypotension, nausea, diarrhea, and fluid retention, all at 1.5 mg/m^2. The maximum tolerated dose of bortezomib was 1.25 mg/m^2 on a schedule of twice-weekly administration for 4 weeks every 6 weeks *(163)*.

5. MULTIDRUG RESISTANCE INHIBITORS

Studies of AML cell lines have shown that resistance to chemotherapeutic agents can be correlated with overexpression of efflux proteins such as P-glycoprotein (Pgp), multidrug resistance (MDR) protein, and the major vault protein (LRP) *(164)*. Pgp is an adenosine-triphosphate-dependent multidrug exporter *(165)*. Its overexpression decreases intracellular accumulation of anthracyclines and is associated with relative in vitro resistance. Drugs such as cyclosporin A, verapamil, and PSC833 inhibit Pgp by competing with chemotherapeutic agents to overcome resistance *(166)*. Multidrug resistance protein 1(MDR1) is overexpressed in elderly patients with AML and is associated with a poor prognosis *(167)*.

5.1. Cyclosporin A

Investigators from the Southwest Oncology Group studied 226 patients with AML who were randomly assigned to receive sequential therapy with cytarabine and infusional daunorubicin with or without intravenous cyclosporin A *(168)*. The cyclosporin A group had a slightly higher CR rate (40% vs 33%; $p = 0.14$) but a significantly lower relapse rate (34% vs 9% at 2 years; $p = 0.031$) and better overall survival (22% vs 12%; $p = 0.046$) *(168)*. The cyclosporin A effect was observed in patient who were MDR1-positive and MDR1-negative patients, but it was more significant in MDR1-positive patients (median survival 12 vs 4 months).

In a randomized controlled trial, the same investigators treated 73 CML-BP patients with cytarabine and infusional daunorubicin with or without intravenous cyclosporin A *(168)*. Addition of cyclosporin A yielded no improvement in outcome as measured by the frequency of induction resistance (68% vs 53%), rate of complete remission or restored chronic phase (CR/CP, 8% vs 30%), and survival (3 vs 5 months). Blast expression of Pgp (63%) and LRP (71%) was common, whereas only Pgp hampered the rate of CR/CP ($p = 0.025$). The authors concluded that Pgp has prognostic relevance in CML-BP but that its modulation with cyclosporin A is ineffective *(168)*.

5.2. PSC833 and Other MDR Modulators

PSC-833 is a potent MDR modifier. It is a cyclosporine analog that increases daunorubicin retention in MDR cells 20 times more than cyclosporine does *(169)*. PSC-833 dose not induce renal toxicity *(170)*. In an early study, the addition of PSC833 to mitoxantrone, etoposide, and ara-C (PSC-MEC) was safe and associated with a CR rate of 29% in relapsed or refractory AML *(171)*.

In a phase III randomized trial by the Cancer and Leukemia Group B investigators, 120 elderly patients with untreated AML were assigned to cytarabine (100 mg/m^2 per day for 7 days), daunorubicin (DNR) (60 mg/m^2 per day for 3 days), and etoposide (ETOP) (100 mg/m^2 per day for 3 days, ADE) or to the same agents at lower doses (DNR at 40 mg/m^2 per day and ETOP at 60 mg/m^2 per day for 3 days) with PSC833 (ADEP) *(172)*. The study was closed early because of a high mortality rate in the ADEP group. There was no difference in disease-free survival or overall survival between the two groups *(172)*.

In another study, the same investigators followed a total of 410 untreated patients with AML, all younger than 60 years *(173)* enrolled in 15 induction regimens containing variable doses of DNR and ETOP and fixed doses of cytarabine evaluated with (ADEP) or without (ADE) a fixed dose of PSC-833. Phase III doses were DNR 90 mg/m^2 and ETOP 100 mg/m^2 in ADE and DNR and ETOP each 40 mg/m^2 in ADEP. Significant mucosal toxicity occurred at higher doses of ADEP. Patients who were 45 year old or younger in the ADEP group showed an apparent advantage with respect to disease-free and overall survival *(173)*. In a randomized trial by Eastern Cooperation Oncology Group in 113 patients with relapsed or refractory AML, no advantage was reported for PSC-MEC over MEC alone *(174)*. Solary et al. conducted a randomized trial in 415 untreated AML patients (15–60 years) examining the addition of quinine to reverse Pgp-mediated drug resistance *(175)*. Quinine had no influence on survival regardless of Pgp or MDR1 expression *(175)*. Van der Holt et al. conducted a randomized trial of 419 untreated patients with AML 60 years and older who received two induction cycles of daunorubicin and cytarabine with or without PSC833 *(176)*. There were no significant differences between the two groups in complete response rate, 5-year event-free survival, disease-free survival, or overall survival *(176)*. More selective and specific MDR modulators, such as the Pipecolinate derivatives VX-710 and VX-853, which target Pgp, MRP-1, and breast cancer resistance protein, are under development *(177)*.

6. OTHER TARGETS

Other therapeutic targets include the steps in the serine–threonine cascades *(137)*. Geldanamycin and derivatives of radicicol destabilize Raf protein and interfere with Raf signaling *(178–180)*. Staurosporine derivatives (UCN-O1, CGP41251, and PKC412) inhibit PKC signaling and have been examined in cell lines and clinical studies *(181–183)*. Aberrant

MEK and ERK activity has been demonstrated in AML and CML *(184–187)*. MEK inhibitors (PD098059, PD184352, and UO126) modulate cellular proliferation, differentiation, and apoptosis *(188–190)*. PD184352 (also called CI-1040) is in phase I evaluation with cancer patients *(191)*. Pharmacological inhibitors of PI3K, wortmannin and LY294002, have shown significant potency in preclinical studies *(192,193)*. The mammalian target of rapamycin (mTOR) is a downstream effector of the PI3K/Akt (protein kinase B) signaling pathway that mediates cell survival and proliferation *(194,195)*. Rapamycin analogs, including CCI-779 and RAD001, and small molecule mTOR inhibitors such as AP23573 are under investigation *(196)*.

7. CONCLUSION

The enhanced understanding of the molecular biological features that are key to the pathophysiology of AML have speeded the discovery of new agents and strategies in the treatment of AML. We anticipate that further research focused on targeted therapies will lead to the development of more potent, less toxic agents that will contribute to the cure of patients with AML.

REFERENCES

1. McCulloch EA. Stem cells in normal and leukemic hemopoiesis. Blood 1983;62(1):1–13.
2. Estey EH, Thall PF. New designs for phase 2 clinical trials. Blood 2003;102:442–448.
3. Parker WB, Shaddix SC, Chang CH, et al. Effects of 2-chloro-9-(2-deoxy-2-fluoro-beta-D-arabinofuranosyl) adenine on K562 cellular metabolism and the inhibition of human ribonucleotide reductase and DNA polymerases by its 5′-triphosphate. Cancer Res 1991;51:2386–2394.
4. Kantarjian HM, Gandhi V, Kozuch P, et al. Phase I clinical and pharmacology study of clofarabine in patients with solid and hematological cancers. J Clin Oncol 2003;21:1167–1173.
5. Kantarjian HM, Gandhi V, Cortes J, et al. Phase II clinical and pharmacology study of clofarabine in patients with refractory or relapsed acute leukemia. Blood 2003;
6. Faderl S, Gandhi V, O'Brien S, et al. Results of a phase 1-2 study of clofarabine in combination with cytarabine (ara-C) in relapsed and refractory acute leukemias. Blood 2005;105(3):940–947.
7. Jeha S, Gandhi V, Chan KW, et al. Clofarabine, a novel nucleoside analog, is active in pediatric patients with advanced leukemia. Blood 2004;103(3):784–789.
8. Tsimberidou AM, Alvarado Y, Giles FJ. Evolving role of ribonucleoside reductase inhibitors in hematological malignancies. Expert Rev Anticancer Ther 2002;2:437–448.
9. Balzarini J, Wedgwood O, Kruining J, et al. Anti-HIV and anti-HBV activity and resistance profile of 2′, 3′-dideoxy-3′-thiacytidine (3TC) and its arylphosphoramidate derivative CF 1109. Biochem Biophys Res Commun 1996;225:363–369.
10. Grove KL, Guo X, Liu SH, et al. Anticancer activity of beta-L-dioxolane-cytidine, a novel nucleoside analogue with the unnatural L configuration. Cancer Res 1995;55:3008–3011.
11. Giles FJ, Cortes JE, Baker SD, et al. Troxacitabine, a novel dioxolane nucleoside analog, has activity in patients with advanced leukemia. J Clin Oncol 2001;19:762–771.
12. Giles FJ, Garcia-Manero G, Cortes JE, et al. Phase II study of troxacitabine, a novel dioxolane nucleoside analog, in patients with refractory leukemia. J Clin Oncol 2002;20:656–664.
13. Giles FJ, Faderl S, Thomas DA, et al. Randomized Phase I/II study of troxacitabine combined with cytarabine, idarubicin, or topotecan in patients with refractory myeloid leukemias. J Clin Oncol 2003;21:1050–1056.
14. Grove KL, Guo X, Liu SH, Gao Z, Chu CK, Cheng YC. Anticancer activity of beta-L-dioxolane-cytidine, a novel nucleoside analogue with the unnatural L configuration. Cancer Res 1995;55:3008–3011.
15. Grove KL, Cheng YC. Uptake and metabolism of the new anticancer compound beta-L-(-)-dioxolane-cytidine in human prostate carcinoma DU-145 cells. Cancer Res 1996;56:4187–4191.
16. Giles FJ, Cortes JE, Baker SD, et al. Troxacitabine, a novel dioxolane nucleoside analog, has activity in patients with advanced leukemia. J Clin Oncol 2001;19:762–771.

17. Giles FJ, Kantarjian HM, Cortes JE, et al. Adaptive randomized study of idarubicin and cytarabine vs troxa-citabine and cytarabine vs troxacitabine and idarubicin in untreated patients 50 years or older with adverse karyotype acute myeloid leukemia. J Clin Oncol 2003;21:1722–1727.

18. Santini V, Kantarjian HM, Issa JP. Changes in DNA methylation in neoplasia: pathophysiology and thera-peutic implications. Ann Intern Med 2001;134:573–586.

19. Singal R, Ginder GD. DNA methylation. Blood 1999;93:4059–4070.

20. Baylin SB, Herman JG, Graff JR, Vertino PM, Issa JP. Alterations in DNA methylation: a fundamental aspect of neoplasia. Adv. Cancer Res 1998;72:141–196.

21. Toyota M, Kopecky KJ, Toyota MO, Jair KW, Willman CL, Issa JP. Methylation profiling in acute myeloid leukemia. Blood 2001;97:2823–2829.

22. Au WY, Fung A, Man C, et al. Aberrant p15 gene promoter methylation in therapy-related myelodysplastic syndrome and acute myeloid leukaemia: clinicopathological and karyotypic associations. Br J Hematol 2003;120:1062–1065.

23. Teofili L, Martini M, Luongo M, et al. Hypermethylation of GpG islands in the promoter region of p15 (INK4b) in acute promyelocytic leukemia represses p15(INK4b) expression and correlates with poor prognosis. Leukemia 2003;17:919–924.

24. Warrell RP, Jr., He LZ, Richon V, Calleja E, Pandolfi PP. Therapeutic targeting of transcription in acute promyelocytic leukemia by use of an inhibitor of histone deacetylase. J Natl Cancer Inst 1998;90:1621–1625.

25. He LZ, Tolentino T, Grayson P, et al. Histone deacetylase inhibitors induce remission in transgenic models of therapy-resistant acute promyelocytic leukemia. J Clin Invest 2001;108:1321–1330.

26. Klisovic MI, Maghraby EA, Parthun MR, et al. Depsipeptide (FR 901228) promotes histone acetylation, gene transcription, apoptosis and its activity is enhanced by DNA methyltransferase inhibitors in AML1/ETO-positive leukemic cells. Leukemia 2003;17(2):350–358.

27. Pinto A, Zagonel V. 5-Aza-2′-deoxycytidine (Decitabine) and 5-azacytidine in the treatment of acute myeloid leukemias and myelodysplastic syndromes: past, present and future trends. Leukemia 1993;7 (suppl 1):51–60.

28. Santi DV, Garrett CE, Barr PJ. On the mechanism of inhibition of DNA-cytosine methyltransferases by cytosine analogs. Cell 1983;33:9–10.

29. Issa JP, Baylin SB, Herman JG. DNA methylation changes in hematological malignancies: biological and clinical implications. Leukemia 1997;11 (suppl 1):S7–11.

30. Momparler RL, Bouchard J, Onetto N, Rivard GE. 5-Aza-2′-deoxycytidine therapy in patients with acute leukemia inhibits DNA methylation. Leuk Res 1984;8:181–185.

31. Rivard GE, Momparler RL, Demers J, et al. Phase I study on 5-aza-2′-deoxycytidine in children with acute leukemia. Leuk Res 1981;5:453–462.

32. Momparler RL, Rivard GE, Gyger M. Clinical trial on 5-aza-2′-deoxycytidine in patients with acute leukemia. Pharmacol Ther 1985;30:277–286.

33. Richel DJ, Colly LP, Kluin-Nelemans JC, Willemze R. The antileukaemic activity of 5-Aza-2 deoxycyti-dine (Aza-dC) in patients with relapsed and resistant leukaemia. Br J Cancer 1991;64:144–148.

34. Kantarjian HM, O'Brien SM, Keating M, et al. Results of decitabine therapy in the accelerated and blastic phases of chronic myelogenous leukemia. Leukemia 1997;11:1617–1620.

35. Kantarjian HM, O'Brien S, Cortes J, et al. Results of decitabine (5-aza-2′deoxycytidine) therapy in 130 patients with chronic myelogenous leukemia. Cancer 2003;98:522–528.

36. Pinto A, Zagonel V. 5-Aza-2′-deoxycytidine (Decitabine) and 5-azacytidine in the treatment of acute myeloid leukemias and myelodysplastic syndromes: past, present and future trends. Leukemia 1993;7 (suppl 1):51–60.

37. Petti MC, Mandelli F, Zagonel V, et al. Pilot study of 5-aza-2′-deoxycytidine (Decitabine) in the treatment of poor prognosis acute myelogenous leukemia patients: preliminary results. Leukemia 1993;7(suppl 1):36–41.

38. Ravandi F, Kantarjian H, Cohen A, et al. Decitabine with allogeneic peripheral blood stem cell transplan-tation in the therapy of leukemia relapse following a prior transplant: results of a phase I study. Bone Marrow Transplant 2001;27:1221–1225.

39. Willemze R, Suciu S, Archimbaud E, et al. A randomized phase II study on the effects of 5-Aza-2′-deoxy-cytidine combined with either amsacrine or idarubicin in patients with relapsed acute leukemia: an EORTC Leukemia Cooperative Group phase II study (06893). Leukemia 1997;11(suppl 1):S24–27.

40. Schwartsmann G, Fernandes MS, Schaan MD, et al. Decitabine (5-aza-2′-deoxycytidine;DAC) plus daunorubicin as a first line treatment in patients with acute myeloid leukemia: preliminary observations. Leukemia 1997;11(suppl 1):S28–31.

41. Issa JP, Garcia-Manero G, Mannari R, et al. Minimal effective dose of the hypomethylating agent decitabine in hematopoietic malignancies. Blood 2001;98:594–595.

42. Issa JP, Garcia-Manero G, Giles FJ, et al. Phase 1 study of low-dose prolonged exposure schedules of the hypomethylating agent 5-aza-2′-deoxycytidine (decitabine) in hematopoietic malignancies. Blood 2004;103(5): 1635–1640.

43. Silverman LR, Demakos EP, Peterson BL, et al. Randomized controlled trial of azacitidine in patients with the myelodysplastic syndrome: a study of the cancer and leukemia group B. J Clin Oncol 2002;20:2429–2440.

44. Kornblith AB, Herndon JE, II, Silverman LR, et al. Impact of azacytidine on the quality of life of patients with myelodysplastic syndrome treated in a randomized phase III trial: a Cancer and Leukemia Group B study. J Clin Oncol 2002;20:2441–2452.

45. Wijermans PW, Krulder JW, Huijgens PC, Neve P. Continuous infusion of low-dose 5-Aza-2′-deoxycytidine in elderly patients with high-risk myelodysplastic syndrome. Leukemia 1997;11 (suppl 1):S19–23.

46. Wijermans P, Lubbert M, Verhoef G, et al. Low-dose 5-aza-2′-deoxycytidine, a DNA hypomethylating agent, for the treatment of high-risk myelodysplastic syndrome: a multicenter phase II study in elderly patients. J Clin Oncol 2000;18:956–962.

47. Lubbert M, Wijermans P, Kunzmann R, et al. Cytogenetic responses in high-risk myelodysplastic syndrome following low-dose treatment with the DNA methylation inhibitor 5-aza-2′-deoxycytidine. Br J Hematol 2001;114:349–357.

48. Daskalakis M, Nguyen TT, Nguyen C, et al. Demethylation of a hypermethylated P15/INK4B gene in patients with myelodysplastic syndrome by 5-aza-2′-deoxycytidine (decitabine) treatment. Blood 2002;100: 2957–2964.

49. Sigalotti L, Altomonte M, Colizzi F, et al. 5-Aza-2′-deoxycytidine (decitabine) treatment of hematopoietic malignancies: a multimechanism therapeutic approach. Blood 2003;101:4644–4646.

50. Wijermans P, Luebbert M, Verhoef G. Low dose decitabine for elderly high-risk MDS patients: who will respond. Blood 2002;100:97a.

51. Saba HI, Rosenfeld CS, Issa JP, Bennett JM, Decastro C, Kantarjian H. Clinical benefit and survival edopoits from a phase III trial comparing decitabine (DAC) VS supportive care (SC) in patients with advanced MDS. J Clin Oncol 2005;

52. Hiebert SW, Lutterbach B, Amann J. Role of co-repressors in transcriptional repression mediated by the t (8;21), t (16;21), t (2;21), and inv (16) fusion proteins. Curr Opin Hematol 2001;8:197–200.

53. Faretta M, Di Croce L, Pelicci PG. Effects of the acute myeloid leukemia–associated fusion proteins on nuclear architecture. Semin Hematol 2001;38:42–53.

54. Ferrara FF, Fazi F, Bianchini A, et al. Histone deacetylase-targeted treatment restores retinoic acid signaling and differentiation in acute myeloid leukemia. Cancer Res 2001;61:2–7.

55. Amann JM, Nip J, Strom DK, et al. ETO, a target of t(8;21) in acute leukemia, makes distinct contacts with multiple histone deacetylases and binds mSin3A through its oligomerization domain. Mol. Cell Biol 2001; 21:6470–6483.

56. Marcucci G, Bruner RJ, Binkley PE, et al. Phase I trial of the histone deacetylase inhibitor depsipeptide (FR901228) in acute myeloid leukemia (AML). Blood 2002;100:86a.

57. Byrd JC, Marcucci G, Parthun MR, et al. A phase 1 and pharmacodynamic study of depsipeptide (FK228) in chronic lymphocytic leukemia and acute myeloid leukemia. Blood 2005;105(3):959–967.

58. Hall AG, Tilby MJ. Mechanisms of action of, and modes of resistance to, alkylating agents used in the treatment of hematological malignancies. Blood Rev 1992;6:63–73.

59. Shyam K, Cosby LA, Sartorelli AC. Synthesis and evaluation of N,N'-bis(arylsulfonyl)hydrazines as antineoplastic agents. J Med Chem 1985;28:525–527.

60. Shyam K, Furubayashi R, Hrubiec RT, Cosby LA, Sartorelli AC. 1,2-Bis(arylsulfonyl)hydrazines. 2. The influence of arylsulfonyl and aralkylsulfonyl substituents on antitumor and alkylating activity. J Med Chem 1986;29:1323–1325.

61. Shyam K, Hrubiec RT, Furubayashi R, Cosby LA, Sartorelli AC. 1,2-Bis(sulfonyl)hydrazines: 3. Effects of structural modification on antineoplastic activity. J Med Chem 1987;30:2157–2161.

62. Shyam K, Penketh PG, Divo AA, Loomis RH, Rose WC, Sartorelli AC. Synthesis and evaluation of 1-acyl-1, 2-bis(methylsulfonyl)-2-(2-chloroethyl)hydrazines as antineoplastic agents. J Med Chem 1993;36:3496–3502.

63. Shyam K, Penketh PG, Loomis RH, Rose WC, Sartorelli AC. Antitumor 2-(aminocarbonyl)-1,2-bis (methylsulfonyl)-1-(2-chloroethyl)-hydrazines. J Med Chem 1996;39:796–801.

64. Pratviel G, Shyam K, Sartorelli AC. Cytotoxic and DNA-damaging effects of 1,2-bis(sulfonyl)hydrazines on human cells of the Mer+ and Mer-phenotype. Cancer Biochem Biophys 1989;10:365–375.

65. Penketh PG, Shyam K, Sartorelli AC. Comparison of DNA lesions produced by tumor-inhibitory 1,2-bis (sulfonyl)hydrazines and chloroethylnitrosoureas. Biochem Pharmacol 2000;59:283–291.

66. Finch RA, Shyam K, Penketh PG, Sartorelli AC. 1,2-Bis(methylsulfonyl)-1-(2-chloroethyl)-2-(methyl-amino)carbonylhydrazine (101M): a novel sulfonylhydrazine prodrug with broad-spectrum antineoplastic activity. Cancer Res 2001;61:3033–3038.

67. Briscoe WT, Duarte SP. Preferential alkylation by 1,3-bis 2-chloroethyl)-1-nitrosourea (BCNU) of guanines with guanines as neighboring bases in DNA. Biochem Pharmacol 1988;37:1061–1066.

68. Lown JW, McLaughlin LW. Nitrosourea-induced DNA single-strand breaks. Biochem Pharmacol 1979;28: 1631–1638.

69. Giles F, Thomas D, Garcia-Manero G, et al. A Phase I and pharmacokinetic study of VNP40101M, a novel sulfonylhydrazine alkylating agent, in patients with refractory leukemia. Clin Cancer Res 2004;10(9): 2908–2917.

70. Tanimoto M, Scheinberg DA, Cordon-Cardo C, Huie D, Clarkson BD, Old LJ. Restricted expression of an early myeloid and monocytic cell surface antigen defined by monoclonal antibody M195. Leukemia 1989;3:339–348.

71. Scheinberg DA, Tanimoto M, McKenzie S, Strife A, Old LJ, Clarkson BD. Monoclonal antibody M195: a diagnostic marker for acute myelogenous leukemia. Leukemia 1989;3:440–445.

72. Winter G, Milstein C. Man-made antibodies. Nature 1991;349:293–299.

73. Caron PC, Scheinberg DA. The biological therapy of acute and chronic leukemia. Cancer Invest 1997;15: 342–352.

74. Caron PC, Co MS, Bull MK, Avdalovic NM, Queen C, Scheinberg DA. Biological and immunological features of humanized M195 (anti-CD33) monoclonal antibodies. Cancer Res 1992;52:6761–6767.

75. Tanimoto M, Scheinberg DA, Cordon-Cardo C, Huie D, Clarkson BD, Old LJ. Restricted expression of an early myeloid and monocytic cell surface antigen defined by monoclonal antibody M195. Leukemia 1989; 3:339–348.

76. Scheinberg DA, Tanimoto M, McKenzie S, Strife A, Old LJ, Clarkson BD. Monoclonal antibody M195: a diagnostic marker for acute myelogenous leukemia. Leukemia 1989;3:440–445.

77. Caron PC, Schwartz MA, Co MS, et al. Murine and humanized constructs of monoclonal antibody M195 (anti-CD33) for the therapy of acute myelogenous leukemia. Cancer 1994;73:1049–1056.

78. Caron PC, Jurcic JG, Scott AM, et al. A phase 1B trial of humanized monoclonal antibody M195 (anti-CD33) in myeloid leukemia: specific targeting without immunogenicity. Blood 1994;83:1760–1768.

79. Jurcic JG, DeBlasio T, Dumont L, Yao TJ, Scheinberg DA. Molecular remission induction with retinoic acid and anti-CD33 monoclonal antibody HuM195 in acute promyelocytic leukemia. Clin Cancer Res 2000;6: 372–380.

80. Feldman E, Kalaycio M, Weiner G, et al. Treatment of relapsed or refractory acute myeloid leukemia with humanized anti-CD33 monoclonal antibody HuM195. Leukemia 2003;17:314–318.

81. Feldman EJ, Brandwein J, Stone R, et al. Phase III randomized multicenter study of a humanized anti-CD33 monoclonal antibody, lintuzumab, in combination with chemotherapy, vs chemotherapy alone in patients with refractory or first-relapsed acute myeloid leukemia. J Clin Oncol 2005;23(18):4110–4116.

82. Sievers EL, Appelbaum FR, Spielberger RT, et al. Selective ablation of acute myeloid leukemia using antibody-targeted chemotherapy: a phase I study of an anti-CD33 calicheamicin immunoconjugate. Blood 1999;93:3678–3684.

83. Sievers EL, Larson RA, Stadtmauer EA, et al. Efficacy and safety of gemtuzumab ozogamicin in patients with CD33-positive acute myeloid leukemia in first relapse. J Clin Oncol 2001;19:3244–3254.

84. Giles FJ, Kantarjian HM, Kornblau SM, et al. Mylotarg (gemtuzumab ozogamicin) therapy is associated with hepatic venoocclusive disease in patients who have not received stem cell transplantation. Cancer 2001;92:406–413.

85. Rajvanshi P, Shulman HM, Sievers EL, McDonald GB. Hepatic sinusoidal obstruction after gemtuzumab ozogamicin (Mylotarg) therapy. Blood 2002;99:2310–2314.

86. Nabhan C, Rundhaugen LM, Riley MB, et al. Phase II pilot trial of gemtuzumab ozogamicin (GO) as first line therapy in acute myeloid leukemia patients age 65 or older. Leuk Res 2005;29(1):53–57.

87. Piccaluga PP, Martinelli G, Rondoni M, et al. Gemtuzumab ozogamicin for relapsed and refractory acute myeloid leukemia and myeloid sarcomas. Leuk Lymphoma 2004;45(9):1791–1795.

88. Estey EH, Thall PF, Giles FJ, et al. Gemtuzumab ozogamicin with or without interleukin 11 in patients 65 years of age or older with untreated acute myeloid leukemia and high-risk myelodysplastic syndrome:

comparison with idarubicin plus continuous-infusion, high-dose cytosine arabinoside. Blood 2002;99: 4343–4349.

89. De Angelo DJ, Schiffer C, Stone R, et al. Interim analysis of a phase II study of the safety and efficacy of gemtuzumab ozogamicin (Mylotarg) given in combination with cytarabine and daunorubicin in patients less than 60 years old with untreated acute myeloid leukemia. Blood 2002;100:198a.

90. Kell JW, Burnett AK, Chopra R, et al. Mylotarg (gemtuzumab ozogamicin) given simultaneously with intensive induction and/or consolidation therapy for AML is feasible and may improve response rate. Blood 2002;100:199a.

91. Piccaluga PP, Martinelli G, Rondoni M, et al. First experience with gemtuzumab ozogamicin plus cytarabine as continuous infusion for elderly acute myeloid leukaemia patients. Leuk Res 2004;28(9): 987–990.

92. McDevitt MR, Ma D, Lai LT, et al. Tumor therapy with targeted atomic nanogenerators. Science 2001;294: 1537–1540.

93. Jurcic JG, Larson SM, Sgouros G, et al. Targeted alpha particle immunotherapy for myeloid leukemia. Blood 2002;100:1233–1239.

94. Pagel JM, Appelbaum FR, Eary JF, et al. 131I-ANTI-CD45 antibody plus busulfan and cyclophosphamide before allogeneic hematopoietic cell transplantation for treatment of acute myeloid leukemia in first remission. Blood 2005;107:2184–2191.

95. Schwartz MA, Lovett DR, Redner A, et al. Dose-escalation trial of M195 labeled with iodine 131 for cyto-reduction and marrow ablation in relapsed or refractory myeloid leukemias. J Clin Oncol 1993;11:294–303.

96. Hall PD, Willingham MC, Kreitman RJ, Frankel AE. DT388-GM-CSF, a novel fusion toxin consisting of a truncated diphtheria toxin fused to human granulocyte-macrophage colony-stimulating factor, prolongs host survival in a SCID mouse model of acute myeloid leukemia. Leukemia 1999;13:629–633.

97. Hogge DE, Willman CL, Kreitman RJ, et al. Malignant progenitors from patients with acute myelogenous leukemia are sensitive to a diphtheria toxin-granulocyte-macrophage colony-stimulating factor fusion protein. Blood 1998;92:589–595.

98. Frankel AE, McCubrey JA, Miller MS, et al. Diphtheria toxin fused to human interleukin-3 is toxic to blasts from patients with myeloid leukemias. Leukemia 2000;14:576–585.

99. Black JH, McCubrey JA, Willingham MC, Ramage J, Hogge DE, Frankel AE. Diphtheria toxin-interleukin-3 fusion protein (DT(388)IL3;prolongs disease-free survival of leukemic immunocompromised mice. Leukemia 2003;17:155–159.

100. Giles FJ, Kantarjian H, Cortes J. Novel therapies for patients with chronic myeloid leukemia. Exp Rev Anticancer Ther 2004;4(2):271–282.

101. Aguayo A, Kantarjian H, Manshouri T, et al. Angiogenesis in acute and chronic leukemias and myelodysplastic syndromes. Blood 2000;96:2240–2245.

102. Hussong JW, Rodgers GM, Shami PJ. Evidence of increased angiogenesis in patients with acute myeloid leukemia. Blood 2000;95:309–313.

103. Giles FJ. Novel agents for the therapy of acute leukemia. Curr Opin Oncol 2002;14:3–9.

104. Karp JE, Gojo I, Pili R, et al. Targeting vascular endothelial growth factor for relapsed and refractory adult acute myelogenous leukemias: therapy with sequential 1-beta-d-arabinofuranosylcytosine, mitoxantrone, and bevacizumab. Clin Cancer Res 2004;10(11):3577–3585.

105. Laird AD, Vajkoczy P, Shawver LK, et al. SU6668 is a potent antiangiogenic and antitumor agent that induces regression of established tumors. Cancer Res 2000;60:4152–4160.

106. Giles FJ, Stopeck AT, Silverman LR, et al. SU5416, a small molecule tyrosine kinase receptor inhibitor, has biological activity in patients with refractory acute myeloid leukemia or myelodysplastic syndromes. Blood 2003;102(3):795–801.

107. Fiedler W, Mesters R, Tinnefeld H, et al. A phase 2 clinical study of SU5416 in patients with refractory acute myeloid leukemia. Blood 2003;102(8):2763–2767.

108. Alberts B, Bray D, Lewis J, Raff M, Roberts K, Watson JD. Molecular biology of the cell. In: Alberts B, Bray D, Lewis J, Raff M, Roberts K, Watson JD, eds. New York: Garland Publishing Inc., 1994:721–785.

109. Ravandi F, Talpaz M, Estrov Z. Modulation of cellular signaling pathways: prospects for targeted therapy in hematological malignancies. Clin Cancer Res 2003;9:535–550.

110. Scheijen B, Griffin JD. Tyrosine kinase oncogenes in normal hematopoiesis and hematological disease. Oncogene 2002;21:3314–3333.

111. Frank DA. STAT signaling in the pathogenesis and treatment of cancer. Mol Med 1999;5:432–456.

112. Cortes J, Giles F, O'Brien S, et al. Results of imatinib mesylate therapy in patients with refractory or recurrent acute myeloid leukemia, high-risk myelodysplastic syndrome, and myeloproliferative disorders. Cancer 2003;97:2760–2766.
113. Kindler T, Breitenbuecher F, Marx A. Efficacy and safety of imatinib in adult patients with c-kit-positive acute myeloid leukemia. Blood 2004;103(10):3644–3654.
114. Tse KF, Mukherjee G, Small D. Constitutive activation of FLT3 stimulates multiple intracellular signal transducers and results in transformation. Leukemia 2000;14:1766–1776.
115. Gilliland DG, Griffin JD. The roles of FLT3 in hematopoiesis and leukemia. Blood 2002;100:1532–1542.
116. Thiede C, Steudel C, Mohr B, et al. Analysis of FLT3-activating mutations in 979 patients with acute myelogenous leukemia: association with FAB subtypes and identification of subgroups with poor prognosis. Blood 2002;99:4326–4335.
117. Gilliland DG, Griffin JD. Role of FLT3 in leukemia. Curr Opin Hematol 2002;9:274–281.
118. Kiyoi H, Ohno R, Ueda R, Saito H, Naoe T. Mechanism of constitutive activation of FLT3 with internal tandem duplication in the juxtamembrane domain. Oncogene 2002;21:2555–2563.
119. Kelly LM, Liu Q, Kutok JL, Williams IR, Boulton CL, Gilliland DG. FLT3 internal tandem duplication mutations associated with human acute myeloid leukemias induce myeloproliferative disease in a murine bone marrow transplant model. Blood 2002;99:310–318.
120. Yamamoto Y, Kiyoi H, Nakano Y, et al. Activating mutation of D835 within the activation loop of FLT3 in human hematological malignancies. Blood 2001;97:2434–2439.
121. Fiedler W, Serve H, Dohner H, et al. A phase 1 study of SU11248 in the treatment of patients with refractory or resistant acute myeloid leukemia (AML) or not amenable to conventional therapy for the disease. Blood 2005;105(3):986–993.
122. O'Farrell AM, Foran JM, Fiedler W, et al. An innovative phase I clinical study demonstrates inhibition of FLT3 phosphorylation by SU11248 in acute myeloid leukemia patients. Clin Cancer Res 2003;9(15): 5465–5476.
123. Stone RM, DeAngelo DJ, Klimek V, et al. Patients with acute myeloid leukemia and an activating mutation in FLT3 respond to a small-molecule FLT3 tyrosine kinase inhibitor, PKC412. Blood 2005;105(1):54–60.
124. Smith BD, Levis M, Beran M, Small D, et al. Single-agent CEP-701, a novel FLT3 inhibitor, shows biological and clinical activity in patients with relapsed or refractory acute myeloid leukemia. Blood 2004;103(10): 3669–3676.
125. O'Farrell AM, Yuen HA, Smolich B, et al. SU5416, a small molecule tyrosine kinase receptor inhibitor, on FLT3 expression and phosphorylation in patients with refractory acute myeloid leukemia. Leuk Res 2004; (7):679–689.
126. Beaupre DM, Kurzrock R. RAS and leukemia: from basic mechanisms to gene-directed therapy. J Clin Oncol 1999;17:1071–1079.
127. Kohl NE, Mosser SD, deSolms SJ, et al. Selective inhibition of ras-dependent transformation by a farnesyl-transferase inhibitor. Science 1993;260:1934–1937.
128. James GL, Goldstein JL, Brown MS, et al. Benzodiazepine peptidomimetics: potent inhibitors of Ras farnesylation in animal cells. Science 1993;260:1937–1942.
129. Gibbs JB. Ras C-terminal processing enzymes-new drug targets? Cell 1991;65:1–4.
130. Karp JE, Lancet JE, Kaufmann SH, et al. Clinical and biological activity of the farnesyltransferase inhibitor R115777 in adults with refractory and relapsed acute leukemias: a phase 1 clinical-laboratory correlative trial. Blood 2001;97:3361–3369.
131. Cortes J, Albitar M, Thomas D, et al. Efficacy of the farnesyl transferase inhibitor R115777 in chronic myeloid leukemia and other hematological malignancies. Blood 2003;101:1692–1697.
132. Kurzrock R, Sebti SM, Kantarjian HM, et al. Phase I study of a farnesyl transferase inhibitor, R115777, in patients with myelodysplastic syndrome. Blood 2001;98:623.
133. Lancet JE, Karp JE, Gotlib J, et al. Zarnestra (R115777) in previously untreated poor-risk AML and MDS: Preliminary results of a phase II trial. Blood 2002;100:560a.
134. Zimmerman TM, Harlin H, Odenike OM, et al. Dose-ranging pharmacodynamic study of tipifarnib (R115777) in patients with relapsed and refractory hematological malignancies. J Clin Oncol 2004;22(23):4816–4822.
135. Kurzrock R, Kantarjian HM, Cortes JE, et al. Farnesyltransferase inhibitor R115777 in myelodysplastic syndrome: clinical and biological activities in the phase I setting. Blood 2003;102(13):4527–4534.
136. Adjei AA, Erlichman C, Davis JN, et al. A Phase I trial of the farnesyl transferase inhibitor SCH66336: evidence for biological and clinical activity. Cancer Res 2000;60:1871–1877.

137. Lee JT Jr., McCubrey JA. The Raf/MEK/ERK signal transduction cascade as a target for chemotherapeutic intervention in leukemia. Leukemia 2002;16:486–507.
138. Cortes J, Albitar M, Thomas D, et al. Efficacy of the farnesyl transferase inhibitor R115777 in chronic myeloid leukemia and other hematological malignancies. Blood 2003;101:1692–1697.
139. Karp JE. Farnesyl protein transferase inhibitors as targeted therapies for hematological malignancies. Semin Hematol 2001;38:16–23.
140. Reed JC. Dysregulation of apoptosis in cancer. J Clin Oncol 1999;17:2941–2953.
141. Reed JC. Bcl-2 family proteins: regulators of apoptosis and chemoresistance in hematological malignancies. Semin Hematol 1997;34:9–19.
142. Marie JP. Drug resistance in hematological malignancies. Curr Opin Oncol 2001;13:463–469.
143. Cotter FE. Antisense therapy of hematological malignancies. Semin Hematol 1999;36:9–14.
144. Gewirtz AM. Antisense oligonucleotide therapeutics for human leukemia. Curr Opin Hematol 1998;5:59–71.
145. Andreeff M, Milella M, Konopleva M. Induction of apoptosis in AML by HA14-1, a small molecule Bcl-2 antagonist is independent of caspase-8 and -9. Blood 2002;100:543a.
146. Marcucci G, Byrd JC, Dai G, et al. Phase 1 and pharmacodynamic studies of G3139, a Bcl-2 antisense oligonucleotide, in combination with chemotherapy in refractory or relapsed acute leukemia. Blood 2003; 101:425–432.
147. Marcucci G, Stock W, Dai G, et al. G3139, a BCL-2 antisense oligo-nucleotide, in AML. Ann. Hematol 2004;83 (suppl 1):S93–94.
148. Ciechanover A. The ubiquitin-proteasome proteolytic pathway. Cell 1994;79:13–21.
149. Almond JB, Cohen GM. The proteasome: a novel target for cancer chemotherapy. Leukemia 2002;16: 433–443.
150. King RW, Deshaies RJ, Peters JM, Kirschner MW. How proteolysis drives the cell cycle. Science 1996;274: 1652–1659.
151. Karin M, Ben-Neriah Y. Phosphorylation meets ubiquitination: the control of NF-(kappa) B activity. Annu Rev Immunol 2000;18:621–663.
152. Chang YC, Lee YS, Tejima T, et al. mdm2 and bax, downstream mediators of the p53 response, are degraded by the ubiquitin-proteasome pathway. Cell Growth Differ 1998;9:79–84.
153. Breitschopf K, Zeiher AM, Dimmeler S. Ubiquitin-mediated degradation of the proapoptotic active form of bid. A functional consequence on apoptosis induction. J Biol Chem 2000;275:21,648–21,652.
154. Li B, Dou QP. Bax degradation by the ubiquitin/proteasome-dependent pathway: involvement in tumor survival and progression. Proc Natl Acad Sci USA 2000;97:3850–3855.
155. Marshansky V, Wang X, Bertrand R, et al. Proteasomes modulate balance among proapoptotic and anti-apoptotic Bcl-2 family members and compromise functioning of the electron transport chain in leukemic cells. J Immunol 2001;166:3130–3142.
156. Gardner RC, Assinder SJ, Christie G, et al. Characterization of peptidyl boronic acid inhibitors of mammalian 20 S and 26 S proteasomes and their inhibition of proteasomes in cultured cells. Biochem J 2000; 346(pt 2):447–454.
157. Almond JB, Snowden RT, Hunter A, Dinsdale D, Cain K, Cohen GM. Proteasome inhibitor-induced apoptosis of B-chronic lymphocytic leukaemia cells involves cytochrome c release and caspase activation, accompanied by formation of an approximately 700 kDa Apaf-1 containing apoptosome complex. Leukemia 2001;15:1388–1397.
158. Masdehors P, Omura S, Merle-Beral H, et al. Increased sensitivity of CLL-derived lymphocytes to apoptotic death activation by the proteasome-specific inhibitor lactacystin. Br J Hematol 1999;105:752–757.
159. Masdehors P, Merle-Beral H, Maloum K, Omura S, Magdelenat H, Delic J. Deregulation of the ubiquitin system and p53 proteolysis modify the apoptotic response in B-CLL lymphocytes. Blood 2000;96:269–274.
160. Chandra J, Niemer I, Gilbreath J, et al. Proteasome inhibitors induce apoptosis in glucocorticoid-resistant chronic lymphocytic leukemic lymphocytes. Blood 1998;92:4220–4229.
161. Adams J, Palombella VJ, Sausville EA, et al. Proteasome inhibitors: a novel class of potent and effective antitumor agents. Cancer Res 1999;59:2615–2622.
162. Cortes JE, Estey E, Giles FJ, et al. Phase I study of Bortezomib (PS-341, VELCADE), a proteasome inhibitor, in patients with refractory or relapsed acute leukemias and myelodysplastic syndromes. Blood 2002;100:560.
163. Cortes J, Thomas D, Koller C, et al. Phase I study of bortezomib in refractory or relapsed acute leukemias. Clin. Cancer Res 2004;10(10):3371–3376. Erratum in: Clin Cancer Res 2004;10(22):7787.

164. Sonneveld P. Multidrug resistance in hematological malignancies. J Intern Med 2000;247:521–534.
165. Ueda K, Cardarelli C, Gottesman MM, Pastan I. Expression of a full-length cDNA for the human "MDR1" gene confers resistance to colchicine, doxorubicin, and vinblastine. Proc Natl Acad Sci USA 1987;84: 3004–3008.
166. Nooter K, Sonneveld P, Oostrum R, Herweijer H, Hagenbeek T, Valerio D. Overexpression of the mdr1 gene in blast cells from patients with acute myelocytic leukemia is associated with decreased anthracycline accumulation that can be restored by cyclosporin-A. Int J Cancer 1990;45:263–268.
167. Leith CP, Kopecky KJ, Godwin J, et al. Acute myeloid leukemia in the elderly: assessment of multidrug resistance (MDR1) and cytogenetics distinguishes biological subgroups with remarkably distinct responses to standard chemotherapy. A Southwest Oncology Group study. Blood 1997;89:3323–3329.
168. List AF, Kopecky KJ, Willman C, et al. Benefit of cyclosporine modulation of drug resistance in patients with poor-risk acute myeloid leukemia: a Southwest Oncology Group study. Blood 2001;98:3212–3220.
169. Boesch D, Gaveriaux C, Jachez B, Pourtier-Manzanedo A, Bollinger P, Loor F. In vivo circumvention of P-glycoprotein-mediated multidrug resistance of tumor cells with SDZ PSC 833. Cancer Res 1991;51: 4226–4233.
170. Tidefelt U, Liliemark J, Gruber A, et al. P-Glycoprotein inhibitor valspodar (PSC 833;increases the intra-cellular concentrations of daunorubicin in vivo in patients with P-glycoprotein-positive acute myeloid leukemia. J Clin Oncol 2000;18:1837–1844.
171. Advani R, Visani G, Milligan D, et al. Treatment of poor prognosis AML patients using PSC833 (valspo-dar) plus mitoxantrone, etoposide, and cytarabine (PSC-MEC). Adv Exp Med Biol 1999;457:47–56.
172. Baer MR, George SL, Dodge RK, et al. Phase 3 study of the multidrug resistance modulator PSC-833 in previously untreated patients 60 years of age and older with acute myeloid leukemia: Cancer and Leukemia Group B Study 9720. Blood 2002;100:1224–1232.
173. Kolitz JE, George SL, Dodge RK, et al. Cancer and Leukemia Group B. Dose escalation studies of cytara-bine, daunorubicin, and etoposide with and without multidrug resistance modulation with PSC-833 in untreated adults with acute myeloid leukemia younger than 60 years: final induction results of Cancer and Leukemia Group B Study 9621. J Clin Oncol 2004;22(21):4290–4301.
174. Greenberg P, Advani R, Tallman M. Treatment of refractory/relapsed AML with PSC833 plus mitoxantrone, etoposide, cytarabine (PSC-MEC) vs MEC: randomized phase III trial (E2995). Blood 1999;94:383a.
175. Solary E, Drenou B, Campos L, et al. Quinine as a multidrug resistance inhibitor: a phase 3 multicentric randomized study in adult de novo acute myelogenous leukemia. Blood 2003;102:1202–1210.
176. Van der Holt B, Lowenberg B, Burnett AK, et al. The value of the MDR1 reversal agent PSC-833 in addi-tion to daunorubicin and cytarabine in the treatment of elderly patients with previously untreated acute myeloid leukemia (AML), in relation to MDR1 status at diagnosis. Blood 2005;106(8): 2646–2654.
177. Baer MR, Suvannasankha A, O'Loughlin KL, Greco WR, Minderman H. The pipecolinate derivatives VX-710 (biricodar; Incel) and VX-853 are effective modulators of drug efflux mediated by the multidrug resistance proteins P-glycoprotein. Blood 2002;100:67.
178. Blagosklonny MV, Fojo T, Bhalla KN, et al. The Hsp90 inhibitor geldanamycin selectively sensitizes Bcr-Abl- expressing leukemia cells to cytotoxic chemotherapy. Leukemia 2001;15:1537–1543.
179. Soga S, Neckers LM, Schulte TW, et al. KF25706, a novel oxime derivative of radicicol, exhibits in vivo antitumor activity via selective depletion of Hsp90 binding signaling molecules. Cancer Res 1999;59: 2931–2938.
180. Shiotsu Y, Neckers LM, Wortman I, et al. Novel oxime derivatives of radicicol induce erythroid differen-tiation associated with preferential G (1) phase accumulation against chronic myelogenous leukemia cells through destabilization of Bcr-Abl with Hsp90 complex. Blood 2000;96:2284–2291.
181. Seynaeve CM, Kazanietz MG, Blumberg PM, Sausville EA, Worland PJ. Differential inhibition of protein kinase C isozymes by UCN-01, a staurosporine analogue. Mol Pharmacol 1994;45:1207–1214.
182. Thavasu P, Propper D, McDonald A, et al. The protein kinase C inhibitor CGP41251 suppresses cytokine release and extracellular signal-regulated kinase 2 expression in cancer patients. Cancer Res 1999;59: 3980–3984.
183. Propper DJ, McDonald AC, Man A, et al. Phase I and pharmacokinetic study of PKC412, an inhibitor of protein kinase C. J Clin Oncol 2001;19:1485–1492.
184. Okuda K, Matulonis U, Salgia R, Kanakura Y, Druker B, Griffin JD. Factor independence of human myeloid leukemia cell lines is associated with increased phosphorylation of the proto-oncogene Raf-1. Exp Hematol 1994;22:1111–1117.

185. Kang CD, Yoo SD, Hwang BW, et al. The inhibition of ERK/MAPK not the activation of JNK/SAPK is primarily required to induce apoptosis in chronic myelogenous leukemic K562 cells. Leuk Res 2000;24: 527–534.

186. Kim SC, Hahn JS, Min YH, Yoo NC, Ko YW, Lee WJ. Constitutive activation of extracellular signal-regulated kinase in human acute leukemias: combined role of activation of MEK, hyperexpression of extracellular signal-regulated kinase, and downregulation of a phosphatase, PAC1. Blood 1999;93:3893–3899.

187. Morgan MA, Dolp O, Reuter CW. Cell-cycle-dependent activation of mitogen-activated protein kinase kinase (MEK-1/2) in myeloid leukemia cell lines and induction of growth inhibition and apoptosis by inhibitors of RAS signaling. Blood 2001;97:1823–1834.

188. Alessi DR, Cuenda A, Cohen P, Dudley DT, Saltiel AR. PD 098059 is a specific inhibitor of the activation of mitogen- activated protein kinase kinase in vitro and in vivo. J Biol Chem 1995;270:27,489–27,494.

189. Dudley DT, Pang L, Decker SJ, Bridges AJ, Saltiel AR. A synthetic inhibitor of the mitogen-activated protein kinase cascade. Proc Natl Acad Sci USA 1995;92:7686–7689.

190. Favata MF, Horiuchi KY, Manos EJ, et al. Identification of a novel inhibitor of mitogen-activated protein kinase kinase. J Biol Chem 1998;273:18,623–18,632.

191. Sebolt-Leopold JS. Development of anticancer drugs targeting the MAP kinase pathway. Oncogene 2000; 19:6594–6599.

192. Powis G, Bonjouklian R, Berggren MM, et al. Wortmannin, a potent and selective inhibitor of phosphat-idylinositol-3- kinase. Cancer Res 1994;54:2419–2423.

193. Vlahos CJ, Matter WF, Hui KY, Brown RF. A specific inhibitor of phosphatidylinositol 3-kinase, 2-(4- morpholinyl)-8-phenyl-4H-1-benzopyran-4-one (LY294002). J Biol Chem 1994;269:5241–5248.

194. Brown EJ, Albers MW, Shin TB, et al. A mammalian protein targeted by G1-arresting rapamycin-receptor complex. Nature 1994;369:756–758.

195. Huang S, Bjornsti MA, Houghton PJ. Rapamycins: mechanism of action and cellular resistance. Cancer Biol Ther 2003;2:222–232.

196. Huang S, Houghton PJ. Targeting mTOR signaling for cancer therapy. Curr Opin Pharmacol 2003;3:371–377.

II   Molecular Foundations of AML Pathogenesis and Physiology

2 Aberrant Transcription Factors in AML

Alan D. Friedman

CONTENTS

Summary

Several transcription factors both play a central role in normal hematopoiesis and are altered in subsets of acute myeloid leukemia (AML). CBF, c-Myb, MLL, HOXA9, WT1, and EVI-1 regulate stem/progenitor cell expansion, C/EBPα, PU.1, and RARα control myeloid development, and GATA-1 is required for erythroid and megakaryocytic development. Chromosomal translocations, point mutations, or indirect effects on expression perturb the normal activities of these factors in myeloid leukemias. The contributions these aberrant transcription factors make to the transformed phenotype are described in this chapter, following a review of the functions of their normal counterparts in hematopoiesis. Targeting transcription factors as a novel mode of AML therapy is also discussed.

Key Words: RUNX1; c-Myb; MLL; HOXA9; WT1; EVI-1; C/EBPα; PU.1; RARα; GATA-1.

1. INTRODUCTION

Transcription factors, proteins that bind genetic regulatory elements and active or repress transcription, play a central role in lineage commitment and maturation within hematopoiesis. Mutations leading to expression of aberrant transcription factors are found in every AML subset. This chapter summarizes our current understanding regarding the role that nine transcription factor oncogene/tumor suppressors play in the pathogenesis of AML. Their biological effects will be reviewed in the context of the role played in hematopoiesis by their normal counterparts. Common themes, including effects on differentiation, cell cycle, and apoptosis and the role of co-repressor interactions will be discussed, as will future experimental directions and opportunities for targeting aberrant transcription factors. Factors stimulating the proliferation of the earliest stages of hematopoiesis (CBF, c-Myb, MLL, HOXA9, WT1, EVI-1) will be considered first, followed by factors active during lineage commitment (C/EBPα, PU.1, RARα, GATA-1). IRF-8, a PU.1 cofactor, will also be discussed. We will not directly address factors broadly involved in carcinogenesis, such as c-Myc or p53. This chapter is meant to complement presentation of the molecular genetic changes that lead to expression of aberrant transcription factors in AML.

The hematopoietic subsets develop from a pluripotent hematopoietic stem cell (HSC). Expression of surface markers allows the isolation of HSC and more committed progenitors *(1,2)*.

From: *Contemporary Hematology: Acute Myelogenous Leukemia*
Edited by: J. E. Karp © Humana Press Inc., Totowa, NJ

Mapping transcription factor expression to these stem cell subsets and their progeny, analysis of regulatory elements for lineage-specific genes, and assessing phenotypes of knockout mice and the effects of factor overexpression *(3–5)* allow us to build a model of the transcriptional regulation of normal hematopoietic development, focused on factors disrupted in AML (Fig. 1). The lymphoid compartment, which branches directly from the HSC, is not included in this diagram.

2. ABERRANT TRANSCRIPTION FACTORS ASSOCIATED WITH AML

2.1. Core Binding Factor

Core binding factor (CBF) is a heterodimeric protein containing CBFα and CBFβ subunits *(6)*. Three genes encode CBFα subunits; their protein products are designated AML1/ RUNX1, AML2/RUNX3, and AML3/RUNX2. Mice lacking AML1 or CBFβ do not develop adult hematopoietic lineages *(7–11)*. AML1 contains a DNA-binding Runt domain at it N-terminus as well as transactivation and transrepression domains. CBFβ does not bind DNA but interacts with the Runt domain to increase DNA affinity *(12,13)*. In addition to its role in HSC, CBF activates several lymphoid and myeloid genes, including those encoding myelo-peroxidase (MPO) and the macrophage-specific colony-stimulating factor (M-CSF) (CSF-1) receptor *(14,15)*.

Point mutations, typically in the Runt domain, inactivate one or both copies of the AML1 gene in 3–5% of AML cases, many of which are FAB M0 *(16)*. The DNA-binding domain of AML1 is fused to ETO by t(8;21) in 12% of AMLs *(17)*. ETO interacts with mSin3A and NCoR/SMRT to mediate transcriptional repression *(18–21)*. In approx 1% of myelodysplastic syndrome (MDS), t(3;21) fuses the Runt domain to MDS1/EVI1, which also inhibits AML1-mediated transactivation *(22,23)*. Additional rare AML1 fusion partners have been identified, and germline deletion of one AML1 allele in familial platelet disorder (FPD) predisposes to AML *(24)*. CBFβ is fused to the rod domain of smooth muscle myosin heavy chain to generate CBFβ-SMMHC as a result of inv(16) or t(16;16) in 8% of AMLs, typically FAB M4eo but also M2 or M5 *(25)*. CBFβ-SMMHC inhibits CBF by sequestering AML1 in filaments, which form via rod domain multimerization and/or by virtue of the ability of AML1:CBFβ-SMMHC heterodimers to bind AML1 target genes and the mSin3A and HDAC8 co-repressors *(26,27)*. A common feature of CBF leukemias is reduction of CBF activity, as supported by the finding that AML1-ETO or CBFβ-SMMHC knockin mice have the same phenotype, lack of definitive hematopoiesis, as AML1 or CBFβ knockout mice *(28–30)*.

In addition to regulating differentiation specific genes, CBF stimulates G1 to S-cell cycle progression and is proapoptotic under stress conditions. CBF thus couples proliferation and differentiation in immature hematopoietic cells. c-Myb likely functions similarly, whereas C/EBPα and GATA-1 link terminal differentiation with proliferation arrest, as will be discussed. The first evidence that CBF (the AML1:CBFβ heterodimer) stimulates proliferation came from the finding that CBFβ-SMMHC blocks G1-to-S progression and elevates hypophospho-rylated Rb in cytokine-dependent hematopoietic cell lines, but not if the CBFβ domain is altered to prevent interaction with AML1 *(31,32)*. AML1-ETO also inhibits G1 progression, dependent upon DNA-binding *(26,33)*. Similar effects are seen in normal myeloid progenitors *(34)*. Induction of cdk4 or cyclin D3 may account for stimulation of G1 progression by AML1 *(35,36)*. CBF inhibition reduces p53 induction and apoptosis in response to DNA damage in murine cell lines lacking p19ARF *(37)*. In addition, CBF directly regulates the human

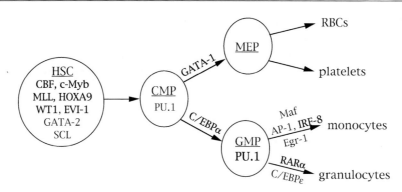

Fig. 1. Transcriptional regulation of hematopoietic lineage commitment. The pluripotent hematopoietic stem cell (HSC) gives rise to a common myeloid progenitor (CMP) that in turn generates both a megakaryocyte/erythroid progenitor (MEP) and a granulocyte-monocyte progenitor (GMP). Not shown is the common lymphoid progenitor (CLP), derived from the HSC, and branches leading to eosinophils, mast cells, and basophils, from the CMP or GMP. Several transcription factors are shown that are required for the formation and proliferation of the HSC. GATA-1 helps specify the MEP, and C/EBPα helps specify the GMP, perhaps via transcriptional induction of PU.1. Several factors are shown that participate in monocyte or granulocyte lineage maturation *(3)*. Transcription factors subject to mutation and/or aberrant expression in AML and discussed herein are highlighted in bold. RBC, red blood cell.

p14ARF promoter, suggesting that inhibition of CBF attenuates p14ARF induction under cytokine or other stress conditions, which in turn is expected to reduce p53 induction and consequent apoptosis *(38)*. Finally, CBF activates the NF-1 gene encoding the RAS-GAP neurofibromin, suggesting that repression of NF-1 by CBF oncoproteins sensitizes leukemic cells to granulocute-macrophage colony-stimulating factor (GM-CSF) and perhaps other cytokines, as in juvenile myelomonocytic leukemia (JMML) cases associated with NF-1 mutation *(39)*.

Inhibition of early differentiation in leukemic stem cells and reduction of apoptosis under stress conditions are expected to contribute to transformation by CBF oncoproteins, whereas G1-to-S blockade seems paradoxical and suggests a requirement for additional mutations that bypass cell cycle inhibition (Fig. 2). In fact, exogenous cdk4, cyclin D, or c-myc prevent G1 inhibition in cell lines, and E7, which degrades Rb, or loss of the p16p19 genes cooperates with CBFβ-SMMHC to generate murine leukemias *(35,40,41)*. Remarkably, a C-terminally truncated AML1-ETO variant, which has reduced ability to slow cell proliferation, rapidly induced murine AML, whereas full-length AML1-ETO did not generate leukemia in the model employed *(42)*. In addition, CBFβ-SMMHC cooperates with PLAG1 or PLAGL2, zinc-finger transcription factors capable of accelerating G1-to-S progression, to induce AML in mice, and PLAGL2 levels are selectively elevated in M4eo AMLs *(43)*.

2.2. c-Myb

c-Myb contains a unique N-terminal DNA-binding domain with conserved tryptophans contributing to a helix-turn-helix structure. c-Myb binds and transactivates multiple lineage-specific genes, regulating MPO synergistically with CBF *(44)*, and mice lacking c-Myb are deficient in lymphoid, erythroid, and myeloid cells *(45)*. Anti-sense inhibition of c-Myb reduces the proliferation of normal hematopoietic progenitors and of AML blasts *(46)*.

v-Myb induces an avian myeloproliferative disease and is activated, unlike c-Myb, by deletion of the C-terminal negative regulatory domain and by additional point mutations *(47)*.

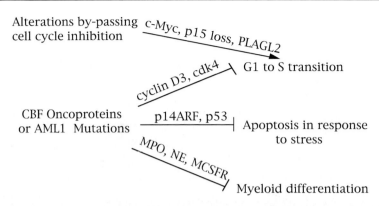

Fig. 2. Model for transformation by CBF oncoproteins and AML1 mutations. These alterations are expected to contribute to myeloid transformation by inhibiting differentiation, via inhibition of target genes such as MPO, NE, and MCSFR, and by inhibiting apoptosis in response to stress conditions such as DNA damage, hypoxia, or excessive cytokine signaling via inhibition of p14ARF-dependent and independent p53 induction. On the other hand, inhibition of G1- to-S progression, potentially via effects on cyclin D3 or cdk4 gene transcription, may be countered by additional genetic changes, such as increased c-myc, loss of p15 because of promoter methylation, and expression of PLAGL2 *(40,43)*.

Analogous mutations have not been found in human cases of AML. However, the transforming ability of v-Myb, the association of increased c-Myb expression with AML in murine models, and the association of c-Myb expression with proliferating myeloid cells lends support to the idea that increased c-Myb, when present in AML stem cells, contributes to AML *(48,49)*.

2.3. MLL

Mixed lineage leukemia (MLL) is a large protein with the capacity to bind AT-rich DNA elements and induce HOX gene expression. Induction of HOX genes requires interaction of the MLL SET domain with Menin, a component of a histone methyltransferase protein complex *(50)*. Use of MLL(−/−) ES cells to generate murine chimeras demonstrates that MLL contributes to HSC expansion and generation of committed lymphoid and myeloid progenitors *(51)*. Transduction of HOXA9, HOXA10, or HOXB4, but not bcl-2, compensates for loss of MLL to allow formation of hematopoietic colonies *(52)*, indicating that HOX genes are critical MLL targets in HSC, consistent with the central role of MLL in the maintenance of HOX gene expression during embryogenesis *(53)*.

The MLL gene, located at 11q23, is involved in multiple chromosomal translocations associated with *de novo* AML, therapy-associated AML, and pediatric ALL, the latter often having both lymphoid and myeloid surface markers *(54)*. These fusion proteins retain the N-terminal MLL DNA binding but lack the histone methyltransferase domain. Nevertheless, MLL oncoproteins apparently have increased transcriptional activation potency compared with MLL *(55–57)*. The ENL domain of MLL-ENL directly activates transcription, whereas the ELL domain of MLL-ELL interacts with the transcriptionally active EAF1 or EAF2 cofactors *(58)*. In an additional set of fusion proteins, such as MLL-GAS7 or MLL-AF1p, the fusion partner appears to primarily mediate formation of MLL domain homodimers, which themselves have increased transactivating potency *(59)*. MLL-ENL was unable to transform myeloid cells lacking either HOXA7 or HOXA9, indicating that MLL fusion oncoproteins stimulate stem cell proliferation via induction of these and other HOX genes *(60)*.

2.4. HOXA9

HOX genes bind DNA via the homeodomain in cooperation with the cofactors Pbx or Meis. HOX knockout mice have diverse phenotypes. For example, HOXA9(–/–) mice have reduced myeloid, erythroid, and B-lymphoid progenitors but normal numbers of long-term repopulating HSC *(61)*; HOXB4(–/–) mice have mildly reduced numbers of hematopoietic stem/progenitor cells, and this effect is increased by simultaneous deletion of HOXB3 *(62)*. On the other hand, HOXB4 has a remarkable capacity to expand HSC without interfering with their ability to differentiate *(63)*, and HOXA9 also expands this cell population *(64)*. Together, these findings indicate that HOX genes are proliferative in one or more marrow stem cell subset but that no single HOX gene is required for lineage commitment.

Increased HOXA9 expression is common in AML, even in the absence of MLL oncoprotein expression, and portends a poor prognosis *(65,66)*. In rare AML subsets, t(7;11) or t(7;17) fuse HOXA9 to NUP98, a nucleoporin, or MSI2, an RNA-binding protein, and NUP98-HOXA9 induces AML in mice *(67–69)*. Fusion to NUP98 appears to increase the transcriptional activity of HOXA9 *(70)*. In addition to *de novo* AML, NUP98-HOXA9 has been associated with CML blast crisis and cooperates with Bcr-abl to induce acute leukemia in a murine model *(71)*. MEIS1 potentiates the ability of HOXA9, HOXB3, NUP98-HOXA9, orNUP98-HOXD13 to induce AML but is not transforming on its own *(72–75)*.

2.5. WT1

Wilms' tumor 1 (WT1) is a zinc finger protein expressed in human CD34$^+$ cells, an immature marrow subset, but not in more mature cells *(76)*. The DNA-binding domain of WT1 is located near its C-terminus, and WT1 can activate or repress transcription depending upon promoter context *(77)*. WT1 is subject to alternative splicing, generating forms with or without a KTS insert in its DNA-binding domain, as well as proteins lacking exon 5. WT1 (–Ex5/–KTS) accelerates whereas WT1(+Ex5/+KTS) blocks the granulocytic differentiation of the 32Dcl3 cell line in response to G-CSF *(78,79)*. WT1 knockout cells generate all the hematopoietic lineages when transplanted into normal recipients, but compete poorly with wild-type cells, suggesting a proliferative or survival defect *(80)*.

WT1, typically the (+Ex5/+KTS) isoform, is elevated as much as 10-fold in the majority of AML patients compared to wild-type CD34$^+$ levels and portends a poor prognosis *(78,81)*. In addition, point mutations expected to generate truncated proteins lacking the DNA-binding domain have been detected in approx 15% of AML patients but only rarely in ALL *(82,83)*. Full-length WT1(+Ex5/+KTS) and these mutants may dominantly inhibit WT1(–Ex5/–KTS) by forming heterodimers via N-terminal interactions *(84)*. In fact, WT1(+Ex5/+KTS) interferes with the ability of WT1(–Ex5/–KTS) to repress the cyclin E promoter, suggesting a means whereby this leukemic isoform may stimulate proliferation *(85)* In addition, global suppression of WT1 using antisense oligonucleotides inhibited the growth of AML blasts, suggesting that WT1 stimulates proliferation by additional pathways as well *(86)*.

2.6. EVI-1

EVI-1 is a zinc finger protein that represses transcription via interaction with the CtBP co-repressor *(87,88)*. An alternatively spliced form, MDS1/EVI1, is extended at its N-terminus by 188 residues, the PR domain, and does not bind CtBP *(89)*. Although detected in human CD34$^+$ cells *(90)*, the function of EVI-1 in normal stem/progenitor cells is uncertain. Translocations involving 3q26 elevate EVI-1 expression in 1–2% of AML cases, most likely as a result of juxtaposition with a more active promoter *(91)*. In an additional 10% of AML cases,

EVI-1 is overexpressed in the absence of evident chromosomal abnormalities and predicts a poor prognosis *(90)*. In this study of 319 patients, elevated MDS1/EVI1 was seen in 5% of cases and did not correlate with outcome. Interaction of transforming growth factor (TGF)-β with its plasma membrane receptor activates the Smad3 transcription factor. EVI-1 may contribute to myeloid transformation by interacting with Smad3, thereby repressing Smad3 target genes and inhibiting the ability of TGF-β to slow myeloid stem cell proliferation *(92,93)*. In addition, EVI-1 prevents granulocytic differentiation in response to G-CSF *(94)*. The AML1-EVI1 fusion protein expressed from t(3;21) in a small proportion of therapy related MDS/AML or CML blast crisis cases shares many of the activities of EVI-1, including inhibition of TGF-β signaling and blockade of granulocytic maturation *(92,93)*.

2.7. C/EBPα

CCAAT/Enhancer binding protein α (C/EBPα) binds DNA via its C-terminal basic region leucine zipper (bZIP) motif and activates transcription via N-terminal transactivation domains (TADs) *(95,96)*. The bZIP domain contains a basic region (BR) that contacts DNA and an adjacent leucine zipper (LZ) that mediates dimerization via its hydrophobic surface. C/EBPα and its family members are expressed in multiple tissues but are largely restricted to the granulocytic and monocytic lineages during hematopoiesis, with C/EBPα predominating in more immature cells *(97,98)*. In contrast to mice lacking C/EBPβ, C/EBPδ, or C/EBPε, C/EBPα(−/−) mice have a severe hematopoietic defect *(99,100)*, with markedly reduced formation of granulocyte-monocyte progenitors (GMP) and their granulocytic and monocytic progeny. In addition to specifying myeloid differentiation, C/EBPα markedly inhibits G1-to-S-cell cycle progression via several mechanisms, including interaction with E2F and cdk2/4 *(101–103)*. Also, we recently found that C/EBPα inhibits apoptosis in hematopoietic cells withdrawn from cytokines, correlated with induction of bcl-2 *(104)*.

Inhibition of C/EBPα expression and activity is a common feature of AML and arises through several mechanisms. The human C/EBPα promoter is directly bound and activated by CBF; therefore, reduction of CBF activities due to point mutation of the AML1 gene or to expression of the AML1-ETO or CBFβ-SMMHC from the t(8;21) or inv(16) chromosomes is expected to reduce C/EBPα gene transcription *(105)*. Signaling from the constitutively active flt3 receptor (flt3ITD) present in 30% of AML cases also represses C/EBPα mRNA expression *(106)*. In Philadelphia chromosome-positive AML, Bcr-abl inhibits C/EBPα translation *(107)*. Finally, in 10% of AMLs the C/EBPα gene is directly mutated within its open reading frame *(108,109)*. In many cases *CEBPA* mutations are monoallelic, although bialleleic mutations occur as well. Many of the genetic changes that affect C/EBPα occur in separate AML subsets: flt3ITD is less common in CBF leukemias or in AMLs with C/EBPα mutations, CBFβ-SMMHC is associated with FAB M4 cases, whereas *CEBPA* mutation is more common in FAB M2 AMLs, and AML1-ETO and C/EBPα point mutations are found to be mutually exclusive in FAB M2 cases. Interestingly, t(8;21), inv(16), and C/EBPα gene mutations are each considered to be favorable prognostic features of AML, further suggesting a mechanistic link among these leukemia subsets *(110–112)*.

Point mutations in the *CEBPA* mainly fall into two categories: two-thirds lead to premature termination of translation in the N-terminal region and reinitiation of translation at an internal ATG, resulting in expression of a 30 kDa C/EBPαp30 protein, and one-third are inframe point mutations in the vicinity of the first leucine of the leucine zipper (Fig. 3A). We term the latter variants C/EBPαLZ oncoproteins. C/EBPαp30 lacks a potent N-terminal TAD and interferes with transactivation by the remaining 42 kDa wild-type allele, potentially via zippering

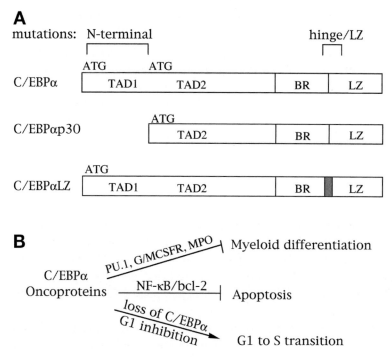

Fig. 3. Transformation by C/EBPα oncoproteins. (**A**) C/EBPα has two transactivation domains (TAD1, TAD2), a basic region (BR), which contacts DNA, and a leucine zipper (LZ), which mediates dimerization required for DNA binding. N-terminal C/EBPα mutations often produce frameshifts and premature stop codons, leading to a ribosome-scanning-mediated increase in translation from an internal ATG and expression of the C/EBPαp30 oncoprotein. Mutations in the BR-LZ are usually inframe and generally occur in the "hinge" region, between the LZ and the BR, or between the first and second leucines of the LZ, generating C/EBPαLZ oncoproteins that cannot bind DNA. (**B**) C/EBPα oncoproteins are expected to contribute to myeloid transformation by inhibiting myeloid differentiation, via reduction of PU.1, cytokine receptors, MPO, and other early myeloid genes, by inhibiting apoptosis, via induction of bcl-2 in cooperation with nuclear factor (NF)-κB p50, and by having reduced ability to inhibit G1-to-S progression.

or by competitively inhibiting binding to *cis* DNA elements. In addition, loss of 119 N-terminal amino acids in C/EBPαp30 has an unexpected effect on the C-terminal bZIP domain, reducing its interaction with a subset of C/EBPα-binding sites, including elements from the G-CSF receptor and PU.1 promoters *(108,113)*. In addition, because the C/EBPα N-terminus is required for inhibition of the cell cycle in fibroblast cells, loss of this region may enable C/EBPαp30 to block differentiation without slowing proliferation. In addition, we find that C/EBPαp30 retains the ability to activate the bcl-2 promoter and inhibit apoptosis. C/EBPαLZ oncoproteins, which cannot bind DNA, also activate the bcl-2 promoter. They may do so by interacting with the p50 subunit of nuclear factor (NF)-κB bound to κB promoter sites. The C/EBPα residues that contact NF-κB p50 lie on the outer surface of the α-helical BR. This finding offers an explanation for why most C/EBPαLZ mutations are inframe and spare the BR *(104)*.

Reduced expression or activity of C/EBPα may contribute to myeloid transformation by impeding differentiation and by diminishing the antiproliferative effect of intact C/EBPα. Inhibition of differentiation may depend upon reduced PU.1 expression, as will be elaborated in the next section. At the same time residual wild-type or mutant C/EBPα may further contribute to transformation by inhibiting apoptosis via induction of bcl-2 (Fig 3B). Our analysis of two published microarray studies *(114,115)* demonstrates that *CEBPA* and Bcl-2 mRNA levels correlate in low-risk patients, with AMLs associated with t(8;21) generally having the lowest, inv(16) intermediate, and t(15;17) the highest levels of each of these mRNAs *(104)*. Induction of bcl-2 by C/EBPα may also have been important during the development of intermediate- or high-risk AMLs, with additional mutations also inhibiting apoptosis by the time these leukemias come to clinical attention. Our analysis also indicates that mutant C/EBPα RNAs are expressed at a higher level than wild-type ones in intermediate-risk patients, consistent with the absence of an antiproliferative effect and selection for an antiapoptotic effect.

2.8. PU.1 and IRF-8

PU.1 is an Ets family transcription factor required for both B lymphoid and myeloid development *(116,117)*. Increased PU.1 levels favor myeloid over lymphoid and monocyte over granulocyte commitment *(118,119)*. Direct activation of the PU.1 gene by C/EBPα may contribute to its increased expression in GMP and thus myeloid commitment *(120,121)*, and PU.1 cofactors such as interferon consensus sequence binding protein/interferon response factor 8 (ICSBP/IRF-8) or c-Jun may account in part for the further commitment of the GMP to the monocytic lineage *(122–124)*.

Point mutations in the PU.1 gene occur only in 1–2% of AML cases *(125–127)*, and most are monoallelic. Nevertheless, two findings in murine models suggest that indirect effects on PU.1 expression are commonly involved in the pathogenesis of AML. First, although PU.1+/− mice do not develop AML, the large majority of mice homozygous for deletion of the PU.1 −14 kb enhancer express 20% of wild-type PU.1 levels and developed AML by 6 months of age *(128)*. Second, radiation-induced murine AML is often associated with deletion of one PU.1 allele and point mutation in the DNA-binding domain of the remaining allele *(129)*. Because both C/EBPα and CBF regulate the PU.1 gene *(121,130)*, inhibition of these transcription factors by various mechanisms may contribute to AML by inhibiting PU.1 expression. In addition AML1-ETO inhibits PU.1 via direct interaction, and flt3ITD suppresses PU.1 transcription *(131,132)*.

IRF-8 binds to ISRE DNA elements in association with IRF-1, IRF-2, or IRF-4, binds to EICE DNA elements in cooperation with PU.1, and binds DNA indirectly via STAT1-binding GAS elements *(133)*. Expression of IRF-8 is undetectable in the majority of AMLs and CMLs *(134)*. This may result in a reduced ability of PU.1 to activate a subset of its target genes and reduced expression of additional genes regulated by ISREs. Interestingly, mice lacking IRF-8 develop a CML-like disease *(135)*, and expression of IRF-8 correlates with responsiveness to IFN-α in human CML cases *(136)*. Downregulation of the bcl-2 promoter via an EICE and GAS element may account in part for the role of IRF-8 as a tumor suppressor in CML and AML *(137)*.

2.9. RARα

Retinoid acid receptors (RARs) bind DNA via their zinc finger domains as heterodimers with RXR proteins. Dominant inhibition of RARα arrests granulocytic maturation at the promyelocyte stage *(138)*, and granulocytic cells lacking both RARα1 and RARγ arrest at the myelocyte stage *(139)*.

The large majority of acute promyelocytic leukemias (APLs) are associated with t(15;17) and express PML-RARα. PLZF-RARα, NPM-RARα, NuMA-RARα, and STAT5b-RARα fusions occur in rare cases *(140)*. The biology of APML is extensively reviewed elsewhere in this volume, and so only key aspects will be discussed here. Each of the RARα fusions retains the RARα DNA-binding and ligand-binding domain. PML provides a coiled-coil domain that allows PML-RARα to bind DNA as a homodimer. The RARα segment of PML-RARα binds the N-CoR histone deacetylase corepressor complex, and this interaction is only relieved by pharmacological doses of retinoic acid (RA) *(141–143)*. Inhibition of RARα target genes by RARα fusion oncoproteins may account for their ability to arrest myeloid differentiation at the promyelocytic stage *(144)*. However, RA target genes required for myeloid differentiation have not been delineated, and so effects on RA-mediated stem cell differentiation, proliferation, or survival may be more relevant to transformation *(145)*. In addition to inhibiting RARα functions, PML-RARα interferes with the functions of PML and PML nuclear bodies, thereby inhibiting apoptosis in response to a variety of stimuli and contributing to genomic instability *(146)*. The reciprocal translocation product RARα-PML accelerates leukemogenesis induced by PML-RARα in a murine model, suggesting that it may also inhibit PML functions and contribute to transformation *(147)*.

2.10. GATA-1

GATA-1 is a monomeric zinc finger transcription required for the development of the erythroid and megakaryocyte lineages. Its DNA-binding zinc finger domain contains N- and C-terminal subdomains. The N-finger interacts with friend-of-GATA-1 (FOG-1), a cofactor that contributes to context-dependent transcriptional activation or repression and, like GATA-1, is required for both erythroid and megakaryocyte maturation *(148)*. GATA-1(−/−) mice die before birth with severe anemia *(149)*. Mice with reduced GATA-1 expression specifically in megakaryocytes, resulting from deletion of a gene-regulatory DNaseI hypersensitivity site, are thrombocytopenic but not anemic *(150)*.

The large majority of transient myeloproliferative disease (TMD) or acute megakaryocytic leukemias (AMKLs) that develop in Down syndrome patients carry mutations in intron 1 or exon 2 of the X-linked GATA-1 gene *(151)*. Similar to N-terminal *CEBPA* mutations, these alterations lead to translation from an internal ATG, corresponding to amino acid 84 of the long isoform. The resulting protein is termed GATA-1s. As with the truncated C/EBPαp30 isoform, GATA-1s lacks an N-terminal transactivation domain. As a result, GATA-1s is expected to have a reduced capacity to transactivate genes required for megakaryocyte development and may also dominantly inhibit GATA-2 by competing for binding to DNA *cis* elements *(4)*. In addition to effects on differentiation, reduced ability of GATA-1 to repress the c-Myc gene may stimulate proliferation in leukemic blasts *(152)*. Association of AMKL with Down syndrome indicates that trisomy of one or more genes on chromosome 21 contributes to transformation. One candidate is the AML1 gene. Perhaps increased AML1 provides a proliferative drive, as occurs in transduced marrow progenitors *(34)*.

3. FUTURE DIRECTIONS/THERAPEUTIC TARGETING

As is evident from the nine examples presented, in addition to contributing to lineage commitment and maturation, many hematopoietic transcription factors are integrated into pathways regulating cell cycle progression and apoptosis. Similarly, cytokine receptors not only provide growth and survival signals but likely also effect transcriptional regulators, although these mechanisms are generally poorly understood. One goal for the future is to develop a better appreciation of how various mutations associated with AML, such as activation of tyrosine kinase receptors, expression of aberrant transcription factors, and alterations in proteins that control cell cycle or apoptosis, cooperate to generate transformed phenotypes. For transcription factors, progress requires elucidation of their genetic targets and characterization of their regulation by protein–protein interactions and by modifications such as phosphorylation and acetylation. A fundamental understanding of oncogene/tumor suppressor cooperation will guide therapeutic efforts to manipulate a complex regulatory system in malignant cells.

Targeting aberrant transcription factors or their interacting co-repressors or co-activators may be an effective approach to therapy, although in most cases this remains to be formally proven using murine models or, preferably, human AML cells. Conceivably, some alterations are important early but not late in the transformation process. Each approach will obviously need to be tailored to relevant AML subsets. For example, HDAC inhibitors are expected to target AML1-ETO and PML-RARα but not MLL fusion oncoproteins, which transactivate HOX genes to induce cell proliferation. And small molecule or anti-sense inhibitors of CBFβ-SMMHC will be useful only for the treatment of AMLs harboring this protein. Attempts to elevate AML1, C/EBPα, or PU.1 expression or activity may have broader application, but need to be evaluated for the possibility that these normal factors will stimulate cell cycle or inhibit apoptosis without inducing differentiation or cell cycle arrest because of the presence of additional genetic changes. Finally, while targeting aberrant transcription factors alone may not be curative, a detailed understanding of the expected effects on apoptosis, cell cycle checkpoints, and other pathways may allow small molecules that target transcription factors and their interactions to be logically combined with other therapeutic modalities.

REFERENCES

1. Akashi K, Traver D, Miyamoto T, Weissman IL. A clonogenic common myeloid progenitor that gives rise to all myeloid lineages. Nature 2000;404:193–197.
2. Traver D, Miyamoto T, Christensen J, Iwasaki-Arai J, Akashi K, Weissman IL. Fetal liver myelopoiesis occurs through distinct, prospectively isolatable progenitor subsets. Blood 2001;98:627–635.
3. Friedman AD. Transcriptional regulation of granulocyte and monocyte development. Oncogene 2002; 1:3377–3390.
4. Crispino JD. GATA1 in normal and malignant hematopoiesis. Semin Cell Dev Biol 2005;16:137–147.
5. Abramovich C, Humphries RK. Hox regulation of normal and leukemic hematopoietic stem cells. Curr Opin Hematol 2005;12:210–216.
6. Friedman AD. Leukemogenesis by CBF oncoproteins. Leukemia 1999;13:1932–1942.
7. Okuda T, van Deursen J, Hiebert SW, Grosveld G, Downing JR. AML-1, the target of multiple chromosomal translocations in human leukemia, is essential for normal murine fetal hematopoiesis. Cell 1996;84:321–330.
8. Wang Q, Stacy T, Binder M, Marin-Padilla M, Sharpe AH, Speck NA. Disruption of the Cbfa2 gene causes necrosis and hemorrhaging in the central nervous system and blocks definitive hematopoiesis. Proc Natl Acad Sci USA 1996;93:3444–3449.
9. Wang Q, Stacy T, Miller JD, et al. The CBFβ subunit is essential for CBFα2(AML1) function in vivo. Cell 1996;87:697–708.
10. Sasaki K, Yagi H, Bronson RT, et al. Absence of fetal liver hematopoiesis in mice deficient in transcriptional coactivator core binding factor β. Proc Natl Acad Sci USA 1996;93:12,359–12,363.
11. Niki M, Okada H, Takano H, et al. Hematopoiesis in the fetal liver is impaired by the targeted mutagenesis of the gene encoding a non-DNA binding subunit of the transcription factor PEBP2/CBF. Proc Natl Acad Sci USA 1997;94:5697–5702.
12. Ogawa E, Inuzuka M, Maruyama M, et al. Molecular cloning and characterization of PEBP2β, the heterodimeric partner of a novel *Drosophila* runt-related DNA binding protein PEBP2α. Virology 1993;194:314–331.
13. Wang S, Wang Q, Crute BE, Melnikova IN, Keller SR, Speck NA. Cloning and characterization of subunits of The T-cell receptor and murine leukemia virus enhancer core-binding factor. Mol Cell Biol 1993;13: 3324–3339.

14. Nuchprayoon I, Meyers S, Scott LM, Suzow J, Hiebert S, Friedman AD. PEBP2/CBF, the murine homolog of the human myeloid AML1 and PEBP2β/CBFβ oncoproteins, regulates the murine myeloperoxidase and neutrophil elastase genes in immature myeloid cells. Mol Cell Biol 1994;14:5558–5568.

15. Zhang DE, Fujioka K, Hetherington CJ, et al. Identification of a region which directs the monocytic activity of the colony-stimulating factor 1 (macrophage colony-stimulating factor) receptor promoter and binds PEBP2/CBF (AML1). Mol Cell Biol 1996;16:1231–1240.

16. Osato M, Asou N, Abdalla E, et al. Biallelic and heterozygous point mutations in the runt domain of the AML1/PEBP2αB gene associated with myeloblastic leukemias. Blood 1999;93:1817–1824.

17. Miyoshi H, Kozu T, Shimizu K, et al. The t(8;21) translocation in acute myeloid leukemia results in production of an AML1-MTG8 fusion transcript. EMBO J 1993;12:2715–2721.

18. Meyers S, Lenny N, Hiebert SW. The t(8;21) fusion protein interferes with AML-1B-dependent transcriptional activation. Mol Cell Biol 1995;15:1974–1982.

19. Wang J, Hishono T, Redner RL, Kajigaya S, Liu JM. ETO, fusion partner in t(8;21) acute myeloid leukemia, represses transcription by interaction with the human N-CoR/mSin3/HDAC1 complex. Proc Natl Acad Sci USA 1998;95:10,860–10,865.

20. Lutterbach B, Westendorf JJ, Linggi B, et al. ETO, a target of t(8;21) in acute leukemia, interacts with N-CoR and mSin3 corepressors. Mol Cell Biol 1998;18:7176–7184.

21. Gelmetti V, Zhang J, Fanelli M, Minucci S, Pelicci P, Lazar MA. Aberrant recruitment of the nuclear receptor corepressor-histone deacetylase complex by the acute myeloid leukemia fusion partner ETO. Mol Cell Biol 1998;18:7185–7191.

22. Tanaka T, Mitani K, Kurokawa M, et al. Dual functions of the AML1/Evi-1 chimeric protein in the mechanism of leukemogenesis in t(3;21) leukemias. Mol Cell Biol 1995;15:2383–2392.

23. Zent CS, Mathieu C, Claxton DF, et al. The chimeric genes AML1/MDS1 and AML1/EAP inhibit AML1B activation of the CSF1R promoter, but only AML1/MDS1 has tumor promoting properties. Proc Natl Acad Sci USA 1996;93:1044–1048.

24. Song WJ, Sullivan MG, Legare RD, et al. Haploinsufficiency of CBFA2 causes familial thrombocytopenia with propensity to develop acute myeloid leukemia. Nat Genet 1999;23:166–175.

25. Liu P, Tarle SA, Hajre A, et al. Fusion between transcription factor CBFβ/PEBP2β and a myosin heavy chain in acute myeloid leukemia. Science 1993;261:1041–1044.

26. Kummalue T, Lou J, Friedman AD. Multimerization via its myosin domain facilitates nuclear localization and inhibition of core binding factor (CBF) by the CBFβ-smooth muscle myosin heavy chain myeloid leukemia oncoprotein. Mol Cell Biol 2002;22:8278–8291.

27. Durst KL, Lutterbach B, Kummalue T, Friedman AD, Hiebert SW. The inv(16) fusion protein associates with corepressors via a smooth muscle myosin heavy-chain domain. Mol Cell Biol 2003;23:607–619.

28. Castilla LH, Wijmenga C, Stacy T, et al. Failure of embryonic hematopoiesis and lethal hemorrhages in mouse embryos heterozygous for a knocked-in leukemia gene CBFB-MYH11. Cell 1996;87:687–696.

29. Yergeau DA, Hetherington CJ, Wang Q, et al. Embryonic lethality and impairment of haematopoiesis in mice heterozygous for an AML1-ETO fusion gene. Nat Genet 1997;15:303–306.

30. Okuda T, Cai Z, Yang S, et al. Expression of a knocked-in AML1-ETO leukemia gene inhibits the establishment of normal definitive hematopoiesis and directly generates dysplastic hematopoietic progenitors. Blood 1998;91:3134–3143.

31. Cao W, Britos-Bray M, Claxton DF, et al. CBFβ-SMMHC, expressed in M4eo AML, reduced CBF DNA-binding and inhibited G1 to S cell cycle transition at the restriction point in myeloid and lymphoid cells. Oncogene 1997;15:1315–1327.

32. Cao W, Adya N, Britos-Bray M, Liu PP, Friedman AD. The core binding factor a interaction domain and the smooth muscle myosin heavy chain segment of CBFβ-SMMHC are both required to slow cell proliferation. J Cell Biol 1998;273:31,534–31,540.

33. Burel SA, Harakawa N, Zhou L, Pabst T, Tenen DG, Zhang DE. Dichotomy of AML1-ETO functions: growth arrest versus block of differentiation. Mol Cell Biol 2001;21:5577–5590.

34. D'Costa J, Chaudhuri S, Civin CI, Friedman AD. CBFβ-SMMHC slows proliferation of primary murine and human myeloid progenitors. Leukemia 2005;19:921–929.

35. Lou J, Cao W, Bernardin F, Ayyanathan K, Rauscher III, FJ, Friedman AD. Exogenous cdk4 overcomes reduced cdk4 RNA and inhibtion of G1 progression in hematoopietic cells expressing a dominant-negative CBF—a model for overcoming inhibition of proliferation by CBF oncoproteins. Oncogene 2000;19: 2695–2703.

36. Bernardin-Fried F, Kummalue T, Leijen S, Collector MI, Ravid K, Friedman AD. AML1/RUNX1 increases during G1 to S cell cycle progression independent of cytokine-dependent phosphorylation and induces cyclin D3 gene expression. J Biol Chem 2004;279:15,678–15,687.
37. Britos-Bray M, Ramirez M, Cao W, et al. CBFβ-SMMHC, expressed in M4eo AML, reduces p53 induction and slows apoptosis in hematopoietic cells exposed to DNA-damaging agents. Blood 1998;92:4344–4352.
38. Linggi B, Muller-Tidow C, van de Locht L, et al. The t(8;21) fusion protein, AML1 ETO, specifically represses the transcription of the p14(ARF) tumor suppressor in acute myeloid leukemia. Nat Med 2002;8: 743–750.
39. Yang G, Khalaf W, van de Locht L, et al. Epigenetic regulation of tumor suppressors in t(8:21)-containing AML. Ann Hematol 2004;83 (suppl 1):S83.
40. Bernardin F, Yang Y, Civin CI, Friedman AD. c-Myc overcomes cell cycle inhibition by CBFβ-SMMHC, a myeloid leukemia oncoprotein. Cancer Biol Ther 2002;1:494–498.
41. Yang Y, Wang W, Cleaves R, et al. Acceleration of G1 cooperates with CBFβ-SMMHC to induce acute leukemia in mice. Cancer Res 2002;62:2232–2235.
42. Yan M, Burel SA, Peterson LF, et al. Deletion of an AML1-ETO C-terminal NcoR/SMRT-interacting region strongly induces leukemia development. Proc Natl Acad Sci USA 2004;101:17,186–17,191.
43. Landrette SF, Kuo Y-H, Hensen K, et al. Plag2 and Plagl2 are oncogenes that induce acute myeloid leukemia in cooperation with Cbfb-MYH11. Blood 2005;105:2900–2907.
44. Britos-Bray M, Friedman AD. Core binding factor cannot synergistically activate the myeloperoxidase proximal enhancer in immature myeloid cells without c-Myb. Mol Cell Biol 1997;17:5127–5135.
45. Mucenski ML, McLain K, Kier AB, et al. A functional c-myb gene is required for normal murine fetal hepatic hematopoiesis. Cell 1991;65:677–689.
46. Calabretta B, Sims RB, Valtieri et al. Normal and leukemic hematopoietic cells manifest differential sensitivity to inhibitory effects of c-myb antisense oligonucleotides: an in vitro study relevant to bone marrow purging. Proc Natl Acad Sci USA 1991;88:2351–2355.
47. Graf T. Leukemogenesis: small differences in Myb have large effects. Curr Biol 1998;8:R353–R355.
48. Gonda TJ, Cory S, Sobieszczuk P, Holtzman D, Adams JM. Generation of altered transcripts by retroviral insertion within the c-myb gene in two monocytic leukemias. J Virol 1987;61:2754–2763.
49. Shen-Ong GL, Wolff L. Moloney murine leukemia virus-induced myeloid tumors in adult BALB/c mice: requirement of c-myb activation but lack of v-abl involvement. J Virol 1987;61:3721–3725.
50. Yokoyama A, Wang Z, Wysocka J, et al. Leukemia proto-oncoprotein MLL forms a SET1-like histone methyltransferase complex with menin to regulate *Hox* gene expression. Mol Cell Biol 2004;24: 5639–5649.
51. Ernst P, Fisher JK, Avery W, Wade S, Foy D, Korsmeyer SJ. Definitive hematopoiesis requires the mixed-lineage leukemia gene. Dev Cell 2004;6:437–443.
52. Ernst P, Mabon M, Davidson AJ, Zon LI, Korsmeyer SJ. An Mll-dependent Hox program drives hematopoietic progenitor expansion. Curr Biol 2004;14:2063–2069
53. Yu BD, Hanson RD, Hess JL, Horning SE, Korsmeyer SJ. MLL, a mammalian trithorax-group gene, functions as a transcriptional maintenance factor in morphogenesis. Proc Natl Acad Sci USA1998;95:10,632–10,636.
54. Ayton PM, Cleary ML. Molecular mechanisms of leukemogenesis mediated by MLL fusion proteins. Oncogene 2001;20:5695–5707.
55. Slany RK, Lavau C, Cleary ML. The oncogenic capacity of HRX-ENL requires the transcriptional transactivation activity of ENL and the DNA binding motif of HRX. Mol Cell Biol 1998;18:122–129.
56. So CW, Cleary ML. MLL-AFX requires the transcriptional effector domains of AFX to transform myeloid progenitors and transdominantly interfere with forkhead protein function. Mol Cell Biol 2002;22:6542–6552.
57. Zeisig BB, Schreiner S, Garcia-Cuellar MP, Slany RK. Transcriptional activation is a key function encoded by MLL fusion partners. Leukemia 2003;17:359–365.
58. Simone F, Luo RT, Polak PE, Kaberlein JJ, Thirman MJ. ELL-associated factor 2 (EAF2), a functional homolog of EAF1 with alternative ELL binding properties. Blood 2003;101:2355–2362.
59. So CW, Cleary ML. Dimerization: a versatile switch in oncogenesis. Blood 2004;104:919–922.
60. Ayton PM, Cleary ML. Transformation of myeloid progenitors by MLL oncoproteins is dependent on Hoxa7 and Hoxa9. Genes Dev 2003;17:2298–2307.
61. Lawrence HJ, Helgason CD, Sauvageau G, et al. Mice bearing targeted interruption of the homeobox gene HOXA9 have defects in myeloid, erythroid, and lymphoid hematopoiesis. Blood 1997;89:1922–1930.
62. Bjornsson JM, Larsson N, Brun AC, et al. Reduced proliferative capacity of hematopoietic stem cells deficient in Hoxb3 and Hoxb4. Mol Cell Biol 2003;23:3872–3883.

63. Antonchuk J, Sauvageau G, Humphries RK. HOXB4 overexpression mediates very rapid stem cell regeneration and competitive hematopoietic repopulation. Exp Hematol 2001;29:1125–1134.

64. Thorsteinsdottir U, Mamo A, Kroon E, et al. Overexpression of the myeloid leukemia-associated *Hoxa9* gene in bone marrow cells induces stem cell expansion. Blood 2002;99:121–129.

65. Golub TR, Slonim DK, Tamayo P, et al. Molecular classification of cancer: class discovery and class prediction by gene expression monitoring. Science 1999;286:531–537.

66. Drabkin HA, Parsy C, Feguson K, et al. Quantitative HOX expression in chromosomally defined subsets of acute myeloid leukemia. Leukemia 2002;16:186–195.

67. Nakamura T, Largaespada DA, Lee MP, et al. Fusion of the nucleoporin gene NUP98 to HOXA9 by the chromosome translocation t(7;11)(p15;p15) in human myeloid leukemia. Nat Genet 1996;12:154–158.

68. Barbouti A, Hoglund M, Johansson B, et al. A novel gene, MS12, encoding a putative RNA-binding protein is recurrently rearranged at disease progression of chronic myeloid leukemia and forms a fusion gene with HOXA9 as a result of cryptic t(7;17)(p15;q23). Cancer Res 2003;63:1202–1206.

69. Kroon E, Thorsteinsdotter U, Mayotte N, et al. NUP98-HOXA9 expression in hemopoietic stem cells induces chronic and acute myeloid leukemias in mice. EMBO J 2001;20:350–361.

70. Ghannam G, Takeda A, Camarata T, et al. The oncogene Nup98-HOXA9 induces gene transcription in myeloid cells. J Biol Chem 2004;279:866–875.

71. Dash AB, Williams IR, Kutok JL, et al. A murine model of CML blast crisis induced by cooperation between BCR/ABL and NUP98/HOXA9. Proc Natl Acad Sci USA 2002;99:7622–7627.

72. Nakamura T, Largaespada DA, Shaughnessy JD Jr, Jenkins NA, Copeland NG. Cooperative activation of Hoxa and Pbx1-related genes in murine myeloid leukemias. Nat Genet 1996;12:149–153.

73. Pineault N, Buske C, Feuring-Buske M, et al. Induction of acute myeloid leukemia in mice by the human leukemia-specific fusion gene NUP98-HOXD13 in concert with Meis1. Blood 2003;101:4529–4538.

74. Pineault N, Abramovich C, Ohta H, et al. Differential and common leukemogenic potentials of multiple NUP98-Hox fusion proteins alone or with Meis1. Mol Cell Biol 2004;24:1907–1917.

75. Thorsteinsdottir U, Kroon E, Jerome L, Blasi F, Sauvageau G. Defining roles for HOX and MEIS1 genes in induction of acute myeloid leukemia. Mol Cell Biol 2001;21:224–234.

76. Maurer U, Brieger J, Weidmann E, Mitrou PS, Hoelzer D, Bergmann L. The Wilms' tumor gene is expressed in a subset of CD34+ progenitors and downregulated early in the course of differentiation in vitro. Proc Natl Acad Sci USA 1997;94:6781–6785.

77. Reddy JC, Licht JD. The WT1 Wilms' tumor suppressor gene: How much do we really know? Biochim Biophys Acta 1996;1287:1–28.

78. Inoue K, Tamaki H, Ogawa H, et al. Wilms' tumor gene (WT1) competes with differentiation-inducing signal in hematopoietic progenitor cells. Blood 1998;91:2969–2976.

79. Loeb DM, Summers JL, Burwell EA, Korz D, Friedman AD, Sukumar S. An isoform of the Wilms' tumor suppressor gene potentiates granulocytic differentiation. Leukemia 2003;17:965–971.

80. Alberta JA, Springett GM, Rayburn, et al. Role of the WT1 tumor suppressor in murine hematopoieis. Blood 2003;101:2570–2574.

81. Inoue K, Sugiyama H, Ogawa H, et al. WT1 as a new prognostic factor and a new marker for the detection of minimal residual disease in acute leukemia. Blood 1994;84:3071–3079.

82. King-Underwood L, Pritchard-Jones, K. Wilms' tumor (WT1) gene mutations occur mainly in acute myeloid leukemia and may confer drug resistance. Blood 1998;91:2961–2968.

83. Miyagawa K, Hayashi Y, Fukuda T, Mitani K, Hirai H, Kamiya K. Mutations of the WT1 gene in childhood nonlymphoid hematological malignancies. Genes Chrom Cancer 1999;25:176–183.

84. Holmes G, Boterashvili S, English M, Wainwright B, Licht J, Little M. Two N-terminal self-association domains are required for the dominant negative transcriptional activity of WT1 Denys-Drash mutant proteins. Biochem Biophys Res Commun 1997;233:723–728.

85. Loeb DM, Korz D, Katsnelson M, Burwell EA, Friedman AD, Sukumar S. Cyclin E is a target of WT1 transcriptional repression. J Biol Chem 2002;277:19,627–19,632.

86. Yamagami T, Sugiyama H, Inoue K, et al. Growth inhibition of human leukemia cells by WT1 (Wilms tumor gene) antisense oligodeoxynucleotides: implications for the involvement of WT1 in leukemogenesis. Blood 1996;87:2878–2884.

87. Izutsu K, Kurokawa M, Imai Y, Maki K, Mitani K, Hirai H. The corepressor CtBP interacts with Evi-1 to repress transforming growth factor β signaling. Blood 2001;97:2815–2822.

88. Palmer S, Brouillet JP, Kilbey A, et al. Evi-1 transforming and repressor activities are mediated by CtBP corepressor protein. J Biol Chem 2001;276:25,834–25,840.

89. Nitta E, Izutsu K, Yamaguchi Y, et al. Oligomerization of Evi-1 regulated by the PR domain contributes to recruitment of corepressor CtBP. Oncogene 2005;24:6165–6173.
90. van Waalwijk van Doorn-Khosrovani SB, Erpelinck C, van Putten WLJ, et al. High EVI1 expression predicts poor survival in acute myeloid leukemia: a study of 319 de novo AML patients. Blood 2003;101:837–845.
91. Morishita K, Parganas E, William CL, et al. Activation of EVI1 gene expression in human acute myelogenous leukemias by translocations spanning 300-400 kilobases on chromosome band 3q26. Proc Natl Acad Sci USA 1992;89:3937–3941.
92. Kurokawa M, Mitani K, Irie K, et al. The oncoprotein Evi-1 represses TGF-β signaling by inhibiting Smad3. Nature 1998;394:92–96.
93. Sood R, Talwar-Trikha A, Chakrabarti SR, Nucifora G. MDS1/EVI1 enhances TGF-β1 signaling and strengthens its growth-inhibitory effect but the leukemia-associated fusion protein AML1/MDS1/EVI1, product of t(3;21), abrogates growth-inhibition in response to TGF-β1. Leukemia 1999;13:348–357.
94. Morishita K, Parganas E, Matsugi T, Ihle J. Expression of the Evi-1 zinc finger gene in 32Dcl3 myeloid cells blocks granulocytic differentiation in response to granulocyte colony-stimulating factor. Mol Cell Biol 1992;12:183–189.
95. Landschulz WH, Johnson PF, McKnight SL. The DNA binding domain of the rat liver protein C/EBP is bipartite. Science 1989;246:1681–1688.
96. Friedman AD, McKnight SL. Identification of two polypeptide segments of CCAAT/enhancer-binding protein required for transcriptional activation of the serum albumin gene. Genes Dev 1990;4:1416–1426.
97. Scott LM, Civin CI, Rorth P, Friedman AD. A novel temporal pattern of three C/EBP family members in differentiating myelomonocytic cells. Blood 1992;80:1725–1735.
98. Antonson P, Stellan B, Yamanaka R, Xanthopoulos KG. A novel human CCAAT/enhancer binding protein gene, C/EBPε, is expressed in cells of lymphoid and myeloid lineages and is localized on chromosome 14q11.2 close to the T cell receptor α/δ locus. Genomics 1996;35:30–38.
99. Zhang DE, Zhang P, Wang N-D, Hetherington CJ, Darlington GJ, Tenen DG. Absence of G-CSF signaling and neutrophil development in CCAAT enhancer binding protein α-deficient mice. Proc Natl Acad Sci USA 1997;94:569–574.
100. Zhang P, Iwasaki-Arai, Iwasaki H, et al. Enhancement of hematopoietic stem cell repopulating capacity and self-renewal in the absence of the transcription factor C/EBPα. Immunity 2004;21:853–863.
101. Umek RH, Friedman AD, McKnight SL. CCAAT/enhancer binding protein: a component of a differentiation switch. Science 1991;25:288–292.
102. Porse BT, Pedersen TA, Xu X, et al. E2F repression by C/EBPα is required for adipogenesis and granulopoiesis in vivo. Cell 2001;107:247–258.
103. Wang H, Iakova P, Wilde M, et al. C/EBPα arrests cell proliferation through direct inhibition of cdk2 and cdk4. Mol Cell 2001;8:817–828.
104. Paz-Priel I, Cai DH, Wang D, et al. C/EBPα and C/EBPα myeloid oncoproteins induce bcl-2 via interaction of their basic regions with nuclear factor-κB p50. Mol Cancer Res 2005;3:585–596.
105. Pabst T, Mueller BU, Harakawa N, et al. AML1-ETO downregulates the granulocytic differentiation factor C/EBPα in t(8;21) myeloid leukemia. Nat Med 2001;7:444–451.
106. Zheng R, Friedman AD, Small D. Internal tandem duplication mutation of FLT3 blocks myeloid differentiation through suppression of C/EBPα expression. Blood 2004;103:1883–1890.
107. Perrotti D, Cesi V, Trotta R, et al. Bcr-abl suppresses C/EBPα expression through inhibitory action of hnRNP E2. Nat Genet 2002;30:48–58.
108. Pabst T, Mueller BU, Zhang P, et al. Dominant-negative mutations of CEBPA, encoding CCAAT/enhancer binding protein-alpha (C/EBPα), in acute myeloid leukemia. Nat Genet 2001;27:263–270.
109. Gombart AF, Hofmann WK, Kawano S, et al. Mutations in the gene encoding the transcription factor CCAAT/enhancer binding protein alpha in myelodysplastic syndromes and acute myeloid leukemias. Blood 2002;99:1332–1340.
110. Marcucci G, Caligiuri MA, Bloomfield CD. Molecular and clinical advances in core binding factor primary acute myeloid leukemia: a paradigm for translational research in malignant hematology. Cancer Invest. 2000;18:768–780.
111. Preudhomme C, Sagot C, Boissel N, et al. Favorable prognostic significance of *CEBPA* mutations in patients with de novo acute myeloid leukemia: a study from the Acute Leukemia French Association (ALFA). Blood 2002;100:2717–2723.
112. Frohling S, Schlenk RF, Stolze I, et al. *CEBPA* mutations in younger adults with acute myeloid leukemia and normal cytogenetics: prognostic relevance and analysis of cooperating mutations. J Clin Onc 2004;22:624–633.

113. Cleaves R, Wang QF, Friedman AD. C/EBPαp30, a myeloid leukemia oncoprotein, limits G-CSF receptor expression but not terminal granulopoiesis via site-selective inhibition of C/EBP DNA binding. Oncogene 2004;23:716–725.

114. Bullinger L, Dohner K, Bair E, et al. Use of gene-expression profiling to identify prognostic subclasses in adult acute myeloid leukemia. N Engl J Med 2004;350:1605–1616.

115. Valk PJM, Verhaak RGW, Beijen MA, et al. Prognostically useful gene-expression profiles in acute myeloid leukemia. N Engl J Med 2004;350:1617–1628.

116. Scott EW, Simon MC, Anastasi J, Singh H. Requirement of transcription factor PU.1 in the development of multiple hematopoietic lineages. Science 1994;265:1573–1577.

117. McKercher SR, Torbett BE, Anderson KL, et al. Targeted disruption of the PU.1 gene results in multiple hematopoietic abnormalities. EMBO J 1996;15:5647–5658.

118. DeKoter RP, Singh H. Regulation of B lymphocyte and macrophage development by graded expression of PU.1. Science 2000;288:1439–1441.

119. Dahl R, Walsh JC, Lancki D, et al. Regulation of macrophage and neutrophil cell fates by the PU.1:C/EBPα ratio and granulocyte colony-stimulating factor. Nat Immunol 2003;4:1029–1036.

120. Wang X, Scott E, Sawyers CL, Friedman AD. C/EBPα by-passes G-CSF signals to rapidly induce PU.1 gene expression, stimulate granulocytic differentiation, and limit proliferation in 32Dcl3 myeloblasts. Blood 1999;94:560–571.

121. Kummalue T, Friedman AD. Cross-talk between regulators of myeloid development: C/EBPα binds and activates the promoter of the PU.1 gene. J Leuk Biol 2003;72:464–470.

122. Tamura T, Nagamura-Inoue T, Shmeltzer Z, Kuwata T, Ozato K. ICSBP directs bipotential myeloid progenitor cells to differentiate into mature macrophages. Immunity 2000;13:155–165.

123. Lord KA, Abdollahi A, Hoffman-Liebermann B, Liebermann DA. Proto-oncogenes of the fos/jun family of transcription factors are positive regulators of myeloid differentiation. Mol Cell Biol 1993;13:841–851.

124. Behre G, Whitmarsh AJ, Coghlan MP, et al. c-Jun is a JNK-independent coactivator of the PU.1 transcription factor. J Biol Chem 1999;274:4939–4946.

125. Mueller BU, Pabst T, Osato M, et al. Heterozygous PU.1 mutations are associated with acute myeloid leukemia. Blood 2002;100:998–1007.

126. Vegesna V, Takeuchi S, Hofmann WK, et al. C/EBP-beta, C/EBP-delta, PU.1, AML1 genes: mutational analysis in 381 samples of hematopoietic and solid malignancies. Leuk Res 2002;26:451–457.

127. Dohner K, Tobis K, Bischof T, et al. Mutation analysis of the transcription factor PU.1 in younger adults (16 to 60 years) with acute myeloid leukemia: a study of the AML Study Group Ulm (AMLSG ULM). Blood 2003;102:3850–3851.

128. Rosenbauer F, Wagner K, Kutok JL, et al. Acute myeloid leukemia induced by graded reduction of a lineage-specific transcription factor, PU.1. Nat Genet 2004;36:624–630.

129. Cook WD, McCaw BJ, Herring C, et al. PU.1 is a suppressor of myeloid leukemia, inactivated in mice by gene deletion and mutation of its DNA binding domain. Blood 2004;3437–3444.

130. Huang G, Zhang P, Koschmieder S, et al. PU.1 is a critical downstream target of AML1. Blood 2004;105a.

131. Vangala RK, Heiss-Neumann M, Rangatia JS, et al. The myeloid master regulator transcription factor PU.1 is inactivated by AML1-ETO in t(8;21) myeloid leukemia. Blood 2003;101:270–277.

132. Mizuki M, Schwable J, Steur C, et al. Suppression of myeloid transcription factors and induction of STAT response genes by AML-specific Flt3 mutations. Blood 2003;101:3164–3173.

133. Tamura T, Ozato K. ICSBP/IRF-8: its regulatory roles in the development of myeloid cells. J Interferon Cytokine Res 2002;22:145–152.

134. Schmidt M, Nagel S, Proba J, et al. Lack of interferon consensus sequence binding protein (ICSBP) transcripts in human myeloid malignancies. Blood 1998;91:22–29.

135. Holtschke T, Lohler J, Kanno Y, et al. Immunodeficiency and chronic myelogenous leukemia-like syndrome in mice with a targeted mutation of the ICSBP gene. Cell 1996;87:307–317.

136. Schmidt M, Hochhaus A, Nitsche A, Hehlmann R, Neubauer A. Expression of nuclear transcription factor interferon consensus sequence binding protein in chronic myeloid leukemia correlates with pretreatment risk features and cytogenetic response to interferon-alpha. Blood 2001;97:3648–3650.

137. Burchert A, Cai D, Hofbauer LC, et al. Interferon consensus sequence binding protein (ICSBP; IRF-8) antagonizes BCR/ABL and down-regulates bcl-2. Blood 2004;103:3480–3489.

138. Tsai S, Collins SJ. A dominant negative retinoic acid receptor blocks neutrophil differentiation at the promyelocyte stage. Proc Natl Acad Sci USA 1993;90:7153–7157.

139. Labrecque J, Allan D, Chambon P, Iscove NN, Lohnes D, Hoang T. Impaired granulocytic differentiation in vitro in hematopoietic cells lacking retinoic acid receptors alpha1 and gamma. Blood 1998;92;607–615.
140. Zelent A, Guidez F, Melnick A, Waxman S, Licht JD. Translocations of the RARα gene in acute promyelocytic leukemia. Oncogene 2001;20:7186–7203.
141. Grignani F, De Matteis S, Nervi C, et al. Fusion proteins of the retinoic acid receptor-alpha recruit histone deacetylase in promyelocytic leukaemia. Nature 1998;19;391:815–818.
142. He LZ, Guidez F, Triboli C, et al. Distinct interactions of PML-RARα and PLZF-RARα with co-repressors determine differential response to RA in APL. Nat Genet 1998;18:126–135.
143. Lin RJ, Nagy L, Inoue S, Shao W, Miller Jr WH, Evans RM. Role of the histone deacetylase complex in acute promyelocytic leukemia. Nature 1998;391:811–814.
144. Grignani F, Valtieri M, Gabbianelli M, et al. PML/RAR alpha fusion protein expression in normal human hematopoietic progenitors dictates myeloid commitment and the promyelocytic phenotype. Blood 2000;96: 1531–1537.
145. Puccetti E, Ruthardt M. Acute promyelocytic leukemia: PML/RARα and the leukemic stem cell. Leukemia 2004;18:1169–1175.
146. Bernardi R, Pandolfi PP. Role of PML and the PML-nuclear body in the control of programmed cell death. Oncogene 2003;22:9048–9057.
147. Pollock JL, Westervelt P, Kurichety AK, Pelicci PG, Grisolano JL, Ley TJ. A bcr-3 isoform of RARα-PML potentiates the development of PML-RARα-driven acute promyelocytic leukemia. Proc Natl Acad Sci USA 1999;96:15,103–15,108.
148. Tsang AP, Visvader JE, Turner CA, et al. FOG, a multitype zinc finger protein, acts as a cofactor for transcription factor GATA-1 in erythroid and megakaryocytic differentiation. Cell 1997;90:109–119.
149. Fujiwara Y, Browne CP, Cunniff K, Goff SC, Orkin SH. Arrested development of embryonic red cell precursors in mouse embryos lacking transcription factor GATA-1. Proc Natl Acad Sci USA 1996;93:12,355–12,358.
150. McDevitt MA, Shivdasani RA, Fujiwara Y, Yang H, Orkin SH. A "knockdown" mutation created by cis-element gene targeting reveals the dependence of erythroid cell maturation on the level of transcription factor GATA-1. Proc Natl Acad Sci USA 1997;94:6781–6785.
151. Wechsler J, Greene M, McDevitt MA, et al. Acquired mutations in GATA1 in the megakaryoblastic leukemia of Down syndrome. Nat Genet 2002;32:148–152.
152. Rylski M, Welch JJ, Chen YY, Letting DL, et al. GATA-1-mediated proliferation arrest during erythroid maturation. Mol Cell Biol 2003;23:5031–5042.

3   Myelodysplasia-Related AML

Jane E. Parker

Summary

The myelodysplastic syndromes (MDSs) comprise a heterogeneous group of clonal stem cell disorders characterized by ineffective hematopoiesis *(1)*. Because progression to acute myeloid leukemia (AML) occurs in one-third of cases, myelodysplasia-related AML (MDS-AML) provides an elegant model for the multistep process of leukemogenesis. This chapter will outline our current understanding of the cellular changes that occur during progression of MDS to AML and discuss the potential molecular lesions underlying these changes.

Key Words: Myelodysplastic syndromes; acute myeloid leukemia; myelodysplasia-related AML; leukemogenesis; apoptosis; proliferation; cell cycle.

1. MYELODYSPLASIA-RELATED AML: CLASSIFICATION

The World Health Organization (WHO) has recently reclassified the myeloid neoplasms *(2)*. By utilizing morphological, genetic, immunophenotypic, biological, and clinical features to define disease entities, this revised classification system attempts to incorporate clinical and biologically relevant features into a useful working nomenclature. The most pertinent changes to AML classification include lowering the blast threshold from 30 to 20% and subdividing AML into distinct subgroups with differing biological features (reviewed in ref. *3*). As such, *de novo* AML associated with multilineage dysplasia and AML evolving from MDS have been grouped together within the subgroup "AML with multilineage dysplasia."

From: *Contemporary Hematology: Acute Myelogenous Leukemia*
Edited by: J. E. Karp © Humana Press Inc., Totowa, NJ

2. THE MULTISTEP PATHOGENESIS OF MYELODYSPLASIA-RELATED AML: AN IMBALANCE BETWEEN SURVIVAL AND DEATH SIGNALS

The pathogenesis of myelodysplasia-related (MDS)-AML differs from that of *de novo* disease in several respects. Balanced chromosomal translocations and mutations are characteristic of *de novo* AML. The resulting abnormal chimeric proteins frequently activate pathways that confer a survival/proliferative advantage to hematopoietic progenitors or alter transcription factors involved in regulating differentiation and survival/proliferation genes. In MDS-AML, however, loss of chromosomal material is commonly observed, suggesting that malignant transformation may arise through deletion of tumor suppressor genes *(4,5)*. The genomic lesions resulting in MDS-AML almost certainly accumulate over a number of years *(6)*. Studies measuring levels of apoptosis and proliferation and the ratio between the two at different disease stages suggest that there are at least four phases in MDS-AML evolution.

1. Very early genetic events almost certainly increase the self-renewal and/or proliferative/survival capacity of primitive hematopoietic stem cells, creating an expanded abnormal clonal stem cell pool. At this stage the disorder is phenotypically silent.
2. Overt, symptomatic early MDS, by contrast, is associated with excessive hematopoietic cell apoptosis, leading to the characteristic cytopenias *(7,8)*. This stage probably arises when the number and/or nature of genetic lesions are sufficient to impair differentiation and trigger DNA damage or immune surveillance mechanisms, with resultant cell death.
3. MDS progression appears initially to be a result of genomic hits that upregulate proliferation, such that the balance between mitotic and apoptotic signals is equalized.
4. Finally, leukemic transformation occurs through the acquisition of lesions that further block differentiation and target apoptotic pathways/checkpoints (Fig. 1) *(9)*.

The ensuing abrogation of programmed cell death (PCD) permits both the illegitimate survival and accumulation of primitive malignant cells and facilitates chemotherapeutic resistance.

3. APOPTOSIS AND PROLIFERATION IN NORMAL HEMATOPOIETIC CELLS

Normal hematopoiesis is dependent upon the precise regulation of complex signaling pathways that control cellular decisions to proliferate, differentiate, arrest cell growth, or undergo apoptosis. In order to unravel the pathogenesis of aberrant cell growth and death in MDS evolution, it is important to understand the mechanisms of apoptosis and proliferation in normal hematopoietic cells.

3.1. Apoptosis

Apoptosis is a tightly controlled form of cell death executed through intrinsic cell suicide machinery. PCD can be triggered when either the extracellular or intracellular milieu is hostile to cell survival/proliferation. Both extrinsic and intrinsic apoptotic stimuli trigger a common effector pathway whereby a cascade of intracellular cysteine aspartate-specific proteases or caspases are activated with resultant cleavage of proteins critical for cell survival (Fig. 2) *(10)*.

3.1.1. EXTRINSIC DEATH SIGNALS

PCD may be triggered when extrinsic death ligands (fas-ligand, tumor necrosis factor [TNF]-α, TNF-related apoptosis-inducing ligand [TRAIL], TNF-like weak inducer of

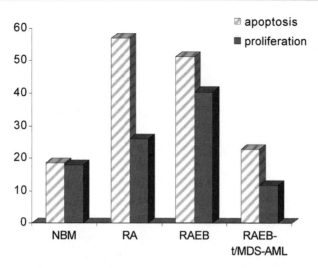

Fig. 1. Flow cytometric evaluation of apoptosis vs proliferation at different stages of myelodysplastic syndrome (MDS) evolution. CD34[+] cell apoptosis was assessed in normal bone marrow (BM) and different MDS categories using phycoerythrin-conjugated anti-CD34 monoclonal antibody (Mab) and fluorescein isothiocyanate (FITC)-conjugated annexin V. Proliferating cells were identified with FITC-conjugated Ki-67 Mab. The bar chart compares median levels of CD34[+] cell apoptosis and proliferation in different diagnostic categories. In normal BM, apoptosis matched proliferation. Conversely, PCD was greatly increased in early MDS (RA, RARS), and the ratio between apoptosis and proliferation (A:P ratio) was >2 in most patients. Progression to RAEB was associated with an increase in Ki-67 positivity such that the A:P ratio equalized. There was a marked fall in both apoptosis and proliferation upon transformation to RAEB-t/MDS-AML in the majority of patients analyzed.

apoptosis [TWEAK]) bind structurally related cell surface transmembrane receptors, causing receptor trimerization *(11–14)*. Trimerization alters the conformation of the cytoplasmic death domain (DD) of the receptor *(12)*, permitting its association with adaptor molecules such as FADD (fas-associated protein with a DD) *(15)* to create a death-inducing signaling complex (DISC) *(16)*. Within the DISC, adaptor molecules recruit and activate procaspases, thereby triggering the caspase cascade (Fig. 2).

3.1.2. INTRINSIC DEATH SIGNALS

Intrinsic stimuli generated following cellular stress can also induce apoptosis. Numerous stress responses (withdrawal of survival stimuli, reactive oxygen species, nitric oxide, calcium ions, genotoxic stress, sphingolipids, proteases) converge on mitochondria and induce alterations in mitochondrial membrane potential *(17)*, triggering the release of several apoptogenic molecules from the mitochondrial intermembrane space *(18)*. Once released into the cytosol, two such proteins, cytochrome c and apoptotic protease-activating factor-1 (Apaf-1), form a complex with procaspase 9. Within this complex, termed an apoptosome, procaspase 9 is activated, which triggers activation of downstream effector caspases *(19,20)*.

Apoptosis may additionally be induced by cell-cycle checkpoints such as p53 and its homologs p51A, p63, and p73, which detect an abnormal cell cycle, genomic damage, or incorrect DNA replication *(21–23)*. Once activated, p53 and its homologs both induce and repress transcription of target genes, which results in cell cycle arrest +/– mitochondrial-induced apoptosis.

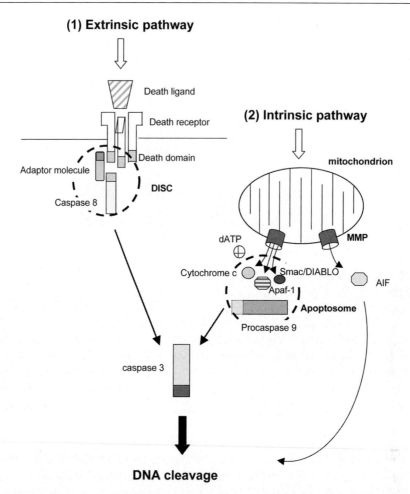

Fig. 2. Apoptotic pathways in normal hematopoietic cells. Apoptosis can be triggered by extrinsic and intrinsic strimuli. **(1)** In the extrinsic pathway, death ligands bind transmembrane receptors, causing receptor trimerization and altered conformation of the cytoplasmic death domain. This triggers binding of secondary adaptor molecules to create a death-inducing signaling complex (DISC). Within the DISC, adaptor molecules recruit and activate procaspase 8. Caspase 8, in turn, directly cleaves and activates effector caspases. **(2)** Intracellular stress responses converge on mitochondria and induce mitochondrial membrane permeabilization (MMP). This results in the release of apoptogenic molecules from the mitochondrial intermembrane space, which can trigger caspase-dependent and caspase-independent apoptotic pathways. Released cytochrome c and Apaf-1 associate with cytosolic procaspase 9 and dATP to form an apoptosome. Within this complex, procaspase 9 becomes activated and subsequently triggers downstream effector caspases. Smac/DIABLO augments this process. Mitochondrial apoptosis-inducing factor (AIF) bypasses the caspases and can directly bind and cleave DNA.

Caspase-independent apoptotic pathways also exist and are triggered by mitochondrial liberation of apoptosis-inducing factor (AIF) (Fig. 2) *(24,25)*.

3.1.3. CELLULAR REGULATION OF APOPTOSIS

The apoptotic apparatus is regulated at several levels. Within the extrinsic pathway, death signaling can be inhibited by the expression of decoy receptors that lack a functional DD *(26,27)* or by molecules that displace secondary adaptor proteins from the DISC, preventing transmission of apoptotic signals *(28,29)*. The intrinsic apoptotic pathway is largely regulated by the Bcl-2 family of proteins. Both pro- and anti-apoptotic molecules exist, and it is the ratio of the two at the level of the mitochondrial membrane that determines the mitochondrion's susceptibility to death signals *(30)*. A separate family of proteins termed the inhibitor of apoptosis protein (IAP) family inhibits both the extrinsic and intrinsic apoptotic pathways by interfering with the activation of caspases *(31)*. IAPs may additionally block caspase-independent mechanisms of apoptosis *(32)*. Several proteins negatively regulate the function of the IAP family. One such antagonist is Smac/DIABLO (second mitochondria-derived activator of caspase/direct inhibitor of apoptosis-binding protein with low pI), which is released from mitochondria into the cytosol during apoptosis *(33,34)*.

3.2. Proliferation

The cell cycle ensures that DNA is accurately replicated and that identical chromosomal copies are distributed equally between two daughter cells. The majority of mammalian cells exist in the nonproliferating state (G0). Entry into the cell cycle is normally stimulated by extra-cellular growth signals such as hematopoietic cytokines and chemokines, which bind to and activate transmembrane receptor tyrosine kinases (RTKs). RTK activation subsequently triggers a branching network of cytoplasmic signal transduction pathways (covered in more detail in Section 4.2.), which ultimately converge on the nuclear machinery. During G1, when cell size, protein, and RNA content increase in preparation for DNA synthesis, cells are responsive to extracellular signals, either advancing toward division, arresting in G1 if conditions are unfavor-able for proliferation, or withdrawing from the cell cycle entirely *(35)*. Commitment to mitosis occurs as cells pass a restriction point (R) in late G1. After this point cells become refractory to regulatory signals and are consigned to the autonomous program of proliferation *(36)*.

3.2.1. Cell Cycle Regulation

Orderly cell cycle progression is dependent upon a family of serine/threonine kinases termed cyclin-dependent kinases (Cdk) bound to a regulatory cyclin molecule. This cyclin/Cdk complex enables the cell to pass through several regulatory transition points. Within the complex, kinase activity is regulated by phosphorylation and dephosphorylation, executed by cyclin-dependent kinase inhibitors (CdkI) and phosphatases, respectively *(37)*. Retinoblastoma (Rb) protein family members—Rb, p107, and p130—are major substrates for the G1/S kinases *(38)*. Rb family members regulate G1 progression by reversibly interacting with the E2F family of transcription factors, which activate transcription of genes whose products are required for entry into the S-phase *(39)*.

3.2.2. Cell Cycle Checkpoints

Several checkpoints are built into the cell cycle, which detect genomic defects or incorrect DNA replication. A major checkpoint involves the tumor supressor p53, which becomes stabi-lized in the presence of DNA damage *(40)*. Its subsequent accumulation induces G1 arrest, allowing repair of DNA before cells become committed to DNA replication *(41)*. Alternatively, if genomic damage is overwhelming, p53 triggers PCD (discussed in Section 3.1.2.).

4. ABERRANT APOPTOSIS/PROLIFERATION IN MYELODYSPLASIA-RELATED AML: PUTATIVE LESIONS

The lesions underlying aberrant apoptosis and proliferation in MDS and MDS-AML remain elusive. Very early genomic hits, occurring before MDS is clinically apparent, pos-sibly target transcription factors, which regulate genes involved in the self-renewal capacity of hematopoietic progenitors. Increased apoptosis in symptomatic early MDS may arise from intrinsic cellular defects such as genomic damage, which trigger PCD through mitochondrial membrane changes. Alternatively, the bone marrow (BM) microenvironment (aberrant cytokine release, increased death ligands, defective stromal function, or immune-mediated changes) might induce cell death via the extrinsic apoptotic pathway, either as a result of a primary microenvironmental defect or as a response to the abnormal MDS clone. Increased proliferation associated with MDS progression may be a result of constitutive activation of signal transduction pathways regulating cell mitosis and/or enhanced survival signals from the bone marrow microenvironment. In contrast, reduced PCD characteristic of MDS-AML might arise from acquired defects in the apoptotic machinery, upregulation of negative regulators of apoptosis, elimination or evasion of clone-directed cytotoxic T-cells, or manipulation of the BM microenvironment by leukemic blasts to support clonal survival.

4.1. Upregulated Apoptosis in Symptomatic Early MDS

4.1.1. EXTRACELLULAR TRIGGERS

4.1.1.1. Abnormal Stroma. The disordered BM architecture characteristic of MDS may reflect an underlying abnormality of the marrow stroma. Certainly, apoptosis in MDS affects both stromal cells and hematopoietic progenitors *(42)*. MDS stroma also has a reduced capacity to support normal CD34$^+$ cell proliferation and differentiation in long-term BM culture systems *(43)*. Moreover, an MDS stromal cell line has been shown to induce PCD of both normal hematopoietic and leukemic cells, possibly mediated via integrins *(44)*.

4.1.1.2. Abnormal Progenitor Cell Adhesion. In normal hematopoiesis, integrin-mediated interactions between progenitors and fibronectin are critical for progenitor cell survival. Delforge et al. *(45)* recently demonstated downregulation of $\alpha4\beta1$ and $\alpha5\beta1$ integrins on CD34$^+$ cells in MDS patients who had at least 25% progenitors ungoing PCD.

4.1.1.3. Increased Death Signals. Increased levels of death ligands and their receptors have been documented in early MDS. Elevated TNF-α levels in early disease are correlated with the degree of anemia and a poor response to erythropoietin (EPO) *(46)*. TNF receptor expression is also upregulated *(47)*. Similarly, increased BM fas mRNA and protein levels have been detected in myelodysplasia *(47,48)*. Constitutive expression of TRAIL and its receptors has also been demonstrated in MDS BM *(49,50)*. Whereas normal marrow was resistant to TRAIL-induced PCD, MDS BM showed significant increases in apoptosis and suppression of colony growth following TRAIL exposure *(50)*. Moreover, TRAIL preferentially eliminated clonally abnormal cells as identified by chromosomal markers. Zang et al. *(49)* hypothesized that this could be a result of high ratios of agonist vs decoy TRAIL receptors on MDS CD34$^+$ cells, the reverse being true for normal CD34$^+$ progenitors. Early MDS has additionally been associated with increased FADD expression in MDS erythroid cells. Moreover, transduction of a dominant negative mutant of FADD into MDS erythroid progenitors inhibited apoptosis and rescued eryhroid colony growth *(51)*. Other studies have demonstrated downregulation of the negative regulators of death receptors—Fap-1 (protein-tyrosine phosphatase-L1) and FLICE inhibitory protein (FLIPL)—in early MDS *(52,53)*.

4.1.1.4. Impaired Growth Signals. Reduced granulocyte colony-stimulating factor receptor (G-CSFR) expression has been reported on MDS CD34$^+$ progenitors *(54)*. Low levels of hematopoietic cytokines such as stem cell factor (SCF) and granulocyte-macrophage CSF (GM-CSF) have also been described *(55,56)*. This may be a result of apoptosis and/or functional abnormalities of stromal cells *(42,57)* or decreased production by MDS monocytes/ macrophages *(56,58)*. Similarly, erythroid response to EPO is reduced in MDS BM. Although

EPO receptor (EpoR) levels are normal and the ligand-binding capacity of the receptor is intact *(59)*, studies have shown impaired activation of the signaling molecule signal transducer and activator of transcription 5 (STAT5) by the EPO receptor upon ligand binding, which results in reduced binding activity of the transcription factor GATA-1, an important regulator of erythropoiesis *(60)*. Likewise, defective megakaryopoiesis in MDS is not caused by reduced thrombopoietin receptor (c-mpl) expression, but by failure of c-mpl-induced activation of STAT3 and STAT5 *(61)*.

4.1.1.5. Immune Insult. Studies showing a high frequency of T-cell receptor V-β skewing in MDS patients, indicating the presence of a clonally expanded T-cell population character-istic of an autoimmune process, suggests that, at least in some cases, apoptosis may be immune-mediated. T-cells inhibitory to autologous granulocyte or erythroid colony growth have also been described. Moreover, removal of T-cells enhances colony formation in some patients *(62)*. An autoimmune pathophysiology appears to be a particular feature of MDS associated with trisomy 8 as a sole karyotypic abnormality. Indeed, Sloand et al. *(63)* have shown that treatment with antithymocyte globulin reverses cytopenias, increases the proportion of trisomy 8 cells, and normalizes the T-cell repertoire in two-thirds of such patients.

4.1.2. Intracellular Triggers

4.1.2.1. Mitochondrial Changes. Mitochondrial pathology has been observed in a number of studies and appears to be a particular feature of the MDS subtype—refractory anemia with ringed sideroblasts *(64)*. Mitochondrial abnormalities include iron accumulation within the mitochondrial matrix of ringed sideroblasts *(65)*, electron-microscopic morphological abnor-malities *(66)*, and mitochondrial DNA mutations *(67)*. The latter have been directly linked to elevated apoptosis *(68)*.

4.1.2.2. DNA Repair Defects. Both inherited disorders of DNA repair *(69)* and exposure to cytotoxic therapy *(70)* or environmental toxins *(71)* predispose to myelodysplasia. A link between MDS and polymorphisms in genes that mediate DNA repair or metabolize environ-mental carcinogens has also been observed *(72,73)*. Moreover, DNA microarray analysis has demonstrated downregulation of genes involved in protecting CD34$^+$ cells from cellular stress induced by mutagens in early MDS *(74)*, indicating that increased sensitivity of hematopoietic progenitors to cellular stress/DNA damage may both facilitate gene mutations and trigger PCD in some cases.

4.2. Increased Proliferation During MDS Progression

Mutations of genes whose products result in activation of signal transduction pathways regulating cell proliferation are the probable initial targets in MDS progression. The most likely culprits are proteins of the ras signaling pathway.

4.2.1. RTKs

At the cell surface, RTKs are normally maintained in an inactive conformation by auto-inhibitory domains, ensuring that intracellular signals are transduced only upon extracellular ligand binding. In leukemic cells, the genes that encode RTKs may undergo mutation, resulting in constitutive receptor activation. The receptors implicated in MDS include members of the class III RTK receptor family: c-kit, fms and FLT3.

The c-kit receptor is found on the majority of CD34$^+$ hematopoietic stem cells *(75)*. Binding of c-kit to its ligand, SCF, induces quiescent stem cells to enter the cell cycle and, in combi-nation with other growth factors, induces progenitor cell proliferation and differentiation *(76)*.

Although elevated c-kit m-RNA and protein has been reported in MDS, especially in advanced disease *(77)*, this may merely reflect the increased numbers of CD34$^+$ cells present in myelodysplastic BM compared to normal controls. More recently, co-expression of c-kit and SCF has been detected in AML cell lines and primary AML samples *(78)*, implying that c-kit might contribute to leukemogenesis through autocrine, paracrine, or intracrine stimulation.

Located at chromosome 5q33 *(79)*, *fms* encodes the receptor for macrophage colony-stimulating factor *(80)*. Activating point mutations at codon 301 or 969 are found in 5–15% of MDS patients and, in some studies, have been associated with more advanced disease and an increased risk of leukemic transformation *(81)*. Other authors have detected *fms* mutations in hematologically normal patients previously treated with cytotoxic agents and healthy individuals with no known mutagenic exposure *(82)*, suggesting that, in some cases, mutation of *fms* may be an early initiating event.

In normal BM, FLT3 (fms-like tyrosine kinase 3) expression is restricted to early progenitors *(83)*. Its ligand, FLT3 ligand, a transmembrane protein that can be released as a soluble homo-dimeric molecule *(84)*, is expressed by cells of the hematopoietic BM microenvironment *(85)*. Both membrane-bound and soluble forms of FLT3 ligand can activate FLT3 tyrosine kinase activity, and they synergize with other hematopoietic growth factors and interleukins to stimulate growth and expansion of immature hematopoietic progenitors *(86–88)*. FLT3 ligand also stimulates proliferation and differentiation of dendritic cells and natural killer cells *(89)*. High FLT3 levels have been detected in over 90% of AML cases *(90)*, indicating that upregulation of FLT3-mediated signaling is likely to play a role in the survival and/or proliferation of leukemic blasts. Two types of FLT3 mutations are also observed in AML and MDS: (1) in-frame, variable-length internal tandem duplications (ITDs) in the juxtamem-brane domain and (2) point mutations at a specific aspartic acid residue, Asp835, which alter the configuration of the activation loop. Both lesions disrupt the autoinhibitory activity of the respective domains and result in constitutive tyrosine kinase activation. FLT3 ITDs are observed in up to 6% of patients with MDS and are restricted to the FAB subtypes RAEB, RAEB-t and CMML. Mutations within the activation loop occur at a lower frequency (1–3%) and are similarly associated with advanced disease *(91–94)*. Paired sequence analysis shows that 14% of MDS patients acquire activating mutations of FLT3 upon AML evolution *(93)*. Although the presence of activation loop mutations does not appear to influence prognosis, FLT3 ITD-positive MDS-AML is associated with an increased relapse rate, a more rapid transformation to AML, and shorter survival compared to FLT3 ITD-negative patients *(92–94)*.

4.2.2. SIGNAL TRANSDUCTION PROTEINS

4.2.2.1. The ras Signaling Pathway. The ras family of proteins (H-, K- and N-ras) serves as the hub of multiple cellular signal transduction pathways, which regulate diverse cellular processes including proliferation, differentiation, and cell death. Binding of ligand to its respective RTK causes receptor dimerization and autophosphorylation. Phosphorylated RTK, in turn, phosphorylates and activates the adaptor protein Grb-2, which subsequently associates with SOS (Son of Sevenless). The Grb-2/SOS complex interacts with inactive, GDP-bound ras, altering its conformation to favor GTP binding. In this active, GTP-bound state, ras recruits and activates downstream signaling molecules such as raf, MAP/ERK kinase, and mitogen-activating protein kinase (MAPK) *(95)*. The ras protein has intrinsic GTPase activity, maintaining it in its inactive form. Ras activation is also tightly controlled by thepositive and negative regulators guanine-nucleotide exchange factors (GEFs) and GTPase activating proteins (GAPs), respectively *(96,97)*. Point mutations at codons 12, 13, or 61 inhibit the intrinsic GTPase activity of the ras protein, resulting in constitutive GTP-binding and downstream signaling regardless of upstream stimuli *(98)*. *Ras* mutations have been detected in 5–24% of MDS patients, preferentially in the FAB subtype CMML (40%) (reviewed in ref. *99*) and in approx 10–30% of AML cases *(100,101)*. The prognostic significance of *ras* mutations in MDS is unclear. As with *fms*, mutant *ras* has been detected in hematologically normal patients previously exposed to cytotoxic therapy as well as in healthy individuals with no known mutagenic exposure *(102)*, suggesting that it may be an early initiating event in leukemogenesis. Other studies indicate that *ras* mutations are associated with advanced disease and a poor prognosis *(81,103)*. Paired sequence analysis, however, although demonstrating that a significant proportion of patients acquires *ras* mutations upon leukemic transformation, found that its presence does not affect time to AML evolution or overall survival *(93)*.

Deregulation of positive (GEFs) and negative (GAPs) ras regulators could theoretically result in constitutive ras signaling. Although deletion of the neurofibromin (NF1) tumor-suppressor gene, a negative ras regulator, is observed in juvenile myelomonocytic leukemia associated with neurofibromatosis, NF1 mutations in sporadic MDS/AML are extremely rare *(104,105)*. Reduced BM NF1 expression has been observed in up to 30% of MDS and AML patients, however. Interestingly, no patient had both mutant *ras* and low NF1 expression, suggesting thatthese lesions may complement each other *(106)*.

The SH2 domain-containing protein-tyrosine phosphatase PTPN11 (Shp2) is an essential component of signaling pathways initiated by growth factors, cytokines, and extracellular matrix and acts upstream of ras *(107)*. About 50% of patients with Noonan syndrome, a genetic condition associated with an increased risk of leukemia *(108)*, have germline PTPN11 gain of function mutations. Moreover, somatic PTPN11 mutations have been detected in children with sporadic juvenile myelomonocytic leukemia, MDS, and AML *(109)*, suggesting that PTPN11 may be a novel oncogene, acting via ras activation. Indeed, Schubert et al. *(110)* recently showed that PTPN11 mutations in murine hematopoietic cells enhanced the growth of immature progenitors and impaired normal differentiation in liquid cultures.

4.2.2.2. The PI3 Kinase/Akt Signaling Pathway. The phosphatidyl-inositide 3 kinase (PI3 kinase)/Akt protein kinase pathway is involved in cell growth, proliferation, and apoptosis *(111)*. PI3 kinase is activated in response to multiple hematopoietic cytokines and chemokines *(112)*, including FLT3 ligand *(113,114)*. Many of the regulatory effects of PI3 kinase are mediated through the serine-threonine kinase protein kinase B (PKB/Akt), whose downstream targets include the pro-apoptotic Bcl-2-related protein Bad, caspase 9, nuclear factor (NF)κB, and Forkhead *(115–117)*. A number of studies have shown that the PI3 kinase/Akt signaling pathway is constitutively active in primary AML cells and contributes to blast survival and proliferation *(118–120)*. Moreover, blockade of this pathway with a selective inibitor, LY294002, increases apoptosis of AML blasts via a reduction in NFκB activity and increased p53-mediated transcription *(121)*. Recently, Sujobert et al. *(122)* have shown that it is the p110δ isoform of PI3 kinase that is consistently overexpressed in AML, indicating that this molecule is a potential therapeutic target.

4.2.3. ALTERED MICROENVIRONMENT

The formation of new blood vessels (angiogenesis) is important for maintaining normal tissue viability. Increased angiogenesis has been associated with the growth, survival, dissemination, and metastasis of solid tumors *(123,124)* and malignant hematopoietic cells *(125)*. Angiogenesis may also play a role in MDS progression. Microvessel density (MVD) is significantly greater in MDS BM compared to normal controls. Moreover, vascularity appears to increase with disease progression, with a direct correlation with blast percentage being observed *(126–128)*.

Angiogenesis is tightly regulated by pro- and anti-angiogeneic proteins. In carcinogenesis this balance is altered, leading to increased vessel formation *(129)*. Furthermore, tumor vessels have an abnormal structure, leading to disorganized blood flow, leakiness, and reduced drug delivery *(130,131)*. Pro-angiogeneic molecules in cancer are derived from tumor cells, stromal cells, endothelial cells, and the extracellular matrix *(132)*. In MDS/AML patients and cell lines, elevated levels of the angiogenic factors vascular endothelial growth factor (VEGF), basic fibroblast growth factor (bFGF), hepatocyte growth factor (HGF), and angiogenin have been detected *(125,127,133,134)*. VEGF receptor (VEGFR) (particularly VEGFR-1) expression is also increased and appears to be associated with a bad prognosis *(135)*. In addition, co-expression of VEGF and VEGFR has been reported, implying that autocrine and paracrine VEGF loops play a role in leukemia pathogenesis *(136)*.

VEGF additionally contributes to hematopoiesis by mechanisms other than angiogenesis, suggesting a wider role for this molecule in leukemogenesis. VEGF mediates hematopoietic stem cell survival and repopulation via an autocrine loop and influences the differentiation of multiple hematopoietic cell lines *(137)*. It also blocks maturation of dendritic cells through inhibition of NFκB activation *(138)*. Moreover, VEGF induces the expression of heat-shock protein 90 (hsp90) and potentiates its binding to Bcl-2 and mitochondrial Apaf-1, thus modulating cellular sensitivity to apoptotic stimuli *(139)*.

4.3. Abrogated Apoptosis in Myelodysplasia-Related AML

4.3.1. DEFECTS IN THE EXTRINSIC AND INTRINSIC APOPTOTIC PATHWAYS

An inverse correlation between fas levels and BM blast percentage has been demonstrated in MDS *(50)*, indicating that fas death signaling is downregulated with disease progression. de Thonel et al. *(140)*, however, showed that although fas is expressed in advanced disease, MDS-AML blasts are frequently resistant to fas agonists, possibly because of failure of DISC formation. Other studies have documented resistance to UV light-induced apoptosis in certain leukemia cell lines, which appears to be due to a deficiency of Apaf-1, a critical member of the apoptosome *(141)*.

4.3.2. UPREGULATION OF NEGATIVE APOPTOSIS REGULATORS

Overexpression of the anti-apoptotic protein Bcl-2 in advanced compared to early MDS has been demonstrated immunohistochemically and by flow cytometry *(9,142–145)*. Sequential biopsies have confirmed that Bcl-2 expression increases and PCD decreases upon leukemic transformation *(146)*. Disease progression has also been associated with a fall in both c-myc: Bcl-2 ratios *(142)* and pro- (Bax, Bad) vs anti- (Bcl-2, Bcl-X) apoptotic Bcl-2-related protein ratios *(9)*, which is predominantly a result of Bcl-2 upregulation (Fig. 3). In the latter study, pro- vs anti-apoptotic Bcl-2 ratio was positively associated with apoptotic index and inversely correlated with BM CD34+ cell counts and IPSS score. When evaluating individual protein levels, only Bcl-2 showed any significant correlation with laboratory characteristics, suggesting that this protein is the main Bcl-2 family member influencing MDS pathogenesis *(9)*. Low pro- vs anti-apoptotic Bcl-2 ratios have also been associated with shorter survival and increased risk of leukemic transformation *(147)*, suggesting that they may be of prognostic value. Similarly, low Bax/Bcl-2 ratios in *de novo* AML have been correlated with CD34 and/or CD117 positivity, markers of blast immaturity, poor-risk cytogenetics, lower complete remission rates, and reduced overall and disease-free survival *(148)*. The molecular mechanisms underlying upregulated Bcl-2 expression in advanced MDS are unclear. Abrogation of p53 function, a transcriptional repressor of Bcl-2, may be responsible. Certainly, Kurotaki and colleagues *(146)* have shown a link between Bcl-2 overexpression and p53 accumulation (a marker of p53 mutation) in advanced disease.

Survivin, a member of the IAP family of proteins, is believed to exert its anti-apoptotic effect by binding to Smac/DIABLO, suggesting that it suppresses caspases indirectly by freeing other IAP family members from the constraints of this protein *(149,150)*. Survivin expression is cell cycle dependent, with levels peaking in the G2/M phase *(151)*, implying that it plays a pivotal role in linking cell death and proliferation *(152)*. Survivin is not detected in differentiated normal tissues, but is strongly expressed in transformed cell lines *(153)*. Increased survivin expression has also been detected in myeloid leukemia cell lines and primary AML samples, although no correlation with prognosis was observed *(154,155)*. Moreover, inhibition of survivin expression in HL-60 cells with a survivin anti-sense oligonucleotide blocked significant numbers of HL-60 cells in G2/M phase, halted cell proliferation, and increased apoptosis *(156)*. Survivin expression has also been detected in MDS patients *(157)* and, in some studies, is associated with advanced disease and evolution to AML, suggesting that survivin upregulation may contribute to leukemic transformation in a proportion of cases *(158)*.

Other inhibitors of apoptosis may similarly be upregulated with disease progression. Indeed, Benesch et al. *(53)* have shown that levels of FLIPL, which inhibits both fas- and TRAIL-mediated apoptotic signals, increase with advancing disease stage.

4.3.3. LESIONS THAT TARGET CELL CYCLE MACHINERY

The frequency with which alterations of cell cycle regulatory genes are observed with AML evolution suggests that a breakdown in the processes that normally tightly regulate proliferation and apoptosis is pivotal in leukemogenesis.

4.3.3.1. Retinoblastoma and Associated Proteins. Deregulation of G1/S transition is frequently observed in human cancers, either through overexpression of cyclin D1, which normally regulates Rb phosphorylation *(159)*, or via inactivation of Rb family members *(160)*. Although rarely observed in MDS *(161)*, low or absent Rb expression is detected in 20–30% patients with AML *(162,163)* and is associated with autonomous in vitro proliferation of clonogenic blasts *(164)*, inferior response to conventional therapy, and reduced survival *(163)*. The mechanism of action of altered Rb expression is unclear but does not appear to be a result of inactivating gene mutations or gene silencing through Rb promoter hypermethylation *(165)*.

Purα is a ubiquitous, sequence-specific DNA- and RNA-binding protein that has been implicated in diverse cellular functions, including transcriptional activation and repression, translation, and cell growth. Purα exerts part of its activity by interacting with cellular proteins, including pRb, E2F, and cyclin A, implying that it plays a crucial role in regulating the cell cycle. Moreover, microinjection studies have shown that Purα causes either a G1 or G2 arrest depending on the cell cycle time of injection (reviewed in ref. *166*). Concurrent deletions of Purα at 5q31, and its dimerization partner PURβ, at 7p13 are observed at a rate nearly 1.5-fold higher than statistically expected in MDS and more than 5-fold higher in AML, suggesting that deletion of both dimeric partners simultaneously may contribute towards AML progression in some cases *(167)*.

Deregulated expression of the Rb-binding transcription factor, E2F, renders hematopoietic cells refractory to terminal differentiation *(168)*. Aberrant E2F expression in cancer is uncommon,

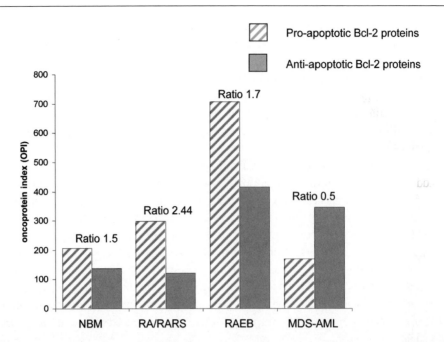

Fig. 3. Pro- vs anti-apoptotic Bcl-2-related protein ratio in myelodysplastic syndrome (MDS)/MDS–acute myeloid leukemia (AML) and normal controls. Expression of two pro-apoptotic (Bax, Bad) and two anti-apoptotic (Bcl-2, Bcl-X) Bcl-2-related proteins within CD34$^+$ bone marrow cells was measured flow cytometrically in different MDS categories and normal controls, and a pro- vs anti-apoptotic Bcl-2 ratio was calculated. Pro-apoptotic Bcl-2 protein expression was elevated in early MDS compared to normal bone marrow (ratio 2.44 vs 1.5). Conversely, progression to MDS-AML was associated with upregulation of anti-apoptotic Bcl-2 proteins, with a reversal of the Bcl-2 ratio (ratio 0.5).

although gene amplification and translocation has been detected in leukemia cell lines *(169)*. Nonetheless, altered expression of the Rb-specific region of E2F has been demonstrated in some MDS patients *(170)*. Such cases were characterized by a higher incidence of hemato-poietic cells simultaneously undergoing proliferation and apoptosis.

4.3.3.2. Cyclin-Dependent Kinase Inhibitors. p15INK4B protein is an inhibitor of cyclin-dependent kinases 4/6 and an upstream regulator of Rb function *(171)*. In MDS, inactivation of the *p15INK4B* gene through promoter hypermethylation has been detected in over 50% cases *(172)*. *p15INK4B* gene methylation is correlated with increased BM blasts *(173)*, increased risk of AML progression, poor prognosis, and possibly chemoresistance *(173–176)*, implying a role for p15INK4B hypermethylation in leukemic transformation. By contrast, some studies have shown increased p15INK4B methylaton in marrows of patients previously treated for lymphoma, suggesting that, at least for secondary hematological disorders, p15INK4B methylation may be an early transforming event *(177)*. The presence of *p15INK4B* gene methylation, however, is not always correlated with absence of expression, nor is expression always present if methylation is absent *(177)*.

Treatment of high-risk MDS patients with the demethylating agent 5-Aza-2′-deoxycyti-dine (decitabine) reverses *p15INK4B* gene methylation and induces normal p15 expression. Moreover, this reversal is correlated with clinical response and delayed progression to leukemia *(172)*, highlighting the importance of *p15INK4B* gene silencing in MDS-AML pathogenesis.

4.3.3.3. p53 Cell Cycle Checkpoint. Loss of function mutations and/or deletions of both alleles of the *p53* gene are observed in 5–15% patients with primary MDS/MDS-AML *(178,179)* and are associated with specific morphological features including dysgranulo-poiesis combining pseudo-Pelger-Huet nuclear hypolobulation and vacuolated cytoplasm *(180)*. Most patients with p53 lesions have advanced disease *(178)* and harbor additional complex chromosomal abnormalities *(181)*. The risk of leukemic transformation is increased *(182)*, response to chemotherapy poor, and overall survival short *(183)*. In multivariate analysis, p53 alterations in MDS patients emerged as the most significant adverse prognostic factor in one study. Moreover, within the intermediate IPSS risk subgroups, the presence of p53 abnor-malities added further significant prognostic information *(184)*. p53 lesions appear to be linked to specific 5q13.3 deletions between the loci D5S672 and D5S620/D5S626, suggesting that a putative tumor suppressor gene at 5q and loss of wild-type p53 function cooperate in myeloid leukemogenesis *(185)*.

Like gene mutations/deletions, p53 protein function can be influenced by posttranscriptional modifications such as phosphorylation or by interactions with other cellular and viral proteins *(186)*. A putative cellular transcription factor, mdm-2 (murine double minute), binds to p53 protein and inhibits its transcriptional activity *(187)*. Amplification of the mdm-2 oncogene, with consequent overabundance of the gene product, has been observed in about 30% of soft-tissue sarcomas *(188)*. Although gene amplification has not been observed in MDS/AML *(189)*, mdm-2 overexpression has been detected in a proportion of patients with AML *(190)* and has been associated with a reduced duration of complete remission and event-free survival *(191)*.

4.3.3.4. P73. p73, an upstream regulator of p21 and a member of the p53 family, is another candidate tumor suppressor gene. Although mutations have not been observed in MDS/AML *(192)*, Schmelz et al. *(193)* recently demonstrated p73 promoter hypermethylation in AML cell lines and primary AML cells. Moreover, the demethylating agent azacitidine induced re-expression of p73 and its downstream target p21, resulting in the arrest of AML cells in G1 phase and activation of the mitochondrial apoptosis pathway through release of cytochrome c and AIF.

4.3.3.5. PI-PLC. Preliminary evidence also suggests that a small group of MDS patients bears a deletion of another cell cycle checkpoint gene, inositide-specific phospholipase C (PI-PLC). Moreover, such patients rapidly evolve to AML, suggesting that PI-PLC may act as a tumor suppressor *(194)*.

4.3.4. Immune Evasion

Upregulation of CD34[+] cell fas-ligand expression has been detected in a significant pro-portion of MDS patients and may represent a means by which neoplastic cells circumvent immunological destruction through the elimination of clone-directed cytotoxic lymphocytes *(195)*. Increased fas-L expression in MDS is associated with greater numbers of abnormal metaphases, progressive disease, and short survival *(196)*. Increased apoptosis of B-lympho-cytes has also been detected *(197)*. Other studies have shown that tumor cell supernatant derived from AML cells inhibited T-cell activation and Th1 cytokine production, prevented activated T-cells from entering the cell cycle, and delayed/inhibited apoptosis of both T- and B-cells, suggesting that immune modulation plays a role in myeloid leukemogenesis *(198,199)*.

4.4. Other Genetic Lesions Implicated in MDS Transformation
4.4.1. AML1/RUNX1

The AML1 (or RUNX1) protein heterodimerizes with core binding factor (CBF)-β to form the core binding factor complex (CBF), an essential transcription factor for normal hematopoieisis *(200)*. The *AML1* gene is one of the most frequent targets for chromosomal translocations in leukemia. Point mutations have also been described *(201)* and, phenotypically, result in immortalized hematopoietic progenitors with impaired differentiation *(5)*. *AML1* point mutations are a particular feature of poorly differentiated AML *(202)* and therapy/irradiation-related MDS/AML *(203)*. *AML1* mutations have also been detected in up to 17% of patients with sporadic MDS or MDS-AML and are associated with more advanced disease and poor prognosis *(204)*. The majority of *AML1* point mutations are clustered within the Runt domain, a highly conserved 128-amino-acid protein motif responsible for both AML1 DNA-binding and CBFβ heterodimerization. These mutations abrogate the DNA-binding potential of AML1, leaving its heterodimerizing properties intact. Thus, this lesion may contribute to leukemic transformation via a dominant negative effect *(205)*. C-terminal mutations have also been described and appear to be specific to sporadic MDS *(204)*. *AML1* mutations alone are not sufficient to cause MDS progression, however. Certainly, sequential analysis has revealed point mutations in early MDS samples, which persisted throughout the disease course *(206)*. Moreover, monoallelic *AML1* germline mutations are found in familial platelet disorder with predisposition to AML *(207)*, suggesting that hematopoietic progenitors with AML1 abnormalities require additional hits for frank leukemic transformation.

4.4.2. MLL

Rearrangement of the mixed lineage leukemia gene *MLL* has been detected in acute lymphoid and myeloid leukemias, MDS, and therapy-related disease, where it is associated with a poor prognosis *(208,209)*. The MLL protein is a methyltransferase that maintains Homeobox *(Hox)* gene expression through direct promoter binding and histone modification *(210,211)*. Hox proteins are important regulators of hematopoiesis and are normally only expressed on early hematopoietic progenitors. *MLL* rearrangements in leukemia, which include *MLL* fusion genes, partial tandem duplications of *MLL*, and *MLL* amplification, upregulate expression of both *Hox* genes (particularly *Hoxa7* and *Hoxa9*) and the Hox cofactor, Meis1 *(212–214)*, resulting in inappropriate maintenance of *Hox* gene expression and a block in hematopoietic differentiation. MLL fusion proteins may further contribute to leukemic transformation through upregulation of other putative oncogenes, including *FLT3* and *N-Myc* *(215)*. Whether MLL fusion proteins are sufficient to induce acute leukemia without additional genetic alterations remains controversial *(215)*. Ono et al. *(216)*, however, recently showed that the fusion product MLL-SEPT6 induced myeloproliferative disease with long latency in mice but not acute leukemia. By contrast, activated FLT3 together with MLL-SEPT6 not only transformed hematopoietic progenitors in vitro but also induced acute biphenotypic or myeloid leukemia with a short latency in vivo, implying that secondary genotoxic events are required to cause AML in patients with a mutated *MLL* gene.

4.4.3. MLF1

The myelodysplasia/myeloid leukemia factor 1 *(MLF1)* gene on chromosome 3 is a novel oncoprotein involved in translocations associated with poor-risk MDS and AML, particularly erythroleukemia *(217,218)*. The most commonly observed translocation, t(3;5)(q25.1;q34), involves fusion of *MLF1* with the nucleophosmin *(NPM)* gene on chromosome 5 *(217)*. Elevated MLF1 expression has also been observed in MDS and AML patients who lack the t(3;5) translocation and has been associated with advanced disease and immature AML subtypes *(219)*. The function of wild-type MLF1 is unclear. MLF1 expression is highest in normal CD34[+] hematopoietic progenitors and decreases during maturation, suggesting that it plays a role in hematopoietic progenitor cell differentiation *(220)*. Indeed, ectopic expression of MLF1 prevented J2E erythroleukemic cells from undergoing maturation in response to EPO in vitro. Furthermore, MLF1 suppressed a rise in the cell cycle inhibitor p27(Kip1) and inhibited EPO-induced cell cycle exit, which is essential for erythroid terminal differentiation *(221)*. The t(3;5) fusion partner NPM may also contribute to leukemogenesis. Certainly, wild-type NPM interacts directly with p53 and regulates the increase in stability and p53 transcriptional activation after different types of cellular stress, suggesting that alterations of NPM function within NPM fusion proteins might lead to deregulation of p53 in tumors *(222)*.

4.4.4. HTIF1α

HTIF1α is a transcriptional coactivator that is encoded by a gene on chromosome 7q32-34, a critical region in AML and MDS. In myeloblastic HL60 and promyelocytic NB4 cells induced to differentiate along the monocytic-macrophage pathway, HTIF1α expression decreased, suggesting that HTIF1α negatively regulates myeloid differentiation *(223)*. Indeed, significantly increased HTIF1α RNA expression has been demonstrated in *de novo* AML and AML secondary to MDS but not myelodysplasia *(223)*, implying that HTIF1α may contribute towards leukemogenesis in some patients.

4.4.5. WT1

The Wilm's tumor gene, *WT1*, encodes a zinc finger transcription factor that regulates the transcription of genes involved in tissue development, proliferation, differentiation, and apoptosis *(224)*. WT1 can both repress and activate gene transcription. WT1 represses the transcription of growth factors (platelet-derived growth factor α chain *[225]*, colony-stimulating factor-1 *[226]*, insulin-like growth factor-II *[227]*, and growth factor receptors), while it upregulates retinoblastoma suppressor-associated protein 46 *(228)* and *bcl-2* *(229)* transcription, thereby modulating the cells sensitivity to apoptotic signals. Inactivation of both *WT1* alleles underlies the pathogenesis of a childhood renal tumor *(230,231)*. Germline mutations are also found in patients with leukemia predisposition syndromes, indicating that WT1 acts as a tumor suppressor. In some cancers, however, WT1 appears to play an onco-geneic rather than a tumor suppressor role. Certainly, increased expression of wild-type WT1 is observed in many leukemias *(233–235)*, while leukemia cell growth can be inhibited by treatment with WT1 antisense oligomers *(236)*. Moreover, transfection of wild-type *WT1* (with subsequent constitutive WT1 expression) into both 32D and normal marrow myeloid cells results in promotion of cell growth, but inhibition of differentiation *(237)*. In MDS, overexpression of WT1 has been associated with advanced disease and progression of MDS to AML *(238,239)*. Certainly, Cilloni et al. (2003) showed a marked increase in WT1 expression in every MDS patient whose disease evolved to AML on sequential analysis. A correlation between WT1 expression, blast percentage, presence of cytogenetic abnormalities, and International Prognostic Scoring System (IPSS) was also observed, suggesting that WT1 expression may be of prognostic value *(240)*. Interestingly, a humoral response against the WT1 protein can be elicited in patients with WT1-expressing hematopoietic malignancies *(241)*, implying that WT1 is a potential target for immunotherapy.

4.4.6. C/EBPα

The CCAAT/enhancer binding protein (C/EBP)α protein is essential for differentiation of a number of tissues, including granulocytes *(242)*. C/EBPα mutations have been detected in 1.1% of patients with MDS and 7.7% of AML samples *(243)*. Some mutations (deletions or nonsense codons) result in a truncated protein with loss of the DNA-binding and dimerization domains, while in-frame deletions and insertion mutations abrogate the transcriptional activation function of C/EBPα on the granulocyte colony-stimulating factor receptor promoter *(243)*.

5. THE PATHOGENESIS OF GENETIC DEFECTS IN MDS AND MYELODYSPLASIA-RELATED AML

A number of genetic lesions have now been implicated in MDS pathogenesis and its subsequent transformation to AML. However, the means by which hematopoietic stem cells derive these defects remains largely unresolved. Potential mechanisms are discussed below.

5.1. Telomere Erosion

Telomeres are specialized nucleoprotein structures that cap the ends of human chromosomes. Together with specific telomere-binding proteins, these terminal elements, composed of simple tandem repeats, protect chromosome ends against degradation and prevent ligation of the ends of DNA by DNA repair enzymes *(244)*. Telomeres are progressively shortened with each cell division, which abrogates their protective function. As a result, chromosomes become unstable, fused, or lost, and the cell loses its capacity to divide. Moreover, if the number and/or nature of DNA defects overwhelm DNA repair mechanisms, cell cycle checkpoints trigger PCD. In theory, the accelerated cell turnover observed in early MDS may lead to telomere shortening and subsequent genomic instability. This, in turn, may facilitate gene deletions or rearrangements with resultant disease progression. Indeed, telomere shortening has been demonstrated in MDS and has been correlated with advanced disease, high IPSS score, an abnormal karyotype, leukemic transformation, and poor prognosis *(245–248)*.

Normal germ cells and early embryonic cells overcome the problem of telomere erosion by means of a complex of proteins and RNA called telomerase. The RNA component of this complex contains a template sequence on which the tandem repeats of telomeres can be synthesized *(249,250)*, thereby maintaining telomere stability and ensuring cell viability. Unlike germ cells and early embryonic cells, most somatic cells switch off telomerase activity after birth. By contrast, many kinds of cancer cells reactivate telomerase, leading to cancer cell immortalization. Indeed, it has been proposed that telomerase reactivation is an essential step in cancer progression *(251)*. Increased telomerase activity is also believed to play a role in MDS progression. Counter et al. *(252)* demonstrated that telomerase activity was enhanced in MDS and more significantly so upon AML evolution. Regardless of telomerase levels, however, telomeres shortened with disease progression. Available evidence therefore suggests that telomere dynamics play an essential role in MDS pathogenesis and its transformation to AML. In early MDS, hematopoietic stem cells lack an efficient mechanism of telomere maintenance, leading to telomere erosion and genomic instability. Telomerase reactivation is a late event in MDS progression, presumably when critical telomere loss generates selective pressure for cell immortality *(252)*.

5.2. Gene Silencing

As discussed earlier, tumor suppressor gene inactivation almost certainly plays a major role in the pathogenesis of AML secondary to MDS. Although inactivation of tumor suppressor genes may occur through mutation or loss of a large portion of their genetic sequence, an equally effective mechanism of eliminating tumor suppressor gene function entails inhibition of gene transcription through chromatin remodeling. Chromatin remodeling represents a powerful mechanism of regulating gene expression and plays an essential role in the normal development of mammalian cells *(253)*. DNA normally exists in a complex configuration with proteins such as histones. These protein–DNA interactions, termed a nucleosome, regulate the packaging of DNA, either maintaining DNA in a compact form, which prevents the access of transcription factors, or alternatively in a relaxed structure, permitting DNA transcription *(254,255)*. Two molecular mechanisms are key to the process of chromatin remodeling: DNA methylation and histone modification *(256,257)*. Both processes appear to work together to block gene transcription in what has been termed a silencing cascade *(258)*. DNA methylation involves the addition of a methyl group to the cytidine residues of cytidine–guanosine (CpG) sequences in the cell genome *(254)*. Mediated via a family of enzymes termed the DNA methyltransferases (DNMTs) *(259)*, methylation of CpG sequences within gene promoter regions causes nucleosomes to become tightly compacted, excluding access by transcription factors and resulting in DNA silencing. DNMTs may additionally contribute to transcriptional repression by mechanisms other than methylation, including recruiting histone deacetylases to gene promoters *(260)*, as discussed below. Nucleosome structure is also regulated by the degree of histone acetylation. This, in turn, is controlled by the opposing activities of two groups of enzymes: the histone acetyl transferases (HATs), which maintain DNA in an active transcribed state, and the histone deacetylases (HDACs), which prevent DNA transcription *(261)*.

Abnormal patterns of DNA methylation in cancer cells have been recognized for more than 20 years *(262)*. Hypermethylation and silencing of multiple genes is a common event in MDS and MDS-AML *(263)* and is a particular feature of advanced disease. As previously discussed, the cyclin-dependent kinase inhibitor P15INK4B is a frequent target of aberrant methylation, and its inactivation is associated with an increased risk of AML progression *(173)*. Other genes may be similarly affected, including those encoding cadherins (CDH1, CDH13), among others *(264)*. The ability of DNA methylation inhibitors (5-azacytidine, 5-aza-2′ –deoxycytidine) to improve cytopenias in MDS and delay leukemic progression illustrates the importance of DNA hypermethylation in the pathogenesis of MDS and its evolution to AML.

6. CONCLUSION

We have come a long way in our understanding of the pathogenesis of MDS and myelodysplasia-related AML since this disease entity was first recognized more than a century ago *(265)*. Although at present allogeneic stem cell transplantation remains the only potentially curative therapeutic strategy *(266)*, a greater insight into the process of leukemogenesis should permit the development of targeted cellular therapies, which will hopefully widen curative options in the future.

REFERENCES

1. Mufti GJ, Galton DA. Myelodysplastic syndromes: natural history and features of prognostic importance. Clin Haematol 1986;15:953–971.
2. Jaffe ES, Harris NL, Stein H, Vardiman JW, eds. World Health Organization Claasification of Tumours: Pathology and Genetics of Tumours of Haematopoietic and Lymphoid Tissues. Lyon, France: IARC Press, 2001.
3. Vardiman JW, Harris NL, Brunning RD. The World Health Organization (WHO) classification of the myeloid neoplasms. Blood 2002;100:2292–2302.
4. Pedersen-Bjergaard J, Rowley JD. The balanced and the unbalanced chromosome aberrations of acute myeloid leukemia may develop in different ways and may contribute differently to malignant transformation. Blood 1994;83:2780–2786.
5. Gilliland DG, Jordan CT, Felix CA. The molecular basis of leukemia. Hematology (Am Soc Hematol Educ Program) 2004:80–97.

6. Wu PS, Hay AE, Thomas GE, Bowen DT. Latency of onset of de novo myelodysplastic syndromes. Haematologica 2004;89:1392–1394.

7. Yoshida Y. Hypothesis: apoptosis may be the mechanism responsible for the premature intramedullary cell death in the myelodysplastic syndrome. Leukemia 1993;7:144–146.

8. Parker JE, Fishlock KL, Mijovic A, Pagliuca A, Mufti GJ. 'Low risk' myelodysplastic syndrome (MDS) is associated with excessive apoptosis and an increased ratio of pro- versus anti-apoptotic Bcl-2 related proteins. Br J Haematol 1998;103:1075–1082.

9. Parker JE, Fishlock KL, Czepulkowski B, Pagliuca A, Mufti GJ. The role of apoptosis, proliferation and the Bcl-2 related proteins in the myelodysplastic syndromes (MDS) and acute myeloid leukaemia (AML) secondary to MDS. Blood 2000;96:3932–3938.

10. Thornberry NA, Lazebnik Y. Caspases: enemies within. Science 1998;281:12.

11. Nagata S, Golstein P. The Fas death factor. Science 1995;267:1449–1456.

12. Banner DW, D'Arcy A, Janes W, et al. Crystal structure of the soluble human 55 kd TNF receptor-human TNF beta complex: implications for TNF receptor activation. Cell 1993;73:431–435.

13. Wiley SR, Schooley K, Smolak PJ, et al. Identification and characterization of a new member of the TNF family that induces apoptosis. Immunity 1995;3:673–682.

14. Chicheportiche Y, Bourdon PR, Xu H, et al. TWEAK, a new secreted ligand in the tumor necrosis factor family that weakly induces apoptosis. J Biol Chem 1997;272:32,401–32,410.

15. Chinnaiyan AM, O'Rourke K, Tewari M, Dixit VM. FADD, a novel death domain-containing protein, interacts with the death domain of Fas and initiates apoptosis. Cell 1995;81:505–512.

16. Kischkel FC, Hellbardt S, Behrmann I, et al. Cytotoxicity-dependent APO-1 (Fas/CD95)-associated proteins form a death-inducing signaling complex (DISC) with the receptor. EMBO J 1995;14:5579–5588.

17. Marchetti P, Castedo M, Susin SA, et al. Mitochondrial permeability transition is a central coordinating event of apoptosis. J Exp Med 1996;184:1155–1160.

18. Liu X, Kim CN, Yang J, Jemmerson R, Wang X. Induction of apoptotic program in cell-free extracts: requirement for dATP and cytochrome c. Cell 1996;86:147–157.

19. Li P, Nijhawan D, Budihardjo I, et al. Cytochome c and dATP-dependent formation of Apaf-1/caspase-9 complex initiates an apoptotic protease cascade. Cell 1997;91:479–489.

20. Zou H, Henzel WJ, Liu XS, Lutschg A, Wang XD. Apaf-1, a human protein homologous to C-elegans CED-4, participates in cytochrome c-dependent activation of caspase-3. Cell 1997;90:405–413.

21. Ryan JJ, Danish R, Gottlieb CA, Clarke MF. Cell cycle analysis of p53-induced cell death in murine erythro-leukemia cells. Mol Cell Biol 1993;13:711–719.

22. Jost CA, Marin MC, Kaelin WG. p73 is a human p53-related protein that can induce apoptosis. Nature 1997;389:191–194.

23. Kaghad M, Bonnet H, Yang A, et al. Monoallelically expressed gene related to p53 at 1p36, a region frequently deleted in neuroblastoma and other human cancers. Cell 1997;90:809–819.

24. Susin SA, Lorenzo HK, Zamzami N, et al. Molecular characterization of mitochondrial apoptosis-inducing factor. Nature 1999;397:441–446.

25. Joza N, Susin SA, Daugas E, et al. Essential role of the mitochondrial apoptosis-inducing factor in programmed cell death. Nature 2001;410:549–554.

26. Pan G, Ni J, Wei YF, Yu G, Gentz R, Dixit VM. An antagonist decoy receptor and a death domain-containing receptor for TRAIL. Science 1997;277:815–818.

27. Pitti RM, Marsters SA, Lawrence DA, et al. Genomic amplification of a decoy receptor for Fas ligand in lung and colon cancer. Nature 1998;396:699–703.

28. Condorelli G, Vigliotta G, Cafieri A, et al. PED/PEA-15: an anti-apoptotic molecule that regulates FAS/TNFR1-induced apoptosis. Oncogene 1999;18:4409–4415.

29. Irmler M, Thome M, Hahne M, et al. Inhibition of death receptor signals by cellular FLIP. Nature 1997;388:190–195.

30. Yang E, Korsmeyer SJ. Molecular thanatopsis: a discourse on the BCL2 family and cell death. Blood 1996;88:386–401.

31. Liston P, Roy N, Tamai K, et al. Suppression of apoptosis in mammalian cells by NAIP and a related family of IAP genes. Nature 1996;379:349–353.

32. Wrzesien-Kus A, Smolewski P, Sobczak-Pluta A, Wierzbowska A, Robak T. The inhibitor of apoptosis protein family and its antagonists in acute leukemias. Apoptosis 2004;9:705–715.

33. Verhagen AM, Ekert PG, Pakusch M, et al. Identification of DIABLO, a mammalian protein that promotes apoptosis by binding to and antagonizing IAP proteins. Cell 2000;102:43–53.

34. Ravagnan L, Roumier T, Kroemer G. Mitochondria, the killer organelles and their weapons. J Cell Physiol 2002;192:131–137.
35. Zetterberg A. Cell growth and cell cycle progression in mammalian cells. In: Thomas NSB, ed. Apoptosis and Cell Cycle Control in Cancer, vol. 2. Oxford: BIOS Scientific Publishers, 1996:17–36.
36. Pardee AB. A restriction point control of normal animal cell proliferation. Proc Natl Acad Sci USA 1974; 71:1286–1290.
37. Grana X, Reddy EP. Cell cycle control in mammalian cells: role of cyclins, cyclin dependent kinases (CDKs), growth suppressor genes and cyclin-dependent kinase inhibitors (CKIs). Oncogene 1995;11:211–219.
38. Kato J, Matsushime H, Hiebert SW, Ewen ME, Sherr CJ. Direct binding of cyclin D to the retinoblastoma gene product (pRb) and pRb phosphorylation by the cyclin D-dependent kinase CDK4. Genes Dev 1993;7: 331–342.
39. Helin K, Harlow E, Fattaey, A. Inhibition of E2F-1 transactivation by direct binding of the retinoblastoma protein. Mol Cell Biol 1993;13:6501–6508.
40. Levine AJ. p53, the cellular gatekeeper for growth and cell division. Cell 1997;88:323–331.
41. Lin D, Shields MT, Ullrich SJ, Appella E, Mercer WE. Growth arrest induced by wild-type p53 protein blocks cells prior to or near the restriction point in late G1 phase. Proc Natl Acad Sci USA 1992;89: 9210–9214.
42. Raza A, Gezer S, Mundle S, et al. Apoptosis in bone marrow biopsy samples involving stromal and hematopoietic cells in 50 patients with myelodysplastic syndromes. Blood 1995;86:268–276.
43. Aizawa S, Nakano M, Iwase O, et al. Bone marrow stroma from refractory anemia of myelodysplastic syndrome is defective in its ability to support normal CD34-positive cell proliferation and differentiation in vitro. Leuk Res 1999;23:239–246.
44. Aizawa S, Hiramoto M, Hoshi H, Toyama K, Shima D, Handa H. Establishment of stromal cell line from an MDS RA patient which induced an apoptotic change in hematopoietic and leukemic cells in vitro. Exp Hematol 2000;28:148–155.
45. Delforge M, Raets V, Van Duppen V, Vandenberghe P, Boogaerts M.CD34+ marrow progenitors from MDS patients with high levels of intramedullary apoptosis have reduced expression of alpha4beta1 and alpha5beta1 integrins. Leukemia 2005;19:1957–1963.
46. Stasi R, Brunetti M, Bussa S, et al. Serum levels of tumour necrosis factor- predict response to recombinant human erythropoietin in patients with myelodysplastic syndrome. Clin Lab Haematol 1997;19:197–201.
47. Gersuk GM, Beckham C, Loken MR, et al. A role for tumour necrosis factor-α, Fas and Fas-Ligand in marrow failure associated with myelodysplastic syndrome. Br J Haematol 1998;103:176–188.
48. Bouscary D, De Vos J, Guesnu M, et al. Fas/Apo-1 (CD95) expression and apoptosis in patients with myelodysplastic syndromes. Leukemia 1997;11:839–845.
49. Zang DY, Goodwin RG, Loken MR, Bryant E, Deeg HJ. Expression of tumor necrosis factor-related apoptosis-inducing ligand, Apo2L, and its receptors in myelodysplastic syndrome: effects on in vitro hemo-poiesis. Blood 2001;98:3058–3065.
50. Plasilova M, Zivny J, Jelinek J, et al. TRAIL (Apo2L) suppresses growth of primary human leukemia and myelodysplasia progenitors. Leukemia 2002;16:67–73.
51. Claessens YE, Park S, Dubart-Kupperschmitt A, et al. Rescue of early stage myelodysplastic syndrome-deriving erythroid precursors by the ectopic expression of a dominant negative form of FADD. Blood 2005 Jan 27; [Epub ahead of print]
52. Mundle SD, Mativi BY, Bagai K, et al. Spontaneous down-regulation of Fas-associated phosphatase-1 may contribute to excessive apoptosis in myelodysplastic marrows. Int J Haematol 1999;70:83–90.
53. Benesch M, Platzbecker U, Ward J, Deeg HJ, Leisenring W. Expression of FLIP(Long) and FLIP(Short) in bone marrow mononuclear and CD34+ cells in patients with myelodysplastic syndrome: correlation with apoptosis. Leukemia 2003;17:2460–2466.
54. Sultana TA, Harada H, Ito K, Tanaka H, Kyo T, Kimura A. Expression and functional analysis of granulo-cyte colony-stimulating factor receptors on CD34++ cells in patients with myelodysplastic syndrome (MDS) and MDS-acute myeloid leukaemia. Br J Haematol 2003;121:63–75.
55. Bowen D, Yancik S, Bennett L, Culligan D, Resser K. Serum stem cell factor concentration in patients with myelodysplastic syndromes. Br J Haematol 1993;85:63–66.
56. Visani G, Zauli G, Tosi P, et al. Impairment of GM-CSF production in myelodysplastic syndromes. Br J Haematol 1993;84:227–231.
57. Gidali J, Feher I, Hollan SR. Blast colony forming cell-binding capacity of bone marrow stroma from myelodysplastic patients. Stem Cells 1996;14:577–583.

58. Greenberg PL, Mackichan ML, Negrin R, Renick M, Ginzton N. Production of granulocyte colony stimulating factor (G-CSF) by normal and myelodysplastic syndrome (MDS) peripheral blood (PB) cells. Blood 1990;76:146a.

59. Backx B, Broeders L, Hoefsloot LH, Wognum B, Löwenberg B. Erythropoiesis in myelodysplastic syndrome: expression of receptors for erythropoietin and kit ligand. Leukemia 1996;10:466–472.

60. Hoefsloot LH, van Amelsvoort MP, Broeders LC, et al. Erythropoietin-induced activation of STAT5 is impaired in the myelodysplastic syndrome. Blood 1997;89:1690–1700.

61. Kalina U, Hofmann WK, Koschmieder S, et al. Alteration of c-mpl-mediated signal transduction in CD34(+) cells from patients with myelodysplastic syndromes. Exp Hematol 2000;28:1158–1163.

62. Molldrem JJ, Jiang YZ, Stetler-Stevenson M, Mavroudis D, Hensel N, Barrett AJ. Hematological response of patients with myelodysplastic syndrome to antithymocyte globulin is associated with a loss of lymphocyte-mediated inhibition of CFU-GM and alterations in T-cell receptor Vβ profiles. Br J Haematol 1998;102: 1314–1322.

63. Sloand EM, Mainwaring L, Fuhrer M, et al. Preferential suppression of trisomy 8 versus normal hematopoietic cell growth by autologous lymphocytes in patients with trisomy 8 myelodysplastic syndrome. Blood 2005 Apr 12; [Epub ahead of print]

64. Tehranchi R, Fadeel B, Forsblom AM, et al. Granulocyte colony-stimulating factor inhibits spontaneous cytochrome c release and mitochondria-dependent apoptosis of myelodysplastic syndrome hematopoietic progenitors. Blood 2003;101:1080–1086.

65. Bessho F, Ohnishi H, Tabuchi K, Kobayashi M, Hayashi Y. Significance of electron-dense deposits in the mitochondrial matrix of erythroid precursors in aplastic anaemia and myelodysplastic syndrome. Br J Haematol 1999;105:149–154.

66. van de Loosdrecht AA, Brada SJ, Blom NR, et al. Mitochondrial disruption and limited apoptosis of erythroblasts are associated with high risk myelodysplasia. an ultrastructural analysis. Leuk Res 2001;25:385–393.

67. Gattermann N, Retzlaff S, Wang YL, et al. Heteroplasmic point mutations of mitochondrial DNA affecting subunit I of cytochrome c oxidase in two patients with acquired idiopathic sideroblastic anemia. Blood 1997;90:4961–4972.

68. Reddy PL, Shetty VT, Dutt D, et al. Increased incidence of mitochondrial cytochrome c-oxidase gene mutations in patients with myelodysplastic syndromes. Br J Haematol 2002;116:564–575.

69. D'Andrea AD, Grompe M. Molecular biology of Fanconi anemia: implications for diagnosis and therapy. Blood 1997;90:1725–1736.

70. Levine EG, Bloomfield CD. Secondary myelodysplastic syndromes and leukaemias. Clin Haematol 1986; 15:1037–1080.

71. West RR, Stafford DA, White DA, Bowen DT, Padua, RA. Cytogenetic abnormalities in the myelodysplastic syndromes and occupational or environmental exposure Blood 2000;95;2093–2097.

72. Chen H, Sandler DP, Taylor JA, et al. Increased risk for myelodysplastic syndromes in individuals with glutathione transferase theta 1 (GSTT1) gene defect. Lancet 1996;347:295–296.

73. Felix CA, Walker AH, Lange BJ, et al. Association of *CYP3A4* genotype with treatment-related leukemia. Proc Natl Acad Sci USA 1998;95:13,176–13,181.

74. Hofmann WK, de Vos S, Komor M, Hoelzer D, Wachsman W, Koeffler HP. Characterization of gene expression of CD34+ cells from normal and myelodysplastic bone marrow. Blood 2002;100:3553–3560.

75. Simmons PJ, Aylett GW, Niutta S, To LB, Juttner CA, Ashman LK. c-kit is expressed by primitive human hematopoietic cells that give rise to colony-forming cells in stroma-dependent or cytokine-supplemented culture. Exp Hematol 1994;22:157–165.

76. Ema H, Takano H, Sudo K, Nakauchi H. In vitro self-renewal division of hematopoietic stem cells. J Exp Med 2000;192:1281–1288.

77. Siitonen T, Savolainen ER, Koistinen P. Expression of the c-kit proto-oncogene in myeloproliferative disorders and myelodysplastic syndromes. Leukemia 1994;8:631–637.

78. Zheng R, Klang K, Gorin NC, Small D. Lack of KIT or FMS internal tandem duplications but co-expression with ligands in AML. Leuk Res 2004;28:121–126.

79. Le Beau MM, Westbrook CA, Diaz MO, et al. Evidence for the involvement of GM-CSF and FMS in the deletion (5q) in myeloid disorders. Science 1986;231:984–987.

80. Sherr CJ, Rettenmier CW, Sacca R, Roussel MF, Look AT, Stanley ER. The c-fms proto-oncogene product is related to the receptor for the mononuclear phagocyte growth factor, CSF-1. Cell 1985;41:665–676.

81. Padua RA, Guinn BA, Al-Sabah AI, et al. RAS, FMS and p53 mutations and poor clinical outcome in myelodysplasias: a 10-year follow-up. Leukemia 1998;12:887–892.

82. Ridge SA, Worwood M, Oscier D, Jacobs A, Padua RA. FMS mutations in myelodysplastic, leukemic, and normal subjects. Proc Natl Acad Sci USA 1990;87:1377–1380.

83. Rosnet O, Buhring HJ, Marchetto S, et al. Human FLT3/FLK2 receptor tyrosine kinase is expressed at the surface of normal and malignant hematopoietic cells. Leukemia 1996;10:238–248.

84. Hannum C, Culpepper J, Campbell D, et al. Ligand for FLT3/FLK2 receptor tyrosine kinase regulates growth of haematopoietic stem cells and is encoded by variant RNAs. Nature 1994;368:643–648.

85. Lisovsky M, Braun SE, Ge Y, et al. Flt3-ligand production by human bone marrow stromal cells. Leukemia 1996;10:1012–1018.

86. Lyman SD, Brasel K, Rousseau AM, Williams DE. The flt3 ligand: a hematopoietic stem cell factor whose activities are distinct from steel factor. Stem Cells 1994;12:99–107.

87. Brasel K, McKenna HJ, Morrissey PJ, et al. Hematologic effects of flt3 ligand in vivo in mice. Blood 1996;88:2004–2012.

88. McKenna HJ, de Vries P, Brasel K, Lyman SD, Williams DE. Effect of flt3 ligand on the ex vivo expansion of human CD34$^+$ hematopoietic progenitor cells. Blood 1995;86:3413–3420.

89. McKenna HJ, Stocking KL, Miller RE, et al. Mice lacking flt3 ligand have deficient hematopoiesis affecting hematopoietic progenitor cells, dendritic cells, and natural killer cells. Blood 2000;95:3489–3497.

90. Birg F, Courcoul M, Rosnet O, et al. Expression of the FMS/KIT-like gene FLT3 in human acute leukemias of the myeloid and lymphoid lineages. Blood 1992;80:2584–2593.

91. Yokota S, Kiyoi H, Nakao M, et al. Internal tandem duplication of the FLT3 gene is preferentially seen in acute myeloid leukemia and myelodysplastic syndrome among various hematological malignancies. A study on a large series of patients and cell lines. Leukemia 1997;11:1605–1609.

92. Schnittger S, Schoch C, Dugas M, et al. Analysis of FLT3 length mutations in 1003 patients with acute myeloid leukemia: correlation to cytogenetics, FAB subtype, and prognosis in the AMLCG study and usefulness as a marker for the detection of minimal residual disease. Blood 2002;100:59–66.

93. Shih LY, Huang CF, Wang PN, et al. Acquisition of FLT3 or N-ras mutations is frequently associated with progression of myelodysplastic syndrome to acute myeloid leukemia. Leukemia 2004;18:466–475.

94. Yamamoto Y, Kiyoi H, Nakano Y, et al. Activating mutation of D835 within the activation loop of FLT3 in human hematologic malignancies. Blood 2001;97:2434–2439.

95. Downward J. Ras signalling and apoptosis. Curr Opin Genet Dev 1998;8:49–54.

96. Quilliam LA, Huff SY, Rabun KM, et al. Membrane-targeting potentiates guanine nucleotide exchange factor CDC25 and SOS1 activation of Ras transforming activity. Proc Nat Acad Sci USA 1994;91:8512–8516.

97. Wittinghofer A, Sceffzek K, Ahmadian MR. The interaction of ras with GTPase-activating proteins. FEBS Lett 1997;410:63–67.

98. Marshall CJ. How does p21ras transform cells? Trends Genet 1991;7:91–95.

99. Parker J, Mufti GJ. Ras and myelodysplasia: lessons from the last decade. Semin Hematol 1996;33:206–224.

100. Bos JL, Verlaan-de Vries M, van der Eb AJ, et al. Mutations in N-ras predominate in acute myeloid leukemia. Blood 1987;69:1237–1241.

101. Farr CJ, Saiki RK, Erlich HA, McCormick F, Marshall CJ. Analysis of RAS gene mutations in acute myeloid leukemia by polymerase chain reaction and oligonucleotide probes. Proc Natl Acad Sci USA 1988; 85:1629–1633.

102. Carter G, Hughes DC, Clark RE, et al. RAS mutations in patients following cytotoxic therapy for lymphoma. Oncogene 1990;5:411–416.

103. Paquette RL, Landaw EM, Pierre RV, et al. N-ras mutations are associated with poor prognosis and increased risk of leukemia in myelodysplastic syndrome. Blood 1993;82:590–599.

104. Ludwig L, Janssen JW, Schulz AS, Bartram CR. Mutations within the FLR exon of NF1 are rare in myelodysplastic syndromes and acute myelocytic leukemias. Leukemia 1993;7:1058–1060.

105. Quesnel B, Preudhomme C, Vanrumbeke M, Vachee A, Lai JL, Fenaux P. Absence of rearrangement of the neurofibromatosis 1 (NF1) gene in myelodysplastic syndromes and acute myeloid leukemia. Leukemia 1994;8:878–880.

106. Lu D, Nounou R, Beran M, et al. The prognostic significance of bone marrow levels of neurofibromatosis-1 protein and ras oncogene mutations in patients with acute myeloid leukemia and myelodysplastic syndrome. Cancer 2003;97:441–449.

107. Dechert U, Duncan AM, Bastien L, Duff C, Adam M, Jirik FR. Protein-tyrosine phosphatase SH-PTP2 (PTPN11) is localized to 12q24.1-24.3. Hum Genet 1995;96:609–615.

108. Johannes JM, Garcia ER, De Vaan GA, Weening RS. Noonan's syndrome in association with acute leukemia. Pediatr Hematol Oncol 1995;12:571–575.

109. Tartaglia M, Niemeyer CM, Fragale A, et al. Somatic mutations in PTPN11 in juvenile myelomonocytic leukemia, myelodysplastic syndromes and acute myeloid leukemia. Nat Genet 2003;34:148–150.
110. Schubbert S, Lieuw K, Rowe SL, et al. Functional analysis of leukemia-associated PTPN11 mutations in primary hematopoietic cells. Blood 2005; [Epub ahead of print]
111. Gold MR, Duronio V, Saxena SP, Schrader JW, Aebersold R. Multiple cytokines activate phosphatidylinositol 3-kinase in hemopoietic cells. Association of the enzyme with various tyrosine-phosphorylated proteins. J Biol Chem 1994;269:5403–5412.
112. Corvera S, Czech MP. Direct targets of phosphoinositide 3-kinase products in membrane traffic and signal transduction. Trends Cell Biol 1998;8:442–446.
113. Beslu N, LaRose J, Casteran N, et al. Phosphatidylinositol-3' kinase is not required for mitogenesis or internalization of the Flt3/Flk2 receptor tyrosine kinase. J Biol Chem 1996;271:20,075–20,081.
114. Dosil M, Wang S, Lemischka IR. Mitogenic signalling and substrate specificity of the Flk2/Flt3 receptor tyrosine kinase in fibroblasts and interleukin 3-dependent hematopoietic cells. Mol Cell Biol 1993;13: 6572–6585.
115. Brunet A, Bonni A, Zigmond MJ, et al. Akt promotes cell survival by phosphorylating and inhibiting a Forkhead transcription factor. Cell 1999;96:857–868.
116. Beraud C, Henzel WJ, Baeuerle PA. Involvement of regulatory and catalytic subunits of phosphoinositide 3-kinase in NF-kappaB activation. Proc Natl Acad Sci USA 1999;96:429–434.
117. Datta SR, Dudek H, Tao X, et al. Akt phosphorylation of BAD couples survival signals to the cell-intrinsic death machinery. Cell 1997;91:231–241.
118. Min YH, Cheong JW, Kim JY, et al. Cytoplasmic mislocalization of p27Kip1 protein is associated with constitutive phosphorylation of Akt or protein kinase B and poor prognosis in acute myelogenous leukemia. Cancer Res 2004;64:5225–5231.
119. Xu Q, Simpson SE, Scialla TJ, Bagg A, Carroll M. Survival of acute myeloid leukemia cells requires PI3 kinase activation. Blood 2003;102:972–980.
120. Zhao S, Konopleva M, Cabreira-Hansen M, et al. Inhibition of phosphatidylinositol 3-kinase dephosphorylates BAD and promotes apoptosis in myeloid leukemias. Leukemia 2004;18:267–275.
121. Grandage VL, Gale RE, Linch DC, Khwaja A. PI3-kinase/Akt is constitutively active in primary acute myeloid leukaemia cells and regulates survival and chemoresistance via NF-kappaB, Mapkinase and p53 pathways. Leukemia 2005;19:586–594.
122. Sujobert P, Bardet V, Cornillet-Lefebvre P, et al. Essential role for the p110 delta isoform in phosphoinositide 3-kinase activation and cell proliferation in acute myeloid leukemia. Blood 2005; [Epub ahead of print]
123. Folkman J. Tumor angiogenesis: therapeutic implications. N Engl J Med 1971;285:1182–1186.
124. Ellis LM, Fidler IJ. Angiogenesis and metastasis. Eur J Cancer 1996;32A:2451–2460.
125. Bellamy WT, Richter L, Frutiger Y, Grogan TM. Expression of vascular endothelial growth factor and its receptors in hematopoietic malignancies. Cancer Res 1999;59:728–733.
126. Pruneri G, Bertolini F, Soligo D, et al. Angiogenesis in myelodysplastic syndromes. Br J Cancer 1999;81: 1398–1401.
127. Aguayo A, Kantarjian H, Manshouri T, et al. Angiogenesis in acute and chronic leukemias and myelodysplastic syndromes. Blood 2000;96:2240–2245.
128. Korkolopoulou P, Apostolidou E, Pavlopoulos PM, et al. Prognostic evaluation of the microvascular network in myelodysplastic syndromes. Leukemia 2001;15:1369–1376.
129. Carmeliet P, Jain RK. Angiogenesis in cancer and other diseases. Nature 2000;407:249–257.
130. Dvorak HF, Nagy JA, Dvorak JT, Dvorak AM. Identification and characterization of the blood vessels of solid tumors that are leaky to circulating macromolecules. Am J Pathol 1988;133:95–109.
131. Morikawa S, Baluk P, Kaidoh T, Haskell A, Jain RK, McDonald DM. Abnormalities in pericytes on blood vessels and endothelial sprouts in tumors. Am J Pathol 2002;160:985–1000.
132. Fukumura D, Xavier R, Sugiura T, et al. Tumor induction of VEGF promoter activity in stromal cells. Cell 1998;94:715–725.
133. Verstovsek S, Kantarjian H, Aguayo A, et al. Significance of angiogenin plasma concentrations in patients with acute myeloid leukaemia and advanced myelodysplastic syndrome. Br J Haematol 2001;114: 290–295.
134. Verstovsek S, Kantarjian H, Estey E, et al. Plasma hepatocyte growth factor is a prognostic factor in patients with acute myeloid leukemia but not in patients with myelodysplastic syndrome. Leukemia 2001;15: 1165–1170.

135. Hu Q, Dey AL, Yang Y, et al. Soluble vascular endothelial growth factor receptor 1, and not receptor 2, is an independent prognostic factor in acute myeloid leukemia and myelodysplastic syndromes. Cancer 2004; 100:1884–1891.

136. Dias S, Hattori K, Heissig B, et al. Inhibition of both paracrine and autocrine VEGF/ VEGFR-2 signaling pathways is essential to induce long-term remission of xenotransplanted human leukemias. Proc Natl Acad Sci USA 2001;98:10,857–10,862.

137. Gerber HP, Malik AK, Solar GP, et al. VEGF regulates haematopoietic stem cell survival by an internal autocrine loop mechanism. Nature 2002;417:954–958.

138. Gabrilovich DI, Chen HL, Girgis KR, et al. Production of vascular endothelial growth factor by human tumors inhibits the functional maturation of dendritic cells. Nat Med 1996;2:1096–1103.

139. Dias S, Shmelkov SV, Lam G, Rafii S. VEGF(165) promotes survival of leukemic cells by Hsp90-mediated induction of Bcl-2 expression and apoptosis inhibition. Blood 2002;99:2532–2540.

140. de Thonel A, Bettaieb A, Jean C, Laurent G, Quillet-Mary A. Role of protein kinase C zeta isoform in Fas resistance of immature myeloid KG1a leukemic cells. Blood. 2001;98:3770–3777.

141. Jia L, Srinivasula SM, Liu FT, et al. Apaf-1 protein deficiency confers resistance to cytochrome c-dependent apoptosis in human leukemic cells. Blood 2001;98:414–421.

142. Rajapaksa R, Ginzton N, Rott LS, Greenberg PL. Altered oncoprotein expression and apoptosis in myelodysplastic syndrome marrow cells. Blood 1996;88:4275–4287.

143. Delia D, Aiello A, Soligo D, et al. bcl-2 proto-oncogene expression in normal and neoplastic human myeloid cells. Blood 1992;79:1291–1298.

144. Davis RE, Greenberg PL. Bcl-2 expression by myeloid precursors in myelodysplastic syndromes: relation to disease progression. Leuk Res 1998;22:767–777.

145. Invernizzi R, Pecci A, Bellotti L, Ascari E. Expression of p53, bcl-2 and ras oncoproteins and apoptosis levels in acute leukaemias and myelodysplastic syndromes. Leuk Lymphoma 2001;42:481–489.

146. Kurotaki H, Tsushima Y, Nagai K, Yagihashi S. Apoptosis, bcl-2 expression and p53 accumulation in myelodysplastic syndrome, myelodysplastic-syndrome-derived acute myelogenous leukemia and de novo acute myelogenous leukemia. Acta Haematol 2000;102:115–123.

147. Boudard D, Vasselon C, Bertheas MF, et al. Expression and prognostic significance of Bcl-2 family proteins in myelodysplastic syndromes. Am J Hematol 2002;70:115–125.

148. Del Poeta G, Venditti A, Del Principe MI, et al. Amount of spontaneous apoptosis detected by Bax/Bcl-2 ratio predicts outcome in acute myeloid leukemia (AML). Blood 2003;101:2125–2131.

149. Du C, Fang M, Li Y, Li L, Wang X. Smac, a mitochondrial protein that promotes cytochrome c-dependent caspase activation by eliminating IAP inhibition. Cell 2000;102:33–42.

150. Verhagen AM, Ekert PG, Pakusch M, et al. Identification of DIABLO, a mammalian protein that promotes apoptosis by binding to and antagonizing IAP proteins. Cell 2000;102:43–53.

151. Li F, Ambrosini G, Chu EY, et al. Control of apoptosis and mitotic spindle checkpoint by survivin. Nature 1998;396:580–584.

152. Altieri DC, Marchisio PC, Marchisio C. Survivin apoptosis: an interloper between cell death and cell proliferation in cancer. Lab Invest 1999;79:1327–1333.

153. Ambrosini G, Adida C, Altieri DC. A novel antiapoptosis gene, survivin, expressed in cancer and lymphoma. Nat Med 1997;3:917–921.

154. Carter BZ, Milella M, Altieri DC, Andreeff M. Cytokine-regulated expression of survivin in myeloid leukemia. Blood 2001;97:2784–2790.

155. Carter BZ, Kornblau SM, Tsao T, et al. Caspase-independent cell death in AML: caspase inhibition in vitro with pan-caspase inhibitors or in vivo by XIAP or Survivin does not affect cell survival or prognosis. Blood 2003;102:4179–4186.

156. Carter BZ, Wang RY, Schober WD, Milella M, Chism D, Andreeff M. Targeting Survivin expression induces cell proliferation defect and subsequent cell death involving mitochondrial pathway in myeloid leukemic cells. Cell Cycle 2003;2:488–493.

157. Badran A, Yoshida A, Wano Y, et al. Expression of the anti-apoptotic gene survivin in myelodysplastic syndrome. Int J Oncol 2003;22:59–64.

158. Invernizzi R, Travaglino E, Lunghi M, et al. Survivin expression in acute leukemias and myelodysplastic syndromes. Leuk Lymphoma 2004;45:2229–2237.

159. Jiang W, Zhang YJ, Kahn SM, et al. Altered expression of the cyclin D1 and retinoblastoma genes in human esophageal cancer. Proc Nat Acad Sci USA 1993;90:9026–9030.

160. Paggi MG, Baldi A, Bonetto F, Giordano A. Retinoblastoma protein family in cell cycle and cancer: a review. J Cell Biochem 1996;62:418–430.
161. Preudhomme C, Vachee A, Lepelley P, et al. Inactivation of the retinoblastoma gene appears to be very uncommon in myelodysplastic syndromes. Br J Haematol 1994;87:61–67.
162. Tang JL, Yeh SH, Chen PJ, Lin MT, Tien HF, Chen YC. Inactivation of the retinoblastoma gene in acute myelogenous leukaemia. Br J Haematol 1992;82:502–507.
163. Kornblau SM, Xu HJ, Zhang W, et al. Levels of retinoblastoma protein expression in newly diagnosed acute myelogenous leukemia. Blood 1994;84:256–261.
164. Zhu YM, Bradbury D, Russell N. Decreased retinoblastoma protein expression in acute myeloblastic leukaemia is associated with the autonomous proliferation of clonogenic blasts. Br J Haematol 1994;86:533–539.
165. Kornblau SM, Qiu YH. Altered expression of retinoblastoma (RB) protein in acute myelogenous leukemia does not result from methylation of the Rb promotor. Leuk Lymphoma 1999;35(3–4):283–288.
166. Gallia GL, Johnson EM, Khalili K. Puralpha: a multifunctional single-stranded DNA- and RNA-binding protein. Nucleic Acids Res 2000;28:3197–3205.
167. Lezon-Geyda K, Najfeld V, Johnson EM. Deletions of PURA, at 5q31, and PURB, at 7p13, in myelodysplastic syndrome and progression to acute myelogenous leukemia. Leukemia 2001;15:954–962.
168. Amanullah A, Hoffman B, Liebermann DA. Deregulated E2F-1 blocks terminal differentiation and loss of leukemogenicity of M1 myeloblastic leukemia cells without abrogating induction of p15(INK4B) and p16. Blood 2000;96:475–482.
169. Saito M, Helin K, Valentine MB, et al. Amplification of the E2F1 transcription factor gene in the HEL erythroleukemia cell line. Genomics 1995;25:130–138.
170. Mundle SD, Mativi BY, Cartlidge JD, et al. Signal antonymy unique to myelodysplastic marrows correlates with altered expression of E2F1. Br J Haematol 2000;109:376–381.
171. Serrano M, Hannon GJ, Beach D. A new regulatory motif in cell-cycle control causing specific inhibition of cyclin D/CDK4. Nature 1993;366:704–707.
172. Daskalakis M, Nguyen TT, Nguyen C, et al. Demethylation of a hypermethylated P15/INK4B gene in patients with myelodysplastic syndrome by 5-Aza-2′-deoxycytidine (decitabine) treatment. Blood 2002; 100:2957–2964.
173. Quesnel B, Guillerm G, Vereecque R, et al. Methylation of the p15(INK4b) gene in myelodysplastic syndromes is frequent and acquired during disease progression. Blood 1998;91:2985–2990.
174. Toyota M, Kopecky KJ, Toyota MO, Jair KW, Willman CL, Issa JP. Methylation profiling in acute myeloid leukemia. Blood 2001;97:2823–2829.
175. Uchida T, Kinoshita T, Nagai H, et al. Hypermethylation of the p15INK4B gene in myelodysplastic syndromes Blood 1997;90:1403–1409.
176. Tien HF, Tang JH, Tsay W, et al. Methylation of the p15(INK4B) gene in myelodysplastic syndrome: it can be detected early at diagnosis or during disease progression and is highly associated with leukaemic transformation. Br J Haematol 2001;112:148–154.
177. Preisler HD, Li B, Chen H, et al. P15INK4B gene methylation and expression in normal, myelodysplastic, and acute myelogenous leukemia cells and in the marrow cells of cured lymphoma patients. Leukemia 2001; 15:1589–1595.
178. Sugimoto K, Hirano N, Toyoshima H, et al. Mutations of the p53 gene in myelodysplastic syndrome (MDS) and MDS-derived leukemia. Blood 1993;81:3022–3026.
179. Soenen V, Preudhomme C, Roumier C, Daudignon A, Lai JL, Fenaux P. 17p Deletion in acute myeloid leukemia and myelodysplastic syndrome. Analysis of breakpoints and deleted segments by fluorescence in situ. Blood 1998;91:1008–1015.
180. Lai JL, Preudhomme C, Zandecki M, et al. Myelodysplastic syndromes and acute myeloid leukemia with 17p deletion. An entity characterized by specific dysgranulopoiesis and a high incidence of P53 mutations. Leukemia 1995;9:370–381.
181. Kaneko H, Misawa S, Horiike S, Nakai H, Kashima K. TP53 mutations emerge at early phase of myelodysplastic syndrome and are associated with complex chromosomal abnormalities. Blood 1995;85: 2189–2193.
182. Kitagawa M, Yoshida S, Kuwata T, Tanizawa T, Kamiyama R. p53 expression in myeloid cells of myelodysplastic syndromes. Association with evolution of overt leukemia. Am J Pathol 1994;145:338–344.
183. Wattel E, Preudhomme C, Hecquet B, et al. p53 mutations are associated with resistance to chemotherapy and short survival in hematologic malignancies. Blood 1994;84:3148–3157.

184. Kita-Sasai Y, Horiike S, Misawa S, et al. International prognostic scoring system and TP53 mutations are independent prognostic indicators for patients with myelodysplastic syndrome. Br J Haematol 2001;115: 309–312.

185. Castro PD, Liang JC, Nagarajan L. Deletions of chromosome 5q13.3 and 17p loci cooperate in myeloid neoplasms. Blood 2000;95:2138–2143.

186. Hupp TR, Meek DW, Midgley CA, Lane DP. Regulation of the specific DNA binding function of p53. Cell 1992;71:875–886.

187. Momand J, Zambetti GP, Olson DC, George D, Levine AJ. The mdm-2 oncogene product forms a complex with the p53 protein and inhibits p53-mediated transactivation. Cell 1992;69:1237–1245.

188. Oliner JD, Kinzler KW, Meltzer PS, George DL, Vogelstein B. Amplification of a gene encoding a p53-associated protein in human sarcomas. Nature 1992;358:80–83.

189. Preudhomme C, Quesnel B, Vachee A, et al. Absence of amplification of MDM2 gene, a regulator of p53 function, in myelodysplastic syndromes. Leukemia 1993;7:1291–1293.

190. Quesnel B, Preudhomme C, Oscier D, et al. Over-expression of the MDM2 gene is found in some cases of haematological malignancies. Br J Haematol 1994;88:415–418.

191. Faderl S, Kantarjian HM, Estey E, et al. The prognostic significance of p16(INK4a)/p14(ARF) locus deletion and MDM-2 protein expression in adult acute myelogenous leukemia. Cancer 2000;89:1976–1982.

192. Stirewalt DL, Clurman B, Appelbaum FR, Willman CL, Radich JP. p73 mutations and expression in adult de novo acute myelogenous leukemia. Leukemia 1999;13:985–990.

193. Schmelz K, Wagner M, Dorken B, Tamm I. 5-Aza-2′-deoxycytidine induces p21(WAF) expression by demethylation of p73 leading to p53-independent apoptosis in myeloid leukemia. Int J Cancer. 2005;114(5): 683–695.

194. Lo Vasco VR, Calabrese G, Manzoli L, et al. Inositide-specific phospholipase c beta1 gene deletion in the progression of myelodysplastic syndrome to acute myeloid leukemia. Leukemia 2004;18:1122–1126

195. Hahne M, Rimoldi D, Schroter M, et al. Melanoma cell expression of Fas(Apo-1/CD95) ligand: implications for tumor immune escape. Science 1996;274:1363–1366.

196. Gupta P, Niehans GA, LeRoy SC, et al. Fas ligand expression in the bone marrow in myelodysplastic syndromes correlates with FAB subtype and anemia, and predicts survival. Leukemia 1999;13:44–53.

197. Amin HM, Jilani I, Estey EH, et al. Increased apoptosis in bone marrow B lymphocytes but not T lymphocytes in myelodysplastic syndrome. Blood 2003;102:1866–1888.

198. Buggins AG, Milojkovic D, Arno MJ, et al. Microenvironment produced by acute myeloid leukemia cells prevents T cell activation and proliferation by inhibition of NF-kappaB, c-Myc, and pRb pathways. J Immunol 2001;167:6021–6030.

199. Milojkovic D, Devereux S, Westwood NB, Mufti GJ, Thomas NS, Buggins AG. Anti-apoptotic microenvironment of acute myeloid leukemia. J Immunol. 2004;173:6745–6752.

200. Speck NA, Gilliland DG. Core-binding factors in haematopoiesis and leukaemia. Nat Rev Cancer 2002;2:502–513.

201. Osato M, Asou N, Abdalla E, et al. Biallelic and heterozygous point mutations in the runt domain of the *AML1/PEBP1B* gene associated with myeloblastic leukemias. Blood 1999;93:1817–1824.

202. Preudhomme C, Warot-Loze D, Roumier C, et al. High incidence of biallelic point mutations in the Runt domain of the AML1/PEBP1B gene in Mo acute myeloid leukemia and in myeloid malignancies with aquired trisomy 21. Blood 2000;96;2862–2869.

203. Harada H, Harada Y, Tanaka H, Kimura A, Inaba T. Implications of somatic mutations in the *AML1* gene in radiation-associated and therapy-related myelodysplastic syndrome/acute myeloid leukemia. Blood 2003; 101:673–680.

204. Harada H, Harada Y, Niimi H, Kyo T, Kimura A, Inaba T. High incidence of somatic mutations in the *AML1/RUNX1* gene in myelodysplastic syndrome and low blast percentage myeloid leukemia with myelodysplasia. Blood 2004;103:2316–2324.

205. Osato M. Point mutations in the RUNX1/AML1 gene: another actor in RUNX leukemia. Oncogene 2004; 23:4284–4296.

206. Nakao M, Horiike S, Fukushima-Nakase Y, et al. Novel loss-of-function mutations of the haematopoiesis-related transcription factor, acute myeloid leukaemia 1/runt-related transcription factor 1, detected in acute myeloblastic leukaemia and myelodysplastic syndrome. Br J Haematol 2004;125:709–719.

207. Song W-J, Sullivan GM, Legare RD, et al. Haploin-sufficiency of *CBFA2* causes familial thrombocytopenia with propensity to develop acute myelogenous leukemia. Nat Genet 1999:23;166–175.

208. Ayton PM, Cleary ML. Molecular mechanisms of leukemogenesis mediated by MLL fusion proteins. Oncogene 2001;20:5695–5707.

209. Schnittger S, Kinkelin U, Schoch C, et al. Screening for MLL tandem duplication in 387 unselected patients with AML identify a prognostically unfavorable subset of AML. Leukemia 2000;14:796–804

210. Milne TA, Briggs SD, Brock HW, et al. MLL targets SET domain methyltransferase activity to Hox gene promoters. Mol Cell 2002;10:1107–1117.

211. Nakamura T, Mori T, Tada S, et al. ALL-1 is a histone methyltransferase that assembles a supercomplex of proteins involved in transcriptional regulation. Mol Cell 2002;10:1119–1128.

212. Ferrando AA, Armstrong SA, Neuberg DS, et al. Gene expression signatures in MLL-rearranged T-lineage and B-precursor acute leukemias: dominance of HOX dysregulation. Blood 2003;102:262–268.

213. Rozovskaia T, Ravid-Amir O, Tillib S, et al. Expression profiles of acute lymphoblastic and myeloblastic leukemias with ALL-1 rearrangements. Proc Natl Acad Sci USA 2003;100:7853–7858.

214. Armstrong SA, Staunton JE, Silverman LB, et al. MLL translocations specify a distinct gene expression profile that distinguishes a unique leukemia. Nat Genet 2002;30:41–47.

215. Zeisig BB, Milne T, García-Cuéllar M-P, et al. *Hoxa9* and *Meis1* are key targets for MLL-ENL-mediated cellular immortalization. Mol Cell Biol 2004;24:617–662.

216. Ono R, Nakajima H, Ozaki K, et al. Dimerization of MLL fusion proteins and FLT3 activation synergize to induce multiple-lineage leukemogenesis. J Clin Invest 2005;115:919–929.

217. Yoneda-Kato N, Look AT, Kirstein MN, et al. The t(3;5)(q25.1;q34) of myelodysplastic syndrome and acute myeloid leukemia produces a novel fusion gene, NPM-MLF1. Oncogene 1996;12:265–275.

218. Kwong YL. Translocation (3;5)(q21;q34) in erythroleukemia: a molecular and in situ hybridization study. Cancer Genet Cytogenet 1998;103:15–19.

219. Matsumoto N, Yoneda-Kato N, Iguchi T, et al. Elevated MLF1 expression correlates with malignant progression from myelodysplastic syndrome. Leukemia 2000;14:1757–1765.

220. Matsumoto N, Yoneda-Kato N, Yamamoto Y, Kishimoto Y, Fukuhara S. Myelodysplasia/myeloid leukemia factor 1, MLF1, as a new marker of prognosis, and leukemia progression from myelodysplastic syndrome. Blood 1997;90:201.

221. Winteringham LN, Kobelke S, Williams JH, Ingley E, Klinken SP. Myeloid leukemia factor 1 inhibits erythropoietin-induced differentiation, cell cycle exit and p27Kip1 accumulation. Oncogene 2004;23:5105–5109.

222. Colombo E, Marine JC, Danovi D, Falini B, Pelicci PG. Nucleophosmin regulates the stability and transcriptional activity of p53. Nat Cell Biol 2002;4:529–533.

223. Gandini D, De Angeli C, Aguiari G. Preferential expression of the transcription coactivator HTIF1alpha gene in acute myeloid leukemia and MDS-related AML. Leukemia 2002;16:886–893.

224. Menke AL, Van der Eb AJ, Jochemsen AG. The Wilms' tumor 1 gene: oncogene or tumor suppressor gene. Int Rev Cytol 1998;181:151–212.

225. Gashler AL, Bonthron DT, Madden SL, Rauscher FJ III, Collins T, Sukhatme VP. Human platelet-derived growth factor A chain is transcriptionally repressed by the Wilms tumor suppressor WT1. Proc Natl Acad Sci USA 1992;89:10,984–10,988.

226. Harrington MA, Konicek B, Song A, Xia XL, Fredericks WJ, Rauscher FJ III. Inhibition of colony-stimulating factor-1 promoter activity by the product of the Wilms' tumor locus. J Biol Chem 1993;268:21,271–21,275.

227. Drummond IA, Madden SL, Rohwer-Nutter P, Bell GI, Sukhatme VP, Rauscher FJ III. Repression of the insulin-like growth factor II gene by the Wilms tumor suppressor WT1. Science 1992;257:674–678.

228. Guan LS, Rauchman M, Wang ZY. Induction of Rb-associated protein (RbAp46) by Wilms' tumor suppressor WT1 mediates growth inhibition. J Biol Chem. 1998;273:27,047–27,050.

229. Mayo MW, Wang CY, Drouin SS. WT1 modulates apoptosis by transcriptionally upregulating the bcl-2 proto-oncogene. EMBO J 1999;18:3990–4003.

230. Call KM, Glaser T, Ito CY, et al. Isolation and characterization of a zinc finger polypeptide gene at the human chromosome 11 Wilms' tumor locus. Cell 1990;60:509–520.

231. Gessler M, Poustka A, Cavenee W, Neve RL, Orkin SH, Bruns GA. Homozygous deletion in Wilms tumours of a zinc-finger gene identified by chromosome jumping. Nature 1990;343:774–778.

232. Little M, Wells C. A clinical overview of WT1 gene mutations. Hum Mutat 1997;9:209–225.

233. Miwa H, Beran M, Saunders GF. Expression of the Wilms' tumor gene (WT1) in human leukemias. Leukemia 1992;6:405–409.

234. Miyagi T, Ahuja H, Kubota T, Kubonishi I, Koeffler HP, Miyoshi I. Expression of the candidate Wilm's tumor gene, WT1, in human leukemia cells. Leukemia 1993;7:970–977.

235. Inoue K, Sugiyama H, Ogawa H, et al. WT1 as a new prognostic factor and a new marker for the detection of minimal residual disease in acute leukemia. Blood 1994;84:3071–3079.

236. Yamagami T, Sugiyama H, Inoue K, et al. Growth inhibition of human leukemic cells by WT1 (Wilms tumor gene) antisense oligodeoxynucleotides: implications for the involvement of WT1 in leukemogenesis. Blood 1996;87:2878–2884.

237. Inoue K, Tamaki H, Ogawa H, et al. Wilms' tumor gene (WT1) competes with differentiation-inducing signal in hematopoietic progenitor cells. Blood 1998;91:2969–2976.

238. Patmasiriwat P, Fraizer G, Kantarjian H, Saunders GF. WT1 and GATA1 expression in myelodysplastic syndrome and acute leukemia. Leukemia 1999;13:891–900.

239. Tamaki H, Ogawa H, Ohyashiki K, et al. The Wilms' tumor gene WT1 is a good marker for diagnosis of disease progression of myelodysplastic syndromes. Leukemia 1999;13:393–399.

240. Cilloni D, Gottardi E, Messa F, et al. Piedmont Study Group on Myelodysplastic Syndromes. Significant correlation between the degree of WT1 expression and the International Prognostic Scoring System Score in patients with myelodysplastic syndromes. J Clin Oncol 2003;21:1988–1995.

241. Elisseeva OA, Oka Y, Tsuboi A, et al. Humoral immune responses against Wilms tumor gene WT1 product in patients with hematopoietic malignancies. Blood 2002;99:3272–3279.

242. Radomska HS, Huettner CS, Zhang P, Cheng T, Scadden DT, Tenen DG. CCAAT/enhancer binding protein alpha is a regulatory switch sufficient for induction of granulocytic development from bipotential myeloid progenitors. Mol Cell Biol 1998;18:4301–4314.

243. Gombart AF, Hofmann WK, Kawano S, et al. Mutations in the gene encoding the transcription factor CCAAT/enhancer binding protein alpha in myelodysplastic syndromes and acute myeloid leukemias. Blood 2002;99:1332–1340.

244. McEachern MJ, Krauskopf A, Blackburn EH. Telomeres and their control. Annu Rev Genet 2000;34: 331–358.

245. Boultwood J, Fidler C, Kusec R, et al. Telomere length in myelodysplastic syndromes. Am J Hematol 1997; 56:266–271.

246. Ohyashiki JH, Iwama H, Yahata N, et al. Telomere stability is frequently impaired in high-risk groups of patients with myelodysplastic syndromes. Clin Cancer Res 1999;5:1155–1160.

247. Sieglova Z, Zilovcova S, Cermak J, et al. Dynamics of telomere erosion and its association with genome instability in myelodysplastic syndromes (MDS) and acute myelogenous leukemia arising from MDS: a marker of disease prognosis? Leuk Res 2004;28:1013–1021.

248. Rigolin GM, Porta MD, Bugli AM, et al. Flow cytometric detection of accelerated telomere shortening in myelodysplastic syndromes: correlations with aetiological and clinical-biological findings. Eur J Haematol 2004;73:351–358.

249. Morin GB. The human telomere terminal transferase enzyme is a ribonucleoprotein that synthesizes TTAGGG repeats. Cell 1989;59:521–529.

250. Feng J, Funk WD, Wang SS, et al. The RNA component of human telomerase. Science 1995;269:1236–1241.

251. Shay JW, Bacchetti S. A survey of telomerase activity in human cancer. Eur J Cancer 1997;33:787–791.

252. Counter CM, Gupta J, Harley CB, Leber B, Bacchetti S. Telomerase activity in normal leukocytes and in hematologic malignancies. Blood 1995;85:2315–2320.

253. Jaenisch R, Bird A. Epigenetic regulation of gene expression: how the genome integrates intrinsic and environmental signals. Nat Genet 2003;33(suppl):245–254.

254. Bird A. DNA methylation patterns and epigenetic memory. Genes Dev 2002;16:6–21.

255. Jones PA, Baylin SB. The fundamental role of epigenetic events in cancer. Nat Rev Genet 2002;3:415–428.

256. Jones PA, Takai D. The role of DNA methylation in mammalian epigenetics. Science 2001;293:1068–1070.

257. Jenuwein T, Allis CD. Translating the histone code. Science 2001;293:1074–1080.

258. Kondo Y, Issa JP. Epigenetic changes in colorectal cancer. Cancer Metastasis Rev 2004;23:29–39.

259. Okano M, Xie S, Li E. Cloning and characterization of a family of novel mammalian DNA (cytosine-5) methyltransferases. Nat Genet 1998;19:219–220.

260. Fuks F, Burgers WA, Godin N, Kasai M, Kouzarides T. Dnmt3a binds deacetylases and is recruited by a sequence-specific repressor to silence transcription. EMBO J 2001;20:2536–2544.

261. Strahl BD, Allis CD. The language of covalent histone modifications. Nature 2000;403:41–45.

262. Laird PW, Jaenisch R. The role of DNA methylation in cancer genetic and epigenetics. Annu Rev Genet 1996;30:441–464.

263. Claus R, Lubbert M. Epigenetic targets in hematopoietic malignancies. Oncogene 2003;22:6489–6496.

264. Esteller M. Profiling aberrant DNA methylation in hematologic neoplasms: a view from the tip of the iceberg. Clin Immunol 2003;109:80–88.
265. Von Leube. Rapid verlaufende schwere Anämie mit gleichzeitiger leukämischer Veränderung des Blutbildes. Berlin Klin Wochenschr 1900;37:85–97.
266. Longmore G, Guinan EC, Weinstein HJ, Gelber RD, Rappeport JM, Antin JH. Bone marrow transplantation for myelodysplasia and secondary acute nonlymphoblastic leukemia. J Clin Oncol 1990;8:1707–1714.

Therapy-Related AML

Lucy A. Godley and Michelle M. Le Beau

CONTENTS

Summary

Patients who have been treated successfully with chemotherapy, radiation therapy, immunosuppressive therapy, or a combination of these modalities are at risk for long-term complications of their treatment. One of the most serious complications is the development of therapy-related myelodysplasia (t-MDS) and therapy-related acute myeloid leukemia (t-AML), which most likely result as a direct consequence of prior cytotoxic therapy. t-MDS/t-AML represent distinct clinical entities as compared to their *de novo* counterparts and confer a poor prognosis. A clearer understanding of the factors that predispose patients to the development of t-MDS and t-AML will help clinicians monitor patients more carefully after treatment for a primary malignancy, during long-term immunosuppression for autoimmune disease, or following solid organ transplants. Ultimately, this knowledge may influence the treatment strategies for those patients with solid tumors and those on long-term immunosuppression, groups that are at increased risk for the development of t-MDS/t-AML. This chapter will review the clinical features and treatment of these disorders, epidemiology, cytogenetic features, and the genetic pathways involved in the pathogenesis of t-MDS/t-AML.

Key Words: Therapy-related myelodysplastic syndrome; therapy-related acute myeloid leukemia; alkylating agent; epipodophyllotoxin; dysplasia; long-term complications.

1. CLINICAL AND MORPHOLOGICAL FEATURES

In general, the diagnosis of t-MDS/t-AML is made after a patient presents with typical symptomatology or laboratory abnormalities. Fatigue, weakness, and occasionally fever are the most frequent patient complaints. Signs of the diseases include bleeding complications caused by thrombocytopenia, anemia, and leukopenia. The anemia is characterized by macrocytosis, and an increased mean corpuscular volume (MCV) is often the first clue as to the diagnosis. Features commonly present in *de novo* acute leukemia, such as hepatomegaly,

From: *Contemporary Hematology: Acute Myelogenous Leukemia*
Edited by: J. E. Karp © Humana Press Inc., Totowa, NJ

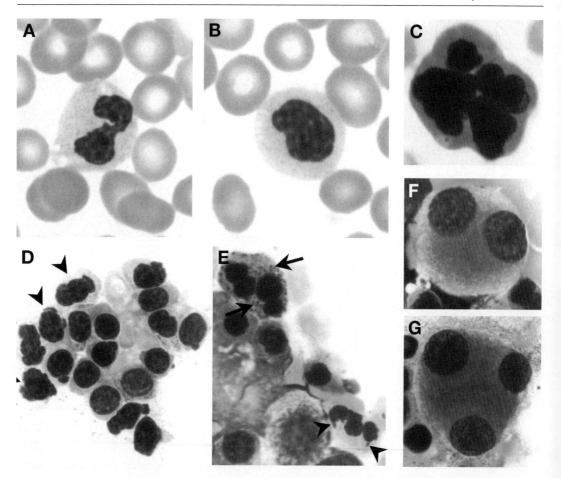

Fig. 1. (Color Plate 1, following page 174) Multilineage dysplasia seen in the peripheral blood and bone marrow aspirate from a 38-year-old survivor of Hodgkin's disease who had been treated with chemotherapy, radiation, and an autologous stem cell transplant. The patient was asymptomatic until presentation with a macrocytic anemia and thrombocytopenia and was found to have therapy-related myelodysplasia. Karyotype analysis revealed a loss of chromosome 7, consistent with alkylating agent-induced t-MDS. **(A–C)** Dysplasia in the peripheral blood. **(A,B)** Dysplastic neutrophils have hypolobated, hypercondensed chromatin and hypogranular cytoplasm. **(C)** A multinucleated abnormal erythroid precursor in the peripheral blood. **(D–G)** Dysplasia in the bone marrow. **(D)** An erythroid colony with apoptotic erythroid cells (arrowheads). **(E)** Erythroid precursors contain irregular nuclear contours and basophilic granules (arrows) derived from improperly processed iron, and dysplastic neutrophils display nuclear excrescences (arrowheads). **(F,G)** Micromegakaryocytes with abnormal separation of nuclear lobes. (Photomicrographs courtesy of Dr. Ozden Ozer, The University of Chicago, Department of Pathology.)

splenomegaly, lymphadenopathy, gingival hyperplasia, skin rash, or neurological complications, are notably absent from the presentations of patients with t-MDS/t-AML. Bone marrow biopsies typically reveal hypercellularity with some degree of marrow fibrosis, although hypocellular and even aplastic marrows can be seen.

Trilineage dysplasia is a hallmark of the therapy-related disorders (Fig. 1; *see* Color Plate 1, following p. 174). Anisopoikilocytosis is found in the peripheral blood, with teardrops, spherocytes, spiculated or nucleated red blood cells, basophilic stippling, circulating erythroblasts, and polychromasia. Granulocytes are commonly hypogranular, with hypo- or hyperlobulated nuclei, nuclear excrescences, and pseudo-Pelger-Huet nuclei. The peripheral blood often shows neutropenia, basophilia, monocytosis, immature myeloid cells, and, ultimately, blasts. Giant or degranulated platelets may appear in the peripheral blood, along with circulating micromegakaryocytes, megakaryoblasts, and megakaryocyte fragments. The bone marrow biopsies also show features of trilineage dysplasia, with periodic acid–Schiff-positive normoblasts, dyserythropoiesis with megaloblastoid changes, erythroid hyperplasia, ringed sideroblasts, nuclear budding, karyorrhexis, binuclearity, and nuclear bridging. Megakaryocyte dysplasia within the bone marrow includes micromegakaryocytes, abnormal nuclear spacings, mononuclear forms, giant compound granules, and hypogranular cytoplasm. Neither t-MDS nor t-AML is easily categorized according to the French–American–British (FAB) classification schema, but the World Health Organization (WHO) classification recognizes them as a distinct entity *(1)*. Morphologically, t-MDS/t-AML most closely resembles acute myeloid leukemia with multilineage dysplasia, also a distinct form of *de novo* AML recognized by the WHO classification. t-AML is distinguished from t-MDS solely based on the blast count being ≥20% in either the peripheral blood or the bone marrow. On the basis of clinical, morphological, and genetic features, t-MDS and t-AML are essentially one disease, each representing different points of the leukemic spectrum. The specific morphological and cytogenetic features of t-MDS/t-AML are largely a function of the type of prior cytotoxic therapy that the patient received for his or her primary medical condition (*see* Section 2).

2. EXPOSURE TO SPECIFIC AGENTS AND CYTOGENETIC FINDINGS

2.1. Alkylator-Induced t-MDS and t-AML

The use of alkylating agents is associated with the development of t-MDS followed by t-AML with characteristic losses of the long arms of chromosomes 5 and/or 7 (Tables 1, 2) *(2,3)*. Alkylating agents vary in their likelihood of causing the development of therapy-related disease (melphalan > cyclophosphamide) *(4,5)*, and there is a dose–response relationship between the amount of alkylating agent received and the risk of disease development *(6–13)*. This form of t-MDS/t-AML typically occurs within 5–7 years after chemotherapy and/or radiotherapy have been given and confers a poor prognosis for patients (*see* Section 7).

2.1.1. MOLECULAR ANALYSIS OF THE DELETED SEGMENT OF CHROMOSOME 5

Loss of a whole chromosome 5 or a deletion of the long arm of this chromosome, –5/del(5q), is observed in 40–50% of patients with t-MDS/t-AML. A commonly deleted segment (CDS) on the long arm of chromosome 5 is predicted to contain a myeloid tumor suppressor gene involved in the pathogenesis of t-MDS/t-AML and cases of *de novo* MDS and AML with abnormalities of chromosome 5 *(3,14–17)*. Using cytogenetic and fluorescence in situ hybridization (FISH) analysis, Le Beau and colleagues have defined a 970-kb CDS within 5q31 flanked by D5S479 and D5S500 *(3)*. The functions of the genes within this CDS cover a spectrum of activities, including the regulation of mitosis and the G2 checkpoint, transcriptional and translational regulators, and cell surface receptors. Analysis of myeloid leukemia cells for inactivating mutations has eliminated all 20 known genes within the CDS, suggesting that a novel myeloid tumor suppressor gene is located in this interval or that other mechanisms, such as haploinsufficiency or gene silencing through promoter methylation, may be involved in the pathogenesis of these disorders *(3,17)*. The CDS identified in patients with t-MDS/t-AML is proximal to the CDS identified within 5q32 in patients with the 5q- syndrome, a form of primary MDS characterized by a del(5q) as the sole karyotypic abnormality, with a female

Table 1
Recurring Cytogenetic Abnormalities in t-MDS/t-AML

Chromosome abnormality	Frequency[a] (%)	Involved genes[b]		Consequence
−7 or del(7q)	50			
−5 or del(5q)	42			
dic(5;17)(q11.1–13; p11.1–p13)	5		TP53	Loss of function, 5q gene unknown
der(1;7)(q10;p10)	3			
t(8;21)(q22;q22)/ t(3;21)(q26.2; q22.1)	3	ETO EAP	RUNX1 RUNX1	RUNX1 fusion protein—altered transcriptional regulation
t(9;11)(p23;q23)/ t(11q23)	3	AF9	MLL	MLL fusion protein—altered transcriptional regulation
inv(16)(p13.1q22)	2	CBFB	MYH11	CBFB fusion protein—altered transcriptional regulation
t(15;17)(q22;q12)	2	PML	RARA	RARA fusion protein—altered transcriptional regulation
t(8;16)(p11.2;p13.3)	<1	MYST3	CBP	MYST3 fusion protein—altered chromatin remodeling and transcriptional regulation
t(11;16)(q23;p13.3)	<1	MLL	CBP	MLL fusion protein—altered transcriptional regulation

[a]Chromosome abnormality frequencies are reported from the University of Chicago series *(42)*.
[b]Genes are listed in order of citation in the karyotype.

predominance, a low rate of leukemic transformation, and a relatively long survival of several years' duration *(18–21)*. In summary, the existing data suggest that there are two nonoverlapping CDSs in 5q31 and 5q32. The proximal segment in 5q31 is likely to contain one or more tumor suppressor gene(s) involved in the pathogenesis of both *de novo* and therapy-related MDS/AML. Band 5q32 is likely to contain an additional myeloid tumor suppressor gene involved in the pathogenesis of the 5q syndrome.

2.1.2. MOLECULAR ANALYSIS OF THE DELETED SEGMENT OF CHROMOSOME 7

The results of cytogenetic, FISH, and loss of heterozygosity (LOH) studies performed in a number of laboratories paint a complex picture of 7q deletions in myeloid malignancies. There is general agreement that 7q22 is involved in the majority of cases. Defining a consistent CDS has been hampered by (1) the relatively low frequency of del(7q) compared to the complete loss of chromosome 7, (2) the use of different techniques to investigate marrow samples, e.g., FISH vs LOH, (3) the wide clinical spectrum of myeloid disorders with alterations in chromosome 7, suggesting genetic heterogeneity, and (4) the existence of multiple and sometimes complex cytogenetic abnormalities in most cases.

Two distinct CDSs on 7q were identified by molecular analysis of 81 patients with *de novo* and therapy-related MDS/AML *(2)*. In 65 patients, the CDS was within q22, whereas in 16 other patients, the CDS involved 7q32-33, a more distal segment. Using FISH analysis, an ~2-Mb CDS in 7q22 was defined, which is consistent with most published data *(2,22–25)*. Tosi et al. *(26)* identified a patient with a complex karyotype and a deletion associated with a t(7;7),

Table 2
Clinical Subgroups of t-MDS/t-AML

Prior treatment with:	Alkylating agents	Topoisomerase II inhibitors	Azathioprine[a]
Preleukemic phase	Yes, MDS	None	Yes, MDS
Cytogenetic abnormalities	−5/del(5q) (21%)	t(11q23) (3%)	Not reported
	−7/del(7q) (26%)	t(21q22) (3%)	
	−5/del(5q) and −7/del(7q) (22%)		
Median latency	5 years	2 years	5–6 years
Long-term survival	−5/del(5q): 7 months	Balanced translocations:	Not reported
	−7/del(7q): 9 months	11 months	
	−5/del(5q) and −7/del(7q): 5 months		

[a]Data from ref. 62.

in which the translocation breakpoint occurred 150 kb proximal to the CDS defined by Le Beau et al. (2). A number of candidate genes have been identified and evaluated for mutations within the CDS at 7q22, although no inactivating mutations have been identified in the remaining allele (27).

2.2. Topoisomerase II Inhibitor-Induced t-AML

t-AML following chemotherapy with topoisomerase II inhibitors is characterized by translocations involving chromosome bands 11q23 or 21q22 (Tables 1, 2) (28–31). These leukemias were first described when t-AML with 11q23 abnormalities developed in children who had received epipodophyllotoxins for the treatment of acute lymphocytic leukemia (ALL), with the highest risk being in children who had received prolonged weekly or twice-weekly etoposide or teniposide (28), and in survivors of non-small-cell lung cancer (29). Balanced translocations may involve the MLL gene at chromosome band 11q23 or the PML/RARA genes in the case of therapy-related acute promyelocytic leukemia. Rearrangements of the core binding factor genes AML1 (RUNX1/CBFA2) at chromosome band 21q22 and CBFB at chromosome band 16q22, as well as the NUP98 gene at chromosome band 11p15.5, have all been described.

In contrast to alkylating agent-associated t-AML, these leukemias are not preceded by t-MDS and occur with a shorter latency, often within 2–3 years of the first cytotoxic therapy and, in some cases, within 12 months. These t-AMLs often present with rapidly progressive leukemia and high white blood cell counts. Although they also have a poor prognosis overall, they are more responsive to initial induction chemotherapy.

Hematopoietic disorders involving rearrangements of the MLL (mixed lineage leukemia) gene (also known as ALL1, HTRX, HRX) usually present as acute myeloid leukemia, and over 50 reciprocal translocations involving MLL have been described (32). Less commonly, patients with MLL rearrangements can present with MDS. In an international workshop on therapy-related diseases, 162 out of 511 patients (32%) had t-MDS/t-AML involving rearrangements of 11q23 (33,34). The translocation partners were 9p22 (48%), 19p13.3 (11%), 19p13.1 (10%), 4q21 (9%), 6q27 (6%), 1p32 (2%), 16p13.1 (2%), 10p13 (1%), and 17q25 (1%). Slightly less than 12% of these patients presented with a t-MDS. One-third

(6/19) of these t-MDS patients had progression to an acute leukemia (5 t-AML, and 1 t-ALL). This study did not find a clear association with FAB subtype. Patients with 11q23 rearrangements had a short median survival of 9 months, compared to 12–31 months for patients with other balanced translocations, even though they were younger and more often received stem cell transplantation.

The t(11;16)(q23;p13.3) is unique among at least 50 recurring translocations of *MLL* in that most patients present with t-MDS *(35)*. In this rearrangement, the *MLL* gene on chromosome 11 is fused with the *CBP* (CREB-binding protein) gene on chromosome 16. The MLL protein is a histone methyltransferase that assembles in protein complexes that regulate gene transcription via chromatin remodeling, e.g., *HOX* genes during embryonic development. CBP is an adapter protein involved in histone acetylation, which mediates chromosome decondensation and thereby facilitates transcription. Both *MLL* and *CBP* have multiple translocation partners in various hematological disorders.

In the international workshop on therapy-related diseases, 79 out of 511 patients (15.5%) had t-MDS/t-AML involving rearrangements of 21q22 *(36)*. Several translocations comprised the majority of cases: t(8;21) (56%), t(3;21) (20%), and t(16;21) (5%). In total, 23 different translocation partners were found for the *AML1/CBFA2/RUNX1* gene located at 21q22. t-MDS/t-AML with 21q22 rearrangements was associated with dysplasia, multiple translocation partners, prior exposure to radiation, epipodophyllotoxins, and anthracyclines, as well as longer latency periods. Patients with t(8;21) had a significantly longer median survival time than did those patients with other 21q22 rearrangements, 19 months vs 7 months, respectively ($p = 0.0007$).

Patients with inv(16), which results in the fusion of the *CBFB* and *MYH11* genes, comprised 48 out of the 511 patients (9%) studied in the international workshop on therapy-related diseases *(37)*. More than half of these patients had additional cytogenetic abnormalities, most commonly +8, +21, +22, and del(7q). Half of the patients with inv(16) had been treated with alkylating agents in addition to topoisomerase II inhibitors, and 21% of the patients had been treated with radiation only. The majority of patients with inv(16) (79%) presented with t-AML, and 85% of the patients achieved a complete response with intensive chemotherapy. The median survival for patients who achieved a complete response was 29 months, with improved survival for those patients younger than 55 years old.

The international workshop on therapy-related diseases identified other rare recurring translocations seen in patients with t-MDS/t-AML *(38)*. These translocations involved 3q21 and/or rearrangements of 3q26.2 (22%), 11p15.5 (22%), t(9;22) (13%), 12p13 (12%), t(8;16) (p11.2;p13.3) (12%), t(6;9)(p23;q34) (4%), t(10;11)(p13;q13-q21) (4%), t(1;17)(p36.3;q21) (2.5%), t(8;14)(q24.3;q32) (2.5%), t(11;19)(q23;p13.3) and t(11;19)(q23;p13.1) (2.5%), and t(1;3)(p36.3;q21) (2.5%). Of patients with these translocations, the only patients who survived longer than 2 years were those with rearrangements of 3q21/3q26.2 (20%) and of 11p15.5 (33%).

2.3. Other Subtypes of t-MDS/t-AML

Patients with therapy-related acute promyelocytic leukemia (t-APL) have the t(15;17) and, consequently, a very similar disease to that which arises *de novo*. Patients with t-APL comprise 8% of all patients with t-MDS/t-AML, according to the international workshop on therapy-related diseases *(37)*. Many of these patients (41%) had additional cytogenetic abnormalities, most commonly −5, +8, and del(16q). Half of the patients with t-APL had been treated with combined chemotherapy and radiation therapy, and 29% of the patients had been treated with radiation only. Although the t(15;17) in t-APL results in the same fusion

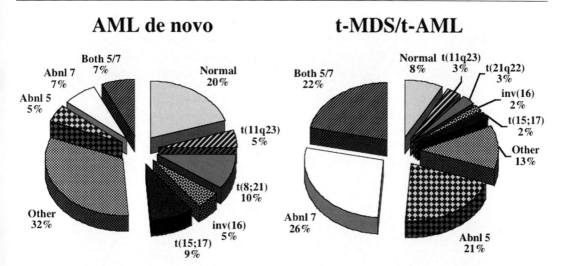

Fig. 2. Recurring chromosomal abnormalities in t-MDS/t-AML **(right)** are contrasted with those found in AML *de novo* **(left)**. Frequencies are reported from the University of Chicago Series *(42)* and unpublished data (Le Beau et al.)

of the *PML* and *RARA* genes as in *de novo* disease and is treated essentially identically, the induction remission rate is not as good. Only 69% of patients with t-APL achieved remission with induction chemotherapy, according to the international workshop. The median survival for patients who achieved a complete response was only 29 months, indicating that t-APL is more aggressive than its *de novo* counterpart.

Although therapy-related leukemias are generally myeloid, therapy-related acute lympho-blastic leukemias (t-ALL) occur, as noted above, albeit more rarely. Numerous case reports have described t-ALL, which universally involve translocations of the *MLL* gene at 11q23 *(39–41)*.

2.4. Clinical Experience

In a series of more than 300 consecutive t-MDS/t-AML patients assessed at The University of Chicago, 78% of patients had received alkylating agents, and 39% had received topoiso-merase II inhibitors prior to the development of their bone marrow malignancy (Fig. 2) *(42)*. Most patients (45%) had received both chemotherapy as well as radiation therapy, although 40% of patients had received only chemotherapy and 14% had undergone only radiation treatment. The overwhelming majority of patients (92%) had a clonal cytogenetic abnormality, with 70% of patients having abnormalities of chromosomes 5, 7, or both. Overall, 21% of patients had an abnormal chromosome 5, 28% had an abnormal chromosome 7, and 22% had abnormalities of both chromosomes 5 and 7. Of the 10% of patients with recurring balanced rearrange-ments, translocations involving 11q23 or 21q22 were each identified in 3% of patients, t(15;17) or inv(16) represented 2% each, and t(8;16) represented 0.3% of the therapy-related malignancies collected in this series. The overall survival in patients was poor, with a median survival of 8 months and 5-year survival of less than 10% (Fig. 3; *see* Color Plate 2, following p. 174).

3. GENETIC PATHWAYS IN t-MDS/t-AML

Extensive experimental evidence indicates that more than one mutation is required for the pathogenesis of hematological malignant diseases *(43,44)*. The expression of translocation-

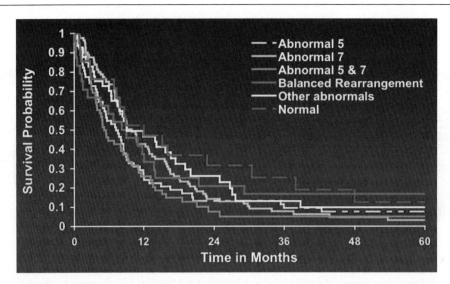

Fig. 3. (Color Plate 2, following p. 174) Survival from diagnosis of t-MDS/t-AML by recurring cytogenetic abnormalities. (From ref 42.)

specific fusion genes or deregulated expression of oncogenes is required, but not sufficient, to induce leukemia. Gilliland and colleagues have described a paradigm in AML involving the cooperation between constitutively-activated tyrosine kinases, such as FLT3, and transcription factor fusion proteins (44). In this model, an activated tyrosine kinase confers a proliferative and/or anti-apoptotic activity, whereas a fusion protein impairs normal differentiation pathways with a limited effect on cellular proliferation. An important aspect of leukemia biology, then, is the elucidation of the spectrum of chromosomal abnormalities and molecular mutations that cooperate in the pathways leading to the development of t-MDS/t-AML (Fig. 4; *see* Color Plate 3, following p. 174) (45).

There is growing evidence that a limited number of molecular pathways may be involved. For example, Christiansen et al. have described therapy-related diseases with a normal karyotype and increased frequency of internal tandem duplications of *FLT3* and *MLL* (46). −7/del(7q) has been associated with activating mutations of the RAS pathway (activating *KRAS1*, *NRAS*, or *PTPN11* mutations, or inactivating mutations of *NF1*), mutation of *RUNX1/ AML1*, as well as methylation silencing of the *CDKN2B* (*p15INK4B*) gene, which is an independent predictor of patient outcome (47–50). *TP53* (*p53*) mutations are uncommon in this subgroup. In contrast, t-MDS associated with −5/del(5q) is associated with *TP53* mutations and a complex karyotype (47,50–52).

Gene expression profiling of *de novo* MDS and t-MDS/t-AML has also provided support for the concept of distinct molecular and genetic subsets. Using expression profiling of CD34+ cells in t-MDS and t-AML, Qian et al. found that patients with a −5/del(5q) have a higher expression of genes involved in cell cycle control (*CCNA2, CCNE2, CDC2*), checkpoints (*BUB1*), or growth (*MYC*), and loss of expression of the gene encoding interferon consensus sequence binding protein (*ICSBP/IRF8*) (53). A second subgroup of t-AML, including patients with −7/del(7q), is characterized by downregulation of transcription factors involved in early hematopoiesis (TAL1, GATA1, and EKLF), and overexpression of proteins involved in signaling pathways in myeloid cells (FLT3) and cell survival (BCL2). Establishing the molecular pathways involved in t-MDS and t-AML may facilitate the identification of selectively expressed genes that can be exploited for the development of urgently needed targeted therapies.

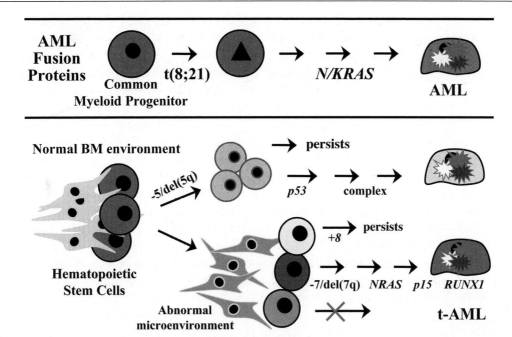

Fig. 4. (Color Plate 3, following p. 174) Models for the genetic pathways leading to t-MDS/t-AML. See text for a full discussion of alternative models. In the lower panel, the examples of the –5/del(5q) and –7/del(7q) are used to illustrate the models of t-MDS/t-AML arising in the setting of a normal bone marrow environment vs an abnormal bone marrow environment, respectively. It is possible that either abnormality can arise in both settings and that each model may occur.

Significant effort has gone into the elucidation of how the balanced translocations occur (reviewed in ref. *54*). Molecular mapping of the genomic breakpoints has revealed an association of the positions of the breakpoints with the location of topoisomerase II cleavage sites *(55–60)*. Recently, Libura et al. provided direct evidence that inhibition of topoisomerase II induces translocations within *MLL (61)*. Libura and colleagues identified rearrangements within the breakpoint cluster region of *MLL* in CD34+ cells exposed to etoposide. Most illegitimate recombination events present in primary CD34+ cells that proliferated for 2–3 days after treatment were translocations, whereas those identified after 10–14 days in culture were internal tandem duplications of the *MLL* gene, suggesting that these events are particularly stable in myeloid precursor cells. What has emerged from these studies is a model in which topoisomerase II-induced double strand breaks are repaired via crossover recombination and nonhomologous end joining of two different chromosomes, producing balanced chromosomal rearrangements. Topoisomerase II inhibitors are thought to interfere with DNA strand passage and religation, increasing the likelihood of producing the illegitimate recombination.

There are still a number of unanswered questions regarding the genetic and molecular pathways involved in the development of therapy-related diseases. For example, we do not yet know the full spectrum of genetic mutations within each pathway, nor do we know the order in which these mutations occur or the prognostic significance associated with various cooperating mutations. A variety of experimental evidence suggests that the recurring chromosomal abnormalities in t-MDS/t-AML are likely to be the initiating event. With respect to the recurring translocations, the rearrangement is likely to occur in a hematopoietic progenitor cell or, in some cases, in a committed myeloid progenitor cell. Leukemogenesis may entail a linear process in which the initiating mutation leads to a specific pattern of stepwise, additional mutations that complete malignant transformation. In t-MDS/t-AML following alkylating agent therapy, the process may vary somewhat in that the initiating mutations may occur in a hemato-poietic stem cell. In the setting of a normal bone marrow microenvironment, the initiating mutation may result in clonal expansion coupled with emerging genetic instability (or the selection of cooperating mutations that lead to instability) and the development of a clonal population. Selective pressures created both by the microenvironment as well as the initiating events could lead to the acquisition of additional mutations necessary to complete malignant transformation. Alternatively, t-MDS/t-AML may arise in the setting of an abnormal bone marrow microenvironment, resulting in the generation of multiple populations with varying initiating events. Some clonal populations may persist, whereas others may undergo cell death, and yet others may go on to acquire additional mutations necessary to complete malignant transformation. The latter model would account for the observation of unrelated cytogenetic clones in the bone marrow of t-MDS/t-AML patients as well as the observation of persistent dysplasia in some t-MDS/t-AML patients following therapy. Emerging technologies, such as the ability to culture stromal cell populations, and proteomics and genomics technologies may facilitate the evaluation of these various models.

4. EPIDEMIOLOGY

To date, the best characterized risk factor for the development of a therapy-related MDS or AML is the type and duration of prior therapy. As noted above, patients who have survived a previous malignancy by treatment with alkylating agents and/or with topoisomerase II inhibitors are at particular risk. Other patients who have undergone transplantation of a solid organ are at risk due to the intensity and duration of immunosuppression *(62)*. The genetic factors that place particular patients at risk for the development of t-MDS/t-AML probably play a critical role as well and are beginning to be elucidated.

Patients with t-MDS/t-AML have a disproportionately high frequency of mutation in NAD(P)H:quinone oxidoreductase (NQO1), a benzene-detoxifying enzyme *(63,64)*. NQO1 converts benzene-derived quinones into hydroquinones, which are less toxic. A point muta-tion, P187S, completely inactivates the enzyme. Larson et al. *(63)* examined nonmalignant lymphoblastoid cells from 56 patients with t-AML and found that 6 (11%) were homozygous and 23 (41%) were heterozygous for the mutant allele. These gene frequencies were higher than the expected numbers given the ethnic mix of the patients. In addition, of 45 patients with abnormalities of chromosomes 5 or 7 (including primary MDS and AML *de novo* patients), 16% were homozygous and 38% were heterozygous for the mutant *NQO1* allele, again both higher than expected. In Japanese individuals, the frequency of a homozygous loss of function mutation at codon 187 was 24% in t-MDS/t-AML patients (14/58) compared to only 16% in AML *de novo* cases and in 11% (16/150) of normal controls *(64)*. Individuals who are homozygous for the mutant allele would be expected to be particularly sensitive to the effects of benzene, since they would be unable to detoxify its byproducts. Patients hetero-zygous for the mutant *NQO1* allele might be represented at a frequency higher than expected if the normal allele undergoes mutation or gene silencing in the malignant clone, or if it is haploinsufficient, theories that have not yet been tested. Furthermore, Wiemels et al. demons-trated an increased incidence of *NQO1* loss of function alleles in pediatric ALL *de novo* cases with *MLL* gene rearrangements *(65)*. The authors of this study postulated that infants with less efficient NQO1 enzymes are predisposed to the development of ALL with *MLL* gene rearrangements through genotoxic exposure *in utero*.

Genetic polymorphisms within the promoter of the cytochrome P450 3A gene (*CYP3A*) have also been identified as a factor in the development of epipodophyllotoxin-associated leukemias, which are characterized by translocations involving the *MLL* gene at 11q23 *(66)*. CYP3A metabolizes the epipodophyllotoxins, generating catechol and quinone metabolites, which can damage DNA. A polymorphism (A/G) exists in the nifedipine-specific response element *(67)*, and Felix et al. found that the wild-type genotype, designated *CYP3A-W*, was significantly associated with the development of therapy-related leukemia *(66)*. The vast majority of patients who developed therapy-related disease had the wild-type genotype, *CYP3A-W* (29/30 = 97%), compared to 81% (80/99) of patients with *de novo* leukemia. Furthermore, 100% (22/22) of t-AML patients with *MLL* rearrangements had the *CYP3A-W* genotype compared to only 79% (33/42) of patients with *de novo* leukemias containing *MLL* rearrangements. Of note, this study did not examine a control population without cancer. In addition, it is not known whether the promoter variant has any functional consequence for the expression of the *CYP3A* gene, e.g., decreased production of CYP3A, leading to diminished intracellular drug oxidation and the production of fewer DNA-damaging intermediates. Nevertheless, this study suggests that patients with the wild-type *CYP3A* promoter may have an increased risk for the development of t-AML and that increased epipodophyllotoxin metabolism by CYP3A may be important in the etiology of t-AML. Notably, no such correlation between leukemia susceptibility and *CYP3A* genotype was seen within the Japanese population *(64)*.

5. THERAPY-RELATED LEUKEMIA AFTER PRIMARY CANCERS

As the survival after treatment for primary cancers has improved, more patients are at risk for the development of long-term complications, including the development of therapy-related bone marrow malignancies. Large numbers of patients who have been treated for specific diseases have been followed to assess the incidence and severity of therapy-related myeloid disorders.

5.1. Therapy-Related Leukemia After Treatment for Hodgkin's Disease

Survivors of Hodgkin's disease represent one of the largest groups studied for long-term complications, including the onset of t-MDS/t-AML *(7,12,13,68–82)*. The incidence of t-MDS/t-AML ranges from less than 1.5 to 10% and varies according to the number of patients studied, their ages, the types of therapies involved, and the length of follow-up. The development of t-MDS/t-AML is rare after treatment with radiation alone (0.4% at 15 years), unless the dose exceeds 2000 cGy *(79,80)* or if extended-field radiation therapy is combined with MOPP chemotherapy *(72,73,77,79)*.

5.2. Therapy-Related Leukemia After Treatment for Non-Hodgkin's Lymphoma (NHL)

Armitage et al. performed a large review of the literature to summarize the findings of many studies that examined the incidence of t-MDS and t-AML following treatment for NHL, including both chemotherapy and radiotherapy regimens, as well as autologous transplantation *(83)*. In this study, Armitage et al. estimated an overall incidence of t-AML of 10%

of NHL patients treated with chemotherapy, radiation therapy, and/or autologous transplantation within 10 years of their primary therapy *(83)*.

5.3. Therapy-Related Leukemia After Treatment for Multiple Myeloma

The Finnish Leukaemia Group observed 14 cases of t-AML in 432 patients treated with chemotherapy for multiple myeloma, giving an overall incidence of 9.8% at 9 years *(83)*. Although patients were followed for an average of 16 years after the administration of chemotherapy, no cases of t-AML were seen after 9 years.

5.4. Therapy-Related Leukemia After Treatment for Breast Cancer

The incidence of t-MDS/t-AML has been studied in survivors of breast cancer. Because breast cancer is a common malignancy and adjuvant chemo-radiotherapy is commonly used for early-stage disease, these women represent a large population at risk for long-term complications. The variance in the incidence rates for the development of t-MDS/t-AML in survivors of breast cancer may reflect the heterogeneity of the patients and their prior treatments.

The National Surgical Adjuvant Breast Project (NSABP) has followed more than 2000 women with a history of breast cancer who were treated with surgery, followed by adjuvant chemotherapy and/or radiotherapy who participated in a three-armed trial in which patients had received four monthly courses of doxorubicin and cyclophosphamide at higher-than-standard doses as well as granulocyte colony-stimualting factor (G-CSF) to decrease toxicity from neutropenia *(84)*. There was a cumulative incidence of 1.68 +/– 0.3% at 10 years for the development of t-MDS/t-AML in patients who received only chemotherapy as adjuvant treatment and an incidence of 1.39 +/– 0.5% at 10 years for patients treated with only regional radiation following surgery. Of five cases of t-AML studied by the NSABP, all had short latency periods, and two displayed 11q23 abnormalities. The rapid appearance of several cases of t-AML in this trial prompted a warning by the National Cancer Institute over concern that the use of growth factors may be synergistic with chemotherapy in inducing t-AML *(85)*. No data outside of this trial have been published to support this association.

Three cases of t-MDS and two cases of leukemia were identified in 2638 patients treated in six Eastern Cooperative Oncology Group (ECOG) clinical trials between 1978 and 1987, yielding an estimated incidence of therapy-related disease to be 26 per 100,000 person-years, not greater than the risk for the general population *(86)*. The first of these cases was t-ALL associated with human T-lymphotropic virus type 1 (HTLV-1), and the second was t-AML, which developed in a patient who had received additional cyclophosphamide for metastatic disease.

Among 13,734 women followed by the Surveillance, Epidemiology, and End Results (SEER) Program, 24 developed t-MDS/t-AML, giving a cumulative incidence of 0.7% at 10 years *(87)*. Carli et al. performed a retrospective analysis of patients registered with hematological malignancies and found that 7.7% (12/156) had a history of breast cancer *(88)*. Ten of these patients had received topoisomerase II inhibitors, and eight of them had received mitoxantrone. In a separate study, 10 cases (0.3%) of t-MDS/t-AML were observed among 3093 women who had been followed for at least 4 years, with a dose-dependent increase in disease incidence in those women who had received mitoxantrone at a dose of >13 mg/m^2 *(89)*. A similar incidence of 0.7% was obtained by Linassier et al. who followed 350 patients who had received mitoxantrone, fluorouracil, and cyclophosphamide, along with regional radiotherapy *(90)*. Within a small series of 24 patients treated with oral etoposide (50 mg or 100 mg per day for 5–7 days at 4-week intervals) for recurrent breast cancer, 3 cases (13%)

of t-MDS/t-AML were diagnosed *(91)*. These patients had been previously treated with anthracyclines, cyclophosphamide, or cisplatin as well as radiotherapy prior to receiving the oral etoposide therapy. No cases of t-MDS/t-AML were observed in 119 similar patients who had not received etoposide.

5.5. Therapy-Related Leukemia After Treatment for Ovarian Cancer

The widespread use of alkylating agents in the treatment of ovarian cancer has led to a careful examination of the incidence of t-MDS/t-AML in this patient population. Among 5455 patients, Reimer et al. observed 13 cases of t-MDS/t-AML (0.2%), all of whom had received alkylating agents, and 9 of whom had also received radiotherapy *(6)*. Among 998 women with ovarian cancer who had received alkylating agents, Greene et al. observed 12 cases of t-MDS/t-AML (1%), an excess risk of 5.8 cases per 1000 women per year *(8)*.

5.6. Therapy-Related Leukemia After Treatment for Germ Cell Tumors

In their original description, Pedersen-Bjergaard et al. observed 5 cases of t-MDS/t-AML out of 212 patients (2%) treated with etoposide, cisplatin, and bleomycin for germ cell tumors *(92)*. More recently, Schneider et al. followed 1132 patients with malignant germ cell tumors prospectively and found a cumulative incidence of 1% at 10 years for patients treated with chemotherapy alone (3/442) and a cumulative incidence of 4.2% for patients treated with chemo-radiotherapy (3/174) *(93)*. Five of these six patients had received epipodophyllotoxins at <2 g/m^2, and four of the patients had received ifosfamide at >20 g/m^2. The incidence of t-MDS/t-AML for survivors of testicular cancer has been estimated at 0.5% at 5 years for patients who have received etoposide at doses of ≤2 g/m^2, whereas the incidence increases to 2% for patients who have received etoposide at doses of >2 g/m^2 *(94)*.

5.7. Therapy-Related Leukemia After Treatment for Childhood Tumors

The incidence of t-AML developing in children who received chemotherapy for Ewing's sarcoma using topoisomerase II inhibitors, alkylating agents, and G-CSF has been estimated at 7.8% +/– 4.7% within 4 years *(95)*. The disease was preceded by a macrocytosis and decreased platelet counts. No cases of t-AML were found in the 32 evaluable patients who were treated on a less chemotherapy-intensive protocol. Unfortunately, in this study the number of patients was insufficient to demonstrate conclusively an association between the use of dose-intensified chemotherapy and the subsequent development of t-MDS/t-AML.

5.8. Therapy-Related Leukemia After Autologous Hematopoietic Stem Cell Transplantation

The use of high-dose, short-duration chemotherapy followed by reinfusion of cryopreserved autologous hematopoietic stem cells has become commonplace in the treatment of relapsed primary malignancies or for high-risk cancers in first remission. The use of autologous stem cell transplant (ASCT) has cured many patients who otherwise would have died from their primary disease, although it has also introduced an alarming rate of t-MDS among these survivors.

Pedersen-Bjergaard et al. reviewed the development of t-MDS/t-AML after the use of high-dose chemotherapy and ASCT *(96)*. Twenty-five percent of t-MDS patients developed their disease within 1 year after ASCT, and another 25% had evidence of t-MDS by 2 years. Ninety-four percent of t-MDS patients developed the disease by 5 years. Similarly, 30% of t-AML patients were diagnosed with leukemia within 1 year of ASCT, with another 30% developing t-AML by 2 years. All cases of t-AML occurred within 5 years after ASCT.

Various risk factors for the development of t-MDS/t-AML include patient age greater than 40 years with Hodgkin's disease *(97,98)* and greater than 35 years with NHL *(99)*, the amount of alkylating agent therapy received prior to ASCT *(12,100–104)*, and a history of radiation *(103)*, especially the use of total body irradiation during the transplant preparative regimen *(98,101)*. Several studies have suggested a higher risk of t-MDS/t-AML for patients who received chemotherapy-primed peripheral blood stem cells, rather than bone marrow-derived stem cells obtained without the use of mobilizing chemotherapy *(99,105)*. Whether this reflects chemotherapy damage to the stem cells in the former case or just different populations of stem cells is not yet clear.

In a study of 230 patients who received cyclophosphamide and total body irradiation followed by ASCT as consolidation therapy for NHL, 27 patients (12%) had developed t-MDS/t-AML (16 t-MDS, 10 t-MDS progressing to t-AML, and 1 t-AML) after a median follow-up of 6 years *(106)*. The median latency time to the development of therapy-related disease was 9 years after the lymphoma diagnosis (range 2.7–21.6 years) and 4.4 years after ASCT (range 11 months to 8.8 years). Karyotype abnormalities most commonly involved chromosomes 5, 7, 13, 18, and 20. The vast majority of these patients received bone marrow-derived stem cells, and only nine patients received peripheral blood progenitor cells. Prior fludarabine therapy and older age were associated with the development of t-MDS/t-AML. Lenz et al. examined 195 patients with a history of low-grade lymphoma who underwent multiagent induction chemotherapy followed by ASCT using myeloablative conditioning and identified five cases of therapy-related diseases, giving an incidence ratio of 3.8% *(107)*.

Twenty-two patients developed t-MDS/t-AML out of 612 patients with either Hodgkin's disease or NHL who underwent high-dose chemotherapy and ASCT using peripheral blood stem cells, giving a cumulative risk of 8.6% +/– 2.1% at 6 years *(108)*. Patients who received etoposide prior to stem cell collection had a 12.3-fold increased risk for developing t-AML with abnormalities of chromosome bands 11q23 or 21q22. The use of etoposide as a means of priming stem cell production and pretransplant radiation were both associated with the development of therapy-related disease in multivariate analysis.

Six cases of t-MDS/t-AML were observed in 649 patients who underwent ASCT at the University of Chicago, an incidence rate of 1% *(109)*. An additional case of t-ALL was also observed. The incidence of developing t-MDS/t-AML was 0.3% for breast cancer (1/354), 6.3% for Hodgkin's disease (5/79), and 1% for NHL (1/103). The median latency periods to develop t-MDS/t-AML after ASCT and after initial diagnosis of the primary disease, respectively, were 1.5 years and 5.5 years for both Hodgkin's and non-Hodgkin's lymphoma, and 2.8 years and 4.4 years for breast cancer. Because these therapy-related leukemias developed approx 4–6 years after primary treatment, i.e., within the same range as the latencies seen for t-AML in other nontransplant settings, it seems most likely that the initial chemotherapy given for the primary malignancy was the predisposing or mutagenic exposure rather than that used for the transplant procedure itself. Alternatively, one might speculate that oligoclonal hematopoiesis occurring during the process of marrow regeneration after ASCT increases the likelihood of the emergence of a neoplastic subclone.

Evidence supporting the hypothesis that the primary chemotherapy given to a patient induces bone marrow damage and predisposes to the development of t-MDS/t-AML comes from a FISH analysis of bone marrow cells obtained from patients with Hodgkin's disease or NHL prior to their ASCT *(110)*. In 9 of 12 cases (75%), the same cytogenetic abnormality ultimately found at the time of the t-MDS/t-AML diagnosis was detectable by FISH in the bone marrow biopsies that had been performed prior to the ASCT. Therefore, it is likely that significant stem cell damage and the initiation of leukemia occur with the initial treatment regimens for Hodgkin's disease and NHL, at least for some patients.

Efforts to identify patients at risk for the development of t-MDS/t-AML after ASCT have not yielded many options for screening or early detection. Legare et al. described one patient in whom a clonal cell population was identified in banked blood samples six months after ASCT and 1 year prior to the clinical recognition of t-AML by analyzing the clonality of the X-linked human androgen receptor (HUMARA) *(111,112)*. This methodology has not yet gained widespread applicability.

A prospective study by Martinez-Climent et al. analyzed the chromosomal abnormalities observed in bone marrow cells of 229 women with high-risk breast cancer who underwent six courses of FAC/FEC chemotherapy followed by high-dose chemotherapy and ASCT *(112)*. No cases of t-AML were identified up to 36 months after ASCT. Out of 60 women who had cytogenetic analysis performed on bone marrow samples 12–59 months after ASCT, three (5%) displayed transient, clonal abnormalities and two (3%) showed nonclonal reciprocal translocations. Thus, in this study, the presence of cytogenetic abnormalities in bone marrow cells was not universally predictive of the development of therapy-related disease. Notably, the incidence of t-AML in this series was less than that reported by other groups and may reflect differences in the specific chemotherapy regimens used.

6. THERAPY-RELATED LEUKEMIA AFTER LONG-TERM IMMUNOSUPPRESSION OR OTHER EXPOSURES

In the past, the description of AML arising in immunosuppressed patients who had received a prior solid organ transplant consisted of rare case reports *(113–115)*. Recently, however, Offman and colleagues have examined an extensive series of more than 170,000 solid organ transplant patients and have shown that they are at significantly increased risk for the development of t-MDS/t-AML *(62)*. Patients who had received heart and/or lung transplants were at the greatest risk, with a relative risk of 5.5 (95% CI 4.0–7.7; $p < 0.0001$). The frequency of therapy-related disease correlated dramatically with azathioprine dosage beginning at 1 year following transplant, when the immunosuppression dosage was relatively stable. Patients who had received kidney transplants were also at an increased risk, with a relative risk of 2.1 (95% CI 1.6–2.7; $p < 0.0001$), and there was a trend to an effect of immunosuppression dosage on t-MDS/t-AML development. The overall incidence of therapy-related disease increased at 4 years posttransplantation, although the authors were not able to comment on the cytogenetic pattern of these diseases. Interestingly, t-MDS/t-AML cells exhibited microsatellite instability in 7 of 7 cases examined, indicating defective DNA mismatch repair, a phenomenon observed with cellular resistance to thiopurines.

In the University of Chicago series, 6% (18/306) of patients who developed t-MDS/t-AML had been treated with chemotherapy and/or radiotherapy for a nonmalignant condition *(42)*, most commonly for a rheumatological disorder. New reports also describe an association between valproic acid, a histone deacetylase inhibitor and an agent that alters the properties of DNA, with the development of t-AML *(116)*. These leukemias have the same chromosomal abnormalities as those described for chemotherapy-associated disease, suggesting a similar pathophysiology.

Recently Uchida et al. have described three patients with a history of non-small-cell lung cancer, treated with chemotherapy with or without radiotherapy and gefitinib (Iressa[TM], AstraZeneca Pharmaceuticals LP), a small molecule inhibitor of the epidermal growth factor receptor, who developed t-APL 15–26 months after gefitinib therapy *(117)*. The authors raised concerns that the incidence of t-APL was much higher than in their clinical experience, and they suggested that gefitinib therapy might predispose to the development of the therapy-related bone marrow malignancy, possibly in combination with prior therapy. A much larger prospective study will help to determine the incidence of t-APL and other therapy-related diseases after gefitinib therapy for non-small-cell lung cancer. However, the concern remains that even molecularly targeted therapies could predispose to t-MDS/t-AML, further emphasizing that a broad spectrum of drugs predisposes to the condition. Thus, it may be that any chemical that alters DNA structure or the growth properties of cells can predispose to the development of myelodysplasia/leukemia.

7. TREATMENT

The treatment of patients with t-MDS/t-AML ranges from supportive care to aggressive chemotherapy and ASCT. The particular treatment plan for an individual patient rests on an assessment of the patient's desire for possible long-term remission/cure and the anticipated toxicities of treatment. A patient's age and performance status as well as the availability of a potential allogeneic donor play significant roles in assessing the suitability of a particular patient for allogeneic transplantation. The outcome of patients treated with chemotherapy and stem cell transplant is difficult to assess from the literature, because most studies have extremely small sample sizes or group patients with t-MDS/t-AML with patients with *de novo* MDS/AML and poor risk features, e.g., poor risk/complex cytogenetic abnormalities, AML arising out of a previous MDS (often called secondary AML), or primary refractory/relapsed AML. Thus, the true response rates of t-MDS/t-AML to any therapeutic intervention are difficult to determine *(118)*.

The survival of patients with t-MDS/t-AML is generally poor despite treatment. In the series of patients who had received autologous transplantation for NHL, 21 out of 27 patients (78%) died from t-MDS/t-AML or their associated treatment at an average of 10 months following diagnosis *(106)*. Of these 21 patients, 16 died without any evidence of their primary diagnosis, NHL. Treatment for most patients was supportive. Three patients, however, were treated with further transplantation: two with a second autologous transplant, and one with an allogeneic transplant. All three patients died from complications arising from the second transplant. Of the six patients living at the time of the paper's publication, two were receiving supportive care, three were treated with antilymphocyte globulin *(119)*, and one underwent nonmyeloablative allogeneic bone marrow transplantation.

7.1. Supportive Care

Most complications from t-MDS/t-AML are the result of the severe cytopenias that can develop. Supportive care covers a range of treatments, including the administration of broad-spectrum oral antibiotics to prevent febrile neutropenia, the administration of packed red blood cell and platelet transfusions when needed, and/or the administration of hematopoietic growth factors to augment patients' own production of blood cells. G-CSF or granulocyte-macrophage (GM)-CSF can be used to stimulate neutrophil production, and erythropoietin can be given to stimulate red blood cell production. Because therapy-related diseases are characterized by trilineage dysplasia, however, the blood cells produced in response to growth factors may not function normally. For example, even patients with normal peripheral platelet counts can have bleeding problems, which may seem paradoxical. Therefore, increasing patients' blood cell counts into the normal range may not completely protect them from infectious or bleeding complications if the cells function poorly.

7.2. Chemotherapy

As noted above, few studies have examined response rates in a large series of patients with t-MDS/t-AML exclusively. However, t-AML generally responds poorly to chemotherapy. Using a retrospective analysis of patients treated with cytarabine/daunorubicin induction chemotherapy, Hoyle et al. found that t-AML patients had a complete remission induction rate of 25%, whereas patients with AML arising from a prior myelodysplastic state or myeloproliferative disorder had remission rates of approx 40% *(120)*. Collectively, these patients had lower remission rates than patients with *de novo* disease, attributed to a higher degree of chemotherapy resistance.

A German multicenter group studied conventional dose combination chemotherapy (idarubicin 10 mg/m^2 on days 1–3, cytarabine 100 mg/m^2 by continuous intravenous infusion on days 1–7, and etoposide 100 mg/m^2 over 1 hour on days 3–7) in six patients with t-AML *(121)*. Four of the patients achieved remission. The survival data were not reported separately for the t-AML patients, but the overall survival for patients who had achieved initial remission was only 21 months.

Several groups have used idarubicin rather than daunorubicin and high-dose cytarabine to increase induction remission rates. Philpot et al. studied five t-AML patients treated with 5 days of idarubicin 5 mg/m^2 (daily, for a total of five doses), cytarabine 2 g/m^2 over 3 hours every 12 hours (for a total of 10 doses), and etoposide 100 mg/m^2 over 1 hour (daily, for a total of five doses), who all achieved remission, without any treatment-related deaths *(122)*. Mehta et al. used the same regimen in five other t-AML patients who all achieved at least initial remission *(123)*. Gardin et al. describe the use of intensive combination chemotherapy using idarubicin 12 mg/m^2 for 3 days along with Ara-C at 1 g/m^2 q12h for 5 days (intermediate-dose) for younger patients and at 100 mg/m^2 via continuous infusion for 7 days in older patients followed by G-CSF support in nine patients with t-AML *(124)*. Five of these patients obtained a complete response initially, and four had received the intermediate-dose Ara-C. However, only one of these patients survived longer than 1 year.

In a nationwide Japanese study of 256 patients with t-MDS/t-AML, the majority of patients (72%) received chemotherapy, either a standard combination of an anthracycline along with cytarabine or low-dose cytarabine, or ATRA in the case of seven patients with t-APL *(125)*. Four of these patients went on to receive an allogeneic stem cell transplant using HLA-identical siblings as donors. A complete response rate of 46% was observed, with a mean duration of 14.6 months. Two of the four transplanted patients maintained their complete response, as did four of the seven patients with t-APL.

7.3. Stem Cell Transplantation

7.3.1. Autologous Stem Cell Transplantation

For patients who do not have an appropriate allogeneic donor or for those who are not candidates for allogeneic transplant because of age, comorbid conditions, or preference, autologous transplant remains a treatment option. Autologous transplant is not considered to be a curative treatment option, however, because therapy-related malignancies are thought to be disorders arising in a bone marrow stem cell. Nonetheless, ASCT has been used as a way of delivering higher doses of chemotherapy to overcome the inherent drug resistance of therapy-related malignancies.

Carella et al. described the use of an idarubicin-containing chemotherapy regimen followed by G-CSF administration to mobilize peripheral stem cells from patients with therapy-related AML (126). Despite each patient having multiple cytogenetic abnormalities prior to chemotherapy, a collection of karyotypically normal peripheral stem cells was obtained for at least some of the patients.

De Witte and colleagues expanded on this approach by examining the effectiveness of ASCT in 21 patients with t-MDS/t-AML (127). The 2-year disease-free survival (DFS) rate after ASCT was 36% for patients with t-MDS/t-AML, compared to 40% for patients with MDS and 30% for patients with AML evolving from a pre-existing MDS. The DFS rates were significantly better for patients less than 40 years old ($p = 0.04$). These results were contrasted to those obtained for matched patients with de novo AML who underwent similar treatment and had a DFS rate of 51%. The relapse rate was 60% for those with therapy-related disease, compared with 40% for those with AML de novo ($p = 0.007$). Thus, although the results are not outstanding, more than one-third of patients with t-MDS/t-AML derive long-term benefit from ASCT.

7.3.2. ALLOGENEIC STEM CELL TRANSPLANTATION

The only potentially curative treatment modality for patients with t-MDS/t-AML is ASCT. Unfortunately, this option is open to few patients with therapy-related disease because of their older age, comorbid conditions, and the availability of a suitable donor. Matched unrelated or umbilical cord donors, available through national and international registries, have increased the donor pool and given more patients with therapy-related malignancies the chance to undergo this potentially life-saving procedure. However, the aggressive nature of therapy-related disease makes long-term remission difficult to achieve. Studies of the effectiveness of allogeneic transplantation suffer from the same issues noted above for studies of chemotherapy, namely, small sample sizes and grouping patients with therapy-related diseases with patients with de novo malignancies or with those AML arising from a myelodysplastic syndrome. In addition, conditioning regimens for allogeneic transplant have changed dramatically in recent years, making the relevance of older studies to current patients questionable. Thus, the effectiveness of ASCT for patients with t-MDS/t-AML is difficult to summarize.

Anderson et al. compared the outcomes of 46 patients (17 with t-AML) who were taken directly to allogeneic transplant vs 20 patients (12 with t-AML) with chemotherapy-sensitive disease who received some chemotherapy followed by allogeneic transplantation (128). There were no survival differences between the two groups. In this study, however, a minority of the patients examined had therapy-related malignancies. All of the other patients had acute leukemias that arose from myelodysplasia. A subgroup analysis of patients with therapy-related disease was not performed because of their small numbers, although there was a trend for therapy-related patients to have shorter disease-free survival and a higher relapse rate.

In an analysis of 31 t-MDS patients and 39 t-AML patients who underwent allogeneic transplantation from 1980 until 1998 in France, poor outcome was associated with age greater than 37 years, male sex, positive recipient cytomegalovirus serology, absence of complete remission at the time of transplantation, and the use of intensive chemotherapy prior to transplantation (129). A variety of stem cell sources and donor types was used: peripheral blood stem cells, 3 patients; bone marrow-derived stem cells, 66; unrelated umbilical cord blood-derived stem cells, 1; and HLA-identical sibling donors, 57; identical twin (syngeneic) donors, 2; HLA-matched unrelated, 5; HLA-mismatched related, 3; and HLA-mismatched unrelated, 3. The estimated 2-year survival rate was 30%, event-free survival rate was 28%, relapse rate was 42%, and transplant-related mortality was 49%. Thus, in patients who have chemotherapy-responsive disease, allogeneic peripheral stem cell transplantation is a viable option but can carry a high risk of treatment-associated morbidity.

Hale et al. obtained similar outcomes in 21 children who had received epipodophyllotoxin-containing regimens for ALL and subsequently developed t-AML *(130)*. Thirteen children received induction chemotherapy prior to allogeneic transplantation, and 7 underwent transplantation immediately after diagnosis. Eleven patients received bone marrow from HLA-identical siblings, whereas 8 received matched unrelated donor marrow and 2 received haploidentical marrow from family members. Three years after transplantation, 4 patients (19%) were alive, whereas 10 patients had succumbed to relapsed disease at a median of 5 months, and 7 patients died of transplant-related causes.

Cesaro et al. reported the use of donor lymphocyte infusion (DLI) in the treatment of one patient who developed t-AML after treatment for anaplastic large cell lymphoma and who relapsed 3 months after allogeneic transplantation *(131)*. The patient was treated successfully with oral etoposide followed by DLI and had 7 months of remission before dying of recurrent anaplastic large cell lymphoma.

8. CONCLUSIONS

Therapy-related myelodysplasia and AML remain one of the most bleak complications of successful therapy for a variety of malignant and nonmalignant conditions. As more agents are associated with this dreaded complication, it appears that virtually any drug or compound that affects cell division or growth can predispose to its development. The factors that place individual patients at risk are beginning to be elucidated and are critical for risk assessment, to allow individualized therapy directed at minimizing its development. Characterizing the pathways that lead to t-MDS/t-AML will lead to a greater understanding of molecular features of the disease and, ultimately, may lead to more targeted therapies for its treatment. In the meantime, chemotherapy and transplantation options must be optimized to help patients overcome the generally dismal prognosis of this disease.

REFERENCES

1. Vardiman JW, Harris NL, Brunning RD. The World Health Organization (WHO) classification of the myeloid neoplasms. Blood 2002;100:2292–2302.
2. Le Beau MM, Espinosa R, 3rd, Davis EM, Eisenbart JD, Larson RA, Green ED. Cytogenetic and molecular delineation of a region of chromosome 7 commonly deleted in malignant myeloid diseases. Blood 1996;88: 1930–1935.
3. Zhao N, Stoffel A, Wang PW, et al. Molecular delineation of the smallest commonly deleted region of chromosome 5 in malignant myeloid diseases to 1-1.5 Mb and preparation of a PAC-based physical map. Proc Natl Acad Sci USA 1997;94:6948–6953.
4. Curtis RE, Boice JD, Jr., Stovall M, et al. Risk of leukemia after chemotherapy and radiation treatment for breast cancer. N Engl J Med 1992;326:1745–1751.
5. Greene MH, Harris EL, Gershenson DM, et al. Melphalan may be a more potent leukemogen than cyclophosphamide. Ann Intern Med 1986;105:360–367.
6. Reimer RR, Hoover R, Fraumeni JF, Jr., Young RC. Acute leukemia after alkylating-agent therapy of ovarian cancer. N Engl J Med 1977;297:177–181.
7. Coltman CA, Jr., Dixon DO. Second malignancies complicating Hodgkin's disease: a Southwest Oncology Group 10-year followup. Cancer Treat Rep 1982;66:1023–1033.
8. Greene MH, Boice JD, Jr., Greer BE, Blessing JA, Dembo AJ. Acute nonlymphocytic leukemia after therapy with alkylating agents for ovarian cancer: a study of five randomized clinical trials. N Engl J Med 1982;307: 1416–1421.

9. Greene MH, Young RC, Merrill JM, DeVita VT. Evidence of a treatment dose response in acute nonlympho-cytic leukemias which occur after therapy of non-Hodgkin's lymphoma. Cancer Res 1983;43:1891–1898.

10. Greene MH, Boice JD, Jr., Strike TA. Carmustine as a cause of acute nonlymphocytic leukemia. N Engl J Med 1985;313:579.

11. Pedersen-Bjergaard J, Ersboll J, Sorensen HM, et al. Risk of acute nonlymphocytic leukemia and preleukemia in patients treated with cyclophosphamide for non-Hodgkin's lymphomas. Comparison with results obtained in patients treated for Hodgkin's disease and ovarian carcinoma with other alkylating agents. Ann Intern Med 1985;103:195–200.

12. Pedersen-Bjergaard J, Specht L, Larsen SO, et al. Risk of therapy-related leukaemia and preleukaemia after Hodgkin's disease. Relation to age, cumulative dose of alkylating agents, and time from chemotherapy. Lancet 1987;2:83–88.

13. van der Velden JW, van Putten WL, Guinee VF, et al. Subsequent development of acute non-lymphocytic leukemia in patients treated for Hodgkin's disease. Int J Cancer 1988;42:252–255.

14. Fairman J, Chumakov I, Chinault AC, Nowell PC, Nagarajan L. Physical mapping of the minimal region of loss in 5q- chromosome. Proc Natl Acad Sci USA 1995;92:7406–7410.

15. Jaju RJ, Boultwood J, Oliver FJ, et al. Molecular cytogenetic delineation of the critical deleted region in the 5q- syndrome. Genes Chromosomes Cancer 1998;22:251–256.

16. Horrigan SK, Arbieva ZH, Xie HY, et al. Delineation of a minimal interval and identification of 9 candidates for a tumor suppressor gene in malignant myeloid disorders on 5q31. Blood 2000;95:2372–2377.

17. Lai F, Godley LA, Joslin J, et al. Transcript map and comparative analysis of the 1.5-Mb commonly deleted segment of human 5q31 in malignant myeloid diseases with a del(5q). Genomics 2001;71:235–245.

18. Boultwood J, Lewis S, Wainscoat JS. The 5q-syndrome. Blood 1994;84:3253–3260.

19. Van den Berghe H, Michaux L. 5q-, twenty-five years later: a synopsis. Cancer Genet Cytogenet 1997; 94: 1–7.

20. Greenberg P, Cox C, LeBeau MM, et al. International scoring system for evaluating prognosis in myelodys-plastic syndromes. Blood 1997;89:2079–2088.

21. Boultwood J, Fidler C, Strickson AJ, et al. Narrowing and genomic annotation of the commonly deleted region of the 5q- syndrome. Blood 2002;99:4638–4641.

22. Kere J. Chromosome 7 long arm deletion breakpoints in preleukemia: mapping by pulsed field gel electro-phoresis. Nucleic Acids Res 1989;17:1511–1520.

23. Lewis S, Abrahamson G, Boultwood J, Fidler C, Potter A, Wainscoat JS. Molecular characterization of the 7q deletion in myeloid disorders. Br J Haematol 1996;93:75–80.

24. Fischer K, Frohling S, Scherer SW, et al. Molecular cytogenetic delineation of deletions and translocations involving chromosome band 7q22 in myeloid leukemias. Blood 1997;89:2036–2041.

25. Dohner K, Brown J, Hehmann U, et al. Molecular cytogenetic characterization of a critical region in bands 7q35-q36 commonly deleted in malignant myeloid disorders. Blood 1998;92:4031–4035.

26. Tosi S, Scherer SW, Giudici G, Czepulkowski B, Biondi A, Kearney L. Delineation of multiple deleted regions in 7q in myeloid disorders. Genes Chromosomes Cancer 1999;25:384–392.

27. Kratz CP, Emerling BM, Donovan S, et al. Candidate gene isolation and comparative analysis of a commonly deleted segment of 7q22 implicated in myeloid malignancies. Genomics 2001;77:171–180.

28. Pui CH, Raimondi SC, Behm FG, et al. Shifts in blast cell phenotype and karyotype at relapse of childhood lymphoblastic leukemia. Blood 1986;68:1306–1310.

29. Ratain MJ, Kaminer LS, Bitran JD, et al. Acute nonlymphocytic leukemia following etoposide and cisplatin combination chemotherapy for advanced non-small-cell carcinoma of the lung. Blood 1987;70:1412–1417.

30. Larson RA, Le Beau MM, Ratain MJ, Rowley JD. Balanced translocations involving chromosome bands 11q23 and 21q22 in therapy-related leukemia. Blood 1992;79:1892–1893.

31. Pedersen-Bjergaard J, Johansson B, Philip P. Translocation (3;21)(q26;q22) in therapy-related myelodysplasia following drugs targeting DNA-topoisomerase II combined with alkylating agents, and in myeloproliferative disorders undergoing spontaneous leukemic transformation. Cancer Genet Cytogenet 1994;76:50–55.

32. Rowley JD. Molecular genetics in acute leukemia. Leukemia 2000;14:513–517.

33. Bloomfield CD, Archer KJ, Mrozek K, et al. 11q23 balanced chromosome aberrations in treatment-related myelodysplastic syndromes and acute leukemia: report from an international workshop. Genes Chromosomes Cancer 2002;33:362–378.

34. Rowley JD, Olney HJ. International workshop on the relationship of prior therapy to balanced chromosome aberrations in therapy-related myelodysplastic syndromes and acute leukemia: overview report. Genes Chromo-somes Cancer 2002;33:331–345.

35. Rowley JD, Reshmi S, Sobulo O, et al. All patients with the T(11;16)(q23;p13.3) that involves MLL and CBP have treatment-related hematologic disorders. Blood 1997;90:535–541.

36. Slovak ML, Bedell V, Popplewell L, Arber DA, Schoch C, Slater R. 21q22 balanced chromosome aberrations in therapy-related hematopoietic disorders: report from an international workshop. Genes Chromosomes Cancer 2002;33:379–394.

37. Andersen MK, Larson RA, Mauritzson N, Schnittger S, Jhanwar SC, Pedersen-Bjergaard J. Balanced chromosome abnormalities inv(16) and t(15;17) in therapy-related myelodysplastic syndromes and acute leukemia: report from an international workshop. Genes Chromosomes Cancer 2002;33:395–400.

38. Block AW, Carroll AJ, Hagemeijer A, et al. Rare recurring balanced chromosome abnormalities in therapy-related myelodysplastic syndromes and acute leukemia: report from an international workshop. Genes Chromosomes Cancer 2002;33:401–412.

39. Secker-Walker LM, Stewart EL, Todd A. Acute lymphoblastic leukaemia with t(4;11) follows neuroblastoma: a late effect of treatment? Med Pediatr Oncol 1985;13:48–50.

40. Archimbaud E, Charrin C, Guyotat D, Magaud JP, Gentilhomme O, Fiere D. Acute leukaemia with t(4;11) in patients previously exposed to carcinogens. Br J Haematol 1988;69:467–470.

41. Jonveaux P, Hillion J, Bernard O, et al. Distinct MLL gene rearrangements associated with successive acute monocytic and lymphoblastic leukemias in the same patient. Leukemia 1994;8:2224–2227.

42. Smith SM, Le Beau MM, Huo D, et al. Clinical-cytogenetic associations in 306 patients with therapy-related myelodysplasia and myeloid leukemia: the University of Chicago series. Blood 2003;102:43–52.

43. Alcalay M, Orleth A, Sebastiani C, et al. Common themes in the pathogenesis of acute myeloid leukemia. Oncogene 2001;20:5680–5694.

44. Kelly L, Clark J, Gilliland DG. Comprehensive genotypic analysis of leukemia: clinical and therapeutic implications. Curr Opin Oncol 2002;14:10–18.

45. Pedersen-Bjergaard J, Andersen MK, Christiansen DH, Nerlov C. Genetic pathways in therapy-related myelodysplasia and acute myeloid leukemia. Blood 2002;99:1909–1912.

46. Christiansen DH, Pedersen-Bjergaard J. Internal tandem duplications of the FLT3 and MLL genes are mainly observed in atypical cases of therapy-related acute myeloid leukemia with a normal karyotype and are unrelated to type of previous therapy. Leukemia 2001;15:1848–1851.

47. Christiansen DH, Andersen MK, Pedersen-Bjergaard J. Methylation of p15INK4B is common, is associated with deletion of genes on chromosome arm 7q and predicts a poor prognosis in therapy-related myelodysplasia and acute myeloid leukemia. Leukemia 2003;17:1813–1819.

48. Christiansen DH, Andersen MK, Pedersen-Bjergaard J. Mutations of AML1 are common in therapy-related myelodysplasia following therapy with alkylating agents and are significantly associated with deletion or loss of chromosome arm 7q and with subsequent leukemic transformation. Blood 2004;104:1474–1481.

49. Loh ML, Vattikuti S, Schubbert S, et al. Mutations in PTPN11 implicate the SHP-2 phosphatase in leukemogenesis. Blood 2004;103:2325–2331.

50. Side LE, Curtiss NP, Teel K, et al. RAS, FLT3, and TP53 mutations in therapy-related myeloid malignancies with abnormalities of chromosomes 5 and 7. Genes Chromosomes Cancer 2004;39:217–223.

51. Andersen MK, Christiansen DH, Pedersen-Bjergaard J. Amplification or duplication of chromosome band 21q22 with multiple copies of the AML1 gene and mutation of the TP53 gene in therapy-related MDS and AML. Leukemia 2005;19:197–200.

52. Andersen MK, Christiansen DH, Pedersen-Bjergaard J. Centromeric breakage and highly rearranged chromosome derivatives associated with mutations of TP53 are common in therapy-related MDS and AML after therapy with alkylating agents: an M-FISH study. Genes Chromosomes Cancer 2005;42:358–371.

53. Qian Z, Fernald AA, Godley LA, Larson RA, Le Beau MM. Expression profiling of CD34+ hematopoietic stem/ progenitor cells reveals distinct subtypes of therapy-related acute myeloid leukemia. Proc Natl Acad Sci USA 2002;99:14,925–14,930.

54. Pedersen-Bjergaard J. Insights into leukemogenesis from therapy-related leukemia. N Engl J Med 2005; 352:1591–1594.

55. Felix CA, Lange BJ, Hosler MR, Fertala J, Bjornsti MA. Chromosome band 11q23 translocation breakpoints are DNA topoisomerase II cleavage sites. Cancer Res 1995;55:4287–4292.

56. Stanulla M, Wang J, Chervinsky DS, Thandla S, Aplan PD. DNA cleavage within the MLL breakpoint cluster region is a specific event which occurs as part of higher-order chromatin fragmentation during the initial stages of apoptosis. Mol Cell Biol 1997;17:4070–4079.

57. Strissel PL, Strick R, Rowley JD, Zeleznik-Le NJ. An in vivo topoisomerase II cleavage site and a DNase I hypersensitive site colocalize near exon 9 in the MLL breakpoint cluster region. Blood 1998;92:3793–3803.

58. Zhang Y, Strissel P, Strick R, et al. Genomic DNA breakpoints in AML1/RUNX1 and ETO cluster with topoisomerase II DNA cleavage and DNase I hypersensitive sites in t(8;21) leukemia. Proc Natl Acad Sci USA 2002;99:3070–3075.

59. Ahuja HG, Felix CA, Aplan PD. Potential role for DNA topoisomerase II poisons in the generation of t(11;20)(p15;q11) translocations. Genes Chromosomes Cancer 2000;29:96–105.

60. Mistry AR, Felix CA, Whitmarsh RJ, et al. DNA topoisomerase II in therapy-related acute promyelocytic leukemia. N Engl J Med 2005;352:1529–1538.

61. Libura J, Slater DJ, Felix CA, Richardson C. Therapy-related acute myeloid leukemia-like MLL rearrangements are induced by etoposide in primary human CD34+ cells and remain stable after clonal expansion. Blood 2005;105:2124–2131.

62. Offman J, Opelz G, Doehler B, et al. Defective DNA mismatch repair in acute myeloid leukemia/myelodysplastic syndrome after organ transplantation. Blood 2004;104:822–828.

63. Larson RA, Wang Y, Banerjee M, et al. Prevalence of the inactivating 609C-->T polymorphism in the NAD(P)H:quinone oxidoreductase (NQO1) gene in patients with primary and therapy-related myeloid leukemia. Blood 1999;94:803–807.

64. Naoe T, Takeyama K, Yokozawa T, et al. Analysis of genetic polymorphism in NQO1, GST-M1, GST-T1, and CYP3A4 in 469 Japanese patients with therapy-related leukemia/ myelodysplastic syndrome and de novo acute myeloid leukemia. Clin Cancer Res 2000;6:4091–4095.

65. Wiemels JL, Pagnamenta A, Taylor GM, Eden OB, Alexander FE, Greaves MF. A lack of a functional NAD(P)H:quinone oxidoreductase allele is selectively associated with pediatric leukemias that have MLL fusions. United Kingdom Childhood Cancer Study Investigators. Cancer Res 1999;59:4095–4099.

66. Felix CA, Walker AH, Lange BJ, et al. Association of CYP3A4 genotype with treatment-related leukemia. Proc Natl Acad Sci USA 1998;95:13,176–13,181.

67. Rebbeck TR, Jaffe JM, Walker AH, Wein AJ, Malkowicz SB. Modification of clinical presentation of prostate tumors by a novel genetic variant in CYP3A4. J Natl Cancer Inst 1998;90:1225–1229.

68. Glicksman AS, Pajak TF, Gottlieb A, Nissen N, Stutzman L, Cooper MR. Second malignant neoplasms in patients successfully treated for Hodgkin's disease: a Cancer and Leukemia Group B study. Cancer Treat Rep 1982;66:1035–1044.

69. Pedersen-Bjergaard J, Larsen SO. Incidence of acute nonlymphocytic leukemia, preleukemia, and acute myeloproliferative syndrome up to 10 years after treatment of Hodgkin's disease. N Engl J Med 1982; 307:965–971.

70. Boivin JF, Hutchison GB, Lyden M, Godbold J, Chorosh J, Schottenfeld D. Second primary cancers following treatment of Hodgkin's disease. J Natl Cancer Inst 1984;72:233–241.

71. Meadows AT, Baum E, Fossati-Bellani F, et al. Second malignant neoplasms in children: an update from the Late Effects Study Group. J Clin Oncol 1985;3:532–538.

72. Valagussa P, Santoro A, Fossati-Bellani F, Banfi A, Bonadonna G. Second acute leukemia and other malignancies following treatment for Hodgkin's disease. J Clin Oncol 1986;4:830–837.

73. Blayney DW, Longo DL, Young RC, et al. Decreasing risk of leukemia with prolonged follow-up after chemotherapy and radiotherapy for Hodgkin's disease. N Engl J Med 1987;316:710–714.

74. Brusamolino E, Papa G, Valagussa P, et al. Treatment-related leukemia in Hodgkin's disease: a multi-institution study on 75 cases. Hematol Oncol 1987;5:83–98.

75. Tucker MA, Coleman CN, Cox RS, Varghese A, Rosenberg SA. Risk of second cancers after treatment for Hodgkin's disease. N Engl J Med 1988;318:76–81.

76. Meadows AT, Obringer AC, Marrero O, et al. Second malignant neoplasms following childhood Hodgkin's disease: treatment and splenectomy as risk factors. Med Pediatr Oncol 1989;17:477–484.

77. Andrieu JM, Ifrah N, Payen C, Fermanian J, Coscas Y, Flandrin G. Increased risk of secondary acute nonlymphocytic leukemia after extended-field radiation therapy combined with MOPP chemotherapy for Hodgkin's disease. J Clin Oncol 1990;8:1148–1154.

78. Devereux S, Selassie TG, Vaughan Hudson G, Vaughan Hudson B, Linch DC. Leukaemia complicating treatment for Hodgkin's disease: the experience of the British National Lymphoma Investigation. Bmj 1990; 301:1077–1080.

79. Henry-Amar M, Aeppli DM, Anderson J, et al. Chapter Workshop statistical report. Part IX: Study of second cancer risk. In: Somers, R., Henry-Amar, M., Meerwaldt, J.H., Carde, P., ed. Treatment strategy in Hodgkin's disease. Colloque Inserm., ed. Somers, R., Henry-Amar, M., Meerwaldt, J.H., Carde, P. Treatment strategy in Hodgkin's disease. Colloque Inserm. 1990;355.

80. Kaldor JM, Day NE, Clarke EA, et al. Leukemia following Hodgkin's disease. N Engl J Med 1990; 322:7–13.
81. Henry-Amar M, Dietrich PY. Acute leukemia after the treatment of Hodgkin's disease. Hematol Oncol Clin North Am 1993;7:369–387.
82. Kaldor JM, Day NE, Band P, et al. Second malignancies following testicular cancer, ovarian cancer and Hodgkin's disease: an international collaborative study among cancer registries. Int J Cancer 1987;39: 571–585.
83. Armitage JO, Carbone PP, Connors JM, Levine A, Bennett JM, Kroll S. Treatment-related myelodysplasia and acute leukemia in non-Hodgkin's lymphoma patients. J Clin Oncol 2003;21:897–906.
84. Fisher B, Rockette H, Fisher ER, Wickerham DL, Redmond C, Brown A. Leukemia in breast cancer patients following adjuvant chemotherapy or postoperative radiation: the NSABP experience. J Clin Oncol 1985;3:1640–1658.
85. Abrams J, Smith M. Acute myeloid leukemia following doxorubicin and cyclophosphamide: increased risk for dose-intensive regimens? Physicians Data Query 1994.
86. Tallman MS, Gray R, Bennett JM, et al. Leukemogenic potential of adjuvant chemotherapy for early-stage breast cancer: the Eastern Cooperative Oncology Group experience. J Clin Oncol 1995;13:1557–1563.
87. Curtis RE, Boice JD, Jr., Moloney WC, Ries LG, Flannery JT. Leukemia following chemotherapy for breast cancer. Cancer Res 1990;50:2741–2746.
88. Carli PM, Sgro C, Parchin-Geneste N, et al. Increase therapy-related leukemia secondary to breast cancer. Leukemia 2000;14:1014–1017.
89. Chaplain G, Milan C, Sgro C, Carli PM, Bonithon-Kopp C. Increased risk of acute leukemia after adjuvant chemotherapy for breast cancer: a population-based study. J Clin Oncol 2000;18:2836–2842.
90. Linassier C, Barin C, Calais G, et al. Early secondary acute myelogenous leukemia in breast cancer patients after treatment with mitoxantrone, cyclophosphamide, fluorouracil and radiation therapy. Ann Oncol 2000; 11:1289–1294.
91. Yagita M, Ieki Y, Onishi R, et al. Therapy-related leukemia and myelodysplasia following oral administration of etoposide for recurrent breast cancer. Int J Oncol 1998;13:91–96.
92. Pedersen-Bjergaard J, Daugaard G, Hansen SW, Philip P, Larsen SO, Rorth M. Increased risk of myelodysplasia and leukaemia after etoposide, cisplatin, and bleomycin for germ-cell tumours. Lancet 1991;338: 359–363.
93. Schneider DT, Hilgenfeld E, Schwabe D, et al. Acute myelogenous leukemia after treatment for malignant germ cell tumors in children. J Clin Oncol 1999;17:3226–3233.
94. Kollmannsberger C, Kuzcyk M, Mayer F, Hartmann JT, Kanz L, Bokemeyer C. Late toxicity following curative treatment of testicular cancer. Semin Surg Oncol 1999;17:275–281.
95. Rodriguez-Galindo C, Poquette CA, Marina NM, et al. Hematologic abnormalities and acute myeloid leukemia in children and adolescents administered intensified chemotherapy for the Ewing sarcoma family of tumors. J Pediatr Hematol Oncol 2000;22:321–329.
96. Pedersen-Bjergaard J, Andersen MK, Christiansen DH. Therapy-related acute myeloid leukemia and myelodysplasia after high-dose chemotherapy and autologous stem cell transplantation. Blood 2000;95:3273–3279.
97. Andre M, Henry-Amar M, Blaise D, et al. Treatment-related deaths and second cancer risk after autologous stem-cell transplantation for Hodgkin's disease. Blood 1998;92:1933–1940.
98. Darrington DL, Vose JM, Anderson JR, et al. Incidence and characterization of secondary myelodysplastic syndrome and acute myelogenous leukemia following high-dose chemoradiotherapy and autologous stem-cell transplantation for lymphoid malignancies. J Clin Oncol 1994;12:2527–2534.
99. Bhatia S, Ramsay NK, Steinbuch M, et al. Malignant neoplasms following bone marrow transplantation. Blood 1996;87:3633–3639.
100. Harrison CN, Gregory W, Hudson GV, et al. High-dose BEAM chemotherapy with autologous haemopoietic stem cell transplantation for Hodgkin's disease is unlikely to be associated with a major increased risk of secondary MDS/AML. Br J Cancer 1999;81:476–483.
101. Stone RM, Neuberg D, Soiffer R, et al. Myelodysplastic syndrome as a late complication following autologous bone marrow transplantation for non-Hodgkin's lymphoma. J Clin Oncol 1994;12:2535–2542.
102. Govindarajan R, Jagannath S, Flick JT, et al. Preceding standard therapy is the likely cause of MDS after autotransplants for multiple myeloma. Br J Haematol 1996;95:349–353.
103. Milligan DW, Ruiz De Elvira MC, Kolb HJ, et al. Secondary leukaemia and myelodysplasia after autografting for lymphoma: results from the EBMT. EBMT Lymphoma and Late Effects Working Parties. European Group for Blood and Marrow Transplantation. Br J Haematol 1999;106:1020–1026.

104. Pedersen-Bjergaard J, Pedersen M, Myhre J, Geisler C. High risk of therapy-related leukemia after BEAM chemotherapy and autologous stem cell transplantation for previously treated lymphomas is mainly related to primary chemotherapy and not to the BEAM-transplantation procedure. Leukemia 1997;11:1654–1660.

105. Miller JS, Arthur DC, Litz CE, Neglia JP, Miller WJ, Weisdorf DJ. Myelodysplastic syndrome after autologous bone marrow transplantation: an additional late complication of curative cancer therapy. Blood 1994;83:3780–3786.

106. Micallef IN, Lillington DM, Apostolidis J, et al. Therapy-related myelodysplasia and secondary acute myelogenous leukemia after high-dose therapy with autologous hematopoietic progenitor-cell support for lymphoid malignancies. J Clin Oncol 2000;18:947–955.

107. Lenz G, Dreyling M, Schiegnitz E, et al. Moderate increase of secondary hematologic malignancies after myeloablative radiochemotherapy and autologous stem-cell transplantation in patients with indolent lymphoma: results of a prospective randomized trial of the German Low Grade Lymphoma Study Group. J Clin Oncol 2004;22:4926–4933.

108. Krishnan A, Bhatia S, Slovak ML, et al. Predictors of therapy-related leukemia and myelodysplasia following autologous transplantation for lymphoma: an assessment of risk factors. Blood 2000;95:1588–1593.

109. Sobecks RM, Le Beau MM, Anastasi J, Williams SF. Myelodysplasia and acute leukemia following high-dose chemotherapy and autologous bone marrow or peripheral blood stem cell transplantation. Bone Marrow Transplant 1999;23:1161–1165.

110. Abruzzese E, Radford JE, Miller JS, et al. Detection of abnormal pretransplant clones in progenitor cells of patients who developed myelodysplasia after autologous transplantation. Blood 1999;94:1814–1819.

111. Legare RD, Gribben JG, Maragh M, et al. Prediction of therapy-related acute myelogenous leukemia (AML) and myelodysplastic syndrome (MDS) after autologous bone marrow transplant (ABMT) for lymphoma. Am J Hematol 1997;56:45–51.

112. Martinez-Climent JA, Comes AM, Vizcarra E, et al. Chromosomal abnormalities in women with breast cancer after autologous stem cell transplantation are infrequent and may not predict development of therapy-related leukemia or myelodysplastic syndrome. Bone Marrow Transplant 2000;25:1203–1208.

113. Doti CA, Gondolesi GE, Sheiner PA, Emre S, Miller CM, Aledort LM. Leukemia after liver transplant. Transplantation 2001;72:1643–1646.

114. Dixit MP, Farias KB, McQuade M, Scott KM. Acute myelo-monocytic infiltrate of the lower esophagus in a 4-year-old renal transplant recipient. Am J Kidney Dis 2003;41:E16.

115. Camos M, Esteve J, Rimola A, et al. Increased incidence of acute myeloid leukemia after liver transplantation? Description of three new cases and review of the literature. Transplantation 2004;77:311–313.

116. Coyle TE, Bair AK, Stein C, Vajpayee N, Mehdi S, Wright J. Acute leukemia associated with valproic acid treatment: a novel mechanism for leukemogenesis? Am J Hematol 2005;78:256–260.

117. Uchida A, Matsuo K, Tanimoto M. APL during gefitinib treatment for non-small-cell lung cancer. N Engl J Med 2005;352:843.

118. Rund D, Ben-Yehuda D. Therapy-related leukemia and myelodysplasia: evolving concepts of pathogenesis and treatment. Hematology 2004;9:179–187.

119. Molldrem JJ, Caples M, Mavroudis D, Plante M, Young NS, Barrett AJ. Antithymocyte globulin for patients with myelodysplastic syndrome. Br J Haematol 1997;99:699–705.

120. Hoyle CF, de Bastos M, Wheatley K, et al. AML associated with previous cytotoxic therapy, MDS or myeloproliferative disorders: results from the MRC's 9th AML trial. Br J Haematol 1989;72:45–53.

121. Ganser A, Heil G, Seipelt G, et al. Intensive chemotherapy with idarubicin, ara-C, etoposide, and m-AMSA followed by immunotherapy with interleukin-2 for myelodysplastic syndromes and high-risk Acute Myeloid Leukemia (AML). Ann Hematol 2000;79:30–35.

122. Philpott N, Mehta J, Treleaven J, Powles R. Idarubicin, high-dose cytarabine and etoposide for remission induction in therapy-related acute myeloid leukemia. Leuk Lymphoma 1994;15:127–130.

123. Mehta J, Powles R, Singhal S, et al. Idarubicin, high-dose cytarabine, and etoposide for induction of remission in acute leukemia. Semin Hematol 1996;33:18–23.

124. Gardin C, Chaibi P, de Revel T, et al. Intensive chemotherapy with idarubicin, cytosine arabinoside, and granulocyte colony-stimulating factor (G-CSF) in patients with secondary and therapy-related acute myelogenous leukemia. Club de Reflexion en Hematologie. Leukemia 1997;11:16–21.

125. Takeyama K, Seto M, Uike N, et al. Therapy-related leukemia and myelodysplastic syndrome: a large-scale Japanese study of clinical and cytogenetic features as well as prognostic factors. Int J Hematol 2000; 71: 144–152.

126. Carella AM, Dejana A, Lerma E, et al. In vivo mobilization of karyotypically normal peripheral blood progenitor cells in high-risk MDS, secondary or therapy-related acute myelogenous leukaemia. Br J Haematol 1996;95:127–130.
127. De Witte T, Van Biezen A, Hermans J, et al. Autologous bone marrow transplantation for patients with myelodysplastic syndrome (MDS) or acute myeloid leukemia following MDS. Chronic and Acute Leukemia Working Parties of the European Group for Blood and Marrow Transplantation. Blood 1997;90:3853–3857.
128. Anderson JE, Gooley TA, Schoch G, et al. Stem cell transplantation for secondary acute myeloid leukemia: evaluation of transplantation as initial therapy or following induction chemotherapy. Blood 1997; 89:2578–2585.
129. Yakoub-Agha I, de La Salmoniere P, Ribaud P, et al. Allogeneic bone marrow transplantation for therapy-related myelodysplastic syndrome and acute myeloid leukemia: a long-term study of 70 patients-report of the French society of bone marrow transplantation. J Clin Oncol 2000;18:963–971.
130. Hale GA, Heslop HE, Bowman LC, et al. Bone marrow transplantation for therapy-induced acute myeloid leukemia in children with previous lymphoid malignancies. Bone Marrow Transplant 1999;24:735–739.
131. Cesaro S, Messina C, Rosolen A, et al. Successful treatment of secondary acute myeloid leukemia relapsing after allogeneic bone marrow transplantation with donor lymphocyte infusion failed to prevent recurrence of primary disease: a case report. Bone Marrow Transplant 1999;23:625–628.

5 The DNA Damage Response, DNA Repair, and AML

David P. Steensma

CONTENTS

Summary

Acute myeloid leukemia (AML)—especially when the condition arises out of a pre-existing melodysplastic syndrome or follows prior therapy with alkylating agents or ionizing radiation—is frequently associated with complex bone marrow karyotypes, including multiple numeric chromosomal abnormalities, diminutive marker chromosomes of uncertain derivation, and interstitial gains and losses of genetic material. In addition, a variety of inherited syndromes with DNA repair defects convey a high risk of myelodysplasia and leukemia. Together, these pieces of evidence suggest that a fundamental defect in the DNA damage recognition and response pathways is an important component of leukemogenesis. Here, the basic DNA damage recognition and repair pathways are reviewed and data on known DNA repair abnormalities in acute leukemia and myelodysplastic syndrome are summarized. In addition, inherited syndromes with a DNA repair defect that predisposes to leukemia are outlined, including Fanconi anemia, Bloom syndrome, ataxia-telangiectasia and ataxia-telangiectasia-like disorder, Nijmegen breakage syndrome, Seckel syndrome, and others.

Key Words: DNA repair; DNA damage recognition; base excision repair; nucleotide excision repair; homologous recombination; nonhomologous end joining; Fanconi anemia; Bloom syndrome; RecQ helicases; inherited syndromes; ataxia-telangiectasia; Nijmegen breakage syndrom; Seckel syndrome; nibrin.

1. INTRODUCTION

Diverse lines of evidence suggest that fundamental alterations in DNA surveillance and repair pathways contribute to leukemogenesis. First, several genetic syndromes that involve DNA repair defects are associated with an increased risk of acute myeloid leukemia (AML)

From: *Contemporary Hematology: Acute Myelogenous Leukemia*
Edited by: J. E. Karp © Humana Press Inc., Totowa, NJ

and/or acute lymphocytic leukemia (ALL). Second, exposure to DNA-damaging agents (carcinogens and chemotherapeutics) enhances the risk of AML. Finally, a subset of AML cases, especially those that arise in the setting of exposure to DNA-damaging agents, such as carcinogenic chemoradiotherapy, exhibits complex clonal karyotypic abnormalities that might indicate DNA damage that was not successfully repaired before the initiating leukemic stem cell divided. To provide a context for understanding these observations, the present chapter reviews the role of DNA repair in maintaining genomic integrity, summarizes current understanding of the biochemical processes that sense and repair DNA damage, and then describes familial syndromes in which diminished DNA repair is associated with an increased risk of AML.

Some investigators consider polymorphisms in enzymes responsible for the breakdown of potentially mutagenic and carcinogenic chemicals that have the potential to harm DNA (e.g., *CYP3A4* [cytochrome P450, family 3, subfamily A, polypeptide 4] or glutathione-S-transferase genotypes) to be germane to the topic of DNA repair. This important issue may indeed be relevant to myeloid neoplasia *(1–4)*, but will not be dealt with further here because of space limitations. In addition, protection of the cell from DNA injury can occur after transcription: DNA mutations that introduce a premature stop codon 5' to the final exon of a gene are frequently detected by cells at the mRNA level by RNA surveillance mechanisms *(5)*. Such transcripts are rapidly eliminated from the cytoplasm by nonsense-mediated decay, reducing the likelihood that cells will inadvertently manufacture a pathogenic truncated polypeptide *(6)*. However, a more detailed discussion of RNA surveillance and "RNA-repair" by mechanisms such as alternative splicing *(7,8)* is also beyond the scope of this review.

2. THE DNA DAMAGE RESPONSE, DNA REPAIR, AND GENOMIC INTEGRITY

Many times each day, cells encounter radiation, environmental chemicals, and internal metabolic mishaps that could alter the structure and sequence of the DNA double helix (Figs. 1 and 2; *see* Color Plates 4 and 5, following p. 174). Without rapid and accurate processes to correct these lesions as soon as they occur, DNA mutations would quickly accumulate, causing impairment of cellular function, neoplastic transformation, or cell death *(9,10)*. The set of processes by which cells monitor themselves for DNA alterations and attempt to restore the wild-type sequence are collectively known as the "DNA damage response" and "DNA repair" pathways *(11)*.

2.1. Mutator Phenotype and Familial Cancer Syndromes

The seriousness with which all cells take the task of genome preservation is demonstrated by both the high degree of evolutionary conservation of the basic DNA surveillance and repair machinery, as well as the complexity and redundancy of the proteins needed to accomplish this mission *(12)*. Studies of simple organisms (especially *Escherichia coli* and *Saccharomyces cerevisiae*) bearing a replication-infidelity "mutator" phenotype led to the identification of dozens of factors important for maintaining basic genomic integrity *(13)*. Almost all of these genes were subsequently found to have human homologs. More than 150 human DNA repair proteins have now been identified; and several additional polypeptides of unknown function localize to damaged DNA, suggesting that there may be other factors yet to be described *(12,14)*.

In addition to in vitro analyses, broad insights into the connections between DNA repair and neoplasia have come from bedside-to-bench studies of families with inherited cancer

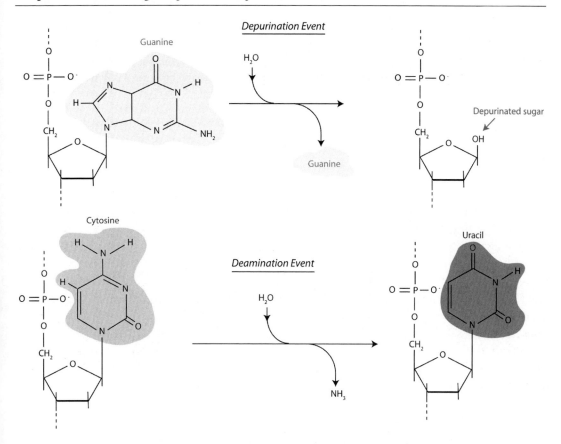

Fig. 1. (Color Plate 4, following p. 174) Common nucleotide anomalies resulting from endogenous cellular metabolism. Depuration **(top)** and deamination **(bottom)** represent two of the most common types of DNA metabolic injuries that take place in the cell. Thousands of adenine or guanines are lost every day from each nucleated human cell by spontaneous hydrolysis of the base–sugar link **(top)**. These result in failure of transcription resulting from stalling of the RNA–polymerase complex. Likewise, more then 100 cytosines are spontaneously deaminated to uracil each day in each nucleated human cell **(bottom)**. Unlike cytosine, uracil preferentially base pairs with adenine, resulting in replication abnormalities. Other depuration events (e.g., adenine) and deamination events (e.g., adenine to hypoxanthine, guanine to xanthine, and 5-methylcytosine to thymine) also occur; the latter is thought to be responsible for the paucity of CpG dinucleotides throughout the eukaryotic genome.

syndromes. Members of these families develop malignancies at a higher rate—and often at a younger age—than the general population *(15)*. These pedigrees often include individuals with characteristic developmental abnormalities, immunodeficiency, or other anomalies in addition to the predisposition to cancer. The repertoire of tumor types in such kindreds often includes acute leukemia, as discussed in greater detail below *(16)*.

While many cancer-prone families have germline mutations in classical oncogenes or tumor suppressors that apparently lack a direct effect on DNA stability (e.g., cell proliferation enhancers or apoptosis inhibitors *[17]*), a subset of cancer-prone kindreds bear mutations in genes directly involved in the DNA damage response and repair pathways, including DNA damage-dependent cell-cycle checkpoint control *(18)*. It is not yet clear why mutations in DNA repair factors are associated with very specific tumor types (e.g., colorectal cancer or

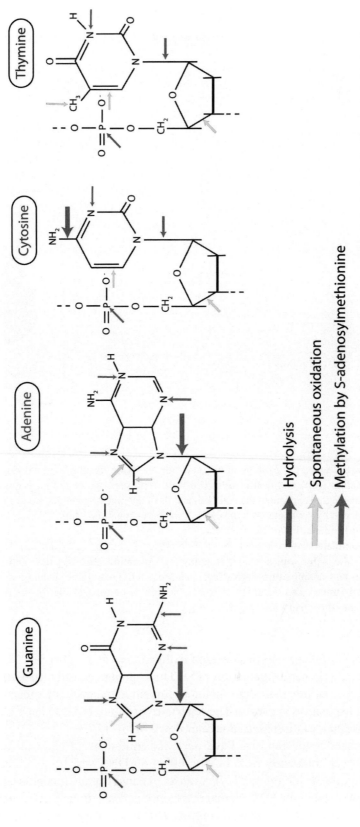

Fig. 2. (Color Plate 5, following p. 174) Chemical loci for endogenous DNA damage. These modifications include hydrolysis (red arrows), oxidative damage (green), and aberrant methylation by S-adenosylmethionine (blue). Arrow thickness gives some measure of the relative frequency of the specific event. (Adapted from refs. 78, 282.)

100

leukemia) but not other kinds of cancers, for most of these genes are ubiquitously expressed. One possibility is that the use of specific repair pathways may be greater in certain cell types. Lymphoid leukemia, for example, may be particularly common in syndromes with defects in repair of DNA double-strand (ds) breaks because of the importance of intact DNA ds break repair mechanisms for normal immunoglobulin V(D)J rearrangement *(19,20)*. The occurrence of myeloid leukemia in the same pedigrees might simply reflect the vast numbers of cell divisions required to sustain lifelong hematopoiesis, but experimental validation of this hypothesis is lacking. Likewise, it is not understood why some familial syndromes with DNA repair defects (e.g., Cockayne syndrome) have clinical findings that are limited to developmental abnormalities and do not generally develop cancer, whereas other families with mutations in other polypeptides in the same pathways (e.g., xeroderma pigmentosum) have a clear-cut neoplasia predisposition *(21)*. Predisposition to cancer of some type would seem a logical consequence of any DNA repair impairment, yet these examples illustrate that many of the details are still poorly understood.

2.2. DNA Damage Repair and Carcinogenesis

Despite the association between some repair defects and cancer, heritable mutations have not yet been described in many human genes encoding core DNA damage response and DNA repair proteins (e.g., the core proteins involved in base excision repair). Such germline mutations would almost certainly be lethal early in development, as they are in murine models *(9,22,23)*. However, the possibility remains that acquired, somatic mutations associated with neoplasia could be detected in any member of this large family of functionally related genes. In contrast, in other cases, murine knockouts have no obvious phenotype, probably because of redundancy in certain repair factors (e.g., the glycosylases involved in base excision repair) *(24)*.

Although inherited cancer syndromes are uncommon, there is growing evidence to support the assertion that changes leading to loss of global genomic integrity are an early, critical event in typical carcinogenesis *(25,26)*. If the multihit hypothesis of cancer is broadly true, impaired DNA surveillance might be critical in order for cells to accumulate the number and spectrum of mutations necessary for transformation. Because replication results in less than 1 error in 10^{10} copy events in normal cells *(27)*, the rate of spontaneous DNA mutations may be insufficient to explain lifelong population cancer acquisition rates unless DNA surveillance mechanisms are impaired.

The evidence for an acquired DNA repair defect commonly contributing to neoplasia is clearest for colorectal cancer, where it has been shown that mutations of genes encoding several proteins involved in DNA mismatch repair (e.g., *MSH2* and *MLH1*) or, more rarely, base excision repair (*MYH*), are an important early step on the pathway to invasive malignancy *(28–30)*. Mutations in these genes presumably contribute to carcinogenesis by facilitating the four or five other key mutations that are needed to turn a healthy epithelial cell into a dedifferentiated, invasive carcinoma with metastatic potential. In other types of neoplastic cells, mismatch repair lesions such as these appear to be uncommon; instead, gross chromosomal instability is seen, with large deletions and rearrangements involving many megabases of DNA *(26)*.

Typical bone marrow karyotypes in patients with therapy-related myelodysplasia (MDS) and AML suggest that abnormalities causing chromosomal instability should be more common than mismatch repair defects. A DNA repair defect is not strictly necessary to produce numerical chromosomal abnormalities and large deletions characteristic of MDS and AML:

Table 1
Human DNA Repair Pathways

DNA repair pathway	Class of DNA damage repaired
Base excision repair	Spontaneous depurination and other hydrolytic cleavage
	Deamination
	Oxidative damage
	Aberrant methylation
	Single-nucleotide single-strand breaks
Nucleotide excision repair and transcription-coupled repair	Bulky and helix-distorting DNA adducts
	Pyrimidine dimers and other photoproducts
	Intrastrand crosslinks
	Lesions causing stalling of RNA polymerase
Nonhomologous end joining	Double-strand breaks
Homologous recombination	Double-strand breaks, DNA crosslinks
Mismatch repair	Replication-mispaired nucleotides
	Small insertion/deletions

abnormal centrosome function or microtubule assembly during mitosis could also play an important role, as might aberrant telomere dynamics (31,32). In addition, while chromosome defects are the most widely recognized lesions in MDS and AML, there is accumulating evidence that point mutations in many genes are also frequent, suggesting that multiple types of genomic instability may be present (33). Interestingly, AML patients with complex karyotypes have characteristic patterns of gene expression that include upregulation of DNA repair genes, but evidently this strategy is not successful in overcoming underlying genomic instability (34).

3. MECHANISMS OF DNA REPAIR

3.1. General Considerations

Biologically important DNA lesions interfere with either transcription or DNA replication. In the former case, the RNA polymerase complex stalls when it encounters an unfamiliar base or helix conformation, and transcription stops abruptly. If this situation is not quickly corrected, the cell dies an apoptotic death (35). In contrast to these transcriptional delays, replication errors can contribute directly to oncogenesis. A specialized class of at least nine DNA polymerases (pol ζ through σ) with looser, more flexible base-pairing properties than canonical DNA polymerases (e.g., DNA pol α, δ, and ε) help overcome DNA damage-related replication stress by translesional DNA synthesis, at the potential cost of mutagenesis (36–40). These alternative, "sloppy copy" polymerases do offer some cellular protection as evidenced, for instance, by the observation that DNA pol η (POLH/XPV/RAD30) mutations result in xeroderma pigmentosum because of failure to bypass ultraviolet (UV)-induced cyclobutane pyrimidine dimers, but a better solution is to fully repair the lesion prior to resuming replication (41,42). Because DNA injury types are diverse, there are multiple, partially overlapping (43) pathways for DNA repair (Figs. 3–7; Table 1). Which one a cell uses depends on the specific type of DNA lesion detected.

3.2. Direct Enzymatic Repair

In rare cases, an abnormal DNA base modification can be repaired directly without involving a complex pathway. For example, O^6-methylguanine-DNA-methyltransferase (O^6-MT, the product of the *MGMT* gene) removes methyl groups that have been added to the 6th position of the purine ring of guanine. O^6-Methylguanine is a particularly dangerous modification because it can lead to mispairing with thymine and because O^6-methylguanine can trick other DNA repair systems into pursuing multiple, futile rounds that simply reincorporate the mutated base *(9)*. The O^6-MT protein is irreversibly inactivated by the process of repairing a single modified guanine, an energy expenditure that demonstrates just how critical this mechanism is for cellular integrity *(9)*.

The functional status of the O^6-MT pathway may be important in patients treated with alkylating agents, for O^6-methylation of guanine appears to be an important effect of some members that class of drugs *(44)*. High levels of O^6-MT are often found in bone marrow stem cells and AML blasts, which are thereby rendered resistant to certain alkylators *(45)*. Conversely, silencing of *MGMT* by mutation or promoter hypermethylation has been associated with a superior response to alkylating agent therapy in certain solid tumors *(46,47)*.

3.3. Single-Strand (ss) vs Double-Strand (ds) Breaks

DNA repair more commonly involves multiple proteins, with excision of a damaged DNA base or segment followed by replacement of damaged nucleotides *(48)*. If DNA damage involves only one strand of the double helix, genome integrity can be restored by base excision repair (BER) or nucleotide excision repair (NER) mechanisms that use the undamaged DNA strand as a template to restore the original sequence (Figs. 3, 4; *see* Color Plates 6 and 7, following p. 174) *(49–51)*. Mismatch repair (MMR) is a special case of single-strand repair that primarily corrects endogenous replication and recombination errors rather than exogenously damaged DNA, but MMR can also be used for special base modifications or for small insertion/deletion loops of up to about 15 base pairs (Fig. 5; *see* Color Plate 8, following p. 174) *(52,53)*. By these three general mechanisms DNA ss lesions can be efficiently corrected.

If both strands of the double helix are disrupted and chromosomal structure itself is at risk, the cell is in grave danger *(54)*. The simplest solution is cleaving residual single-stranded overhanging segments (Fig. 6; *see* Color Plate 9, following p. 174) and religating the severed ends of any adjacent double-stranded DNA molecules that are unprotected by a telomeric repeat, a process known as nonhomologous end joining (NHEJ) *(55)*. This stopgap repair technique may seem a rather shoddy solution, since genetic information is almost invariably lost, but so much of the human genome is noncoding DNA and genes with limited expression that the phenotypic consequences of minor deletions are often negligible. Moreover, NHEJ can be useful: it is the source of immunoglobulin diversity in V(D)J recombination, mentioned above *(19,55)*. Homologous end joining (homologous recombination, HR) is a higher quality repair mechanism that requires the use of general recombination mechanisms similar in principle to those that take place in normal meiosis, with information transfer from an intact chromosomal homolog *(56,57)*. This is the most complex mechanism for DNA repair from a molecular standpoint, and an intact complementary chromosomal strand is necessary. HR has the advantage of offering repair with no or minimal loss of genomic information, but there can be functionally important loss of heterozygosity. While HR predominates in the S and G2 phases of the cell cycle, when a freshly synthesized sister chromatid is available as a repair template, cells must instead settle for NHEJ in G1, when they lack a second copy to use as a template *(58)*.

All of these repair processes are described in greater detail below.

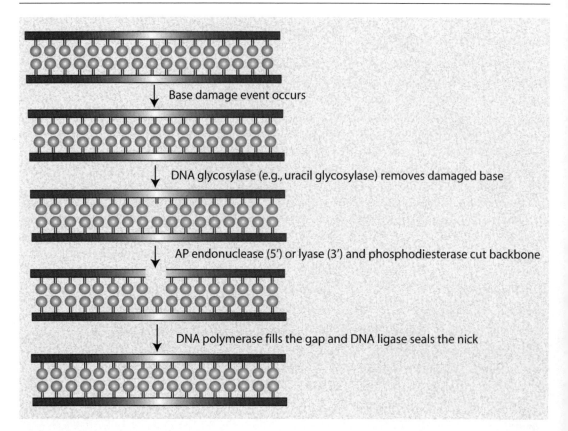

Fig. 3. (Color Plate 6, following p. 174) Base excision repair (BER) mechanisms specialize in responding to DNA damage from normal metabolism, including base modifications via hydrolysis, oxidation, or methylation. Single-strand breaks can also be repaired (not shown). BER is initiated by one of a set of glycosylases that recognize specific altered or inappropriate bases (orange), and then, if necessary, cleave the base from its sugar moiety in the DNA backbone. This results in an apurinic/apyrimidinic (AP) site. The sugar at this AP site is removed by either AP endonuclease or AP lyase. A phosphorylase excises the remaining deoxyribose phosphate residue. The gap is then filled by a DNA polymerase, usually DNA pol β. DNA ligase seals the nick, and DNA integrity is restored (**bottom**). Mice deficient in the core enzymes (e.g., AP endonuclease) needed for appropriate base excision repair usually have embryonic lethal phenotypes, but survival without individual glycosylases is possible.

3.4. DNA Damage Recognition

Before DNA damage can be repaired, it must be recognized. Without high-quality nucleic acid surveillance systems and an efficient "alarm" system, the integrity of specific repair mechanisms is irrelevant (59–61). In addition, DNA repair takes time, and injured cells must also be induced to slow their progression through the normal cell cycle until DNA lesions are corrected. Single-strand lesions are generally signaled by mechanisms that recognize conformation changes in the DNA helix, specific chemically modified bases, or stalling of RNA pol II at transcription sites. Although the precise trigger for recognition of transcriptional complex stalling is not understood, the process is facilitated by RNA pol II ubiquitination (62–64). DNA ds breaks, in contrast, are recognized by specific proteins, including Ku70/Ku80 and the MRE11 complex that can sense loose DNA ends unprotected by telomeres (65).

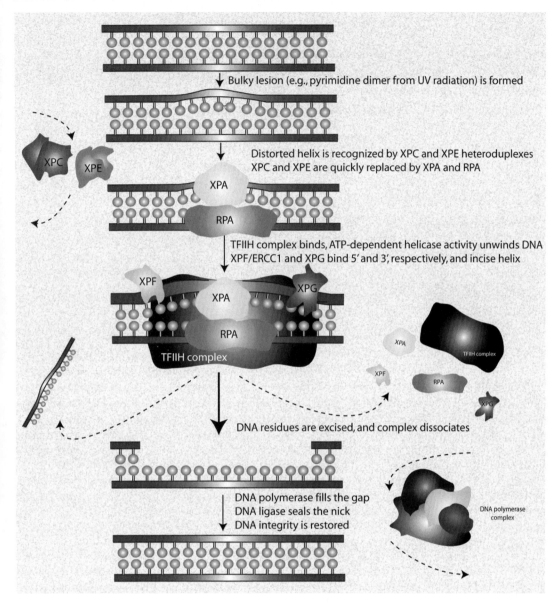

Fig. 4. (Color Plate 7, following p. 174) Nucleotide excision repair (NER) is an extremely versatile mechanism for correction of defects involving bulky DNA damage, such as adducts or dimers. NER is coupled to transcription: transcriptionally active genes are preferentially repaired, and a subpathway called transcription-coupled repair is initiated by specific factors, including CSA and CSB (not shown). Recognition of the lesion involves XPE and XPC-HR23B heteroduplexes, which recognize an abnormal conformation of the DNA backbone that then quickly recruits a complex including XPA and RPA1 and the large multiprotein complex TFIIH. The TFIIH cluster in turn recruits XPG and XPF, and these latter two molecules incise the damaged strand, after which the complex dissociates. A number of proteins, including DNA polymerase and ligase, are then involved in the final steps of repair. Typically, 25–30 nucleotides are excised in an NER cycle, so the drawing here is not quite to scale.

Other participants in the DNA damage recognition and signaling process include ATM (ataxia-telangiectasia mutated), ATR (ataxia-telangiectasia- and Rad3-related), the BRCA1-associated genome surveillance complex (BASC), and p53 (Fig. 7; *see* Color Plate 10,

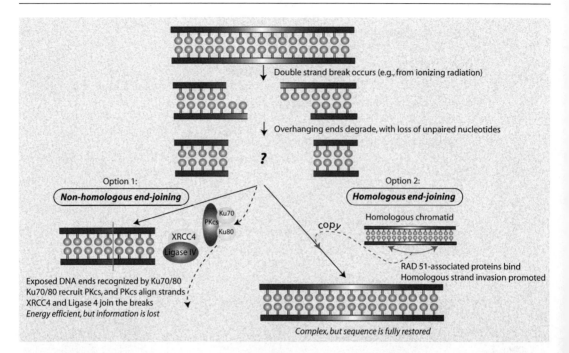

Fig. 5. (Color Plate 8, following p. 174) Pathways for repair of DNA double-strand breaks: double-strand breaks represent a particularly dangerous lesion for the cell because of the lack of adjacent template to facilitate repair. Repair can be carried out by two mechanisms, depending on the cell cycle phase. Most commonly, nonhomologous end joining (NHEJ) occurs **(left)** with loss of several nucleotides. Homologous recombination (HR) **(right)** occurs in G2 and S phases when a pristine sister chromatid may be available. After a DNA double-strand break occurs—for instance, in the presence of ionizing radiation—any over-hanging nucleotides are quickly degraded. The exposed DNA ends that are not protected by telomeres are recognized by a Ku70/Ku80 heterodimer that recruits DNA-dependent protein catalytic proteins (DNA-PKcs). In turn, an NHEJ-specific ligase (ligase IV) and XRCC4 quickly join these breaks. DNA polymerase and other ligases are not required. HR allows restoration of DNA injury with high fidelity and resolution of genomic integrity. Strand invasion and branch migration from the homologous chromosome include replication and formation of a topologically complex Holliday junction (not shown) and are mediated by RAD52, which recruits RAD51 and other proteins. This DNA pathway also involves a complex of RAD50/MRE11/NBN as well as a number of other proteins, including BLM (which helps resolve the Holliday junction) and BRCA1-associated factors. This system is costly in terms of energy exposure and requires an undamaged sister molecule to serve as template for resynthesis of missing nucleotides.

following p. 174) *(66–69)*. p53 is so fundamental to global genomic integrity that it has been dubbed the "guardian of the genome"*(70)*, but the phenotypes associated with ATM, ATR, and BASC mutations suggest that they are also critical. Acquired mutations in this group of surveillance and checkpoint control proteins are among the most common abnormalities in many types of cancer. Moreover, familial syndromes involving these polypeptides have been described, including those with an AML predisposition *(71)*.

How these molecules participate in DNA damage-induced signaling and cell cycle checkpoint control is becoming increasingly well understood. While a review of the cell cycle and its regulation is beyond the scope of the current chapter, a few comments will illustrate how these molecules function to regulate the cell cycle and DNA repair. To take one example, when replication is inhibited (as is the case after treatment with hydroxyurea or cytarabine),

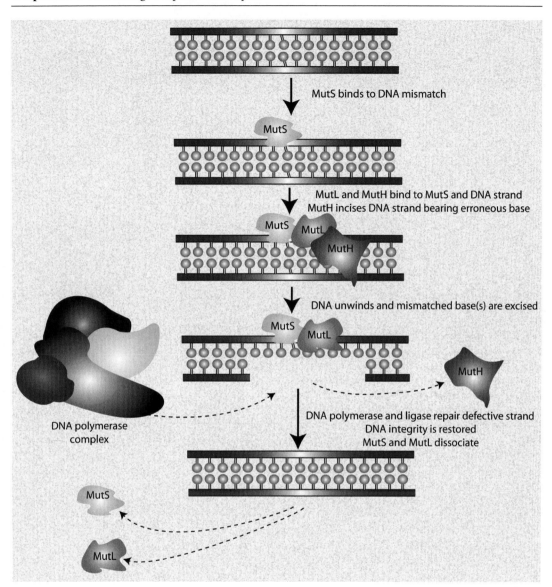

MutS binds to DNA mismatch

MutL and MutH bind to MutS and DNA strand
MutH incises DNA strand bearing erroneous base

DNA unwinds and mismatched base(s) are excised

DNA polymerase and ligase repair defective strand
DNA integrity is restored
MutS and MutL dissociate

DNA polymerase
complex

Fig. 6. (Color Plate 9, following p. 174) DNA mismatch repair (MMR) is responsible for repairing replication errors (orange, top) and small insertion-deletion loops (not shown) resulting from DNA polymerase slippage, particularly at repetitive DNA elements. Heterodimers of hMSH2/6 (single base) or hMSH2/3 (insertion-deletion loops), both homologs of *E. coli* MutS, recognize mismatches that distort the DNA helix. MutL-like protein complexes, including hMLH1/PMS2 and hMLH1/PMS1, join MutS and interact with other proteins (MutH in *E. coli*) that incise the newly replicated, erroneous strand. The new strand may be recognized by its proximity to adjacent replication proteins or perhaps by its methylation status. Once the erroneous strand is excised, resynthesis and ligation occur.

replication forks stall but DNA helicases continue to pry apart the DNA strands ahead of the replication machinery *(72)*. The result is an extended stretch of ss DNA that binds the ss DNA-binding protein replication protein A (RPA), which in turn helps load two complexes. The first consists of the protein kinase ATR and its binding partner ATRIP (ATR-interacting protein). The second consists of Rad17 and the four small RFC subunits, which collectively

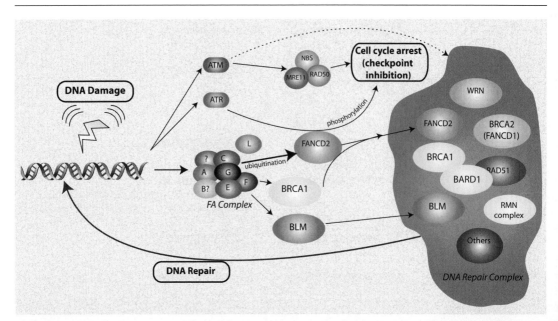

Fig. 7. (Color Plate 10, following p. 174) Fanconi anemia (FA) and BRCA protein complexes and the DNA damage response pathway: DNA damage caused by radiation or by crosslinking agents causes activation of the FA–protein complex. This then leads to monoubiquitination of FANCD2 at lysine 561 by either FANCB or FANCL; FANCD2 subsequently interacts with BRCA1. BRCA1, in turn, is part of a complex that promotes the actual DNA repair. In parallel, damage, especially that caused by ionizing radiation, activates ataxia-telangiectasia mutation (ATM), which phosphorylates FANCD2 instead of ubiquitinating it. This leads to activation of checkpoint response proteins. The ATR protein, as well as the RAD50/MRE11/NBN complex, appear to be important for this signaling. The functions of several proteins in this pathway are incompletely understood, and FANCI and FANCJ have not yet been identified.

form a clamp loader that loads a heterotrimeric clamp consisting of Rad1, Rad9, and Hus1 onto the DNA. In a manner that is poorly understood, this clamp facilitates the action of ATR on a number of substrates, including checkpoint kinase 1 (Chk1). Chk1 in turn phosphorylates and inactivates the phosphatases Cdc25A and Cdc25C, which are required for cyclin-dependent kinase activation to drive initiation of DNA synthesis at origins of replication (S phase) and the G_2/M transition, respectively. In addition, Chk1 phosphorylates Rad51 *(73)*, which is involved in DNA repair and also an unknown substrate involved in replication fork stabilization. At the same time, ATR also phosphorylates the tumor suppressor protein p53. The normally rapid turnover of p53 is slowed by this phosphorylation, resulting in elevated levels of p53, which upon subsequent modification is able to act as a transcription factor that facilitates expression of scores of genes, including the gene encoding p21$^{\text{waf1/cip1}}$, a molecule that inhibits cyclin-dependent kinases and further enforces the cell cycle arrest induced by phosphorylation and inactivation of Cdc25A and Cdc25C.

DNA ds breaks, e.g., after ionizing radiation, result in binding of a complex consisting of MRE11 (meiotic recombination 11A homolog), NBN (nibrin, NBS1), and Rad50 (Rad50 homolog) to DNA *(74)*. NBN in turn binds and activates ATM *(75)*, which phosphorylates a variety of substrates *(72)*, including checkpoint kinase 2 (Chk2) and p53. Chk2 then phosphorylates Cdc25A and Cdc25C on the same sites as Chk1, with identical consequences, whereas p53 again transactivates the same genes. Although similar reactions are triggered after replication stress and DNA ds breaks, the signaling appears to be subtly different, for replication stress typically results in S-phase slowing ("activation of the replication checkpoint"), whereas DNA ds breaks result in a G_1 and/or G_2 arrest ("activation of the DNA damage checkpoint"). This difference might reflect, at least in part, the fact that the Ku70/Ku80 heterodimer, which activates DNA-DKss (the catalytic subunit of DNA-activated protein kinase; PRKDC), also binds DNA ds breaks but not the stalled replication forks. Alternatively, the different response might reflect differences in substrate phosphorylation by ATR vs ATM. In either case, the net result of this signaling is inhibition of cell cycle progression, stabilization of DNA at sites of damage, and activation of the DNA repair machinery.

Interestingly, defects in these DNA damage recognition pathways are occasionally observed in the human population. In particular, germline mutations in ATM (ataxia telangiectasia), ATR (Seckel syndrome), NBN (Nijmegen breakage syndrome), MRE11 (ataxis-telangiectasia-like disorder), and BCRCA2 (Fanconi anemia complementation group D1) have all been associated with familial cancer syndromes, described in more detail below.

3.5. Base Excision Repair

It is estimated that as a byproduct of normal oxidative cellular metabolism, adverse events leading to DNA damage occur on the order of 10,000–20,000 times per cell per day *(76)*. Common events such as generation of reactive oxygen species result in "minor" base modifications with potentially major consequences for disruption of DNA transcription and replication. Examples include deamination of 5-methylcytosine to uracil, spontaneous depurination of guanine and adenine (i.e., hydrolytic attack resulting in cleavage of the *N*-glycosyl linkage of the purine base to the deoxyribose sugar; Figs. 1, 2), uncontrolled methylation of any base by the methyl group donor S-adenosylmethionine, and oxidative damage leading to the creation of the major oxidized purine 8-oxo-7,8-dihydroguanine (8-oxoguanine, a potent mutagen) or disruptive oxidized pyrimidines (thymine glycol, 5-hydroxycytosine, and the formamidopyrimidines) (Figs. 1, 2) *(77,78)*. Cellular antioxidant mechanisms designed to prevent these lesions are elaborate and include glutathione and other radical scavengers, superoxide dismutase, glutathione peroxidase, peroxyredoxins, and catalase *(79)*. Once the damage is done, however, it is the BER process (Fig. 3) that is responsible for the lion's share of the enormous task of fixing this class of ubiquitous lesions *(49)*.

There are at least nine different BER DNA glycosylases, each of which recognizes a specific type or narrow spectrum of modified base, which is then hydrolytically excised from the helix (Table 2) *(80)*. For obvious reasons, repair of spontaneous hydrolytic depurination (Fig. 1), where the base itself is already lost and only the sugar-phosphate backbone remains, requires no such glycosylase activity. Following a glycosylase reaction or spontaneous depurination event, the core BER reaction begins. The apurininc/apyrimidinic (AP) site is opened by a specific endonuclease (AP endonuclease 1 or AP lyase), which cuts the DNA backbone 5′ or 3′ to the decapitated nucleotide, respectively *(9,16,49)*. Then (in mammals) a deoxyribophosphodiesterase removes the sugar-phosphate residue, a DNA polymerase (usually DNA pol β, which has some intrinsic phosphodiesterase activity itself) fills the gap in the DNA strand, and DNA ligase III complexed with XRCC1 (X-ray repair complementing defective repair in Chinese hamster cells 1), a polypeptide of uncertain function, seals the nick to complete the repair.

Most cells are capable of several different variations on this core BER reaction. In the event of DNA ss breaks that remove an entire nucleotide strand yet leave the other strand intact (e.g., from irradiation), the core reaction is the same, but poly(ADP-ribose) polymerase

Table 2
Human DNA Glycosylases Involved in Base Excision Repair

Gene[a]	Enzyme	Primary substrates
MBD4	Methyl-CpG-binding domain protein 4	Uracil or thymine in a U/TpG dinucleotide that is complementary to CpG dinucleotides
MPG	*N*-Methylpurine-DNA-glycosylase	Hypoxanthine, 3-methyl-adenine or -guanine, 7-methyl-adenine or -guanine
MUTYH (MYH)	MutY homolog	Adenine opposite guanine or 8-oxo-7,8-dihyrdoguanine
NTHL1 (NTH1)	nth endonuclease III-like 1	Fragmented or ring-saturated (oxidized) pyrimidines such as thymine glycol
OGG1	8-Oxoguanine DNA-glycosylase 1	8-oxo-7,8-dihydroguanine
SMUG1	Single-strand selective monofunctional uracil DNA glycosylase	Single-stranded uracil, uracil complementary to guanine or adenine
TDG	Thymine DNA glycosylase	Uracil, ethenocytosine, or thymine opposite guanine
UNG1	Uracil DNA glycosylase 1	Single-stranded uracil, uracil complementary to adenine or guanine
UNG2	Uracil DNA glycosylase 2	Uracil opposite adenine

[a]Unlike AP endonuclease, DNA polymerase β, XRCC1, and DNA ligase III, where murine knockout is lethal, knockout of individual glycosylases is associated with a normal phenotype, suggesting that there is some functional redundancy in these activities.

and polynucleotide kinase protect and trim the broken DNA ends before the core BER apparatus takes over *(9,81)*. A slightly different "long patch" BER pathway that employs proliferating cell nuclear antigen (PCNA), flap endonuclease 1 (FEN1), and DNA ligase I in addition to DNA pol β can address larger lesions (2–11 base pairs) than the "short-patch" pathway described above *(82)*. There are also some data suggesting involvement of p53 in some variations of BER. In particular, p53-deficient cells, which lack DNA pol β, have difficulty repairing lesions induced by the base-damaging agent methyl methanesulfonate *(83–85)*.

BER is so essential for cellular survival that mouse knockout models for the fundamental enzymes in this pathway are invariably associated with embryonic lethality *(86,87)*. In humans, germline mutations have been reported in only a single member of this pathway (*MYH* [MutY homolog]), where a base pair change predisposes to colorectal cancer and is associated with a DNA transversion in the *APC* (adenomatous polyposis coli) gene *(29,88)*. A few polymorphisms in other BER elements, possibly leading to increased cancer susceptibility, have also been described *(89)*. The specific importance of BER for AML, however, is unclear.

3.6. Nucleotide Excision Repair

NER pathways specialize in removing DNA damage that is bulky or distorts the normal DNA helical structure, such as DNA crosslinks, pyrimidine dimers (often caused by UV light), and large chemical adducts (e.g., from carcinogenic chemicals such as those found in tobacco smoke) *(90)*. This versatile mechanism removes not only the abnormal base or bases themselves, but also usually resects and replaces a large stretch of adjacent normal nucleotides.

The first step in the NER process is recognition of DNA damage by DDB1 (damage-specific DNA binding protein 1, XPE) and XPC/RAD23B (HR23B, Rad23 homolog B) complexes. This particular recognition may take place on the basis of physical conformation changes of the helix induced by disrupted base pairing rather than the specific chemical recognition that characterizes BER *(91)*. Lesions such as cyclobutane pyrimidine dimers, for example, are not particularly distorting and are ineffectively recognized by NER *(91)*. In any case, binding of the XPC complex results in DNA bending *(92)*, which is followed by recruitment of RPA1/XPA (replication protein A1) and associated proteins. If the appropriate abnormal backbone structure is not present, RPA1/XPA aborts NER *(93)*. If the appropriate backbone structure is present, the large GTF2H4 (TFIIH)–ERCC5 (XPG)–ERCC4 (XPF)–ERCC1 complex then binds RPA1/XPA. This multiunit complex includes helicases such as ERCC3 (excision repair cross-complementing rodent repair deficiency complementation group 3, also known as XPB) and ERCC2 (XPD), which relax the tightly-wound DNA. The complex also includes proteins that incise the damaged DNA strand at some distance on either side of the defect, generating a single-strand stretch about 30 base pairs in length. It is notable that GTF2H4 (general transcription factor IIH polypeptide 4, TFIIH), which is an important part of the NER pathway, is also key part of the core transcription initiation complex *(94)*. This suggests the possibility that the phenotype in patients with NER defects may in part be a consequence of defective transcription. In any case, once the damaged stretch is removed, repair replication based on the normal DNA template can occur, followed by DNA ligation to finish the job—and then the whole complex dissociates (Fig. 4) *(95)*.

More than two dozen polypeptides participate in NER, and they are tightly regulated *(9,96)*. The "XP" designation in the official symbol or the alternative name of many of these proteins stands for xeroderma pigmentosum, an autosomal recessive clinical condition caused by defects in this pathway; and the various letters (XPA, XPB, etc.) designate distinct complementation groups first defined by cell fusion studies that corrected the associated defect. The XP syndrome that results when these polypeptides are defective is characterized by photosensitivity and development of multiple skin tumors *(21)*, highlighting the essential role of NER in repairing UV-associated DNA damage. Patients with XP do not develop leukemia and appear to be at low risk for solid tumors, possibly because of the low internal penetration of UV light.

3.7. Transcription-Coupled Repair (TCR)

Sometimes a bulky, unrepaired DNA lesion best addressed by NER pathways will first be encountered during the process of transcription *(62,64,97,98)*. When RNA pol II stalls because it encounters such a lesion before DDB1/XPE and XPC/RAD23B/HR23B have had a chance to find it and recruit the usual NER machinery, a dedicated TCR pathway comes into play *(62,98)*. The TCR complex, including proteins CSA (Cockayne syndrome A) and CSB, displaces the stalled RNA polymerase and repairs the defect using the NER machinery described above, allowing transcription to resume *(97,99)*. Although the TCR pathway is highly conserved in evolution, defects in the TCR-specific factors (i.e., those not already discussed above under NER generally) have not been proven to be associated with neoplastic transformation. Instead, mutations in CSA and CSB result in Cockayne syndrome, an autosomal recessive disease characterized by mental retardation, growth retardation, and photosensitivity, but not cancer. Other pathway defects result in trichothiodystrophy, which has similar features to Cockayne syndrome, with the addition of brittle hair and nails due to a deficiency in protein sulfur content *(21)*. In addition to *ERCC8* (*CSA*) and *ERCC6* (*CSB*), genes involved in TCR include *ERCC3* (*XPB*), *ERCC2* (*XPD*), *ERCC5* (*XPG*), and genes encoding currently unidentified pathway components that lead to trichothiodystrophy *(100,101)*.

3.8. Mismatch Repair

No enzyme is perfect at what it does, and the DNA polymerases are no exception. During normal replication, nucleotides are occasionally mismatched. In addition, the polymerases can occasionally "slip" and replicate the same nucleotide twice or miss a nucleotide entirely. Such slippage leads to small insertions and deletions, creating small loops of ss DNA. Cellular MMR mechanisms are responsible for recognizing and removing these nucleotides, which are structurally normal, yet out of place. Mice engineered to have inborn MMR deficiencies generally develop normally, but are cancer-prone *(102)*.

MMR pathways follow a pattern similar to that already described with other excision repair mechanisms *(52)*. The mammalian proteins involved are homologs of *E. coli* prototypes MutS, MutL, and MutH (Fig. 6) or *S. cerevisiae* PMS and are named accordingly *(103)*. The initating step in MMR occurs when a DNA mismatch is recognized by specialized recognition proteins: the heterodimer hMSH2/hMSH6 (human mutS homologs 2 and 6, collectively called hMutSα) for single base-pair mismatches, and the comparable hMSH2/MSH3 (hMutSβ) for short loops. As with NER, the basis of this recognition appears to be DNA kinking *(104)*. After recognition, hMLH1/PMS2 (mutL homolog 1/postmeiotic segregation increased 2, collectively called hMutLα) and hMLH1/PMS1 (hMutLβ) heterodimers are recruited. Based on methylation patterns or interactions with nearby replication machinery *(9)*, these polypeptides help determine which DNA strand is the newly synthesized strand containing the error and which is the template. Together, these MutL-homolog heterodimers excise a short oligonucleotide containing the aberrant DNA causing the mismatch. DNA polymerases and ligases then finish the job of restoring the proper DNA sequence *(105)*.

This MMR mechanism appears to be especially important for maintaining the integrity of highly repetitive DNA, as evidenced by the observation that spontaneous mutations occur in repetitive segments with a high frequency when MMR function is impaired *(106,107)*. This phenomenon, known as "microsatellite instability," is well described in several types of solid tumors but is rare in *de novo* AML and MDS (<10% of cases) *(108–113)*. However, MMR defects may be much more common in MDS and AML cases that occur after prior exposure to alkylating agents, radiation, or thiopurines administered as immunosuppressants following solid-organ transplantation *(114–117)*. Microsatellite instability has been reported in more than 90% of therapy-related AML in some series *(118)*. Point mutations in core MMR factors do not appear to be common in these AML cases, but expression changes may be widespread *(119)*. Unlike the case with solid tumors, these expression changes in AML do not appear to be due to hypermethylation and silencing of relevant MMR gene promoters *(113,115,120,121)*, and their basis requires further study.

MMR defects are thought to drive the neoplastic process by causing inactivating mutations in microsatellite-bearing growth-suppressive genes and activating mutations in growth-promoting genes *(122)*. The target genes mutated as a consequence of defective MMR in solid tumors include *BAX* (BCL2-associated X protein), *TGFBR2 (*transforming growth factor, β receptor II)*, E2F4 (*E2F transcription factor 4)*, IGF2R* (insulin-like growth factor 2 receptor), *APC*, *CASP5* (caspase 5), *PTEN* (phosphatase and tensin homolog), and *MBD4* (methyl-CpG binding domain protein 4). In AML the target genes are less well defined *(16)*. *BAX* is mutated in some AML cell lines *(122)*, but *E2F4 (123)*, *TGFBR2*, *IGF2R* and others are not usually mutated either in cell lines or patient samples *(113)*. P53 mutations, rare in AML in general (<15% of cases), are more common in the presence of microsatellite instability *(118,119)*.

In addition to recognizing the products of polymerase infidelity, the MMR machinery can also recognize certain forms of damaged DNA and trigger apoptosis when alkylated DNA bases or other chemical adducts are detected. As a result, intact MMR may be important in sensitivity to certain chemotherapeutic agents such as alkylators *(124)*. Conversely, loss of MMR in therapy-related AML may have implications for cellular sensitivity to various chemotherapeutic agents. For instance, the drug 6-thioguanine, sometimes used in AML induction or salvage regimens, is incorporated into DNA and modified to S^6-methyl-thioguanine, an abnormal base that can pair with either cytosine or thymine *(125)*. Because cytotoxicity results only if this aberrant pairing is recognized by MMR, MMR-deficient cells are resistant to 6-thioguanine *(126)*.

3.9. Homologous and Nonhomologous End Joining

DNA ds breaks can result from ionizing radiation, volatile chemicals, or replication of an unrepaired DNA ss break *(54)*. In HR, which has substantial overlap with general mechanisms of DNA recombination, DNA ds breaks are repaired by directing a single strand from an intact homologous chromosome or sister chromatid to invade the injured DNA (Fig. 5).

An early event in HR is recruitment of ATM, which phosphorylates the MRE11/ RAD50/ NBN complex *(59)*. In parallel with this, chromatin structure is altered by ATM-dependent phosphorylation of histone H2AX (H2A histone family, member X) over a large range of DNA adjacent to the break, and phosphorylated H2AX facilitates recruitment of additional repair factors *(127)*.

The MRE11/NBN/RAD50 complex, which has exonuclease activity, exposes 3′ ends of DNA to promote homologous strand invasion *(128)*. RPA1/XPA then facilitates assembly of a large complex, including several RAD51-related proteins, XRCC2, XRCC3, and others, at the site of the break *(129)*. Full HR function also depends on BRCA1 (breast cancer 1) *(130)*, a substrate of the Chk2 and ATM kinases *(131)*, and the FA (Fanconi anemia) protein complex, including BRCA2 (Fig. 7) *(132,133)*. A large cohesin complex, with its assembly dependent on histone conformation, is also necessary to ensure appropriate alignment of the homologous strand *(134,135)*.

Once the sister chromatid is identified and aligned, copying of the homologous element can take place, resulting in a transient, topologically complex four-way Holliday junction with strands from both the damaged and intact DNA molecules and their replicates *(136)*. Proteins such as BLM1 (Bloom syndrome 1), topoisomerases, and others are necessary to resolve this tangle *(137,138)*.

Where an intact homologous chromosome or sister chromatid is not readily available (e.g., in G0/G1 phase), the cell must resort to direct ligation of the broken ends of DNA. The NHEJ pathway is simpler than HR and requires no complementary template. A Ku70 and Ku80 protein heterodimer binds to broken DNA ends, along with DNA-PKcs, which appears to have a signaling function *(54)*. Direct ligation by XRCC4 and DNA ligase IV follows. This ligation may be most efficient when the DNA ends are still held together by nucleosomes *(9)*.

4. FAMILIAL SYNDROMES WITH LEUKEMIA RISK AND DNA DAMAGE RESPONSE OR REPAIR DEFECTS

A number of well-described human disorders are characterized by inherited defects in the DNA damage response and repair pathways leading to genomic instability *(18,139,140)*. Several of these syndromes include an inherent predisposition to hematologic malignancies, including AML *(16)*. Immunodeficiency is also common in these syndromes *(141)*, presumably because of the important role of DNA repair in rearrangements of normal immunoglobulin and T-cell receptor genes. Defects in the rearrangements of these genes may underlie the predisposition to lymphoblastic leukemia, as mentioned above *(19)*.

The neoplasia pattern and the leukemia risk vary depending on the specific syndrome, specific mutation, and penetrance within a given pedigree. In some syndromes the cancer risk is overwhelmingly restricted to a single tumor type (e.g., lymphoma and lymphoid leukemia in Nijmegen breakage syndrome *[142]* or skin cancer in XP *[100]*), whereas in other syndromes the cancer spectrum is very broad (e.g., Li-Fraumeni syndrome *[143]*). In some syndromes, the overall malignancy risk is dramatically elevated above the background rate (e.g., ataxia-telangiectasia, or AT *[144]*), whereas in other settings the risk is only slightly greater than that of the general population (e.g., heterozygotes for Bloom syndrome *[145]*). The reasons for these variations are not currently understood.

In general, the inherited DNA repair syndromes can be detected in cytogenetic assays as an increase in the risk of chromosomal breakage or exchange between sister chromatids—either spontaneously or in response to low-intensity exposure to clastogens (e.g., mitomycin C, diepoxybutane, irradiation) that would not normally result in widespread chromosomal breakage *(146)*. Clinicians should consider an undiagnosed DNA repair disorder when a patient presents with leukemia and has either unexplained short stature, long-standing immunodeficiency, or dysmorphic features.

The clinical features and molecular characteristics of several of the familial syndromes with a leukemia risk are described below. In some settings the development of leukemia requires special therapeutic approaches, including dose modification (e.g., the extreme chemoradiosensitivity of Fanconi anemia). Accordingly, readers are encouraged to consult up-to-date reviews of specific disorders for the latest management principles.

4.1. Fanconi Anemia

FA (Mendelian Inheritance in Man [MIM] cat. no. 277650 and others) is an autosomal recessive and rarely X-linked syndrome that may be the most common form of congenital bone marrow failure *(147)*. Because infants usually have normal blood counts, neonatal screening for FA is ineffective. While FA usually presents in childhood (median age at diagnosis 7 years), a few cases are not recognized until early adulthood, sometimes when affected individuals present with MDS or AML *(148)*.

The precise prevalence of FA is not known. It has been suggested that FA affects approximately three births in a million, and the heterozygote frequency (for all complementation groups combined) in the general American and Western European population is estimated at 1 in 300 *(149,150)*. Since the first description in a Swiss family by Guido Fanconi in 1927 *(151)*, approx 1300 cases have been reported in the medical literature *(152)*, and the International Fanconi Anemia Registry begun in 1982 now includes more than 700 patients *(148)*. If the birth incidence is truly three births in a million, this implies that most cases are unreported to registries or in the medical literature. No particular ethnic group is at risk, although there are founder mutations in Ashkenazi Jews, Afrikaaners, South African blacks, and Romani (Gypsy) groups in Spain *(153–156)*.

About two-thirds of FA patients have one or more physical anomalies *(135)*. The most common of these are hypo- or hyperpigmented areas of the skin, including large freckles and café-au-lait spots; growth retardation (with short adult stature); and skeletal abnormalities, especially of the upper limbs (e.g., hypoplastic thumbs and other radial ray or digital anomalies). Patients with radial abnormalities have a higher risk of marrow failure *(157)*. A minority of patients have other features such as microcephaly, neck deformity, genital abnormalities (especially undescended testes, testicular agenesis, hypospadias, or bicornuate uterus with associated infertility), neurodevelopmental delay, a wide spectrum of kidney anomalies, various gastrointestinal and cardiac anomalies, or abnormal development of the eyes or ears, including microphthalmia, strabismus, ptosis, and low-set deformed ears. About one-third of patients have no such physical abnormalities, however, and may not be easily recognizable as having FA, especially if there is no history of childhood marrow failure *(158)*. Such individuals may be diagnosed when a sibling is found to have more typical FA features or when they develop hematological problems themselves as adolescents or young adults. Elevated serum α-fetoprotein levels, which are observed in these patients regardless of their liver status, may be a simple screening test, although it is not specific for FA *(159)*.

FA homozygotes/compound heterozygotes have a striking predisposition to malignancy. AML is the most common neoplasm observed, with an incidence more than 700 times that of the general population *(152,160)*. All AML types are represented with the exception of progranulocytic leukemia *(152)*. A review of the International FA Registry estimated an actuarial risk of at least 33% for developing AML or myelodysplasia by age 40, and almost all Registry patients developed progressive bone marrow failure by adulthood *(148,161)*. Ascertainment bias, however, may affect these and other registry statistics. Other series have put the cumulative AML risk in FA at closer to 10% and MDS risk at 5–10% *(152)*, with an increase in this risk if patients develop clonal abnormalities of chromosome 3q in the marrow *(162)*. There is also a greatly increased incidence of solid tumors, especially vulvar, esophageal, and head and neck cancers *(148,152, 160,163)*. This tumor pattern may reflect the poor ability of FA patients to control papillomaviruses *(164)*. Hepatic tumors are also increased, probably because androgen therapy (a known risk factor for hepatoma) is commonly prescribed to palliate disease-associated anemia. It is not clear whether heterozygous carriers of an FA-associated gene have an increased risk of malignancy.

The diagnosis of FA is usually confirmed by demonstrating an increased sensitivity of patients' cells to DNA crosslinking agents such as mitomycin C or diepoxybutane in vitro *(165)*. The chromosome breakage pattern with these agents is usually characteristic, but somatic mosaicism may make test interpretation difficult *(166)*. The same clastogenic agents cause G2 delay or arrest that can be measured by flow cytometry in cycling cells from FA patients *(167)*.

Cell fusion experiments and somatic genetic work have demonstrated at least 11 different FA complementation groups, designated FA-A, FA-B, FA-C, FA-D1, FA-D2, FA-E, FA-F, FA-G, FA-I, FA-J, and FA-L *(168,169)*. FA-H was found to be a variant of FA-A and is no longer discussed *(170)*. Eight of the associated genes have been cloned, the first two (FA-A and FA-C) in 1996 *(171,172)* and the most recent (FA-B) in 2005 *(168,173)*. The gene most commonly mutated is *FANCA*, at chromosome 16q24.3, which is altered in 60–65% of FA patients *(171)*. *FANCC* and *FANCG* mutations account for most of the remaining cases.

There is mounting evidence that the FA genes are involved in coupling certain types of DNA damage to HR (Fig. 7). When FANCD1 was found to be identical to BRCA2, interest in this obscure hematopoietic disorder skyrocketed because of the link of BRCA2 to breast and ovarian cancer and the much greater general incidence of those conditions *(148)*. Damage of DNA by bifunctional alkylating agents leads to activation of the FA complex by unknown mechanisms. Within this activated complex, FANCB monoubiquitinates FANCD2 at lysine residue 561, triggering an interaction of FANCD2 directly with BRCA1 *(174,175)*. BRCA1, in turn, is part of a complex that produces the actual DNA repair, as described above.

New evidence suggests that the FA pathway can become involved in DNA repair by a second mechanism: ionizing radiation activates ATM and ATR, which phosphorylates FANCD2 instead of ubiquitinating it (Fig. 7) *(176)*. This leads to activation of an S-phase checkpoint response, which is also dependent on the MRE11/RAD50/NBN complex *(177)*.

For unclear reasons, telomere shortening is also accelerated in FA compared with age-matched healthy controls *(178)*. Although the neoplasia predisposition in FA makes sense in view of the inability to efficiently repair DNA damage, it is not presently known whether the telomerase shortening and associated senescence also contribute to the compromised hematopoiesis before causing MDS or AML.

4.2. Bloom Syndrome and Related Conditions

Bloom syndrome (BS, MIM cat. no. 210900), described by Donald Bloom in 1954 *(179)* and linked to chromosomal instability by James German in 1965 *(180)*, is an autosomal recessive disorder that is most commonly found in the Ashkenazi Jewish population resulting from a founder mutation *(181)*. The same mutation ("blmAsh") has now been described at low frequency in a number of ethnic groups. The true incidence of the disorder is unknown, but it is clearly very rare. The BS Registry *(182)* maintained by German includes several hundred patients, and the carrier rate in Israel is estimated at approx 1 in 1100 (perhaps as high as 1 in 100 in Ashkenazim) *(183)*. Afflicted patients are characterized by predisposition to early development of a wide variety of neoplasms, including AML *(184)*.

BS is linked to the *BLM* (Bloom syndrome; RECQ3L, RECQ2) gene at chromosome 15q26.1 *(185)*. This gene encodes a member of the RecQ helicase family (BLM) that is important in maintaining appropriate DNA conformation during chromosomal recombination and repair *(186)*. Together with topoisomerase III *(187)*, BLM resolves Holliday junctions during HR by a mechanism called double-junction dissolution that is distinct from classical Holliday junction resolution and that prevents erroneous exchange of flanking sequences *(137,188)*.

Other members of the RecQ helicase group that are associated with a predispostion to neoplasia include *WRN* (RECQ3, RECQL2), the gene that is linked to the progeria and varied cancer risk of Werner syndrome (MIM cat. no. 277700), and *RECQL4*, linked to Rothmund-Thomson syndrome (familial osteosarcoma, MIM cat. no. 268400) *(186,189)*. Rare cases of AML have been reported in Werner syndrome, and there is a report of AML in Rothmund-Thomson as well, but BS has a more striking predisposition to this specific malignancy *(190–192)*.

In BS, photosensitivity, immunodeficiency, and growth abnormalities are almost universal, and infertility is common *(185,193)*. Characteristic facial features, often described as a "keel-shaped face," include malar hypoplasia, a prominent nose, and a small mandible with protuberant ears *(194)*. In the full syndrome, upper lateral incisors are missing.

Photosensitivity is typical and may be mild or frankly disfiguring. Telangiectasias have been described *(195)*. Pigmentation abnormalities are common, especially on the trunk. Intellectual development is often (but not inevitably) subnormal. For unclear reasons, patients have a predisposition to diabetes *(196)*. They also frequently die from recurrent infections of the respiratory system *(184)*. Most patients have decreased immunoglobulin levels, athough the immunodeficiency is quite variable in severity *(141,197,198)*.

The typical BS patient is diagnosed in childhood, but some individuals may not be recognized until adulthood, as the growth retardation is not specific and can be mistaken for other forms of dwarfism *(193)*. Development of a neoplasm such as leukemia can belatedly lead to the proper diagnosis.

By age 25, approximately half of patients with BS have developed neoplasia *(184)*. Non-Hodgkin's lymphoma and AML predominate, but there are also case reports of various carcinomas, especially as patients age *(184)*. The exact incidence of AML is unknown; and there does not seem to be a predisposition to any specific subtype. The relative contributions of the underlying immunodeficiency and consequent impaired tumor surveillance vs the DNA repair defect itself to the neoplasia risk are unclear. Heterozygote carriers do not have syndromal features, but do have chromosomal breakage in spermatozoa *(199)* and possibly a slightly increased risk of malignancy (heterozygote mice certainly do get cancer at an increased rate over *BLM* wild type mice) *(145,200,201)*.

The diagnosis of BS is made by observing a markedly increased number of sister chromatid exchanges during karyotyping, which can be performed on prenatal specimens *(202,203)*. Despite all of the potentially serious problems from BS, life expectancy is now reasonably long, with many patients surviving well into adulthood *(194)*. Accordingly, when the adult hematologist encounters a leukemia patient with short stature or abnormal facial features, it seems prudent to consider the possibility of BS as well as FA, as a fraction of cases will represent a new diagnosis.

4.3. Nijmegen Breakage Syndrome

First described by a Dutch group in 1981, Nijmegen breakage syndrome (NBS, MIM cat. no. 251260), like BS and FA, is an autosomal recessive disorder *(142,204)*. NBS patients generally live in Eastern Europe or are descendants of immigrants from Eastern Europe. In the Czech Republic, the heterozygote frequency is estimated at 1 in 130, leading to a birth rate of 1 in 90,000 *(205)*. Nonetheless, the NBS registry includes fewer than 100 cases *(206)*.

NBS is caused by abnormalities in the *NBN* gene at 8p21 *(207,208)*, which encodes the protein NBN (NBS1). Complete loss of this polypeptide is lethal; the disease-causing gene encodes a hypomorphic allele. The NBN polypeptide forms a complex with MRE11 and RAD50 (Fig. 6) that localizes to DNA ds breaks and is involved in DNA damage-induced signaling and HR as described above *(74,209)*.

NBS children have short stature, microcephaly, and immunodeficiency *(210)*. The short stature is often accompanied by rather striking microcephaly and what is sometimes called a "bird-like face," including a long sloping forehead and nose, a small mandible, and abnormal slanting of the palpebral fissures *(211)*. The frontal lobe of the brain is markedly underdeveloped *(210,212)*. A number of other serious malformations, including limb malformations and gastrointestinal narrowing, have also been described. Hypopigmented skin lesions are commonly seen, as are café-au-lait spots.

Neoplasia, the most common cause of death for NBS patients, often develops in the first decade of life and has occurred in 40% of patients by age 21 *(206)*. Although the predominant neoplasm is lymphoma, both lymphoid and myeloid leukemia have been reported *(213)*, as have a few solid tumors. Heterozygotes have no developmental abnormalities, but chromosome instability is present and there is probably an increased malignancy risk *(214–216)*. Acquired mutations in NBS1 do not appear to be common in AML cells *(208,217)*.

As with BS, immunodeficiency is the second most common cause of death in NBS, usually from recurrent respiratory tract infections *(206)*. These patients generally have hypogamma-globulinemia or sometimes complete agammaglobulinemia (described in about one-third of cases) *(218)*. The patients exhibit lymphopenia and, at autopsy, a hypoplastic thymus *(212)*. Overall, life expectancy is markedly reduced *(206)*.

Even in the absence of malignancy, conventional cytogenetic studies indicate that the blood karyotype is often abnormal in NBS, with structural chromosomal abnormalities reported in about one-third of cases *(219)*. These most commonly involve chromosomes 7 and 14 at the sites of T-cell receptor and immunoglobulin genes, respectively, and may be a consequence of immunodevelopmental gene rearrangement proceeding in a faulty manner *(204,219)*. NBS patients' chromosomes are generally hypersensitive to irradiation, an observation that can be used diagnostically, but occasional cases have normal chromosome stability *(204,220)*. Almost all cases have an identical point mutation of *NBN* (657del5) *(208,221)*. Testing for this mutation can help eliminate any confusion with AT or ataxia-telangiectasia-like disorder (ATLD). Other features that distinguish NBS from AT include the lack of neurodegeneration and normal serum α-fetoprotein levels in NBS. NBS cases have also been confused with FA, in part because of the associated short stature and other overlapping features, including aplastic anemia *(222,223)*.

4.4. Ataxia-Telangiectasia and Ataxia-Telangiectasia-Like Disorder

AT (MIM cat. no. 208900) is an autosomal recessive disorder with no particular population predisposition. Patients exhibit characteristic cutaneous and ocular telangiectasias, progressive cerebellar ataxia, immunodeficiency, and an increased incidence of malignancy, especially lymphoid neoplasms *(144,224–226)*. The homozygous form of the disorder (actually compound heterozygous in most cases, unlike NBS and BS) was first described in the French literature in 1926 and named AT in 1958 *(227,228)*. Although AT is rare (11 patients per million births), heterozygosity is common, with approx 1 in 50 Americans of European descent having a mutation in the *ATM* gene *(229,230)*. A registry is maintained at the Karolinska Institute in Stockholm (http://www.biosci.ki.se/ATbase/). Like NBS sufferers, AT patients are hypersensitive to ionizing radiation, both clinically and at a karyotypic level *(224)*. Like BS and FA patients, AT patients develop diabetes mellitus as a result of insulin resistance *(231)*.

The *ATM* (ataxia-telangiectasia-mutated) gene at chromosome 11q22.3 *(232)* encodes a protein kinase that, as described above, plays a critical role in DNA damage detection and in halting cell cycle progression until repair is completed *(67,68)*. When ATM is dysfunctional or absent, cells are able to progress from G1 to S phase and initiate DNA replication in the presence of DNA damage. While the mechanism of ATM activation remains the subject of current investigation *(75,233)*, it is clear that activated ATM phosphorylates a number of polypeptides that contribute to cell cycle arrest and DNA repair, including BRCA1, NBN, the c-ABL tyrosine kinase, and p53 *(72,234)*. In addition, ATM phosphorylates eIF-4E-binding protein 1, which does not appear to have any specific DNA repair function, but instead contributes to insulin-induced cell protein synthesis. Failure to phosphorylate this latter polypeptide may explain the diabetes risk and perhaps some of the growth retardation seen in AT patients *(235)*.

AT patients are typically identified in the first few years of life. After uncomplicated perinatal and early developmental periods, their walking skills do not progress normally, and oculomotor function is noticeably abnormal *(236,237)*. They have a peculiar weaving gait, yet rarely fall. Many patients are mistakenly diagnosed with cerebral palsy until the degenerative nature of the disease and the associated anomalies are appreciated *(238)*. Skin findings are primarily scattered telangiectasias, but it is important to note that these generally do not appear until the preschool period. The diagnosis can be made before telangiectasias are present; and AT should be considered as part of the differential diagnosis of infantile ataxia *(238)*.

AT is accompanied by characteristic but nonspecific laboratory abnormalities. AT patients usually have elevation of α-fetoprotein, a finding that is present from the first year of life, does not correlate with the severity of disease, and is of unclear etiology *(239)*. As with NBS, chromosomes 7 and 14 seem to be particularly common areas of chromosomal translocations and rearrangements *(240,241)*. Serum IgA levels are usually low in AT. Published diagnostic criteria for AT incorporate the clinical findings described above, low IgA levels, elevated serum α-fetoprotein, and increased irradiation-induced and spontaneous chromosomal fragility in cultured cells *(242)*.

The median age of AT patients at death is about 20 years. Immunodeficiency, which may include hypogammaglobulinemia, IgG and IgA subclass deficiency, and/or lymphopenia *(243–245)*, is associated with recurrent sinopulmonary and other infections. Even though this immunodeficiency is variable, the associated infections represent the leading cause of death in AT *(226)*.

Neoplasms are also quite common in AT patients, representing the second most common cause of death. While almost all of these are lymphomas and lymphoid leukemias, AML has also been reported *(246,247)*. It is important to recognize the underlying AT in patients with these malignancies because administration of conventional doses of ionizing radiation and chemotherapy can be catastrophic, as with FA *(248–250)*. Even patients who are given reduced doses (or are simple heterozygotes) may have an increased risk for acute and late complications of chemoradiotherapy *(251)*. Because radiosensitivity may vary from patient to patient, however, dosing decisions are complex *(252)*.

There is controversy over whether heterozygosity for an ATM mutation also predisposes to cancer, especially breast cancer *(225)*. One study of 161 families with AT (performed before the gene was cloned) suggested a 3.5- to 6.4-fold increase in overall cancer rate *(230,253)*. In addition, genealogical records showed that AT carrier grandparents died approx 8 years earlier than grandparents of matched families without AT, primarily from cancer *(254)*. Another analysis of 1423 AT patient blood relatives showed a more modest increase for breast cancer and no increase other tumors *(255)*, and a similar population-based study of 1218 Scandinavian patients from 50 AT families suggested a slight increase in breast cancer that was not statistically significant *(256)*. The precise cancer risk may depend on the specific *ATM* mutation present *(257)*.

An AT-related condition called ataxia telangiectasia-like disorder (ATLD, MIM cat. no. 604391) was first clinically identified in the United Kingdom as a degenerative ataxia that failed to link to chromosome 11q22-23, where the AT locus had been placed even before the *ATM* gene was cloned *(258)*. ATLD is now known to be caused by mutations in the *MRE11A* gene at 11q21, which encodes another member of the MRE11/RAD50/NBN complex that is so important for HR *(259)*. ATLD has only been diagnosed in a few families, but some experts believe that a proportion of AT cases not studied genetically are actually ATLD that has been misdiagnosed. ATLD patients have progressive ataxia and oculomotor apraxia, but lack telangiectasia, α-fetoprotein elevation, and hypogammaglobulins *(258,260)*. The paucity of characteristic features means a high index of suspicion is necessary for the proper diagnosis to be made. Lymphocytes demonstrate the same chromosomal breaks, both spontaneous and radiation-induced, that are seen in AT. Because the overall frequency of this rare condition is unknown, it is not clear whether it also predisposes to AML.

4.5. Seckel Syndrome and Others

There are a number of other familial leukemia syndromes that are, as of yet, unexplained. Given the complexity of DNA repair pathways, it is possible that some of these are to the result of fundamental DNA repair defects that have not yet been detected, including private mutations. For instance, a new syndrome due to mutations in DNA ligase IV at 13q22-34 (LIG4 syndrome, MIM cat. no. 606593) was described in 2001 *(261)*. Like FA, LIG4 syndrome is associated with pancytopenia. Only time will tell if patients with this NHEJ abnormality develop MDS or AML *(262)*.

Another illustrative example is Seckel syndrome ("bird-headed dwarfism," MIM cat. no. 210600 and others), named for Hans Seckel, who in 1960 wrote a pioneering book on 13 such cases in the published literature or in his clinic. One form of Seckel syndrome was recently linked to splicing mutations in *ATR* at 3q22-24, which encodes the ATR kinase that responds to replication stress by phosphorylating Chk1 and activating the S-phase checkpoint as described above (Fig. 7) *(263)*. Only a few dozen cases of this obscure malady have been reported, and the causes for cases that link to chromosomes 18 and 14 remain unknown. These individuals have chromosomal instability at fragile sites, a peculiar type of genomic instability that has been traced to defective ATR function *(264)*. Despite the extreme rarity of the syndrome, there is now a report of Seckel syndrome-associated AML with multiple karyotypic abnormalities *(265)*. As might be expected in a syndrome in which responses to replicative stresses are abnormal *(72)*, treatment of this patient with chemotherapy led to prolonged marrow aplasia and death.

It is also important to point out that not all defects in checkpoint and repair pathways lead to an increased risk of acute leukemia. Mosaic variegated aneuploidy syndrome (MIM cat. no. 257300), a rare autosomal recessive condition characterized by short stature, chromosomal aneuploidy, and cancer risk, initially seemed a likely candidate for a DNA repair defect, especially when a 3-year-old child with the condition developed MDS *(266)*. However, chromosomal instability was not present, and the syndrome was soon thereafter linked to mutations in the *BUB1B* (budding uninhibited by benzimidazoles 1) gene, which encodes a key regulator of the mitotic spindle checkpoint and chromosome segregation *(267,268)*. In addition, several proteins such as BRCA1 that directly interact with a number of factors that clearly do cause AML do not themselves appear to carry an increased leukemia risk when mutated. Accordingly, many pages in the story of leukemia and DNA repair have yet to be written.

5. KARYOTYPIC ABNORMALITIES IN THERAPY-RELATED MDS AND AML: FAILURE OF DNA REPAIR OR PHENOCOPY?

One of the striking features of therapy-related MDS and AML, particularly after alkylator therapy, is the presence of frequent large chromosomal deletions and translocations *(269)*. It is tempting to speculate that these chromosomal abnormalities reflect a failure in the mechanism of DNA ds repair. Aside from some defects in mismatch repair, which have not been associated with chromosomal abnormalities in other neoplasms (e.g., colon cancer), however, defects in DNA repair have not generally been found in therapy-related AML.

It is also important to recognize that gross chromosome structural abnormalities like those seen in therapy-related AML and MDS may also result when cells have divided so many times that their telomeres (long $(TTAGGG)_n$ repeats) have shortened to the point where they can no longer faithfully mark chromosome ends *(270)*. Because of rapid cell division, telomeres in neoplastic cells are often shorter than normal, even though telomerase, a specialized reverse transcriptase normally active only in germ cells and a few other specialized cells, is often reactivated in neoplastic cells *(270)*. If the telomeres get too short, genomic chaos with inhibition of DNA repair may result, causing a "telomere crisis" *(271–273)*. Ku proteins, which can easily tell the difference between broken DNA and telomeres, do not initiate NHEJ when the flailing end of a DNA segment that they encounter is actually a telomere *(274)*.

Although the telomere failure mechanism of genomic instability may be operative in MDS and AML, more work needs to be done to prove this hypothesis *(32,275)*. Telomeres in these conditions are shorter than normal—especially in patients with an abnormal karyotype—and telomerase expression is sometimes (but not always) abnormal *(276–281)*. Specific mutations in the gene encoding telomerase, however, have not been found.

6. CONCLUSION

Failure of cells to recognize and efficiently repair damaged DNA is an important component of the neoplastic phenotype. Abnormalities in DNA response and repair pathways can be either inherited or acquired. The relevant molecular pathways are extraordinarily complex; and considerable work is ongoing to define them more fully. Investigative efforts into the role of these systems specifically in AML are only in their infancy. While it is clear that certain defects in these pathways can create a genetic predisposition to AML, the vast majority of AML patients do not have familial syndromes with repair defects. Nonetheless, existing evidence suggests that genomic instability is relevant, particularly for therapy-related leukemia and MDS.

ACKNOWLEDGMENTS

Supported in part by K12 CA90628. I thank Scott Kaufmann for helpful comments on the manuscript and Deb Strauss for editorial assistance.

REFERENCES

1. Blanco JG, Edick MJ, Hancock ML, et al. Genetic polymorphisms in CYP3A5, CYP3A4 and NQO1 in children who developed therapy-related myeloid malignancies. Pharmacogenetics 2002;12(8):605–611.
2. Collado M, Barragan E, Bolufer P, et al. Lack of association of CYP3A4-V polymorphism with the risk of treatment-related leukemia. Leuk Res 2005;29(5):595–597.
3. Naoe T, Takeyama K, Yokozawa T, et al. Analysis of genetic polymorphism in NQO1, GST-M1, GST-T1, and CYP3A4 in 469 Japanese patients with therapy-related leukemia/ myelodysplastic syndrome and de novo acute myeloid leukemia. Clin Cancer Res 2000;6(10):4091–4095.
4. Felix CA, Walker AH, Lange BJ, et al. Association of CYP3A4 genotype with treatment-related leukemia. Proc Natl Acad Sci USA 1998;95(22):13176–13181.
5. Weischenfeldt J, Lykke-Andersen J, Porse B. Messenger RNA surveillance: neutralizing natural nonsense. Curr Biol 2005;15(14):R559–R562.
6. Conti E, Izaurralde E. Nonsense-mediated mRNA decay: molecular insights and mechanistic variations across species. Curr Opin Cell Biol 2005;17(3):316–325.

7. Mansfield SG, Chao H, Walsh CE. RNA repair using spliceosome-mediated RNA trans-splicing. Trends Mol Med 2004;10(6):263–268.
8. Matlin AJ, Clark F, Smith CW. Understanding alternative splicing: towards a cellular code. Nat Rev Mol Cell Biol 2005;6(5):386–398.
9. Hoeijmakers JH. Genome maintenance mechanisms for preventing cancer. Nature 2001;411(6835):366–374.
10. Lindahl T, Wood RD. Quality control by DNA repair. Science 1999;286(5446):1897–1905.
11. Sancar A, Lindsey-Boltz LA, Unsal-Kacmaz K, Linn S. Molecular mechanisms of mammalian DNA repair and the DNA damage checkpoints. Annu Rev Biochem 2004;73:39–85.
12. Wood RD, Mitchell M, Lindahl T. Human DNA repair genes, 2005. Mutat Res 2005;577(1–2):275–283.
13. Bielas JH, Loeb LA. Mutator phenotype in cancer: timing and perspectives. Environ Mol Mutagen 2005;45(2–3):206–213.
14. Kalogeraki VS, Tornaletti S, Hanawalt PC. Transcription arrest at a lesion in the transcribed DNA strand in vitro is not affected by a nearby lesion in the opposite strand. J Biol Chem 2003;278(21):19,558–19,564.
15. Garber JE, Offit K. Hereditary cancer predisposition syndromes. J Clin Oncol 2005;23(2):276–292.
16. Das-Gupta EP, Seedhouse CH, Russell NH. DNA repair mechanisms and acute myeloblastic leukemia. Hematol Oncol 2000;18(3):99–110.
17. Evan GI, Vousden KH. Proliferation, cell cycle and apoptosis in cancer. Nature 2001;411(6835):342–348.
18. Ford JM, Hanawalt PC. Role of DNA excision repair gene defects in the etiology of cancer. Curr Top Microbiol Immunol 1997;221:47–70.
19. O'Driscoll M, Jeggo P. Immunological disorders and DNA repair. Mutat Res 2002;509(1–2):109–126.
20. Storb U, Peters A, Kim N, et al. Molecular aspects of somatic hypermutation of immunoglobulin genes. Cold Spring Harb Symp Quant Biol 1999;64:227–234.
21. Lehmann AR. The xeroderma pigmentosum group D (XPD) gene: one gene, two functions, three diseases. Genes Dev 2001;15(1):15–23.
22. Hoogervorst EM, van Steeg H, de Vries A. Nucleotide excision repair- and p53-deficient mouse models in cancer research. Mutat Res 2005;574(1–2):3–21.
23. Ishikawa T, Zhang SS, Qin X, et al. DNA repair and cancer: lessons from mutant mouse models. Cancer Sci 2004;95(2):112–117.
24. Wilson DM, 3rd, Thompson LH. Life without DNA repair. Proc Natl Acad Sci USA 1997;94(24):12,754–12,757.
25. Loeb LA. Cancer cells exhibit a mutator phenotype. Adv Cancer Res 1998;72:25–56.
26. Loeb KR, Loeb LA. Significance of multiple mutations in cancer. Carcinogenesis 2000;21(3):379–385.
27. Loeb LA. Mutator phenotype may be required for multistage carcinogenesis. Cancer Res 1991;51(12):3075–3079.
28. Peltomaki P. Role of DNA mismatch repair defects in the pathogenesis of human cancer. J Clin Oncol 2003;21(6):1174–1179.
29. Sampson JR, Jones S, Dolwani S, Cheadle JP. MutYH (MYH) and colorectal cancer. Biochem Soc Trans 2005;33(pt 4):679–683.
30. Rowley PT. Inherited susceptibility to colorectal cancer. Annu Rev Med 2005;56:539–554.
31. Kramer A, Neben K, Ho AD. Centrosome aberrations in hematological malignancies. Cell Biol Int 2005;29(5):375–383.
32. Ohyashiki JH, Ohyashiki K, Fujimura T, et al. Telomere shortening associated with disease evolution patterns in myelodysplastic syndromes. Cancer Res 1994;54(13):3557–3560.
33. Steensma DP, List AF. Genetic testing in the myelodysplastic syndromes: molecular insights into hemato-logic diversity. Mayo Clin Proc 2005;80(5):681–698.
34. Schoch C, Kern W, Kohlmann A, Hiddemann W, Schnittger S, Haferlach T. Acute myeloid leukemia with a complex aberrant karyotype is a distinct biological entity characterized by genomic imbalances and a specific gene expression profile. Genes Chromosomes Cancer 2005;43(3):227–238.
35. Yamaizumi M, Sugano T. U.v.-induced nuclear accumulation of p53 is evoked through DNA damage of actively transcribed genes independent of the cell cycle. Oncogene 1994;9(10):2775–2784.
36. Friedberg EC, Wagner R, Radman M. Specialized DNA polymerases, cellular survival, and the genesis of mutations. Science 2002;296(5573):1627–1630.
37. Kunkel TA, Pavlov YI, Bebenek K. Functions of human DNA polymerases eta, kappa and iota suggested by their properties, including fidelity with undamaged DNA templates. DNA Repair (Amst) 2003;2(2):135–149.
38. Kunkel TA. Considering the cancer consequences of altered DNA polymerase function. Cancer Cell 2003;3(2):105–110.

39. Shcherbakova PV, Bebenek K, Kunkel TA. Functions of eukaryotic DNA polymerases. Sci Aging Knowledge Environ 2003;2003(8):RE3.
40. Goodman MF, Tippin B. Sloppier copier DNA polymerases involved in genome repair. Curr Opin Genet Dev 2000;10(2):162–168.
41. Masutani C, Kusumoto R, Yamada A, et al. The XPV (xeroderma pigmentosum variant) gene encodes human DNA polymerase eta. Nature 1999;399(6737):700–704.
42. Johnson RE, Kondratick CM, Prakash S, Prakash L. hRAD30 mutations in the variant form of xeroderma pigmentosum. Science 1999;285(5425):263–265.
43. Vidakovic M, Poznanovic G, Bode J. DNA break repair: refined rules of an already complicated game. Biochem Cell Biol 2005;83(3):365–373.
44. Kaina B, Christmann M. DNA repair in resistance to alkylating anticancer drugs. Int J Clin Pharmacol Ther 2002;40(8):354–367.
45. Gerson SL, Trey JE. Modulation of nitrosourea resistance in myeloid leukemias. Blood 1988;71(5):1487–1494.
46. Kohonen-Corish MR, Daniel JJ, Chan C, et al. Low microsatellite instability is associated with poor prognosis in stage C colon cancer. J Clin Oncol 2005;23(10):2318–2324.
47. Hegi ME, Diserens AC, Gorlia T, et al. MGMT gene silencing and benefit from temozolomide in glioblastoma. N Engl J Med 2005;352(10):997–1003.
48. Ford JM. DNA damage response pathways and cancer. In: Abeloff MD, Armitage JO, Niederhuber JE, Kastan MB, McKenna WG, eds. Clinical Oncology (3rd edition). Philadelphia: Churchill Livingstone; 2004:191–205.
49. Seeberg E, Eide L, Bjoras M. The base excision repair pathway. Trends Biochem Sci 1995;20(10):391–397.
50. Batty DP, Wood RD. Damage recognition in nucleotide excision repair of DNA. Gene 2000;241(2):193–204.
51. de Laat WL, Jaspers NG, Hoeijmakers JH. Molecular mechanism of nucleotide excision repair. Genes Dev 1999;13(7):768–785.
52. Kolodner RD, Marsischky GT. Eukaryotic DNA mismatch repair. Curr Opin Genet Dev 1999;9(1):89–96.
53. Kunkel TA, Erie DA. DNA Mismatch Repair. Annu Rev Biochem 2004.
54. Khanna KK, Jackson SP. DNA double-strand breaks: signaling, repair and the cancer connection. Nat Genet 2001;27(3):247–254.
55. Weterings E, van Gent DC. The mechanism of non-homologous end-joining: a synopsis of synapsis. DNA Repair (Amst) 2004;3(11):1425–1435.
56. Helleday T. Pathways for mitotic homologous recombination in mammalian cells. Mutat Res 2003;532(1–2):103–115.
57. Dudas A, Chovanec M. DNA double-strand break repair by homologous recombination. Mutat Res 2004;566(2):131–167.
58. Takata M, Sasaki MS, Sonoda E, et al. Homologous recombination and non-homologous end-joining pathways of DNA double-strand break repair have overlapping roles in the maintenance of chromosomal integrity in vertebrate cells. EMBO J 1998;17(18):5497–5508.
59. Jackson SP. Sensing and repairing DNA double-strand breaks. Carcinogenesis 2002;23(5):687–696.
60. Bradbury JM, Jackson SP. The complex matter of DNA double-strand break detection. Biochem Soc Trans 2003;31(pt 1):40–44.
61. Cline SD, Hanawalt PC. Who's on first in the cellular response to DNA damage? Nat Rev Mol Cell Biol 2003;4(5):361–372.
62. van Hoffen A, Balajee AS, van Zeeland AA, Mullenders LH. Nucleotide excision repair and its interplay with transcription. Toxicology 2003;193(1–2):79–90.
63. Yang LY, Jiang H, Rangel KM. RNA polymerase II stalled on a DNA template during transcription elongation is ubiquitinated and the ubiquitination facilitates displacement of the elongation complex. Int J Oncol 2003;22(3):683–689.
64. van den Boom V, Jaspers NG, Vermeulen W. When machines get stuck—obstructed RNA polymerase II: displacement, degradation or suicide. Bioessays 2002;24(9):780–784.
65. Lisby M, Rothstein R. DNA damage checkpoint and repair centers. Curr Opin Cell Biol 2004;16(3):328–334.
66. Shiloh Y. ATM: sounding the double-strand break alarm. Cold Spring Harb Symp Quant Biol 2000;65:527–533.
67. Shiloh Y. ATM and related protein kinases: safeguarding genome integrity. Nat Rev Cancer 2003;3(3):155–168.

68. Khanna KK, Lavin MF, Jackson SP, Mulhern TD. ATM, a central controller of cellular responses to DNA damage. Cell Death Differ 2001;8(11):1052–1065.
69. Jhanwar-Uniyal M. BRCA1 in cancer, cell cycle and genomic stability. Front Biosci 2003;8:s1107–1117.
70. Janus F, Albrechtsen N, Dornreiter I, Wiesmuller L, Grosse F, Deppert W. The dual role model for p53 in maintaining genomic integrity. Cell Mol Life Sci 1999;55(1):12–27.
71. Sigal A, Rotter V. Oncogenic mutations of the p53 tumor suppressor: the demons of the guardian of the genome. Cancer Res 2000;60(24):6788–6793.
72. Kastan MB, Bartek J. Cell-cycle checkpoints and cancer. Nature 2004;432(7015):316–323.
73. Sorensen CS, Hansen LT, Dziegielewski J, et al. The cell-cycle checkpoint kinase Chk1 is required for mammalian homologous recombination repair. Nat Cell Biol 2005;7(2):195–201.
74. Connelly JC, Leach DR. Tethering on the brink: the evolutionarily conserved Mre11-Rad50 complex. Trends Biochem Sci 2002;27(8):410–418.
75. Falck J, Coates J, Jackson SP. Conserved modes of recruitment of ATM, ATR and DNA-PKcs to sites of DNA damage. Nature 2005;434(7033):605–611.
76. Fortini P, Pascucci B, Parlanti E, D'Errico M, Simonelli V, Dogliotti E. The base excision repair: mechanisms and its relevance for cancer susceptibility. Biochimie 2003;85(11):1053–1071.
77. Cadet J, Berger M, Douki T, Ravanat JL. Oxidative damage to DNA: formation, measurement, and biological significance. Rev Physiol Biochem Pharmacol 1997;131:1–87.
78. Lindahl T. Instability and decay of the primary structure of DNA. Nature 1993;362(6422):709–715.
79. Finkel T, Holbrook NJ. Oxidants, oxidative stress and the biology of ageing. Nature 2000;408(6809):239–247.
80. Dizdaroglu M. Base-excision repair of oxidative DNA damage by DNA glycosylases. Mutat Res 2005; 591(1–2):45–59.
81. Whitehouse CJ, Taylor RM, Thistlethwaite A, et al. XRCC1 stimulates human polynucleotide kinase activity at damaged DNA termini and accelerates DNA single-strand break repair. Cell 2001;104(1):107–117.
82. Liu Y, Beard WA, Shock DD, Prasad R, Hou EW, Wilson SH. DNA polymerase beta and flap endonuclease 1 enzymatic specificities sustain DNA synthesis for long patch base excision repair. J Biol Chem 2005; 280(5):3665–3674.
83. Seo YR, Fishel ML, Amundson S, Kelley MR, Smith ML. Implication of p53 in base excision DNA repair: in vivo evidence. Oncogene 2002;21(5):731–737.
84. Smith ML, Seo YR. p53 regulation of DNA excision repair pathways. Mutagenesis 2002;17(2):149–156.
85. Seo YR, Jung HJ. The potential roles of p53 tumor suppressor in nucleotide excision repair (NER) and base excision repair (BER). Exp Mol Med 2004;36(6):505–509.
86. Xanthoudakis S, Smeyne RJ, Wallace JD, Curran T. The redox/DNA repair protein, Ref-1, is essential for early embryonic development in mice. Proc Natl Acad Sci USA 1996;93(17):8919–8923.
87. Gu H, Marth JD, Orban PC, Mossmann H, Rajewsky K. Deletion of a DNA polymerase beta gene segment in T cells using cell type-specific gene targeting. Science 1994;265(5168):103–106.
88. Al-Tassan N, Chmiel NH, Maynard J, et al. Inherited variants of MYH associated with somatic G:C>->T:A mutations in colorectal tumors. Nat Genet 2002;30(2):227–232.
89. Zhang X, Miao X, Liang G, et al. Polymorphisms in DNA base excision repair genes ADPRT and XRCC1 and risk of lung cancer. Cancer Res 2005;65(3):722–726.
90. Hutsell SQ, Sancar A. Nucleotide excision repair, oxidative damage, DNA sequence polymorphisms, and cancer treatment. Clin Cancer Res 2005;11(4):1355–1357.
91. Sugasawa K, Okamoto T, Shimizu Y, Masutani C, Iwai S, Hanaoka F. A multistep damage recognition mechanism for global genomic nucleotide excision repair. Genes Dev 2001;15(5):507–521.
92. Janicijevic A, Sugasawa K, Shimizu Y, et al. DNA bending by the human damage recognition complex XPC-HR23B. DNA Repair (Amst) 2003;2(3):325–336.
93. Buschta-Hedayat N, Buterin T, Hess MT, Missura M, Naegeli H. Recognition of nonhybridizing base pairs during nucleotide excision repair of DNA. Proc Natl Acad Sci USA 1999;96(11):6090–6095.
94. Liu J, Akoulitchev S, Weber A, et al. Defective interplay of activators and repressors with TFIH in xeroderma pigmentosum. Cell 2001;104(3):353–363.
95. Houtsmuller AB, Rademakers S, Nigg AL, Hoogstraten D, Hoeijmakers JH, Vermeulen W. Action of DNA repair endonuclease ERCC1/XPF in living cells. Science 1999;284(5416):958–961.
96. Ford JM. Regulation of DNA damage recognition and nucleotide excision repair: Another role for p53. Mutat Res 2005;577(1–2):195–202.
97. Mellon I. Transcription-coupled repair: A complex affair. Mutat Res 2005;577(1–2):155–161.
98. Tornaletti S, Hanawalt PC. Effect of DNA lesions on transcription elongation. Biochimie 1999;81(1–2):139–146.

99. Le Page F, Kwoh EE, Avrutskaya A, et al. Transcription-coupled repair of 8-oxoguanine: requirement for XPG, TFIIH, and CSB and implications for Cockayne syndrome. Cell 2000;101(2):159–171.

100. Lehmann AR. DNA repair-deficient diseases, xeroderma pigmentosum, Cockayne syndrome and trichothiodystrophy. Biochimie 2003;85(11):1101–1111.

101. Itin PH, Sarasin A, Pittelkow MR. Trichothiodystrophy: update on the sulfur-deficient brittle hair syndromes. J Am Acad Dermatol 2001;44(6):891–920; quiz 1–4.

102. Heyer J, Yang K, Lipkin M, Edelmann W, Kucherlapati R. Mouse models for colorectal cancer. Oncogene 1999;18(38):5325–5333.

103. Harfe BD, Jinks-Robertson S. DNA mismatch repair and genetic instability. Annu Rev Genet 2000;34: 359–399.

104. Lamers MH, Perrakis A, Enzlin JH, Winterwerp HH, de Wind N, Sixma TK. The crystal structure of DNA mismatch repair protein MutS binding to a G x T mismatch. Nature 2000;407(6805):711–717.

105. Jiricny J, Nystrom-Lahti M. Mismatch repair defects in cancer. Curr Opin Genet Dev 2000;10(2):157–161.

106. Jiricny J. Eukaryotic mismatch repair: an update. Mutat Res 1998;409(3):107–121.

107. Jiricny J. Replication errors: cha(lle)nging the genome. EMBO J 1998;17(22):6427–6436.

108. Olipitz W, Tilz GP, Beham-Schmid C, Eibinger C, Kerzina P, Sill H. Microsatellite analysis in acute myeloid leukaemia evolving from myelodysplastic syndrome. Br J Haematol 2001;112(1):248–249.

109. Ribeiro EM, Rodriguez JM, Coser VM, et al. Microsatellite instability and cytogenetic survey in myeloid leukemias. Braz J Med Biol Res 2002;35(2):153–159.

110. Rimsza LM, Kopecky KJ, Ruschulte J, et al. Microsatellite instability is not a defining genetic feature of acute myeloid leukemogenesis in adults: results of a retrospective study of 132 patients and review of the literature. Leukemia 2000;14(6):1044–1051.

111. Sill H, Goldman JM, Cross NC. Rarity of microsatellite alterations in acute myeloid leukaemia. Br J Cancer 1996;74(2):255–257.

112. Tasak T, Lee S, Spira S, et al. Infrequent microsatellite instability during the evolution of myelodysplastic syndrome to acute myelocytic leukemia. Leuk Res 1996;20(2):113–117.

113. Nomdedeu JF, Perea G, Estivill C, et al. Microsatellite instability is not an uncommon finding in adult de novo acute myeloid leukemia. Ann Hematol 2005;84(6):368–375.

114. Das-Gupta EP, Seedhouse CH, Russell NH. Microsatellite instability occurs in defined subsets of patients with acute myeloblastic leukaemia. Br J Haematol 2001;114(2):307–312.

115. Sheikhha MH, Tobal K, Liu Yin JA. High level of microsatellite instability but not hypermethylation of mismatch repair genes in therapy-related and secondary acute myeloid leukaemia and myelodysplastic syndrome. Br J Haematol 2002;117(2):359–365.

116. Casorelli I, Offman J, Mele L, et al. Drug treatment in the development of mismatch repair defective acute leukemia and myelodysplastic syndrome. DNA Repair (Amst) 2003;2(5):547–559.

117. Offman J, Opelz G, Doehler B, et al. Defective DNA mismatch repair in acute myeloid leukemia/myelodysplastic syndrome after organ transplantation. Blood 2004;104(3):822–828.

118. Ben-Yehuda D, Krichevsky S, Caspi O, et al. Microsatellite instability and p53 mutations in therapy-related leukemia suggest mutator phenotype. Blood 1996;88(11):4296–4303.

119. Zhu YM, Das-Gupta EP, Russell NH. Microsatellite instability and p53 mutations are associated with abnormal expression of the MSH2 gene in adult acute leukemia. Blood 1999;94(2):733–740.

120. Scott S, Kimura T, Ichinohasama R, et al. Microsatellite mutations of transforming growth factor-beta receptor type II and caspase-5 occur in human precursor T-cell lymphoblastic lymphomas/leukemias in vivo but are not associated with hMSH2 or hMLH1 promoter methylation. Leuk Res 2003;27(1):23–34.

121. Matsushita M, Takeuchi S, Yang Y, et al. Methylation of the MLH1 gene in hematological malignancies. Oncol Rep 2005;14(1):191–194.

122. Meijerink JP, Mensink EJ, Wang K, et al. Hematopoietic malignancies demonstrate loss-of-function mutations of BAX. Blood 1998;91(8):2991–2997.

123. Komatsu N, Takeuchi S, Ikezoe T, et al. Mutations of the E2F4 gene in hematological malignancies having microsatellite instability. Blood 2000;95(4):1509–1510.

124. Karran P, Offman J, Bignami M. Human mismatch repair, drug-induced DNA damage, and secondary cancer. Biochimie 2003;85(11):1149–1160.

125. Swann PF, Waters TR, Moulton DC, et al. Role of postreplicative DNA mismatch repair in the cytotoxic action of thioguanine. Science 1996;273(5278):1109–1111.

126. Aebi S, Fink D, Gordon R, et al. Resistance to cytotoxic drugs in DNA mismatch repair-deficient cells. Clin Cancer Res 1997;3(10):1763–1767.

127. Paull TT, Rogakou EP, Yamazaki V, Kirchgessner CU, Gellert M, Bonner WM. A critical role for histone H2AX in recruitment of repair factors to nuclear foci after DNA damage. Curr Biol 2000;10(15):886–895.
128. Petrini JH. The Mre11 complex and ATM: collaborating to navigate S phase. Curr Opin Cell Biol 2000; 12(3):293–296.
129. Thacker J. The RAD51 gene family, genetic instability and cancer. Cancer Lett 2005;219(2):125–135.
130. Bhattacharyya A, Ear US, Koller BH, Weichselbaum RR, Bishop DK. The breast cancer susceptibility gene BRCA1 is required for subnuclear assembly of Rad51 and survival following treatment with the DNA cross-linking agent cisplatin. J Biol Chem 2000;275(31):23,899–23,8903.
131. Ting NS, Lee WH. The DNA double-strand break response pathway: becoming more BRCAish than ever. DNA Repair (Amst) 2004;3(8–9):935–944.
132. Davies AA, Masson JY, McIlwraith MJ, et al. Role of BRCA2 in control of the RAD51 recombination and DNA repair protein. Mol Cell 2001;7(2):273–282.
133. Zhang J, Willers H, Feng Z, et al. Chk2 phosphorylation of BRCA1 regulates DNA double-strand break repair. Mol Cell Biol 2004;24(2):708–718.
134. Unal E, Arbel-Eden A, Sattler U, et al. DNA damage response pathway uses histone modification to assemble a double-strand break-specific cohesin domain. Mol Cell 2004;16(6):991–1002.
135. Tischkowitz M, Dokal I. Fanconi anaemia and leukaemia—clinical and molecular aspects. Br J Haematol 2004;126(2):176–191.
136. van Gent DC, Hoeijmakers JH, Kanaar R. Chromosomal stability and the DNA double-stranded break connection. Nat Rev Genet 2001;2(3):196–206.
137. Wu L, Hickson ID. The Bloom's syndrome helicase suppresses crossing over during homologous recombination. Nature 2003;426(6968):870–874.
138. Johnson FB, Lombard DB, Neff NF, et al. Association of the Bloom syndrome protein with topoisomerase IIIalpha in somatic and meiotic cells. Cancer Res 2000;60(5):1162–1167.
139. Bohr VA, Sander M, Kraemer KH. Rare diseases provide rare insights into DNA repair pathways, TFIIH, aging and cancer center. DNA Repair (Amst) 2005;4(2):293–302.
140. van Brabant AJ, Stan R, Ellis NA. DNA helicases, genomic instability, and human genetic disease. Annu Rev Genomics Hum Genet 2000;1:409–459.
141. Gennery AR, Cant AJ, Jeggo PA. Immunodeficiency associated with DNA repair defects. Clin Exp Immunol 2000;121(1):1–7.
142. Weemaes CM, Smeets DF, van der Burgt CJ. Nijmegen Breakage syndrome: a progress report. Int J Radiat Biol 1994;66(6 Suppl):S185–188.
143. Olivier M, Goldgar DE, Sodha N, et al. Li-Fraumeni and related syndromes: correlation between tumor type, family structure, and TP53 genotype. Cancer Res 2003;63(20):6643–6650.
144. Stankovic T, Kidd AM, Sutcliffe A, et al. ATM mutations and phenotypes in ataxia-telangiectasia families in the British Isles: expression of mutant ATM and the risk of leukemia, lymphoma, and breast cancer. Am J Hum Genet 1998;62(2):334–345.
145. Gruber SB, Ellis NA, Scott KK, et al. BLM heterozygosity and the risk of colorectal cancer. Science 2002;297(5589):2013.
146. Howell RT. Sister chromatid exchange evaluation as an aid to the diagnosis and exclusion of Fanconi's anaemia by induced chromosome damage analysis. J Med Genet 1991;28(7):468–471.
147. Sieff CA, Nisbet-Brown E, Nathan DG. Congenital bone marrow failure syndromes. Br J Haematol 2000; 111(1):30–42.
148. Kutler DI, Singh B, Satagopan J, et al. A 20-year perspective on the International Fanconi Anemia Registry (IFAR). Blood 2003;101(4):1249–1256.
149. Schroeder TM, Tilgen D, Kruger J, Vogel F. Formal genetics of Fanconi's anemia. Hum Genet 1976;32(3):257–288.
150. Swift M. Fanconi's anaemia in the genetics of neoplasia. Nature 1971;230(5293):370–373.
151. Fanconi G. Familiaere infantile perniziosaartige Anaemie (pernizioeses Blutbild und Konstitution). Jahrbuch Kinderheil 1927;117:257–280.
152. Alter BP. Cancer in Fanconi anemia, 1927–2001. Cancer 2003;97(2):425–440.
153. Verlander PC, Kaporis A, Liu Q, Zhang Q, Seligsohn U, Auerbach AD. Carrier frequency of the IVS4 + 4 A—>T mutation of the Fanconi anemia gene FAC in the Ashkenazi Jewish population. Blood 1995; 86(11):4034–4038.
154. Rosendorff J, Bernstein R, Macdougall L, Jenkins T. Fanconi anemia: another disease of unusually high prevalence in the Afrikaans population of South Africa. Am J Med Genet 1987;27(4):793–797.

155. Morgan NV, Essop F, Demuth I, et al. A common Fanconi anemia mutation in black populations of sub-Saharan Africa. Blood 2005;105(9):3542–3544.
156. Callen E, Casado JA, Tischkowitz MD, et al. A common founder mutation in FANCA underlies the world's highest prevalence of Fanconi anemia in Gypsy families from Spain. Blood 2005;105(5):1946–1949.
157. Rosenberg PS, Huang Y, Alter BP. Individualized risks of first adverse events in patients with Fanconi anemia. Blood 2004;104(2):350–355.
158. Giampietro PF, Verlander PC, Davis JG, Auerbach AD. Diagnosis of Fanconi anemia in patients without congenital malformations: an international Fanconi Anemia Registry Study. Am J Med Genet 1997;68(1):58–61.
159. Cassinat B, Guardiola P, Chevret S, et al. Constitutive elevation of serum alpha-fetoprotein in Fanconi anemia. Blood 2000;96(3):859–863.
160. Rosenberg PS, Greene MH, Alter BP. Cancer incidence in persons with Fanconi anemia. Blood 2003;101(3):822–826.
161. Butturini A, Gale RP, Verlander PC, Adler-Brecher B, Gillio AP, Auerbach AD. Hematologic abnormalities in Fanconi anemia: an International Fanconi Anemia Registry study. Blood 1994;84(5):1650–1655.
162. Tonnies H, Huber S, Kuhl JS, Gerlach A, Ebell W, Neitzel H. Clonal chromosomal aberrations in bone marrow cells of Fanconi anemia patients: gains of the chromosomal segment 3q26q29 as an adverse risk factor. Blood 2003;101(10):3872–3874.
163. Kutler DI, Auerbach AD, Satagopan J, et al. High incidence of head and neck squamous cell carcinoma in patients with Fanconi anemia. Arch Otolaryngol Head Neck Surg 2003;129(1):106–112.
164. Lowy DR, Gillison ML. A new link between Fanconi anemia and human papillomavirus-associated malignancies. J Natl Cancer Inst 2003;95(22):1648–1650.
165. Auerbach AD. Fanconi anemia diagnosis and the diepoxybutane (DEB) test. Exp Hematol 1993;21(6):731–733.
166. Dokal I, Chase A, Morgan NV, et al. Positive diepoxybutane test in only one of two brothers found to be compound heterozygotes for Fanconi's anaemia complementation group C mutations. Br J Haematol 1996;93(4):813–816.
167. Seyschab H, Friedl R, Sun Y, et al. Comparative evaluation of diepoxybutane sensitivity and cell cycle blockage in the diagnosis of Fanconi anemia. Blood 1995;85(8):2233–2237.
168. Meetei AR, Levitus M, Xue Y, et al. X-linked inheritance of Fanconi anemia complementation group B. Nat Genet 2004;36(11):1219–1224.
169. Levitus M, Rooimans MA, Steltenpool J, et al. Heterogeneity in Fanconi anemia: evidence for 2 new genetic subtypes. Blood 2004;103(7):2498–2503.
170. Joenje H, Levitus M, Waisfisz Q, et al. Complementation analysis in Fanconi anemia: assignment of the reference FA-H patient to group A. Am J Hum Genet 2000;67(3):759–762.
171. Positional cloning of the Fanconi anaemia group A gene. The Fanconi anaemia/breast cancer consortium. Nat Genet 1996;14(3):324–328.
172. Lo Ten Foe JR, Rooimans MA, Bosnoyan-Collins L, et al. Expression cloning of a cDNA for the major Fanconi anaemia gene, FAA. Nat Genet 1996;14(3):320–323.
173. Fei P, Yin J, Wang W. New advances in the DNA damage response network of Fanconi anemia and BRCA proteins. FAAP95 replaces BRCA2 as the true FANCB protein. Cell Cycle 2005;4(1):80–86.
174. Hussain S, Wilson JB, Medhurst AL, et al. Direct interaction of FANCD2 with BRCA2 in DNA damage response pathways. Hum Mol Genet 2004;13(12):1241–1248.
175. Nakanishi K, Yang YG, Pierce AJ, et al. Human Fanconi anemia monoubiquitination pathway promotes homologous DNA repair. Proc Natl Acad Sci USA 2005;102(4):1110–1115.
176. Pichierri P, Rosselli F. The DNA crosslink-induced S-phase checkpoint depends on ATR-CHK1 and ATR-NBS1-FANCD2 pathways. EMBO J 2004;23(5):1178–1187.
177. Matsuura S, Kobayashi J, Tauchi H, Komatsu K. Nijmegen breakage syndrome and DNA double strand break repair by NBS1 complex. Adv Biophys 2004;38:65–80.
178. Leteurtre F, Li X, Guardiola P, et al. Accelerated telomere shortening and telomerase activation in Fanconi's anaemia. Br J Haematol 1999;105(4):883–893.
179. Bloom D. Congenital telangiectatic erythema resembling lupus erythematosus in dwarfs; probably a syndrome entity. AMA Am J Dis Child 1954;88(6):754–758.
180. German J, Archibald R, Bloom D. Chromosomal Breakage in a Rare and Probably Genetically Determined Syndrome of Man. Science 1965;148:506–507.

181. Ellis NA, Ciocci S, Proytcheva M, Lennon D, Groden J, German J. The Ashkenazic Jewish Bloom syndrome mutation blmAsh is present in non-Jewish Americans of Spanish ancestry. Am J Hum Genet 1998; 63(6):1685–1693.

182. German J, Bloom D, Passarge E. Bloom's syndrome XI. Progress report for 1983. Clin Genet 1984;25(2): 166–174.

183. Peleg L, Pesso R, Goldman B, et al. Bloom syndrome and Fanconi's anemia: rate and ethnic origin of mutation carriers in Israel. Isr Med Assoc J 2002;4(2):95–97.

184. German J. Bloom's syndrome. XX. The first 100 cancers. Cancer Genet Cytogenet 1997;93(1):100–106.

185. Ellis NA, German J. Molecular genetics of Bloom's syndrome. Hum Mol Genet 1996;5 Spec No:1457–1463.

186. Hickson ID. RecQ helicases: caretakers of the genome. Nat Rev Cancer 2003;3(3):169–178.

187. Wu L, Davies SL, North PS, et al. The Bloom's syndrome gene product interacts with topoisomerase III. J Biol Chem 2000;275(13):9636–9644.

188. Wu L, Lung Chan K, Ralf C, et al. The HRDC domain of BLM is required for the dissolution of double Holliday junctions. EMBO J 2005;24(14):2679–2687.

189. Mankouri HW, Hickson ID. Understanding the roles of RecQ helicases in the maintenance of genome integrity and suppression of tumorigenesis. Biochem Soc Trans 2004;32(Pt 6):957–958.

190. Bartal C, Yerushalmi R, Zilberman D, Yermiyahu T. A patient with Werner's syndrome and erythroleukemia: just coincidence? Leuk Lymphoma 1996;21(5–6):509–513.

191. Tao LC, Stecker E, Gardner HA. Werner's syndrome and acute myeloid leukemia. Can Med Assoc J 1971;105(9):951 passim.

192. Porter WM, Hardman CM, Abdalla SH, Powles AV. Haematological disease in siblings with Rothmund-Thomson syndrome. Clin Exp Dermatol 1999;24(6):452–454.

193. Kaneko H, Kondo N. Clinical features of Bloom syndrome and function of the causative gene, BLM helicase. Expert Rev Mol Diagn 2004;4(3):393–401.

194. German J. Bloom syndrome: a mendelian prototype of somatic mutational disease. Medicine (Baltimore) 1993;72(6):393–406.

195. Sahn EE, Hussey RH, 3rd, Christmann LM. A case of Bloom syndrome with conjunctival telangiectasia. Pediatr Dermatol 1997;14(2):120–124.

196. Kondo N, Asano J, Kimura S, Asano T, Orii T. Insulin-dependent diabetes developed in a young man with Bloom's syndrome. Clin Genet 1991;40(3):251–252.

197. Van Kerckhove CW, Ceuppens JL, Vanderschueren-Lodeweyckx M, Eggermont E, Vertessen S, Stevens EA. Bloom's syndrome. Clinical features and immunologic abnormalities of four patients. Am J Dis Child 1988;142(10):1089–1093.

198. Taniguchi N, Mukai M, Nagaoki T, et al. Impaired B-cell differentiation and T-cell regulatory function in four patients with Bloom's syndrome. Clin Immunol Immunopathol 1982;22(2):247–258.

199. Martin RH, Rademaker A, German J. Chromosomal breakage in human spermatozoa, a heterozygous effect of the Bloom syndrome mutation. Am J Hum Genet 1994;55(6):1242–1246.

200. Goss KH, Risinger MA, Kordich JJ, et al. Enhanced tumor formation in mice heterozygous for Blm mutation. Science 2002;297(5589):2051–2053.

201. Fodde R, Smits R. Cancer biology. A matter of dosage. Science 2002;298(5594):761–763.

202. Shulman LP, Li LR, Tharapel AT, Simpson JL, Elias S. Sister chromatid exchange (SCE) frequencies differ between directly prepared cytotrophoblasts and cultured mesenchymal core cells. Hum Genet 1991;87(6): 734–736.

203. Howell RT, Davies T. Diagnosis of Bloom's syndrome by sister chromatid exchange evaluation in chorionic villus cultures. Prenat Diagn 1994;14(11):1071–1073.

204. Weemaes CM, Hustinx TW, Scheres JM, van Munster PJ, Bakkeren JA, Taalman RD. A new chromosomal instability disorder: the Nijmegen breakage syndrome. Acta Paediatr Scand 1981;70(4):557–564.

205. Seeman P, Gebertova K, Paderova K, Sperling K, Seemanova E. Nijmegen breakage syndrome in 13% of age-matched Czech children with primary microcephaly. Pediatr Neurol 2004;30(3):195–200.

206. Nijmegen breakage syndrome. The International Nijmegen Breakage Syndrome Study Group. Arch Dis Child 2000;82(5):400–406.

207. Varon R, Vissinga C, Platzer M, et al. Nibrin, a novel DNA double-strand break repair protein, is mutated in Nijmegen breakage syndrome. Cell 1998;93(3):467–476.

208. Varon R, Schoch C, Reis A, Hiddemann WC, Sperling K, Schnittger S. Mutation analysis of the Nijmegen breakage syndrome gene (NBS1) in nineteen patients with acute myeloid leukemia with complex karyotypes. Leuk Lymphoma 2003;44(11):1931–1934.

209. Kobayashi J, Antoccia A, Tauchi H, Matsuura S, Komatsu K. NBS1 and its functional role in the DNA damage response. DNA Repair (Amst) 2004;3(8–9):855–861.
210. Bekiesinska-Figatowska M, Chrzanowska KH, Jurkiewicz E, et al. Magnetic resonance imaging of brain abnormalities in patients with the Nijmegen breakage syndrome. Acta Neurobiol Exp (Wars) 2004;64(4): 503–509.
211. van der Burgt I, Chrzanowska KH, Smeets D, Weemaes C. Nijmegen breakage syndrome. J Med Genet 1996;33(2):153–156.
212. Van de Kaa CA, Weemaes CM, Wesseling P, Schaafsma HE, Haraldsson A, De Weger RA. Postmortem findings in the Nijmegen breakage syndrome. Pediatr Pathol 1994;14(5):787–796.
213. Resnick IB, Kondratenko I, Togoev O, et al. Nijmegen breakage syndrome: clinical characteristics and mutation analysis in eight unrelated Russian families. J Pediatr 2002;140(3):355–361.
214. Tanzanella C, Antoccia A, Spadoni E, et al. Chromosome instability and nibrin protein variants in NBS heterozygotes. Eur J Hum Genet 2003;11(4):297–303.
215. Steffen J, Varon R, Mosor M, et al. Increased cancer risk of heterozygotes with NBS1 germline mutations in Poland. Int J Cancer 2004;111(1):67–71.
216. Seemanova E. An increased risk for malignant neoplasms in heterozygotes for a syndrome of microcephaly, normal intelligence, growth retardation, remarkable facies, immunodeficiency and chromosomal instability. Mutat Res 1990;238(3):321–324.
217. Taylor GM, O'Brien HP, Greaves MF, Ravetto PF, Eden OB. Correspondence re: R. Varon et al., Mutations in the Nijmegen breakage syndrome gene (NBS1) in childhood acute lymphoblastic leukemia. Cancer Res., 61: 3570–3572, 2001. Cancer Res 2003;63(19):6563–6564; author reply 5.
218. Chrzanowska KH, Kleijer WJ, Krajewska-Walasek M, et al. Eleven Polish patients with microcephaly, immunodeficiency, and chromosomal instability: the Nijmegen breakage syndrome. Am J Med Genet 1995; 57(3):462–471.
219. Taalman RD, Hustinx TW, Weemaes CM, et al. Further delineation of the Nijmegen breakage syndrome. Am J Med Genet 1989;32(3):425–431.
220. Seemanova E, Sperling K, Neitzel H, et al. Nijmegen Breakage Syndrome (NBS) with neurological abnormalities and without chromosomal instability. J Med Genet 2005;43(3):218–224.
221. Resnick IB, Kondratenko I, Pashanov E, et al. 657del5 mutation in the gene for Nijmegen breakage syndrome (NBS1) in a cohort of Russian children with lymphoid tissue malignancies and controls. Am J Med Genet A 2003;120(2):174–179.
222. New HV, Cale CM, Tischkowitz M, et al. Nijmegen breakage syndrome diagnosed as Fanconi anaemia. Pediatr Blood Cancer 2005;44(5):494–499.
223. Pasic S. Aplastic anemia in Nijmegen breakage syndrome. J Pediatr 2002;141(5):742.
224. Bundey S. Clinical and genetic features of ataxia-telangiectasia. Int J Radiat Biol 1994;66(6 Suppl): S23–29.
225. Khanna KK. Cancer risk and the ATM gene: a continuing debate. J Natl Cancer Inst 2000;92(10):795–802.
226. Nowak-Wegrzyn A, Crawford TO, Winkelstein JA, Carson KA, Lederman HM. Immunodeficiency and infections in ataxia-telangiectasia. J Pediatr 2004;144(4):505–511.
227. Centerwall WR, Miller MM. Ataxia, telangiectasia, and sinopulmonary infections; a syndrome of slowly progressive deterioration in childhood. AMA J Dis Child 1958;95(4):385–396.
228. Boder E, Sedgwick RP. Ataxia-telangiectasia; a familial syndrome of progressive cerebellar ataxia, oculocutaneous telangiectasia and frequent pulmonary infection. Pediatrics 1958;21(4):526–554.
229. Swift M, Morrell D, Cromartie E, Chamberlin AR, Skolnick MH, Bishop DT. The incidence and gene frequency of ataxia-telangiectasia in the United States. Am J Hum Genet 1986;39(5):573–583.
230. Swift M, Reitnauer PJ, Morrell D, Chase CL. Breast and other cancers in families with ataxia-telangiectasia. N Engl J Med 1987;316(21):1289–1294.
231. Morrell D, Chase CL, Kupper LL, Swift M. Diabetes mellitus in ataxia-telangiectasia, Fanconi anemia, xeroderma pigmentosum, common variable immune deficiency, and severe combined immune deficiency families. Diabetes 1986;35(2):143–147.
232. Savitsky K, Bar-Shira A, Gilad S, et al. A single ataxia telangiectasia gene with a product similar to PI-3 kinase. Science 1995;268(5218):1749–1753.
233. Bakkenist CJ, Kastan MB. DNA damage activates ATM through intermolecular autophosphorylation and dimer dissociation. Nature 2003;421(6922):499–506.
234. Khanna KK, Keating KE, Kozlov S, et al. ATM associates with and phosphorylates p53: mapping the region of interaction. Nat Genet 1998;20(4):398–400.

235. Yang DQ, Kastan MB. Participation of ATM in insulin signalling through phosphorylation of eIF-4E-binding protein 1. Nat Cell Biol 2000;2(12):893–898.

236. Crawford TO. Ataxia telangiectasia. Semin Pediatr Neurol 1998;5(4):287–294.

237. Lewis RF, Lederman HM, Crawford TO. Ocular motor abnormalities in ataxia telangiectasia. Ann Neurol 1999;46(3):287–295.

238. Cabana MD, Crawford TO, Winkelstein JA, Christensen JR, Lederman HM. Consequences of the delayed diagnosis of ataxia-telangiectasia. Pediatrics 1998;102(1 pt 1):98–100.

239. Waldmann TA, McIntire KR. Serum-alpha-fetoprotein levels in patients with ataxia-telangiectasia. Lancet 1972;2(7787):1112–1115.

240. Taylor AM, Oxford JM, Metcalfe JA. Spontaneous cytogenetic abnormalities in lymphocytes from thirteen patients with ataxia telangiectasia. Int J Cancer 1981;27(3):311–319.

241. Aurias A, Dutrillaux B, Buriot D, Lejeune J. High frequencies of inversions and translocations of chromosomes 7 and 14 in ataxia telangiectasia. Mutat Res 1980;69(2):369–374.

242. Conley ME, Notarangelo LD, Etzioni A. Diagnostic criteria for primary immunodeficiencies. Representing PAGID (Pan-American Group for Immunodeficiency) and ESID (European Society for Immunodeficiencies). Clin Immunol 1999;93(3):190–197.

243. Fiorilli M, Businco L, Pandolfi F, Paganelli R, Russo G, Aiuti F. Heterogeneity of immunological abnormalities in ataxia-telangiectasia. J Clin Immunol 1983;3(2):135–141.

244. Rivat-Peran L, Buriot D, Salier JP, Rivat C, Dumitresco SM, Griscelli C. Immunoglobulins in ataxia-telangiectasia: evidence for IgG4 and IgA2 subclass deficiencies. Clin Immunol Immunopathol 1981;20(1): 99–110.

245. Giovannetti A, Mazzetta F, Caprini E, et al. Skewed T-cell receptor repertoire, decreased thymic output, and predominance of terminally differentiated T cells in ataxia telangiectasia. Blood 2002;100(12):4082–4089.

246. Viniou N, Terpos E, Rombos J, et al. Acute myeloid leukemia in a patient with ataxia-telangiectasia: a case report and review of the literature. Leukemia 2001;15(10):1668–1670.

247. Taylor AM, Metcalfe JA, Thick J, Mak YF. Leukemia and lymphoma in ataxia telangiectasia. Blood 1996;87(2):423–438.

248. Morgan JL, Holcomb TM, Morrissey RW. Radiation reaction in ataxia telangiectasia. Am J Dis Child 1968;116(5):557–558.

249. Sandoval C, Swift M. Commentary: appropriate cancer chemotherapy for ataxia-telangiectasia patients. Med Pediatr Oncol 2000;34(1):65–66.

250. Sandoval C, Swift M. Treatment of lymphoid malignancies in patients with ataxia-telangiectasia. Med Pediatr Oncol 1998;31(6):491–497.

251. Cesaretti JA, Stock RG, Lehrer S, et al. ATM sequence variants are predictive of adverse radiotherapy response among patients treated for prostate cancer. Int J Radiat Oncol Biol Phys 2005;61(1):196–202.

252. Chessa L, Petrinelli P, Antonelli A, et al. Heterogeneity in ataxia-telangiectasia: classical phenotype associated with intermediate cellular radiosensitivity. Am J Med Genet 1992;42(5):741–746.

253. Swift M, Morrell D, Massey RB, Chase CL. Incidence of cancer in 161 families affected by ataxia-telangiectasia. N Engl J Med 1991;325(26):1831–1836.

254. Su Y, Swift M. Mortality rates among carriers of ataxia-telangiectasia mutant alleles. Ann Intern Med 2000;133(10):770–778.

255. Geoffroy-Perez B, Janin N, Ossian K, et al. Cancer risk in heterozygotes for ataxia-telangiectasia. Int J Cancer 2001;93(2):288–293.

256. Olsen JH, Hahnemann JM, Borresen-Dale AL, et al. Cancer in patients with ataxia-telangiectasia and in their relatives in the nordic countries. J Natl Cancer Inst 2001;93(2):121–127.

257. Bernstein JL, Bernstein L, Thompson WD, et al. ATM variants 7271T>G and IVS10-6T>G among women with unilateral and bilateral breast cancer. Br J Cancer 2003;89(8):1513–1516.

258. Hernandez D, McConville CM, Stacey M, et al. A family showing no evidence of linkage between the ataxia telangiectasia gene and chromosome 11q22-23. J Med Genet 1993;30(2):135–140.

259. Stewart GS, Maser RS, Stankovic T, et al. The DNA double-strand break repair gene hMRE11 is mutated in individuals with an ataxia-telangiectasia-like disorder. Cell 1999;99(6):577–587.

260. Klein C, Wenning GK, Quinn NP, Marsden CD. Ataxia without telangiectasia masquerading as benign hereditary chorea. Mov Disord 1996;11(2):217–220.

261. O'Driscoll M, Cerosaletti KM, Girard PM, et al. DNA ligase IV mutations identified in patients exhibiting developmental delay and immunodeficiency. Mol Cell 2001;8(6):1175–1185.

262. O'Driscoll M, Gennery AR, Seidel J, Concannon P, Jeggo PA. An overview of three new disorders associated with genetic instability: LIG4 syndrome, RS-SCID and ATR-Seckel syndrome. DNA Repair (Amst) 2004; 3(8–9):1227–1235.
263. O'Driscoll M, Ruiz-Perez VL, Woods CG, Jeggo PA, Goodship JA. A splicing mutation affecting expression of ataxia-telangiectasia and Rad3-related protein (ATR) results in Seckel syndrome. Nat Genet 2003; 33(4):497–501.
264. Casper AM, Nghiem P, Arlt MF, Glover TW. ATR regulates fragile site stability. Cell 2002;111(6):779–789.
265. Hayani A, Suarez CR, Molnar Z, LeBeau M, Godwin J. Acute myeloid leukaemia in a patient with Seckel syndrome. J Med Genet 1994;31(2):148–149.
266. Jacquemont S, Boceno M, Rival JM, Mechinaud F, David A. High risk of malignancy in mosaic variegated aneuploidy syndrome. Am J Med Genet 2002;109(1):17–21.
267. Hanks S, Rahman N. Aneuploidy-cancer predisposition syndromes: a new link between the mitotic spindle checkpoint and cancer. Cell Cycle 2005;4(2):225–227.
268. Hanks S, Coleman K, Reid S, et al. Constitutional aneuploidy and cancer predisposition caused by biallelic mutations in BUB1B. Nat Genet 2004;36(11):1159–1161.
269. Pedersen-Bjergaard J, Pedersen M, Roulston D, Philip P. Different genetic pathways in leukemogenesis for patients presenting with therapy-related myelodysplasia and therapy-related acute myeloid leukemia. Blood 1995;86(9):3542–3552.
270. Maser RS, DePinho RA. Keeping telomerase in its place. Nat Med 2002;8(9):934–936.
271. Wong KK, Chang S, Weiler SR, et al. Telomere dysfunction impairs DNA repair and enhances sensitivity to ionizing radiation. Nat Genet 2000;26(1):85–88.
272. DePinho RA. The age of cancer. Nature 2000;408(6809):248–254.
273. O'Hagan RC, Chang S, Maser RS, et al. Telomere dysfunction provokes regional amplification and deletion in cancer genomes. Cancer Cell 2002;2(2):149–155.
274. Hsu HL, Gilley D, Galande SA, et al. Ku acts in a unique way at the mammalian telomere to prevent end joining. Genes Dev 2000;14(22):2807–2812.
275. Engelhardt M, Wasch R, Guo Y. Telomeres and telomerase in normal and leukemic hematopoietic cells. Leuk Res 2004;28(10):1001–1004.
276. Ohyashiki K, Shay JW, Ohyashiki JH. Lack of mutations of the human telomerase RNA gene (hTERC) in myelodysplastic syndrome. Haematologica 2005;90(5):691.
277. Sashida G, Ohyashiki JH, Nakajima A, et al. Telomere dynamics in myelodysplastic syndrome determined by telomere measurement of marrow metaphases. Clin Cancer Res 2003;9(4):1489–1496.
278. Ohyashiki K, Iwama H, Yahata N, et al. Telomere dynamics in myelodysplastic syndromes and acute leukemic transformation. Leuk Lymphoma 2001;42(3):291–299.
279. Ohyashiki JH, Iwama H, Yahata N, et al. Telomere stability is frequently impaired in high-risk groups of patients with myelodysplastic syndromes. Clin Cancer Res 1999;5(5):1155–1160.
280. Hartmann U, Brummendorf TH, Balabanov S, Thiede C, Illme T, Schaich M. Telomere length and hTERT expression in patients with acute myeloid leukemia correlates with chromosomal abnormalities. Haematologica 2005;90(3):307–316.
281. Roth A, Vercauteren S, Sutherland HJ, Lansdorp PM. Telomerase is limiting the growth of acute myeloid leukemia cells. Leukemia 2003;17(12):2410–2417.
282. Alberts B, Johnson A, Lewis J, Raff M, Roberts K, Walter P. Molecular Biology of the Cell. New York: Garland Science, 2002.

6 Altered Apoptosis in AML

Potential Implications for Pathogenesis and Therapeutic Response

Ruben A. Mesa and Scott H. Kaufmann

Summary

Apoptosis is a highly regulated, biochemically distinct cell death process that is tightly linked to cell growth and differentiation. Alterations in the ability of cells to undergo apoptosis have been implicated in the pathogenesis of acute myeloid leukemia (AML) and resistance to currently available therapy. Factors that might contribute to apoptotic resistance in AML include increased expression of Bcl-2 and related anti-apoptotic proteins, loss of p53 function, mutation of *Ras* alleles (stimulating the Raf/MEK/ERK and PI3k/Akt pathways) or *FLT3*, and increased expression of the anti-apoptotic regulator XIAP. Based on improved understanding of apoptotic pathways and their alteration in AML, three different approaches for overcoming apaptotic resistance have been proposed: (1) administering "pro-apoptotic" agents that directly inhibit anti-apoptotic molecules such as Bcl-2 or XIAP; (2) using signal transduction inhibitors to modulate anti-apoptotic signaling pathways; and (3) employing cytotoxic cytolines that, in contrast to most currectly employed antileukemic agents, trigger apoptosis through the death receptor pathway. Whether any of these approaches will improve current therapy of AML remains to be determined.

Key Words: Apoptosis; acute myeloid leukemia; drug resistance; myeloid malignancy; Bcl-2; Mcl-1; XIAP; bone marrow microenvironment; Ras; Flt3.

1. INTRODUCTION

Studies performed over the past two decades have demonstrated that virtually all antileukemic drugs are capable of inducing apoptosis in susceptible leukemia cell lines in vitro *(1,2)* and in acute myeloid leukemia (AML) cells after drug administration in vivo *(3,4)*. Conversely, it has also been suggested that alterations in the ability of leukemia cells to undergo apoptosis

From: *Contemporary Hematology: Acute Myelogenous Leukemia*
Edited by: J. E. Karp © Humana Press Inc., Totowa, NJ

might cause a unique form of broad-spectrum drug resistance *(5–7)*. In the sections that follow, we briefly review the current understanding of apoptotic pathways, summarize the evidence that alterations in these pathways contribute to the pathogenesis and/or drug resistance in AML, and outline investigational strategies for overcoming this resistance.

1.1. Two Apoptotic Pathways

Originally identified as a morphologically distinct form of cell death *(8)*, apoptosis has subsequently been shown to reflect a stereotypic series of biochemical changes *(9,10)*. Over the past decade, many hallmarks of this process have been traced to activation of caspases, a family of cysteine proteases that cleave on the C-terminal side of aspartate residues *(11,12)*. Like other proteases (e.g., the blood coagulation factors), caspases are synthesized as zymogens that are then activated by specific biochemical processes. The presence of caspase inhibitors and antagonists of the inhibitors *(9,13)* further heightens the parallel between intracellular caspase cascades and extracellular blood coagulation. As is the case with blood coagulation, two distinct but related pathways lead to caspase activation within cells undergoing apoptosis (Fig. 1) *(14–16)*.

The "intrinsic" or "mitochondrial" pathway *(15,17)* is utilized by cells to respond to various types cellular stress *(18)*. This pathway involves the regulated release of mitochondrial inter-membrane polypeptides to the cytoplasm, where cytochrome c facilitates a dATP *(19)*- or ATP *(20)*-dependent conformational change in the adaptor protein Apaf-1 (apoptotic protease activating factor-1), which acquires the ability to bind and activate procaspase 9 in a manner that remains incompletely understood *(21)*. Activated caspase 9 proteolytically activates the caspase 3 zymogen, and caspase 3 in turn catalyzes many of the substrate cleavages that result in the biochemical and morphological changes recognized as apoptosis *(11,12)*. In cells that express high levels of X-linked inhibitor of apoptosis protein (XIAP), which inhibits caspases 3, 7, and 9 *(22,23)*, signaling through this pathway is blocked unless other polypeptides released from mitochondria (typified by the polypeptide now known as Smac *[24,25]*) compete for XIAP binding and release the caspases as described below.

The extrinsic or death receptor (DR) pathway (reviewed in refs. *26,27–30*) is activated when certain members of the tumor necrosis factor (TNF)-α family, including Fas ligand (FasL), TNF-α-related apoptosis-inducing ligand (TRAIL), and TNF-α itself, bind certain receptors at the cell surface *(31,32)*. These ligand–receptor interactions play critical roles in the ability of cytotoxic T-cells to kill their targets *(27,33,34)*, the regulation of lympho-hematopoietic cell number, and the elimination of neoplastically transformed cells by natural killer cells *(29,35–37)*. Each of the active receptors for a cytotoxic TNF-α family ligand contains a so-called death domain (DD) near its cytoplasmic terminus. In the case of Fas and the TRAIL receptors DR4 and DR5, ligand binding enhances affinity of the DD for the cytoplasmic adaptor protein FADD (Fas-associated protein with death domain). Bound FADD in turn recruits the monomeric cytoplasmic zymogen procaspase 8 *(38)*, which under-goes presumed FADD-mediated oligomerization *(21)* and activation *(39,40)*. Although less intensively studied, procaspase 10 appears to be activated similarly *(41,42)*. Fully mature caspases 8 and 10 are released to the cytoplasm, where they cleave a handful of substrates, including procaspase 3 and Bid. In so-called type I cells *(43)*, the caspase 3 activity that is generated is sufficient to induce cellular disassembly. In type II cells, which are postulated to initially exhibit caspase 3 inhibition as a consequence of higher levels of XIAP *(44)*, cleavage of the BH3-only polypeptide Bid leads to permeabilization of the outer mitochondrial mem-brane *(45,46)*, which releases not only cytochrome c, but also Smac (second mitochondrial

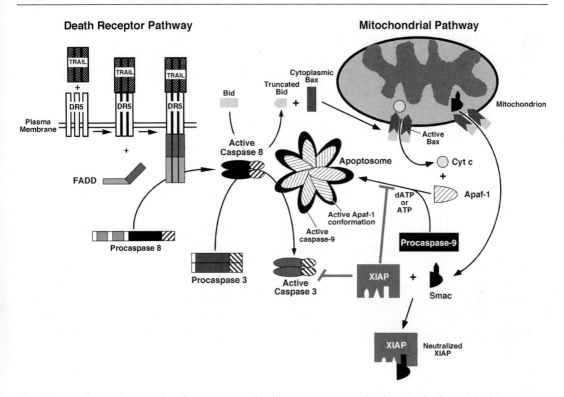

Fig. 1. Two distinct but overlapping pathways leading to caspase activation. As indicated in the text, two different but intersecting protease cascades lead to activation of the major effector caspase, caspase 3. One pathway starts with ligation of tumor necrosis factor (TNF)-α family receptors, recruitment of adaptor proteins, and presumed oligomerization-induced activation of caspase 8 and caspase 10. The other is initiated by Bcl-2 family member-regulated release of cytochrome c from the mitochondrial intermembrane space. Once in the cytosol, cytochrome c acts as a cofactor for Apaf-1-mediated oligomerization, which facilitates caspase 9 activation. Also depicted in this figure are XIAP, which inhibits procaspase 9 oligomerization and caspase 3 activity, as well as Smac, the XIAP antagonist that is released along with cytochrome c from the mitochondrial intermembrane space.

activator of caspases) and other polypeptides that can antagonize XIAP, thereby facilitating caspase 3-mediated cleavages.

1.2. Regulation of Apoptotic Pathways by Bcl-2 Family Members

As the two apoptotic signaling pathways described above have been elucidated, various mechanisms of regulation have also been identified. This regulation is widely acknowledged to occur at multiple different levels.

Release of cytochrome c from mitochondria is regulated by members of the Bcl-2 family *(9,14,47)*. The approx 20 polypeptides in this family can be divided into three groups *(48–50)*. Group I includes Bcl-2, Bcl-x_L, Bcl-w, Mcl-1, A1/Bfl1, Boo/Diva, Nrf3, and Bcl-B, all of which are anti-apoptotic polypeptides that localize at the cytoplasmic surfaces of various intracellular membranes, including the outer mitochondrial membrane and the endoplasmic reticulum. Group II includes Bax, Bak, and Bok/Mtd, all of which are pro-apoptotic and appear to directly regulate cytochrome c release as described below. Group III, which includes Bid, Bad, Bik, Bim, Blk, Bmf, Hrk, Bnip3, Nix, Noxa, PUMA, and Bcl-G, encompasses a more heterogeneous collection of polypeptides that display sequence homology only in their

15-amino-acid BH3 domains, which are involved in binding and regulating the function of group I and group II polypeptides *(47,49,51)*.

According to current understanding, which is summarized in Fig. 2, the group II family members Bax and Bak directly mediate cytochrome c release *(17,52)*. When the mitochondrial pathway is triggered, Bax, which is ordinarily found in the cytoplasm or loosely bound to the mitochondrial surface *(53)*, is inserted into the mitochondrial outer membrane *(54)* as a consequence of changes in its conformation and oligomerization state *(55–57)*. Bak, which normally is associated with the outer mitochondrial membrane, likewise undergoes a conformational change that results in its deeper membrane insertion *(58–60)*. In a manner that remains incompletely understood but likely involves formation of a Bax- and/or Bak-containing pore in the outer mitochondrial membrane, mitochondrial intermembrane proteins are then released.

Insertion of Bax and Bak into the outer mitochondrial membrane is thought to be regulated by group III Bcl-2 family members in at least two ways *(61)*. Some of the group III polypeptides, including Puma and a caspase 8-generated fragment of Bid, have been reported to directly interact with Bax *(62)*, thereby inducing the conformation change required for Bax insertion into the outer mitochondrial membrane *(61)*. In contrast, the other group III polypeptides participate in Bax/Bak activation by binding and neutralizing various group I (anti-apoptotic) Bcl-2 family members *(61,63)*, including Bcl-2, Bcl-x_L and Mcl-1, which otherwise would bind Bax and Bak, preventing their insertion into the outer mitochondrial membrane *(54,56,64–66)*.

Studies performed over the past decade have demonstrated that interactions between Bcl-2 family members vary dynamically in response to the conditions that cells encounter. In particular, BH3-only polypeptides appear to monitor various types of cellular stress *(18)*. Bid is cleaved to an active fragment by caspase-8 *(45,46)*, granzyme B *(67)*, or lysosomal cathepsins *(68)*; Bad is dephosphorylated and released from cytoplasmic 14-3-3 protein-binding sites upon cytokine withdrawal *(69)*; Bim is detached from microtubules upon treatment of cells with paclitaxel *(70–72)*; and Bmf is released from actin filaments when cell-substrate attachment is disrupted *(73)*. In contrast, Noxa and Puma are synthesized in a p53-dependent manner in response to DNA damage *(74,75)*, providing a potential explanation for the ability of DNA lesions within nuclei to signal mitochondrial cytochrome c release *(76–78)*. In addition, Puma is synthesized in a p53-independent manner in response to certain cytotoxic agents such as glucocorticoids *(77)*.

Once activated, the group III polypeptides specifically interact with distinct subsets of group I polypeptides. Bad and Bmf, for example, bind Bcl-x_L and Bcl-w with nanomolar affinity but have lower affinity for Mcl-1 and A1 *(63)*. Conversely, Noxa binds Mcl-1 and A1 avidly but has low affinity for Bcl-x_L and Bcl-w. Bim and Puma, on the other hand, appear to bind all group I family members fairly equally. When the stresses that activate these BH3-only polypeptides (*see* preceding paragraph) are considered in light of observed tissue-specific differences in expression of the anti-apoptotic Bcl-2 family members *(79,80)*, it becomes clear how the ability of divers stimuli to induce cytochrome c release can vary widely from cell type to cell type.

1.3. Regulation of Bcl-2 Family Members by Kinases and Phosphatases

As might be expected for polypeptides that are the final arbiters of cytochrome c release by various stresses, expression and activity of the group I Bcl-2 family members are also regulated. Control of these processes occurs at several levels and typically involves the action of a number of anti-apoptotic signal transduction pathways, including the mitogen-activated

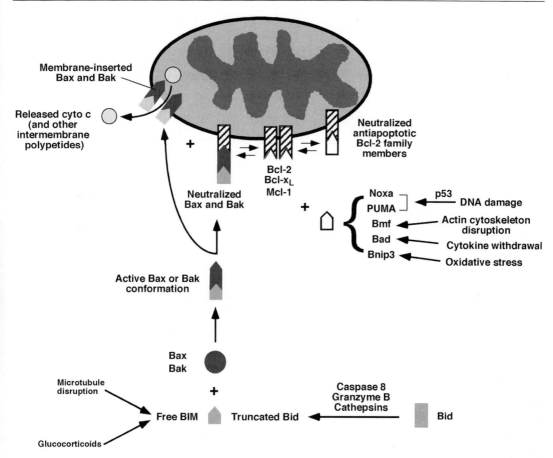

Fig. 2. Regulation of the mitochondrial pathway by Bcl-2 family members. As indicated in the text, group II Bcl-2 family members such as Bax or Bak (dark grey) can assume an active conformation that results in their insertion into the outer mitochondrial membrane, where they facilitate release of cytochrome c and other intermembrane proteins. Antiapoptotic Bcl-2 family members (crosshatched) bind the active conformations of Bax and Bak, preventing this breach in the outer mitochondrial membrane. On the other hand, group III polypeptides are thought to facilitate Bax or Bak action in two distinct ways. Bim and caspase 8-cleaved Bid (light grey) are reported to directly bind Bax and facilitate release of cytochrome c. Other BH3-only polypeptides (white) bind and neutralize group I Bcl-2 family members, thereby facilitating Bax and/or Bak insertion into the outer mitochondrial membrane.

protein (MAP) kinase pathway, the phosphatidylinositol-3 kinase (PI3k)/Akt pathway, and the Janus kinase (Jak)/signal tranducer and activator of transcription (Stat) pathway (Fig. 3).

A complete description of these signal transduction pathways is provided in recent reviews and is beyond the scope of this chapter. In broad stroke, the MAP kinase pathway (reviewed in refs. *81–83*) is activated when a number of growth factors, including the hematopoietic cytokines c-kit ligand, granulocyte-macrophage colony-stimulating factor (GM-CSF), inter-leukin (IL)-3, and IL-5, bind to their cell surface receptors *(84,85)*. Autophosphorylation of the ligated receptor tyrosine kinases results in binding of adaptor proteins, which in turn bind and activate guanine nucleotide exchange factors that facilitate GTP binding to the Ras proteins, notably c-H-Ras. In its GTP-bound (activated) state, Ras assumes a conformation that binds and activates Raf kinases, leading to phosphorylation and activation of the MAP kinase kinases MEK1 and MEK2, which then phosphorylate and activate extracellular-regulated kinases

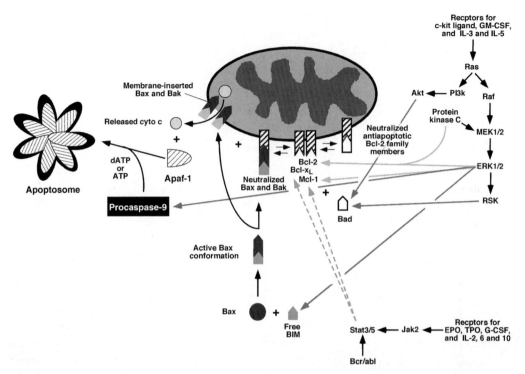

Fig. 3. Regulation of the mitochondrial pathway by kinase cascades. As indicated in the text, three kinase cascades inhibit apoptosis. A partial schematic of effects of those signal transduction pathways is shown. Green and red solid arrows indicate activating and inactivating phosphorylations, respectively. Dashed arrows indicate elevated protein levels as a consequence of transcriptional activation.

Signaling through the mitogen activated protein (MAP) kinase pathway leads to phosphorylation of Bcl-2 and Mcl-1 by extracellular-regulated kinase (ERK)1/2. These phosphorylations activate Bcl-2 and stabilize Mcl-1. At the same time, ERK-mediated phosphorylation of procaspase 9 inhibits activation of this zymogen. RSK, which is downstream of ERK1/2, catalyzes inactivating phosphorylation of Bad.

Signaling through the Akt pathway leads to phosphorylation of Bad (on different residues), facilitating its sequestration by cytoplasmic 14-3-3 proteins. Akt has also been reported to inhibit cytochrome c release in a Bad-independent manner and to facilitate expression of antiapoptotic Bcl-2 family members through its effects on nuclear factor (NF)κB.

STAT3 and STAT5 are known to act as transcription factors for the genes encoding Bcl-x$_L$ and Mcl-1. These transcription factors are activated as a consequence of phosphorylation by receptor-bound Jak2, by constitutively active mutant Jak2 or by Bcr/abl.

(ERKs) 1 and 2. Once activated by dual phosphorylation on a threonine and nearby tyrosine, the ERKs in turn phosphorylate and activate a number of substrates, including the transcription factors Elk-1, c-jun, and c-myc *(86–88)* as well as the p90 ribosomal S6 kinase (RSK) *(89)*.

Another molecule that is bound by activated Ras is the p85 regulatory subunit of PI3k. Upon binding, this regulatory subunit activates the catalytic subunit of PI3k, which then phosphorylates the lipid intermediate phosphatidylinositol-4,5-biphosphosphate to form phosphatidylinosil-3,4,5-trisphosphate (PI3). PI3 in turn activates several kinases, including 3-phosphoinositide-dependent kinase 1, which catalyzes one of the phosphorylation events required to activate the anti-apoptotic kinase Akt *(90–93)*. Akt in turn phosphorylates a number of polypeptides involved in the regulation of apoptosis, including the caspase inhibitor XIAP *(94)*; the forkhead family transcription factor FOXO3a, which activates the genes for CD95/Fas and Bim in its unphosphorylated state but becomes sequestered in the cytoplasm upon phosphorylation *(95,96)*; and the transcription factor nuclear factor (NF)κB *(97,98)*, which turns on the genes for anti-apoptotic polypeptides such as XIAP and c-FLIP (described below) upon activation by this phosphorylation *(99)*.

Finally, another group of cytokines, including type I and type II interferons (IFNs), erythropoietin, thrombopoetin, granulocyte-colony stimulating factor (G-CSF), GM-CSF, and IL-2, -6, and -10, all activate Jak/Stat pathways (reviewed in refs. *100–102*). In brief, ligand binding is thought to result in a conformational change in the dimeric receptors for these cytokines. Jak kinases, which are noncovalently attached to the cytoplasmic domains of these receptors, are brought into apposition by this conformational change, allowing them to phosphorylate and activate each other. The activated Jaks then phosphorylate critical tyrosine residues on the cytoplasmic Stat molecules, allowing them to dimerize, translocate to the nucleus, and transactivate critical target genes involved in proliferation, differentiation, and the regulation of apoptosis *(101,103)*.

Collectively, these signal transduction cascades regulate Bcl-2 family members in a number of ways. The genes encoding Bcl-2, Bcl-x_L and Mcl-1 are activated by MAP kinase signaling in some cell types *(104,105)*, cytokine-mediated STAT activation in others *(106–108)*, and PI3k/Akt signaling, possibly acting through the transcription factor NF-κB, in others *(109– 112)*. In each case, gene activation results in increased expression at the polypeptide level.

The activity of group I polypeptides is also regulated posttranslationally by phosphorylation. Bcl-2 is activated by protein kinase Cα or ERK-mediated phosphorylation on Ser^{70} *(113,114)* and other sites *(115)*. Mcl-1 is likewise phosphorylated and stabilized in an ERK-dependent manner *(116–118)* as well as an ERK-independent manner involving the kinase Akt and possibly others *(112,119)*. These observations, along with the gene expression results described above, provide at least a partial explanation for the anti-apoptotic effect of MAP kinase signaling *(81,120)*.

Whereas anti-apoptotic group I Bcl-2 family members are stabilized or activated by MAP kinase- or Akt-initiated phosphorylation, the same kinase pathways repress, destabilize, or inactivate pro-apoptotic group III polypeptides. Bim represents a particularly informative example. In different cell types, transcription of the Bim gene is inhibited by activation of the ERK *(121–123)* or Akt pathways *(124,125)*. ERK also directly phosphorylates the extra-long isoform of Bim on multiple sites *(126–129)*, reportedly inhibiting its interaction with Bax *(129)* and promoting its proteasome-mediated turnover *(72,126,127,130)*. In a somewhat analogous fashion, cytokine-induced Akt activation results in phosphorylation of Bad, which is then sequestered in the cytoplasm by a 14-3-3 protein *(131–133)*. Phosphorylation of Bad on different residues by protein kinase A *(134)* or RSK also inhibits its function *(135,136)*.

While the phosphorylation events described above activate group I Bcl-2 family members and inactivate group III family members, there are exceptions to this paradigm. A variety of earlier studies demonstrated that stimulation of Jun N-terminal kinase (Jnk) isoforms contributes to activation of the mitochondrial pathway *(120,137,138)*. More recent results have suggested that Jnk phosphorylates Bim *(139,140)* and Bmf *(139)*, leading to their release from cytoskeletal binding sites and subsequent activation of Bax and Bak. In addition, it has been reported that Jnk phosphorylates a cytoplasmic 14-3-3 protein, causing it to release Bax, which then translocates to the mitochondrial outer membrane *(141)*. Future studies will undoubtedly reveal additional ways in which kinase pathways regulate Bcl-2 family members.

1.4. Regulation of Apoptosis by XIAP and XIAP Antagonists

Apoptotic pathways are also regulated by members of the inhibitor of apoptosis (IAP) family *(142)*. This group of polypeptides, which includes XIAP (X-linked IAP), cIAP1 (cellular IAP1), cIAP2, and ML-IAP (melanoma-associated IAP), regulates apoptosis by modulating caspase activity *(142)*.

XIAP, the best understood of the IAPs, contains three zinc finger-like baculovirus inhibitor repeat (BIR) domains. The third BIR domain of XIAP is capable of binding caspase 9 and preventing the dimerization that activates it *(143,144)*. In addition the second BIR of XIAP binds caspases 3 and 7, orienting the molecules so that a short peptide immediately upstream from BIR2 can block access to the active sites of these caspases *(142,145)*. Based on these observations, it has been suggested that XIAP constitutes a buffer that prevents inadvertent caspase activation in cells destined to live.

If the action of XIAP were left unchecked, caspase 3 might be inactivated as quickly as it is activated. The polypeptide Smac/DIABLO (second mitochondrial activator of caspases/ direct IAP binding polypeptide with low pI) has been proposed as nature's solution to this problem. This mitochondrial intermembrane protein, which is usually released to the cytoplasm under conditions that allow cytochrome c release, binds to XIAP and disrupts its binding to caspases *(24,25,146,147)*.

As is the case with the clotting cascade, there are not only a caspase inhibitor and an antagonist of the inhibitor, but also regulators of the antagonist. The XIAP homologs cIAP1, cIAP2, and ML-IAP exhibit low affinity for active caspases *(148,149)* but nonetheless inhibit apoptosis under certain conditions. Recent experiments have suggested that these other IAP proteins avidly bind Smac, thereby freeing XIAP from Smac and allowing XIAP-mediated caspase inhibition *(149,150)*.

The existence of additional molecules with Smac-like function would add another potential layer of complexity to this regulation *(13)*. Current data suggest that mammalian cells contain at least four additional polypeptides that are cleaved under various conditions to species that could bind XIAP *(13,151)*. Gene targeting studies in mice, however, have failed to reveal any evidence of inhibited apoptosis when the genes encoding Smac and HtRA2/Omi, the other widely studied IAP-binding protein, are individually deleted (reviewed in ref. *152*). Accordingly, further study is required to determine whether the elegant in vitro studies implicating these molecules in XIAP regulation were misleading or the redundancy of these polypeptides accounts for the lack of an apoptotic phenotype when only one gene is deleted.

1.5. Regulation of the Death Receptor Pathway

Like the mitochondrial pathway, the DR pathway is also regulated at several levels *(153,154)*. At the cell surface, ligand binding reflects a competition between agonistic receptors, some of which are transcriptionally regulated *(155,156)*, and receptor homologs known as "decoy receptors," which compete for ligand but cannot signal to FADD *(28,157)*. At the cytoplasmic surface of the active receptors, the ability of FADD to activate procaspase 8 (and presumably procaspase 10) is regulated by c-FLIP, an enzymatically inactive caspase 8 homolog *(158,159)* that enhances *(40,160,161)* or inhibits *(162)* procaspase 8 activation depending on the cellular context, the precise splice variant of c-FLIP expressed, and the relative levels of c-FLIP vs procaspase 8. Finally, as mentioned above, the ability of caspase 8 to directly trigger apoptosis is also thought to be regulated by cellular XIAP levels. In type II cells, cleavage of Bid to activate the mitochondrial pathway plays a critical role in death ligand signaling, as indicated by studies showing that overexpression of Bcl-2, Bcl-x_L, or Mcl-1 renders certain cells resistant to death ligands *(43,44,111,163–166)*.

2. APOPTOTIC RESISTANCE AND MYELOID NEOPLASMS

2.1. The Role of Apoptosis in Normal Myeloid Differentiation and Survival

Current models suggest that apoptosis plays an important role in the genesis and function myeloid of cells. Key regulatory cytokines such as erythropoietin (EPO), stem cell factor (SCF), and GM-CSF increase the number of their target cells, at least in part, by inhibiting apoptosis in progenitor populations *(167)*. Moreover, the survival of neutrophils, the terminally differentiated cell of the myeloid lineage, is modulated by regulating apoptosis. When not needed, these cells have a half-life in the circulation of only a few hours and then spontaneously undergo apoptosis *(168)*. During inflammation, a variety of cytokines (IL-1β, IL-2, IL-15, IFN-γ, G-CSF, GM-CSF) as well as bacterial lipopolysaccharide can prolong neutrophil survival, in part, by blocking apoptosis *(169)*. TNF-α appears to play a dual role, with short incubations (<8 h) at high concentrations being found to stimulate neutrophil apoptosis, whereas long exposures (>12 h) to lower concentrations may inhibit it *(170)*.

2.2. Apoptotic Resistance and Chronic Myeloid Neoplasms

Aberrations in any of the pathways regulating apoptosis can give a cell a selective survival advantage. Accordingly, dysregulated apoptosis is felt to be integral to the pathogenesis of a variety of malignancies and their resistance to therapy *(171,172)*. Consistent with this hypothesis, alterations in the control of apoptosis have been found in a wide range of hematological malignancies, including those of myeloid origin. It is important to emphasize, however, that much of this work is correlative and that definitive experiments showing a contribution of these alterations to neoplastic transformation in many cases remain to be performed *(10)*.

The chronic myeloid disorders are a spectrum of diseases that historically include both myelodysplastic syndrome (MDS) and the myeloproliferative disorders. Although it has been suggested that increased apoptosis contributes to the pathogenesis of MDS *(173)*, it has also been reported that MDS cells exhibit resistance to apoptosis. While a variety of mechanisms are involved, particularly prominent is increased expression of Bcl-2 *(174,175)*. Similarly, chronic myelomonocytic leukemia (CMML), a unique myeloid disorder with both proliferative and dysplastic phenotypic features, is reportedly resistant to induction of apoptosis as a consequence of activation of Ras-initiated signaling pathways *(176)*.

Resistance to apoptosis is also a prominent feature of chronic myeloproliferative disorders, a group of conditions that includes chronic myeloid leukemia (CML), polycythemia vera (PV), and agnogenic myeloid metaplasia (AMM). CML, the best understood of these, is caused by a translocation that results in fusion of the *BCR* (breakpoint cluster region) gene on chromosome 22 and the *ABL* (Abelson kinase) gene on chromosome 9. The resulting p210[Bcr/abl] fusion product appears to cause CML through decreased apoptosis as well as increased cell proliferation *(177,178)*. The decreased apoptosis reflects, at least in part, p210[Bcr/abl]-mediated phosphorylation of Stat5 *(179)*, which transcriptionally activates the genes encoding Bcl-x_L *(107)* and Mcl-1 *(108,180)*.

Like CML, PV appears to result, at least in part, from impairment of apoptosis. Unlike their normal counterparts, PV erythroid precursors can survive and proliferate in the absence of EPO *(181)*. Moreover, they are hypersensitive to other growth factors such as IL-3,

GM-CSF, stem cell factor (SCF), and thrombopoietin *(182)*. In >70% of PV patients, this cytokine hypersensitivity can be traced to an activating amino acid substitution (Val617Phe) in Jak2 kinase *(183,184)*, leading to ligand-independent STAT3 phosphorylation *(185)* and STAT-mediated Bcl-x$_L$ overexpression *(186)*. The same Val617Phe mutation is also present in 35% of AMM patients *(183,184)* and is thought to contribute to the cytokine-independent activation of STAT5 and NFκB *(187)* that results in cytokine-independent growth of megakaryocytes and other myeloid progenitors. Consistent with current understanding of the signal transduction pathways described in Section 1.3., our group has reported that neutrophils isolated from many AMM patients exhibit less spontaneous or Fas-stimulated apoptosis than normal neutrophils in vitro *(188)* and is currently attempting to correlate this finding with Jak2 mutations and constitutive STAT activation.

Resistance to apoptosis in these chronic myeloid disorders is pertinent to AML in a number of ways. First, the resistance to apoptosis seen in the chronic phase of these disorders appears to provide a favorable platform for the selection of cells with a more malignant phenotype. As a result, all of the chronic myeloid disorders have a potential (in some cases inevitable) transformation to AML. Second, AML arising in the setting of a preexisting chronic myeloid disorder has an extremely poor prognosis, usually related to its resistance to current chemotherapeutic agents *(189)*. While multiple mechanisms undoubtedly play a role in this drug resistance, accumulating evidence suggests that alterations in apoptotic pathways might contribute.

2.3. Apoptotic Resistance in AML: Possible Mechanisms

In addition to AML arising in the setting of a preexisting myeloid disorder, some cases of de novo AML also exhibit resistance to apoptosis *(190)*. Indeed, the concept of altered cell death in AML dates to early studies of AML blasts by McCulloch and coworkers, who demonstrated an imbalance between proliferation and differentiation *(191)*. Although only a minority of AML blasts are cycling, they remain in the proliferative pool in part as a result of decreased cell death *(191)*. Subsequent studies have identified a number of different alterations in apoptotic pathways (Table 1) that might contribute to apoptotic resistance in AML.

2.3.1. CASPASES

If the final common pathway of apoptosis involves caspase activation, the first question is whether there is an obvious problem with caspase expression or function in AML cells? Schimmer and colleagues evaluated this question by adding proapoptotic polypeptides to the cytosol of primary AML samples (cytochrome c for the intrinsic pathway and activated caspase 8 for the extrinsic pathway) and analyzing caspase activation under cell-free conditions *(192)*. A block in one of the pathways was observed in samples from the majority of patients and was not predictive of response. In contrast, a block in both apoptotic pathways was seen in a smaller fraction of samples and was predictive of clinical chemoresistance and decreased survival. These results suggested the possibility that effector caspases are inhibited at some point after the confluence of the two pathways in resistant AML cells.

Several studies have assessed the possibility that this block might reflect diminished expression of caspases, especially caspase 3 (reviewed in ref. *193*). These studies demonstrated that levels of Apaf-1 and caspase zymogens in clinical AML samples, while heterogeneous, do not correlate with clinical outcome *(193)*. Accordingly, the block observed by Schimmer and coworkers is currently unexplained but appears to reflect altered regulation of the caspase activation pathways rather than a simple change in caspase or Apaf-1 expression.

Table 1
Alterations in Apoptotic Pathways Described in AML Cells

Molecule	Function	Change in AML	Ref.
Bcl-2	Anti-apoptotic regulator	Overexpression	198
Bcl-x$_L$	Anti-apoptotic regulator	Overexpression	198
BAD	Pro-apoptotic regulator	Inhibited by constitutive phosphorylation	219
XIAP	Inhibitor of apoptosis	Upregulated by PI3k and M-CSF	233
Ras	Couples receptor occupation with activation of Raf/MEK/ERK and PI3k/Akt pathways	Activating mutations in 20–30% of AML	204
ERK	Survival signal	Constitutive activation	105
PI3K	Survival signal	Constitutive activation	275
NFκB	Anti-apoptotic transcription factor	Constitutive activation	221,222
FLT-3 ITD	Factor-independent activation of STAT5 leading to Bcl-x$_L$ overexpression	Activating mutations in 20–30% of AML	207,210
Stromal cells	Maintain marrow micro-environment	Induce increased expression of Bcl-2 and Bcl-x$_L$	229

2.3.2. BCL-2 FAMILY MEMBERS

As indicated in Section 1.3. and Fig. 2, Bcl-2 family members play critical roles in the regulation of caspase activation. In addition, Bcl-2 overexpression inhibits proliferation *(194)*, most likely by downregulating reactive oxygen species *(195,196)* that ordinarily act as proliferation-inducing second messengers by inhibiting protein tyrosine phosphatases *(197)*.

Consistent with the dual role of Bcl-2 as a prosurvival and anti-proliferative polypeptide, it has been reported that Bcl-2 and Bcl-x$_L$ are expressed at higher levels in quiescent CD34$^+$ cells than in proliferating CD34$^+$ cells from AML patients *(198)*. In addition to its effect on cytochrome c release, Bcl-2 might be contributing to resistance of these CD34$^+$ cells by diminishing their entry into S phase of the cell cycle, where a variety of antileukemic agents are exclusively or preferentially toxic.

Some groups have found that high Bcl-2 expression is associated with a poor response of AML to antileukemic therapy *(199,200)*. Others, however, have reported that Bcl-2 expression alone is not predictive of a poor prognosis in AML *(201,202)*, but co-expression of Bcl-2 with another marker of drug resistance (e.g., P-glycoprotein) is associated with a significantly lower probability of remission and survival *(202)*. These disparate observations might reflect differences in patient populations or therapies administered.

2.3.3. ACTIVATION OF THE MAP KINASE AND PI3K/AKT SURVIVAL PATHWAYS

The correlation between expression of Bcl-2 family members and prognosis, when observed, might reflect alterations in the antiapoptotic signaling pathways that regulate expression of these polypeptides (*see* Section 1.3.). The Ras family of GTP-regulated switches, which couple signals from receptors of stimulatory cytokines such as IL-3 and GM-CSF to downstream signal transduction pathways *(203)*, are constitutively activated by point mutations (mainly in *N-Ras* genes) in 20–30% of AML cases *(204)*. These mutant Ras alleles activate a variety of growth stimulatory pathways, including the Raf/MEK/

ERK and PI3k/Akt pathways, which then inhibit apoptosis as summarized in Section 1.3. and Fig. 3.

It is important to emphasize, however, that *Ras* mutations are not the only way to activate these pathways. FLT3 (*fms*-like tyrosine kinase-3) is a receptor tyrosine kinase that plays an important role in normal hematopoiesis and leukemogenesis *(205)*. Activation of this receptor by its ligand, which occurs in up to 70% of AMLs expressing the normal receptor *(206)*, inhibits apoptosis *(207)*. In addition, up to 25% of AMLs harbor activating mutations of the *FLT3* gene, including internal tandem duplications (ITDs) and point mutations in the activation loop *(208,209)*. These activating mutations result in ligand-independent FLT3 tyrosine kinase activity, which in turn produces activation of (nonmutant) Ras and the downstream MAP kinase pathway as well as constitutive activation of STAT5 *(210)* leading to upregulation of the serine/threonine kinase Pim-1 *(211)* and Bcl-x$_L$ *(212)*. Not surprisingly, these *FLT3* mutations, like *Ras* mutations, have been associated with resistance to apoptotic stimuli in vitro *(210,213)* and a poorer prognosis *(208,209)*.

Whether activated by point mutations, constitutive signaling from mutated FLT3, or by other means, Ras acts as a switch that turns on the Raf/MEK/ERK pathway. A number of studies demonstrated that this pathway is activated, as assessed by ERK1/2 phosphorylation or measurements of ERK1/2 enzymatic activity, in 40–70% of primary AML specimens *(105,117,214,215)*. The observation that AML samples with constitutive activation of this pathway undergo apoptosis upon prolonged exposure to MEK inhibitors such as PD098059 or CI-1040 highlights the importance of this pathway for survival of blasts from some patients *(105)*.

PI3k/Akt pathway activation has also been implicated in the apoptotic resistance of leukemia cell lines and primary AML cells *(216)*. Indeed, the PI3K/Akt pathway has been shown to be constitutively activated in a majority of primary AML samples *(217,218)*. Moreover, blockade of this pathway (e.g., using the PI3k inhibitor LY294002) results in dephosphorylation of the pro-apoptotic regulator BAD *(219)*, increased apoptosis *(220)*, and decreased cytarabine resistance *(218)*.

One of the downstream targets of activated Akt (*see* Section 1.3.) is the transcription factor NFκB *(97,98)*, which induces transcription of genes encoding anti-apoptotic polypeptides such as c-FLIP and XIAP. NFκB is constitutively activated in as many as 75% of AML cases *(221,222)*. While Akt contributes to NFκB transcriptional activity, this transcription factor must first be activated by liberation from its cytoplasmic binding partner IκB and translocated to the nucleus, a process that involves phosphorylation of IκB by the IκB kinase (IKK) complex *(223,224)*. The potential importance of these events in AML was recently underscored by the demonstration that (1) NFκB activation correlates with diminished spontaneous apoptosis in AML samples and (2) SN-50, a peptide that inhibits nuclear import of NFκB, enhances etoposide-induced apoptosis in vitro *(222)*. Curiously, activation of the PI3k/Akt pathway was explained by activating *Ras* or *FLT3* mutations in fewer than 50% of cases examined *(222)*, suggesting that further dissection of the changes leading to activation of this pathway is required.

2.3.4. XIAP

A number of anti-apoptotic genes are regulated by NFκB *(99)*. Of primary importance to the present discussion is the gene encoding XIAP, the principal endogenous inhibitor of caspases 3, 7, and 9 (Section 1.4.). Macrophage colony stimulating factor (M-CSF), a cytokine that can rescue myeloid blasts from apoptosis *(225)*, enhances XIAP expression in myeloid leukemia cells *(226)*. Conversely, treatment with caffeic acid phenylethyl ester (CAPE), which is postulated to inhibit NFκB-mediated XIAP transcription, enhances apoptosis despite M-CSF treatment in vitro.

Additional studies have demonstrated that XIAP expression in AML correlates with PI3k and MAPK activation *(227)*. The potential importance of this XIAP expression is highlighted by the demonstration that XIAP antisense oligonucleotides enhance cytarabine sensitivity in HL-60 cells *(227)*. Whether a similar effect is observed in primary AML samples remains to be determined.

2.3.5. Stromal Cell Contributions

Recent studies suggest that, in addition to the effects of leukemia cell-intrinsic processes, the bone marrow microenvironment can also contribute to resistance to apoptosis in hematological malignancies. Co-culture of AML samples with the H5 human bone marrow stromal line increases short-term viability and resistance to cytarabine or daunorubicin in colony-forming assays in vitro *(228)*. Co-culture of leukemia cells lines and clinical AML isolates with stromal cells also induces expression of Bcl-2 and Bcl-x_L in vitro *(229)*. Interestingly, stroma-induced Bcl-2 upregulation is reportedly observed only in chemotherapy-resistant AML samples. How this fits with previous observations that Bcl-2 levels in primary AML specimens assayed directly after aspiration harvest fail to predict outcome *(201,202)* is at present unclear. Nonetheless, these observations offer a glimpse into an area that is ripe for future investigation and potential therapeutic intervention.

3. MEASUREMENT AND PROGNOSTIC IMPLICATIONS OF APOPTOTIC RESISTANCE IN AML

Because AML is a very heterogeneous disease in terms of causality, molecular pathogenesis, and response to therapy, it should come as no surprise that intrinsic sensitivity to apoptosis (either spontaneous or in response to therapy) is also quite variable. The critical issue is whether assays of apoptotic sensitivity are able to discriminate among prognostically heterogeneous patients.

Work of Smith and coworkers suggests that the amount of spontaneous apoptosis observed when AML blasts are cultured ex vivo correlates with sensitivity of the leukemia to induction chemotherapy in vivo *(190)*. Subsequent work also provides evidence that a block in both the intrinsic and extrinsic pathways is predictive of chemoresistance and decreased patient survival *(192)*. On the other hand, these conclusions have not been universally confirmed. Others have reported that the mitochondrial pathway can be trigged by etoposide or cytarabine in blasts from AML patients regardless of karyotype (unfavorable vs favorable prognosis) or clinical response to therapy *(230)*. Whether these divergent results reflect methodological differences, variations in patient populations studied, or other factors remains to be sorted out. Nonetheless, divergent results such as these explain why neither baseline measurements of apoptotic regulators nor assays of in vitro apoptotic sensitivity are routinely performed at present.

Acting on the presumption that apoptotic susceptibility will ultimately translate into improved therapeutic response, a number of groups have begun to examine the correlation between expression of various apoptotic regulators and response to therapy. For example, expression of Bcl-2, Bcl-x_L, Mcl-1, and Bax at diagnosis and at the time of minimal residual disease (either after consolidation 3 or stem cell transplant) has been assessed using four-color flow cytometry *(231).* Interestingly, patients who had detectable residual disease after chemotherapy had higher levels of group I Bcl-2 polypeptides at the time of diagnosis; and this anti-apoptotic phenotype simply persisted after the therapy *(231,232).* These results not only demonstrate the feasibility of simultaneously assaying multiple apoptotic regulators, but also raise the possibility that failure to simultaneously take into account levels of multiple polypeptides might explain the inability of some previous studies to demonstrate a relationship between Bcl-2 family member expression and clinical outcome. These types of observations also raise the possibility that the failure of previous studies to find a correlation between prognosis and endogenous XIAP levels *(233)* might likewise reflect the need to assay multiple polypeptides, e.g., XIAP, cIAP1, cIAP2, Smac, and HtRA2.

It has also been suggested that the particularly poor prognosis of elderly AML patients, while multifactorial, might reflect resistance of AML blasts to apoptosis. In support of this hypothesis, both spontaneous and cytarabine- or daunorubicin-induced apoptosis is reportedly decreased in circulating blasts from "elderly" (>age 55) compared to young AML patients *(234).* In addition, blasts from elderly AML patients were observed to express higher levels of Bcl-2 (and P-glycoprotein) than blasts from younger patients, although this might reflect the maturation state of the blasts (less maturation of the blasts in older patients) rather than any intrinsic age-related difference in gene expression *per se (235).* Whether these types of observations can be translated into therapeutic benefit for elderly and high-risk patients is a matter of substantial current investigation.

4. THERAPEUTIC STRATEGIES FOR OVERCOMING APOPTOTIC RESISTANCE IN AML

The hypothesis that intrinsic differences in sensitivity to apoptotic stimuli can affect therapeutic outcome in AML has several important implications (Table 2). First, it should be possible to demonstrate that cells become more resistant to apoptosis with each relapse. To our knowledge, a longitudinal study examining blasts from the same patients over time has not been completed. Second, it should be possible to demonstrate changes in the apoptotic machinery in sequential samples of blasts from individual patients. Consistent with this hypothesis, it has been shown that Mcl-1 is frequently upregulated at the time of relapse *(201),* whereas levels of caspases *(193)* and XIAP (P. Svingen and S. Kaufmann, unpublished observations) do not change in sequential samples. Third, as the alterations that contribute to diminished apoptosis in the clinical setting are identified, it might be possible to devise strategies to target these alterations. Whether these strategies will improve the therapeutic outcome, however, will depend on whether normal tissues are sensitive to the same to treatments or not. Nonetheless, three different approaches have been suggested based on improved understanding of the apoptotic pathways and their alterations in AML: (1) administering "pro-apoptotic" agents that directly inhibit components of the apoptotic machinery such as Bcl-2 family members or XIAP; (2) using signal transduction inhibitors to modulate anti-apoptotic signaling pathways; and (3) employing cytotoxic cytokines that, in contrast to most currently employed antileukemic agents *(236),* trigger apoptosis through the DR pathway. The current status of each of these approaches is summarized below.

4.1. Antagonizing Antiapoptotic Proteins: Targeting Bcl-2 and XIAP

In view of reports that Bcl-2 overexpression correlates with drug resistance in at least some studies (*see* Section 2.5.), targeting Bcl-2 is a logical approach for overcoming the inhibition

Table 2
Therapeutic Strategies for Overcoming Apoptotic Resistance in AML Cells

Target	Agent(s)	Class	Status	Ref.
Inhibitors of Anti-Apoptotic Proteins				
Bcl-2	G3139	Antisense nucleotide	Phase I AML	239
Bcl-2, Bcl-x_L,	ABT-737	Inhibitors of BH3	Preclinical	244
and Bcl-w	(−)Gossypol	protein binding	Preclinical	235,247
Bcl-x_L	ATRA	Retinoid	Combination phase II AML	198
XIAP	AEG 35156	Antisense nucleotide	Phase I solid tumors	249
XIAP	Small molecule antagonists	Small molecule	Preclinical	251,254, 256–258
Inhibitors of Survival Pathways				
Target	Agent(s)	Class	Status	Ref.
Raf (and others)	Sorfenib	Multitargeted kinase inhibitor	Phase III solid tumor Phase I leukemia	276
MEK	CI-1040	Selective small molecule inhibitors	Phase II solid tumor	105,119,264
	U0126		Preclinical	
PI3k	LY294002	PI3k inhibitor	Preclinical	217,218
	CCI-779	mTOR inhibitor	Phase II lymphoma	277
	RAD001	mTOR inhibitor	Phase I lymphoma	
FLT3 mutations	SU5416	Selective small molecule inhibitors	Phase II AML	268,269,278
	SU11248		Phase II AML	270,271
	CEP 701		Phase II AML	267
	PKC 412		Phase II AML	272
Death Receptor Ligands				
TRAIL	TRAIL	Cytotoxic cytokine	Phase I solid tumor	
TRAIL	Anti-DR4	Agonistic anti-receptor antibodies	Phase I	
	Anti-DR5		Phase II lymphoma	

of apoptosis in AML. G3139, an 18-mer antisense oligonucleotide directed against the first six codons of the Bcl-2 mRNA *(237)*, interrupts Bcl-2 production in vitro *(238)*. Two phase I clinical trials of G3139 in AML patients have been published. The first, which combined G3139 with FLAG (fludarabine, cytarabine, and G-CSF), demonstrated responses and successful Bcl-2 downregulation in 75% of patients with relapsed/refractory AML *(239)*. A subsequent trial of G3139 in combination with "standard" acute leukemia therapy (induction with cytarabine and daunorubicin, consolidation with high-dose cytarabine) in older patients with untreated AML demonstrated a CR rate of 50% with a median duration of remission of 1 year in those achieving a CR *(240)*. In the latter study, G3139 decreased Bcl-2 levels in responders but not nonresponders.

Although these preliminary studies are intriguing, it remains to be demonstrated that this strategy provides clinical benefit beyond standard therapy. Moreover, recent results have raised the possibility that any therapeutic benefit of G3139 might be related to off-target effects rather than Bcl-2 downregulation. In particular, it has been reported that G3139 retains its effects (inhibition of cellular growth and upregulation of reactive oxygen species) even in cells in which Bcl-2 has been downregulated *(241)*. In addition, it appears that the G3139 sequence is particularly effective at inducing an IFN-like response in cells treated in vitro *(242)*. These results will make it very difficult to determine what effect Bcl-2 downregulation by itself has on AML.

In another series of studies, treatment of cells with all-*trans*-retinoic acid (ATRA) has been shown to decrease levels of Bcl-2 and Bcl-X_L in AML samples, with concomitant enhancement of cytarabine-induced apoptosis *(198)*. Consistent with these observations, a clinical trial utilizing ATRA to enhance sensitivity of AML to cytotoxic agents has proven preliminarily encouraging *(243)*, although it remains to be shown that ATRA actually induced Bcl-2 or Bcl-x_L downregulation in the clinical setting.

An alternative approach for circumventing the anti-apoptotic action of Bcl-2 and its kin was recently described by Oltersdorf et al. *(244)*. In brief, these investigators reported that the ability of Bcl-2, Bcl-x_L, and Bcl-w to bind and neutralize proapoptotic Bcl-2 family members could be inhibited by ABT-737, a small molecule designed to fit into the cleft where antiapoptotic Bcl-2 homologs bind the BH3 domains of Bax, Bak, and group III polypeptides. ABT-737 not only induced apoptosis in lymphoma and small-cell lung cancer cells that overexpress Bcl-2, but also enhanced apoptosis induced by cytotoxic chemotherapeutic agents in vitro and in xenograft models. Studies in AML cells were not reported but are undoubtedly ongoing.

These types of effects are not limited to ABT-737. Gossypol, an agent previously studied as a male contraceptive, and some of its derivatives also bind the BH3 receptor on Bcl-2 and Bcl-x_L *(245,246)*. Additional studies have indicated that the negative enantiomer of gossypol induces cytochrome c release from isolated mitochondria *(247)*, enhances the cytotoxic effects of a number of pro-apoptotic treatments in vitro, and increases the efficacy of CHOP chemotherapy in a diffuse large cell lymphoma xenograft model *(248)*. In view of the evidence for selectivity in vivo, results of the ongoing phase I trials of (–)gossypol and its derivatives are awaited with interest.

Similar approaches have been devised to inhibit the expression or action of XIAP. In particular, an antisense oligonucleotide that downregulates XIAP (AEG 35156) has been developed and is now undergoing phase I clinical testing *(249)*. Results with this agent as well as XIAP small interfering RNA (siRNA) demonstrate that XIAP downregulation results in enhanced sensitivity to killing by TRAIL as well as some cytotoxic chemotherapeutic agents, but not others *(250)*. Further preclinical studies of these agents in AML cell lines and clinical AML samples are awaited with interest.

An alternative approach again involves the identification of small molecule antagonists. As indicated in Section 1.4., the Smac polypeptide binds and neutralizes XIAP, preventing the inhibition of caspases. Structural analyses (reviewed in refs. *251,252*) have demonstrated that four amino acids at the N-terminus of the mature Smac polypeptide are responsible for the inhibition of XIAP. Subsequent studies have demonstrated that introduction of Smac or its N-terminal tetrapeptide can, like XIAP antisense oligonucleotides, enhance TRAIL-induced apoptosis in the Jurkat human leukemia cell line *(253)* and anticancer drug-induced apoptosis in various models (reviewed in refs. *251,252*). Based on these results, several groups have identified XIAP antagonists using structure-based synthesis *(254,255)* or high-throughput screening *(256,257)*. One of the most promising leads, polyphenylurea 1396-12, reportedly induces apoptosis of AML samples in vitro in a Bcl-2-independent manner *(258)*. Additional preclinical and clinical studies of several of these XIAP antagonists are currently ongoing.

4.2. Inhibiting Prosurvival Signaling

As indicated in Section 1.3. and Fig. 3, signaling through the Raf/MEK/ERK, PI3K/Akt, and Jak/Stat pathways inhibits apoptosis, at least in part, by affecting the expression and action of Bcl-2 family members. Accordingly, blockade of these signal transduction pathways is another appealing approach for overcoming apoptotic resistance in AML.

Several components of the PI3k/Akt pathway have been examined as potential targets with this in mind. Inhibition of PI3k by LY294002 results in dephosphorylation of both Akt and BAD as well as increased AML cell apoptosis *(220)*. In addition, LY294002 markedly reduces NFκB activation and enhances the cytotoxicity of cytarabine in AML cells *(218)*.

An alternative approach involves inhibition of the same pathway downstream of Akt at the level of mTOR (mammalian target of rapamycin), an intermediary kinase that regulates protein synthesis and a variety of other cellular processes *(259,260)*. Elegant studies have demonstrated that the mTOR inhibitor rapamycin enhances the effectiveness of DNA-damaging chemotherapy in vivo in murine lymphoma cells containing activated Akt *(261)*. Consistent with these results, the rapamycin analog RAD001 has been shown to induce apoptosis in AML blasts and enhance cytarabine sensitivity in vitro *(217)*.

A number of agents that inhibit the Raf/MEK/ERK pathway have also been tested in preclinical studies. BAY 43-9006 (sorafenib), which inhibits Raf as well as other kinases *(262)*, has been shown to induce apoptosis in human leukemia cell lines, most likely through Mcl-1 downregulation, and to enhance the cytotoxic effects of DNA damage *(119,263)*. Likewise, the MEK inhibitors PD09859, CI-1040, and U0126 have been shown to induce apoptosis in AML cell lines and clinical AML samples in vitro *(105,117,264)*. Consistent with their proposed effects on anti-apoptotic Bcl-2 family members, the MEK inhibitors also sensitize AML cells to drug-induced apoptosis *(105)*.

Although JAK inhibitors are not yet available for testing in AML, it has been reported that the kinase inhibitor flavopiridol exerts its cytotoxic effects, at least in part, by inhibiting Stat3 binding to DNA *(265)*. A phase I study has demonstrated that flavopiridol exhibits single-agent activity against AML *(266)*.

Finally, constitutive signaling by mutant FLT3 receptors has been targeted by a number of tyrosine kinase inhibitors. Four agents that target this receptor with varying degrees of specificity, CEP-701 *(267)*, SU5416 *(268,269)*, SU11248 *(270,271)* and PKC 412 *(272)*, are currently in clinical development and are extensively reviewed elsewhere in this monograph.

4.3. Activating the Death Receptor Pathway

All of the strategies described above either activate or modulate the mitochondrial pathway. An alterative approach would be to activate the DR pathway. Among the death ligands, TRAIL has received the most extensive preclinical evaluation as a potential antineoplastic agent *(29,153,273)*. In addition to TRAIL itself, agonistic antibodies that activate the TRAIL receptors DR4 and DR5 have recently entered clinical testing.

For reasons that remain incompletely understood, TRAIL is selectively toxic to a variety of neoplastic cells in vitro and in vivo. A number of studies (reviewed in ref. *274*) have not only demonstrated that AML blasts express receptors for this cytokine, but also confirmed that TRAIL, which has little or no toxicity in normal marrow in vitro or in vivo, kills blasts from a subset of AML patients ex vivo. While these observations provide the impetus for further preclinical and possible clinical study of TRAIL or the agonistic antibodies in AML, three issues need to be addressed by further preclinical study. First, it is unclear whether AML blasts are type I cells, in which case TRAIL-induced killing would proceed independent of Bcl-2 status, or type II cells, in which case Bcl-2 status might have a profound impact on sensitivity to these agents. Second, it is unclear which receptor, DR4 or DR5, is the predominant receptor mediating TRAIL-induced killing of AML blasts. Earlier studies suggested that DR5 is the predominant receptor mediating all TRAIL-induced killing, but recent results in clinical samples of chronic lymphocytic leukemia have called this conclusion into question (reviewed in ref. *274*). Finally, because TRAIL does not kill logs of blasts, at least not in vitro (reviewed in ref. *274*), further preclinical studies that better define the determinants of sensitivity to these agents and possibly modulate that sensitivity appear to be needed. Results of these studies are awaited with interest.

5. SUMMARY

The suggestion that antileukemic agents kill blasts, at least in part, by activating intrinsic cell death pathways *(1,8)* has led to the hypothesis that therapeutic drug resistance might reflect alterations in the apoptotic machinery (reviewed in refs. *7,10*). At the present time this hypothesis is being extensively tested. At the same time, elucidation of the apoptotic machinery and the signal transduction pathways that regulate it has identified new targets for possible therapeutic intervention. It remains to be determined whether agents that target this apoptotic machinery will truly improve the efficacy of antileukemic therapy.

ACKNOWLEDGMENTS

Work in the authors' laboratories is supported by K23 CA96780 (R.A.M.) and R01 CA69008 (S.H.K.). The authors also acknowledge stimulating conversations with David Vaux, William C. Earnshaw, Greg Gores, O. Michael Colin, and Gary Kruh, as well as the editorial assistance of Deb Strauss.

REFERENCES

1. Kaufmann SH. Induction of endonucleolytic DNA cleavage in human acute myelogenous leukemia cells by etoposide, camptothecin, and other cytotoxic anticancer drugs: a cautionary note. Cancer Res 1989;49: 5870–5878.
2. Kaufmann SH, Earnshaw WC. Induction of apoptosis by cancer chemotherapy. Exp Cell Res 2000;256:42–49.
3. Li X, Gong J, Feldman E, Seiter K, Traganos F, Darzynkiewicz Z. Apoptotic cell death during treatment of leukemias. Leuk Lymph 1994;13:65–70.
4. Seiter K, Feldman EJ, Halicka HD, et al. Phase I clinical and laboratory evaluation of topotecan and cytarabine in patients with acute leukemia. J Clin Oncol 1997;15:44–51.
5. Green DR, Bissonnette RP, Cotter TG. Apoptosis and cancer. Import Adv Oncol 1994;1994:37–52.
6. Hannun YA. Apoptosis and the dilemma of cancer chemotherapy. Blood 1997;89:1845–1853.
7. Johnstone RW, Ruefli AA, Lowe SW. Apoptosis. A link between cancer genetics and chemotherapy. Cell 2002;108:153–164.
8. Wyllie AH, Kerr JFR, Currie AR. Cell death: the significance of apoptosis. Int Rev Cytol 1980;68:251–306.
9. Hengartner MO. The biochemistry of apoptosis. Nature 2000;407:770–776.
10. Kaufmann SH, Vaux DL. Alterations in the apoptotic machinery and their Potential role in anticancer drug resistance. Oncogene 2003;22:7414–7430.
11. Earnshaw WC, Martins LM, Kaufmann SH. Mammalian caspases: structure, activation, substrates and functions during apoptosis. Ann Rev Biochem 1999;68:383–424.
12. Fischer U, Janicke RU, Schulze-Osthoff K. Many cuts to ruin: a comprehensive update of caspase substrates. Cell Death Diff 2003;10:76–100.
13. Vaux DL, Silke J. Mammalian mitochondrial IAP binding proteins. Biochem Biophys Res Comm 2003; 304:499–504.
14. Danial NN, Korsmeyer SJ. Cell death: critical control points. Cell 2004;116:205–219.
15. Jiang X, Wang X. Cytochrome c-mediated apoptosis. Ann Rev Biochem 2004;73:87–106.
16. Green Dr. Apoptotic pathways: ten minutes to dead. Cell 2005;121:671–674.

17. Green DR, Kroemer G. The pathophysiology of mitochondrial cell death. Science 2004;305:626–629.
18. Cory S, Adams JM. The Bcl2 family: regulators of the cellular life-or-death switch. Nat Rev Cancer 2002;2: 647–656.
19. Liu X, Kim CN, Yang J, Jemmerson R, Wang X. Induction of apoptotic program in cell-free extracts: requirement for dATP and cytochrome c. Cell 1996;86:147–157.
20. Mesner PW, Jr., Bible KC, Martins LM, et al. Characterization of caspase processing and activation of HL-60 cell cytosol under cell-free conditions: nucleotide requirement and inhibitor profile. J Biol Chem 1999;274: 22,635–22,645.
21. Shi Y. Caspase activation: revisiting the induced proximity model. Cell 2004;117:855–858.
22. Deveraux QL, Takahashi R, Salvesen GS, Reed JC. X-Linked IAP is a direct inhibitor of cell-death proteases. Nature 1997;388:300–304.
23. Deveraux QL, Leo E, Stennicke HR, Welsh K, Salvesen GS, Reed JC. Cleavage of human inhibitor of apoptosis protein XIAP results in fragments with distinct specificities for caspases. EMBO J 1999;18:5242–5251.
24. Verhagen AM, Ekert PG, Pakusch M, et al. Identification of DIABLO, a mammalian protein that promotes apoptosis by binding to and antagonizing IAP proteins. Cell 2000;102:45–53.
25. Du C, Fang M, Li Y, Li L, Wang X. Smac, a mitochondrial protein that promotes cytochrome c-dependent caspase activation by eliminating IAP inhibition. Cell 2000;102:33–42.
26. Walczak H, Krammer PH. The CD95 (APO-1/Fas) and the TRAIL (APO-2L) apoptosis systems. Exp Cell Res 2000;256:58–66.
27. Krammer PH. CD95's deadly mission in the immune system. Nature 2000;407:789–795.
28. Ashkenazi A. Targeting death and decoy receptors of the tumour-necrosis factor superfamily. Nat Rev Cancer 2002;2:420–430.
29. Smyth MJ, Takeda K, Hayakawa Y, Peschon JJ, van den Brink MR, Yagita H. Nature's TRAIL—on a path to cancer immunotherapy. Immunity 2003;18:1–6.
30. Thorburn A. Death receptor-induced cell killing. Cell Signal 2004;16:139–144.
31. Aggarwal BB. Signalling pathways of the TNF superfamily: a double-edged sword. Nat Rev Immunol 2003; 3:745–756.
32. Wajant H. Death receptors. Essays Biochem 2003;39:53–71.
33. Nagata S. Apoptosis by death factor. Cell 1997;88:355–365.
34. Green DR, Ferguson TA. The role of Fas ligand in immune privilege. Nat Rev Mol Cell Biol 2001;2: 917–924.
35. Takeda K, Smyth MJ, Cretney E, et al. Critical role for tumor necrosis factor-related apoptosis-inducing ligand in immune surveillance against tumor development. J Exp Med 2002;195:161–169.
36. Takeda K, Hayakawa Y, Smyth MJ, et al. Involvement of tumor necrosis factor-related apoptosis-inducing ligand in surveillance of tumor metastasis by liver natural killer cells. Nature Med 2001;7:94–100.
37. Smyth MJ, Cretney E, Takeda K, et al. Tumor necrosis factor-related apoptosis-inducing ligand (TRAIL) contributes to interferon gamma-dependent natural killer cell protection from tumor metastasis. J Exp Med 2001;193:661–670.
38. Boatright KM, Renatus M, Scott FL, et al. A unified model for apical caspase activation. Mol Cell 2003; 11:529–541.
39. Chang DW, Xing Z, Capacio VL, Peter ME, Yang X. Interdimer processing mechanism of procaspase-8 activation. EMBO J 2003;22:4132–4142.
40. Chang DW, Xing Z, Pan Y, et al. c-FLIP(L) is a dual function regulator for caspase-8 activation and CD95-mediated apoptosis. EMBO J 2002;21:3704–3714.
41. Kischkel FC, Lawrence DA, Tinel A, et al. Death receptor recruitment of dndogenous caspase-10 and apoptosis initiation in the absence of caspase-8. J Biol Chem 2001;276:46,639–46,646.
42. Boatright KM, Deis C, Denault JB, Sutherlin DP, Salvesen GS. Activation of caspases-8 and -10 by FLIP(L). Biochem J 2004;382:651–657.
43. Scaffidi C, Fulda S, Srinivasan A, et al. Two CD95 (APO-1)/Fas signaling pathways. EMBO J 1998; 17:1675–1687.
44. Sun XM, Bratton SB, Butterworth M, MacFarlane M, Cohen GM. Bcl-2 and Bcl-xL inhibit CD95-mediated apoptosis by mitochondrial release of Smac/DIABLO and subsequentinactivation of X-linked inhibitor-of-apoptosis rrotein. J Biol Chem 2002;277:11,345–11,351.
45. Li H, Zhu H, Xu CJ, Yuan J. Cleavage of BID by caspase 8 mediates the mitochondrial damage in the Fas pathway of apoptosis. Cell 1998;94:491–501.

46. Luo X, Budihardjo I, Zou H, Slaughter C, Wang X. Bid, a Bcl2 interacting protein, mediates cytochrome c release from mitochondria in response to activation of cell surface death receptors. Cell 1998;94:481–490.

47. Karp JE, Passaniti A, Gojo I, et al. Phase I and pharmacokinetic study of flavopiridol followed by 1-beta-D-arabinofuranosylcytoine and mitoxantrone in relapsed and refractory adult acute leukemias. Clin Cancer Res 2005;11:8403–8412.

48. Gross A, McDonnell JM, Korsmeyer SJ. BCL-2 family members and the mitochondria in apoptosis. Genes Dev 1999;13:1899–1911.

49. Cory S, Huang DC, Adams JM. The Bcl-2 family: roles in cell survival and oncogenesis. Oncogene 2003; 22:8590–8607.

50. Coultas L, Strasser A. The role of the Bcl-2 protein family in cancer. Semin Cancer Biol 2003;13:115–123.

51. Kaufmann SH, Steensma DP. On the TRAIL of a new therapy for leukemia. Leukemia 2005;19:2195–2202.

52. Newmeyer DD, Ferguson-Miller S. Mitochondria: releasing power for life and unleashing the machineries of death. Cell 2003;112:481–490.

53. Wolter KG, Hsu YT, Smith CL, Nechushtan A, Xi XG, Youle RJ. Movements of bax from cytosol to mitochondria during apoptosis. J Cell Biol 1997;139:1281–1292.

54. Antonsson B, Montessuit S, Sanchez B, Martinou JC. Bax is present as a high molecular weight oligomer/complex in the mitochondrial membrane of apoptotic cells. J Biol Chem 2001;276:11,615–11,623.

55. Desagher S, Osen-Sand A, Nichols A, et al. Bid-induced conformational change of Bax is responsible for mitochondrial cytochrome c release during apoptosis. J Cell Biol 1999;144:891–901.

56. Eskes R, Desagher S, Antonsson B, Martinou JC. Bid induces the oligomerization and insertion of Bax into the outer mitochondrial membrane. Mol Cell Biol 2000;20:929–935.

57. Makin GWJ, Corfe BM, Griffiths GJ, Thistlethwaite A, Hickman JA, Dive C. Damage-induced Bax N-terminal change, translocation to mitochondria and formation of Bax dimers/complexes occur regardless of cell fate. EMBO J 2001;20:6306–6315.

58. Griffiths GJ, Dubrez L, Morgan CP, et al. Cell damage-induced conformational changes of the pro-apoptotic protein Bak in vivo precede the onset of apoptosis. J Cell Biol 1999;144:903–914.

59. Wei MC, Zong WX, Cheng EH, et al. Proapoptotic BAX and BAK: A Requisite Gateway to Mitochondrial Dysfunction and Death. Science 2001;292:727–730.

60. Cheng EH, Wei MC, Weiler S, et al. BCL-2, BCL-X(L) Sequester BH3 Domain-Only Molecules Preventing BAX- and BAK-Mediated Mitochondrial Apoptosis. Mol Cell 2001;8:705–711.

61. Kuwana T, Bouchier-Hayes L, Chipuk JE, et al. BH3 Domains of BH3-only proteins differentially regulate Bax-mediated mitochondrial membrane permeabilization both directly and indirectly. Mol Cell 2005;17:525–535.

62. Cartron P-F, Gallenne T, Bougras G, et al. The first helix of Bax plays a necessary role in its ligand-induced activation by the BH3-only proteins Bid and PUMA. Mol Cell 2004;16:807–818.

63. Chen L, Willis SN, Wei A, et al. Differential targeting of prosurvival Bcl-2 proteins by their BH3-only ligands allows complementary apoptotic function. Mol Cell 2005;17:393–403.

64. Cuconati A, Mukherjee C, Perez D, White E. DNA damage response and MCL-1 destruction initiate apoptosis in adenovirus-infected cells. Genes Dev 2003;17:2922–2932.

65. Mikhailov V, Mikhailova M, Degenhardt K, Venkatachalam MA, White E, Saikumar P. Association of Bax and Bak homo-oligomers in mitochondria. Bax requirement for Bak reorganization and cytochrome c release. J Biol Chem 2003;278:5367–5376.

66. Willis SN, Chen L, Dewson G, et al. Proapoptotic Bak is sequestered by Mcl-1 and Bcl-xL, but not Bcl-2, until displaced by BH3-only proteins. Genes Dev 2005;19:1294–1305.

67. Barry M, Heibein JA, Pinkoski MJ, et al. Granzyme B short-circuits the need for caspase 8 activity during granule-mediated cytotoxic T-lymphocyte killing by directly cleaving Bid. Mol Cell Biol 2000;20:3781–3794.

68. Stoka V, Turk B, Schendel SL, et al. Lysosomal protease pathways to apoptosis. Cleavage of bid, not pro-caspases, is the most likely route. J Biol Chem 2001;276:3149–3157.

69. Gajewski TF, Thompson CG. Apoptosis meets signal transduction: elimination of a BAD influence. Cell 1996;87:589–592.

70. Puthalakath H, Huang DCS, O'Reilly LA, King SM, Strasser A. The proapoptotic activity of the Bcl-2 family member Bim is regulated by interaction with the dynein motor complex. Mol Cell 1999;3:287–296.

71. Bouillet P, Metcalf D, Huang DC, et al. Proapoptotic Bcl-2 relative Bim required for certain apoptotic responses, leukocyte homeostasis, and to preclude autoimmunity. Science 1999;286:1735–1738.

72. Tan T-T, Degenhardt K, Nelson DA, et al. Key roles of BIM-driven apoptosis in epithelial tumors and rational chemotherapy. Cancer Cell 2005;7:227–238.

73. Puthalakath H, Villunger A, O'Reilly LA, et al. Bmf: A proapoptotic BH3-only protein regulated by interaction with the myosin V actin motor complex, activated by anoikis. Science 2001;293:1829–1832.

74. Yu JJ, Zhang L, Hwang PM, Kinzler KW, Vogelstein B. PUMA induces the rapid apoptosis of colorectal cancer cells. Mol Cell 2001;7:673–682.

75. Oda E, Ohki R, Murasawa H, et al. Noxa, a BH3-only member of the Bcl-2 family and candidate mediator of p53-induced apoptosis. Science 2000;288:1053–1058.

76. Yu J, Wang Z, Kinzler KW, Vogelstein B, Zhang L. PUMA mediates the apoptotic response to p53 in colorectal cancer cells. Proc Natl Acad Sci USA 2003;100:1931–1936.

77. Villunger A, Michalak EM, Coultas L, et al. p53- and drug-induced apoptotic responses mediated by BH3-only proteins puma and noxa. Science 2003;302:1036–1038.

78. Jeffers JR, Parganas E, Lee Y, et al. PUMA is an essential mediator of p53-dependent and -independent apoptotic pathways. Cancer Cell 2003;4:321–328.

79. Krajewski S, Krajewska M, Shabaik A, et al. Immunohistochemical analysis of in vivo patterns of Bcl-X expression. Cancer Res 1994;54:5501–5507.

80. Krajewski S, Bodrug S, Krajewska M, et al. Immunohistochemical analysis of Mcl-1 protein in human tissues. Am J Pathol 1995;146:1309–1319.

81. Dent P, Grant S. Pharmacologic interruption of the mitogen-activated extracellular-regulated kinase/mitogen-activated protein kinase signal transduction pathway: potential role of promoting cytotoxic arug action. Clin Cancer Res 2001;7:775–783.

82. Allen LF, Sebolt-Leopold J, Meyer MB. CI-1040 (PD184352), a targeted signal transduction inhibitor of MEK (MAPKK). Semin Oncol 2003;30:105–116.

83. Repasky GA, Chenette EJ, Der CJ. Renewing the conspiracy theory debate: does Raf function alone to mediate Ras oncogenesis? Trends Cell Biol 2004;14:639–647.

84. Okuda K, Sanghera JS, Pelech SL, et al. Granulocyte-macrophage colony-stimulating factor, interleukin-3 and stell factor induce rapid tyrosine phosphorylation of p42 and p44 MAP kinase. Blood 1992;79:2880–2887.

85. Welham MJ, Duronio V, Sanghera JS, Pelech SL, Schrader JW. Multiple hemopoietic growth factors stimulate activation of mitogen-activated protein kinase family members. J Immunol 1992;149:1683–1693.

86. Pulverer BJ, Kyriakis JM, Avruch J, Nikolakaki E, Woodgett JR. Phosphorylation of c-jun mediated by MAP kinases. Nature 1991;353:670–674.

87. Marais R, Wynne J, Treisman R. The SRF accessory protein Elk-1 contains a growth factor-regulated transcriptional activation domain. Cell 1993;73:381–393.

88. Seth A, Alvarez E, Gupta S, Davis RJ. A phosphorylation site located in the NH2-terminal domain of c-Myc increases transactivation of gene expression. J Biol Chem 1991;266:23,521–23,524.

89. Frodin M, Gammeltoft S. Role and regulation of 90 kDa ribosomal S6 kinase (RSK) in signal transduction. Mol Cell Endocrinol 1999;151:65–77.

90. Datta SR, Brunet A, Greenberg ME. Cellular survival: a play in three Akts. Genes Dev 1999;13:2905–2927.

91. Downward J. PI 3-kinase, Akt and cell survival. Semin Cell Biol 2004;15:177–182.

92. Amaravadi R, Thompson CB. The survival kinases Akt and Pim as potential pharmacological targets. J Clin Invest 2005;115:2618–2624.

93. Woodgett JR. Recent advances in the protein kinase B signaling pathway. Curr Opin Cell Biol 2005;17:150–157.

94. Dan HC, Sun M, Kaneko S, et al. Akt phosphorylation and stabilization of X-linked inhibitor of apoptosis protein (XIAP). J Biol Chem 2004;279:5405–5412.

95. Brunet A, Bonni A, Zigmond MJ, et al. Akt promotes cell survival by phosphorylating and inhibiting a forkhead transcription factor. Cell 1999;96:857–868.

96. Gilley J, Coffer PJ, Ham J. FOXO transcription factors directly activate bim gene expression and promote apoptosis in sympathetic neurons. J Cell Biol 2003;162:613–622.

97. Sizemore N, Leung S, Stark GR. Activation of phosphatidylinositol 3-kinase in response to interleukin-1 leads to phosphorylation and activation of the NF-kappaB p65/RelA subunit. Mol Cell Biol 1999;19:4798–4805.

98. Ozes ON, Mayo LD, Gustin JA, Pfeffer SR, Pfeffer LM, Donner DB. NF-kappaB activation by tumour necrosis factor requires the Akt serine-threonine kinase. Nature 1999;401:82–85.

99. Karin M, Lin A. NF-kappaB at the crossroads of life and death. Nat Immunol 2002;3:221–227.

100. Aaronson DS, Horvath CM. A road map for those who don't know JAK-STAT. Science 2002;296:1653–1655.

101. Shuai K, Liu B. Regulation of JAK-STAT signalling in the immune system. Nat Rev Immunol 2003;3:900–911.

102. Schindler CW. JAK-STAT signaling in human disease. J Clin Invest 2002;109:1133–1137.

103. Rane SG, Reddy EP. JAKs, STATs and Src kinases in hematopoiesis. Oncogene 2002;21:3334–3358.

104. Boucher MJ, Morisset J, Vachon PH, Reed JC, Laine J, Rivard N. MEK/ERK signaling pathway regulates the expression of Bcl-2, Bcl-X(L), and Mcl-1 and promotes survival of human pancreatic cancer cells. J Cell Biochem 2000;79:355–369.
105. Milella M, Kornblau SM, Estrov Z, et al. Therapeutic targeting of the MEK/MAPK signal transduction module in acute myeloid leukemia. J Clin Invest 2001;108:851–859.
106. Catlett-Falcone R, Landowski TH, Oshiro MM, et al. Constitutive activation of Stat3 signaling confers resistance to apoptosis in human U266 myeloma cells. Immunity 1999;10:105–115.
107. Horita M, Andreu EJ, Benito A, et al. Blockade of the Bcr-Abl kinase activity induces apoptosis of chronic myelogenous leukemia cells by suppressing signal transducer and cctivator of transcription 5-dependent expression of Bcl-xL. J Exp Med 2000;191:977–984.
108. Epling-Burnette PK, Liu JH, Catlett-Falcone R, et al. Inhibition of STAT3 signaling leads to apoptosis of leukemic large granular lymphocytes and decreased Mcl-1 expression. J Clin Invest 2001;107:351–362.
109. Wang JM, Chao JR, Chen WS, Kuo ML, Yen JJ, Yang-Yen H-F. The antiapoptotic gene mcl-1 is up-regulated by the phosphatidylinositol 3-kinase/Akt signaling pathway through a transcription factor complex containing CREB. Mol Cell Biol 1999;19:6195–6206.
110. Bernal A, Pastore RD, Asgary Z, et al. Survival of leukemic B cells promoted by engagement of the antigen receptor. Blood 2001;98:3050–3057.
111. Henson ES, Gibson EM, Villanueva J, Bristow NA, Haney N, Gibson SB. Increased expression of Mcl-1 is responsible for the blockage of TRAIL-induced apoptosis mediated by EGF/ErbB1 signaling pathway. J Cell Biochem 2003;89:1177–1192.
112. Kobayashi S, Werneburg NW, Bronk SF, Kaufmann SH, Gores GJ. Interleukin-6 contributes to myeloid cell leukemia-1 upregulation (Mcl-1) and TRAIL resistance vis an Akt signaling pathway in cholangiocarcinoma cells. Gastroenterology 2005;128:2054–2065.
113. Ruvolo PP, Deng X, Carr BK, May WS. A functional role for mitochondrial protein kinase C alpha in Bcl2 phosphorylation and suppression of apoptosis. J Biol Chem 1998;273:25,436–25,442.
114. Deng X, Ruvolo P, Carr B, May WS, Jr. Survival function of ERK1/2 as IL-3-activated, staurosporine-resistant Bcl2 kinases. Proc Natl Acad Sci USA 2000;97:1578–1583.
115. Deng X, Gao F, Flagg T, May WS, Jr. Mono- and multisite phosphorylation enhances Bcl2′s antiapoptotic function and inhibition of cell cycle entry functions. Proc Natl Acad Sci USA 2004;101:153–158.
116. Domina AM, Smith JH, Craig RW. Myeloid cell leukemia 1 is phosphorylated through two distinct pathways, one associated with extracellular signal-regulated kinase activation and the other with G2/M accumulation or protein phosphatase 1/2A inhibition. J Biol Chem 2000;275:21,688–21,694.
117. Meng X, Chandra J, Loegering D, et al. Central role of FADD in apoptosis induction by the mitogen activated protein kinase inhibitor CI1040 (PD184352) in acute lymphocytic leukemia cell lines in vitro. J Biol Chem 2003;278:47,236–47,339.
118. Domina AM, Vrana JA, Gregory MA, Hann SR, Craig RW. MCL1 is phosphorylated in the PEST region and stabilized upon ERK activation in viable cells, and at additional sites with cytotoxic okadaic acid or taxol. Oncogene 2004;23:5301–5315.
119. Lee YK, Isham CR, Kaufman SH, Bible KC. Flavopiridol disrupts STAT3/DNA interactions, attenuates STAT3-directed transcription, and combines with the Jak kinase inhibitor AG490 to achieve cytotoxic synergy. Mol Cancer Ther 2006;5:138–148.
120. Xia Z, Dickens M, Raingeaud J, Davis RJ, Greenberg ME. Opposing effects of ERK and JNK-p38 MAP kinases on apoptosis. Science 1995;270:1326–1331.
121. Marani M, Hancock D, Lopes R, Tenev T, Downard J, Lemoine NR. Role of Bim in the survival pathway induced by Raf in epithelial cells. Oncogene 2004;23:2431–2441.
122. Shinjyo T, Kuribara R, Inukai T, et al. Downregulation of Bim, a proapoptotic relative of Bcl-2, is a pivotal step in cytokine-initiated survival signaling in murine hematopoietic progenitors. Mol Cell Biol 2001;21:854–864.
123. Collins NL, Reginato MJ, Paulus JK, Sgroi DC, Labaer J, Brugge JS. G1/S cell cycle arrest provides anoikis resistance through Erk-mediated Bim suppression. Mol Cell Biol 2005;25:5282–5291.
124. Stahl M, Dijkers PF, Kops GJ, et al. The forkhead transcription factor FoxO regulates transcription of p27Kip1 and Bim in response to IL-2. J Immunol 2002;168:5024–5031.
125. Levine RL, Wadleigh M, Cools J, et al. Activating mutation in the tyrosine kinase JAK2 in polycythemia vera, essential thrombocythemia, and myeloid metaplasia with myelofibrosis. Cancer Cell 2005;7:387–397.
126. Ley R, Balmanno K, Hadfield K, Weston C, Cook SJ. Activation of the ERK1/2 signaling pathway promotes phosphorylation and proteasome-dependent degradation of the BH3-only protein, Bim. J Biol Chem 2003;278:18,811–18,816.

127. Luciano F, Jacquel A, Colosetti P, et al. Phosphorylation of Bim-El by Erk1/2 on serine 69 promotes its degradation via the proteasome pathway and regulates its proapoptotic function. Oncogene 2003;22: 6785–6793.

128. Ley R, Ewings KE, Hadfield K, Howes E, Balmanno K, Cook SJ. Extracellular signal-regulated kinases 1/2 are serum-stimulated Bim$_{EL}$ causing its phosphorylation and turnover. J Biol Chem 2004;279:8837–8847.

129. Harada H, Quearry B, Ruiz-Vela A, Korsmeyer SJ. Survival factor-induced extracellular signal-regulated kinase phosphorylates BIM, inhibiting its association with BAX and proapoptotic activity. Proc Natl Acad Sci USA 2004;101:15,313–15,317.

130. Ley R, Hadfield K, Howes E, Cook SJ. Identification of a DEF-type docking domain for extracellular signal-regulated kinases 1/2 that directs phosphorylation and turnover of the BH3-only protein BimEL. J Biol Chem 2005;280:17,657–17,663.

131. Zha J, Harada H, Yang E, Jockel J, Korsmeyer SJ. Serine phosphorylation of death agonist BAD in response to survival factor results in binding to 14-3-3 not Bcl-XL. Cell 1996;87:619–628.

132. Datta SR, Dudek H, Tao X, et al. Akt phosphorylation of BAD couples survival signals to the cell-intrinsic death machinery. Cell 1997;91:231–241.

133. del Peso L, Gonzalez-Garcia M, Page C, Herrera R, Nunez G. Interleukin-3-induced phosphorylation of BAD through the protein kinase Akt. Science 1997;278:687–689.

134. Harada H, Becknell B, Wilm M, et al. Phosphorylation and inactivation of BAD by mitochondria-anchored protein kinase A. Mol Cell 1999;3:413–422.

135. Tan Y, Ruan H, Demeter MR, Comb MJ. p90(RSK) blocks bad-mediated cell death via a protein kinase C-dependent pathway. J Biol Chem 1999;274:34,859–34,867.

136. Eisenmann KM, VanBrocklin MW, Staffend NA, Kitchen SM, Koo HM. Mitogen-activated protein kinase pathway-dependent tumor-specific survival signaling in melanoma cells through inactivation of the proapoptotic protein bad. Cancer Res 2003;63:8330–8337.

137. Tournier C, Hess P, Yang DD, et al. Requirement of JNK for stress-induced activation of the cytochrome c-mediated death rathway. Science 2000;288:870–874.

138. Lei K, Nimnual A, Zong WX, et al. The Bax subfamily of Bcl2-related proteins is essential for apoptotic signal transduction by c-Jun NH(2)-terminal kinase. Mol Cell Biol 2002;22:4929–4942.

139. Lei K, Davis RJ. JNK phosphorylation of Bim-related members of the Bcl2 family induces Bax-dependent apoptosis. Proc Natl Acad Sci USA 2003;100:2432–2437.

140. Putcha GV, Le S, Frank S, et al. JNK-mediated BIM phosphorylation potentiates BAX-dependent apoptosis. Neuron 2003;38:899–914.

141. Tsuruta F, Sunayama J, Mori Y, et al. JNK promotes Bax translocation to mitochondria through phosphorylation of 14-3-3 proteins. EMBO J 2004;23:1889–1899.

142. Salvesen GS, Duckett CS. IAP Proteins: Blocking the road to death's door. Nat Rev Cell Mol Biol 2002; 3:401–410.

143. Srinivasula SM, Hegde R, Saleh A, et al. A conserved XIAP-interaction motif in caspase-9 and Smac/DIABLO regulates caspase activity and apoptosis. Nature 2001;410:112–116.

144. Shiozaki EN, Chai J, Rigotti DJ, et al. Mechanism of XIAP-mediated inhibition of caspase-9. Mol Cell 2003;11:519–527.

145. Scott FL, Denault JB, Riedl SJ, Shin H, Renatus M, Salvesen GS. XIAP inhibits caspase-3 and -7 using two binding sites: evolutionarily conserved mechanism of IAPs. EMBO J 2005;24:645–655.

146. Wilkinson JC, Wilkinson AS, Scott FL, Csomos RA, Salvesen GS, Duckett CS. Neutralization of Smac/Diablo by inhibitors of apoptosis (IAPs). A caspase-independent mechanism for apoptotic inhibition. J Biol Chem 2004;279:51,082–51,090.

147. Ekert PG, Silke J, Hawkins CJ, Verhagen AM, Vaux DL. DIABLO promotes apoptosis by removing MIHA/XIAP from processed caspase 9. J Cell Biol 2001;152:483–490.

148. Roy N, Deveraux QL, Takahashi R, Salvesen GS, Reed JC. The c-IAP-1 and c-IAP-2 proteins are direct inhibitors of specific caspases. EMBO J 1997;16:6914–6925.

149. Hwain S, Renatus M, Eckelman BP, Nunes VA, Sampaio CAM, Salvesen GS. The BIR domain of IAP-like protein 2 is conformationally unstable: implications for caspase inhibition. Biochem J 2005;385:1–10.

150. Vucic D, Franklin MC, Wallweber HJA, et al. Engineering ML-IAP to produce an extraordinarily potent caspase 9 inhibitor: implications for Smac-dependent anti-apoptotic activity of ML-IAP. Biochem J 2005; 385:11–20.

151. Hegde R, Srinivasula SM, Datta P, et al. The polypeptide chain-releasing factor GSPT1/eRF3 is proteolytically processed into an IAP-binding protein. J Biol Chem 2003;278:38,699–38,706.

152. Ekert PG, Vaux DL. The mitochondrial death squad—hardened killers or innocent bystanders? Curr Opin Cell Biol 2005;17:in press.

153. Wang S, El-Deiry WS. TRAIL and apoptosis induction by TNF-family death receptors. Oncogene 2003;22: 8628–8633.

154. Puthalakath H, Strasser A. Keeping killers on a tight leash: transcriptional and post-translational control of the pro-apoptotic activity of BH3-only proteins. Cell Death Differ 2002;9:505–512.

155. Wu GS, Burns TF, McDonald ER, et al. KILLER/DR5 is a DNA damage-inducible p53-regulated death receptor gene. Nat Genet 1997;17:141–143.

156. Wen J, Ramadevi N, Nguyen D, Perkins CL, Worthington E, Bhalla KN. Antileukemic drugs increase death receptor 5 levels and enhance apo-2L-induced apoptosis of human acute leukemia cells. Blood 2000;96: 3900–3906.

157. Ozoren N, El-Deiry WS. Cell surface death receptor signaling in normal and cancer cells. Semin Cancer Biol 2003;13:135–147.

158. Krueger A, Baumann S, Krammer PH, Kirchhoff S. FLICE-inhibitory proteins: regulators of death receptor-mediated apoptosis. Mol Cell Biol 2001;21:8247–8254.

159. Thome M, Tschopp J. Regulation of lymphocyte proliferation and death by FLIP. Nat Rev Immunol 2001;1:50–58.

160. Micheau O, Thome M, Schneider P, et al. The long form of FLIP is an activator of caspase-8 at the Fas death-inducing signaling complex. J Biol Chem 2002;277:45,162–45,171.

161. Dohrman A, Russell JQ, Cuenin S, Fortner K, Tschopp J, Budd RC. Cellular FLIP long form augments caspase activity and death of T cells through heterodimerization with and activation of caspase-8. J Immunol 2005; 175:311–318.

162. Sharp DA, Lawrence DA, Ashkenazi A. Selective knockdown of the long variant of cellular FLICE inhibitory protein augments death receptor-mediated caspase-8 activation and apoptosis. J Biol Chem 2005;280: 19,401–19,409.

163. Taniai M, Grambihler A, Higuchi H, et al. Mcl-1 mediates tumor necrosis factor-related apoptosis-inducing ligand resistance in human cholangiocarcinoma cells. Cancer Res 2004;64:3517–3524.

164. Zhang XD, Borrow JM, Zhang XY, Nguyen T, Hersey P. Activation of ERK1/2 protects melanoma cells from TRAIL-induced apoptosis by inhibiting Smac/DIABLO release from mitochondria. Oncogene 2003; 22:2869–2881.

165. Zhang L, Fang B. Mechanisms of resistance to TRAIL-induced apoptosis in cancer. Cancer Gene Ther 2005;12:228–237.

166. Schulze-Bergkamen H, Brenner D, Krueger A, et al. Hepatocyte growth factor induces Mcl-1 in primary human hepatocytes and inhibits CD95-mediated apoptosis via Akt. Hepatology 2004;39:645–654.

167. Muta K, Krantz SB. Apoptosis of human erythroid colony-forming cells is decreased by stem cell factor and insulin-like growth factor I as well as erythropoietin. J Cell Physiol 1993;156:264–271.

168. Savill JS, Wyllie AH, Henson JE, Walport MJ, Henson PM, Haslett C. Macrophage phagocytosis of aging neutrophils in inflammation. Programmed cell death in the neutrophil leads to its recognition by macrophages. J Clin Invest 1989;83:865–875.

169. Akgul C, Moulding DA, Edwards SW. Molecular control of neutrophil apoptosis. FEBS Lett 2001;487: 318–322.

170. Murray J, Barbara JA, Dunkley SA, et al. Regulation of neutrophil apoptosis by tumor necrosis factor-alpha: requirement for TNFR55 and TNFR75 for induction of apoptosis in vitro. Blood 1997;90:2772–2783.

171. Hanahan D, Weinberg RA. The hallmarks of cancer. Cell 2000;100:57–70.

172. Evan GI, Vousden KH. Proliferation, cell cycle and apoptosis in cancer. Nature 2001;411:342–348.

173. Mundle SD, Ali A, Cartlidge JD, et al. Evidence for involvement of tumor necrosis factor-alpha in apoptotic death of bone marrow cells in myelodysplastic syndromes. Am J Hematol 1999;60:36–47.

174. Horikawa K, Nakakuma H, Kawaguchi T, et al. Apoptosis resistance of blood cells from patients with paroxysmal nocturnal hemoglobinuria, aplastic anemia, and myelodysplastic syndrome. Blood 1997;90: 2716–2722.

175. Suarez L, Vidriales MB, Garcia-Larana J, et al. CD34+ cells from acute myeloid leukemia, myelodysplastic syndromes, and normal bone marrow display different apoptosis and drug resistance-associated phenotypes. Clin Cancer Res 2004;10:7599–7606.

176. Cambier N, Baruchel A, Schlageter MH, et al. Chronic myelomonocytic leukemia: from biology to therapy. Hematol Cell Ther 1997;39:41–48.

177. McGahon A, Bissonnette R, Schmitt M, Cotter KM, Green DR, Cotter TG. Bcr-Abl maintains resistance of chronic myelogenous leukemia cells to apoptotic cell death. Blood 1994;83:1179–1187.
178. Bedi A, Zehnbauer BA, Barber JP, Sharkis SJ, Jones RJ. Inhibition of apoptosis by Bcr-Abl in chronic mlyeloid leukemia. Blood 1994;83:2038–2044.
179. Carlesso N, Frank DA, Griffin JD. Tyrosyl phosphorylation and DNA binding activity of signal transducers and activators of transcription (STAT) proteins in hematopoietic cell lines transformed by Bcr/Abl. J Exp Med 1996;183:811–820.
180. Aichberger KJ, Mayerhofer M, Krauth MT, et al. Identification of mcl-1 as a BCR/ABL-dependent target in chronic myeloid leukemia (CML): evidence for cooperative antileukemic effects of imatinib and mcl-1 antisense oligonucleotides. Blood 2005;105:3303–3311.
181. Prchal JF, Axelrad AA. Letter: Bone-marrow responses in polycythemia vera. N Engl J Med 1974;290:1382.
182. Pahl HL. Towards a molecular understanding of polycythemia rubra vera. Eur J Biochem 2000;267:3395–3401.
183. Baxter EJ, Scott LM, Campbell PJ, et al. Acquired mutation of the tyrosine kinase JAK2 in human myeloproliferative disorders. Lancet 2005;365:1054–1061.
184. Rahmani M, Davis EM, Bauer C, Dent P, Grant S. Apoptosis induced by the kinase inhibitor BAY 43-9006 in human leukemia cells involves down-regulation of Mcl-1 through inhibition of translation. J Biol Chem 2005;280:35,217–35,227.
185. Roder S, Steimle C, Meinhardt G, Pahl HL. STAT3 is constitutively active in some patients with Polycythemia rubra vera. Exp Hematol 2001;29:694–702.
186. Silva M, Richard C, Benito A, Sanz C, Olalla I, Fernandez-Luna JL. Expression of Bcl-x in erythroid precursors from patients with polycythemia vera. N Engl J Med 1998;338:564–571.
187. Komura E, Debili N, Vainchenker W, Giraudier S. Activation of STAT5 and NFkB through FKBP51 are involved in the spontaneous growth of megakaryocytes in primary myelofibrosis (PMF). Blood 2002;100:a531.
188. Mesa RA, Tefferi A, Gray LA, Reeder T, Schroeder G, Kaufmann SH. In vitro antiproliferative activity of the farnesyltransferase inhibitor R115777 in hematopoietic progenitors from patients with myelofibrosis with myeloid metaplasia. Leukemia 2003;17:849–855.
189. Mesa RA, Li CY, Ketterling RP, Schroeder GS, Knudson RA, Tefferi A. Leukemic transformation in myelofibrosis with myeloid metaplasia: a single-institution experience with 91 cases. Blood 2005;105:973–977.
190. Smith BD, Bambach BJ, Vala MS, et al. Inhibited apoptosis and drug resistance in acute myeloid leukaemia. Brit J Haematol 1998;102:1042–1049.
191. McCulloch EA. Stem cells in normal and leukemic hemopoiesis (Henry Stratton Lecture, 1982). Blood 1983;62:1–13.
192. Schimmer AD, Pedersen IM, Kitada S, et al. Functional blocks in caspase activation pathways are common in leukemia and predict patient response to induction chemotherapy. Cancer Res 2003;63:1242–1248.
193. Svingen PA, Karp JE, Krajewski S, et al. Evaluation of the prognostic significance of Apaf-1 and caspases -2, -3, -7, -8 and -9 in acute leukemia. Blood 2000;96:3922–3931.
194. Borner C. Diminished cell proliferation associated with the death-protective activity of Bcl-2. J Biol Chem 1996;271:12,695–12,698.
195. Hockenbery DM, Oltvai ZN, Yin X-M, Milliman CL, Korsmeyer SJ. Bcl-2 Functions in an antioxidant pathway to prevent apoptosis. Cell 1993;75:241–252.
196. Deng X, Gao F, May WS, Jr. Bcl2 retards G1/S cell cycle transition by regulating intracellular ROS. Blood 2003;102:3179–3185.
197. Denu JM, Tanner KG. Specific and reversible inactivation of protein tyrosine phosphatases by hydrogen peroxide: evidence for a sulfenic acid intermediate and implications for redox regulation. Biochemistry 1998;37:5633–5642.
198. Konopleva M, Zhao S, Hu W, et al. The anti-apoptotic genes Bcl-X(L) and Bcl-2 are over-expressed and contribute to chemoresistance of non-proliferating leukaemic CD34+ cells. Br J Cancer 2002;118:521–534.
199. Campos L, Rouault JP, Sabido O, et al. High expression of Bcl-2 protein in acute myeloid-leukemia cells is associated with poor response to chemotherapy. Blood 1993;81:3091–3096.
200. Maung ZT, MacLean FR, Reid MM, et al. The relationship between *bcl-2* expression and response to chemotherapy in acute leukaemia. Brit J Haematol 1994;88:105–109.
201. Kaufmann SH, Karp JE, Svingen PA, Krajewski S, Burke PJ, Gore SD. Elevated expression of the apoptotic regulator Mcl-1 at the time of leukemic relapse. Blood 1998;91:991–1000.
202. Kasimir-Bauer S, Beelen D, Flasshove M, Noppeney R, Seeber S, Scheulen ME. Impact of the expression of P glycoprotein, the multidrug resistance-related protein, bcl-2, mutant p53, and heat shock protein 27 on

response to induction therapy and long-term survival in patients with de novo acute myeloid leukemia. Exp Hematol 2002;30:1302–1308.

203. Chida D, Miura O, Yoshimura A, Miyajima A. Role of cytokine signaling molecules in erythroid differentiation of mouse fetal liver hematopoietic cells: functional analysis of signaling molecules by retrovirus-mediated expression. Blood 1999;93:1567–1578.

204. Appelbaum FR, Rowe JM, Radich J, Dick JE. Acute myeloid leukemia. Hematology (Am Soc Hematol Educ Program) 2001:62–86.

205. Drexler HG, Meyer C, Quentmeier H. Effects of FLT3 ligand on proliferation and survival of myeloid leukemia cells. Leuk Lymphoma 1999;33:83–91.

206. Zheng R, Levis M, Piloto O, et al. FLT3 ligand causes autocrine signaling in acute myeloid leukemia cells. Blood 2004;103:267–274.

207. Lisovsky M, Estrov Z, Zhang X, et al. Flt3 ligand stimulates proliferation and inhibits apoptosis of acute myeloid leukemia cells: regulation of Bcl-2 and Bax. Blood 1996;88:3987–3997.

208. Gilliland DG. Molecular genetics of human leukemias: new insights into therapy. Sem Hematol 2002;39:6–11.

209. Levis M, Small D. FLT3: it does matter in leukemia. Leukemia 2003;17:1738–1752.

210. Mizuki M, Fenski R, Halfter H, et al. Flt3 mutations from patients with acute myeloid leukemia induce transformation of 32D cells mediated by the Ras and STAT5 pathways. Blood 2000;96:3907–3914.

211. Kim KT, Baird K, Ahn JY, et al. Pim-1 is up-regulated by constitutively activated FLT3 and plays a role in FLT3-mediated cell survival. Blood 2005;105:1759–1767.

212. Bagrintseva K, Geisenhof S, Kern R, et al. FLT3-ITD-TKD dual mutants associated with AML confer resistance to FLT3 PTK inhibitors and cytotoxic agents by overexpression of Bcl-x(L). Blood 2005;105: 3679–3685.

213. Minami Y, Yamamoto K, Kiyoi H, Ueda R, Saito H, Naoe T. Different antiapoptotic pathways between wild-type and mutated FLT3: insights into therapeutic targets in leukemia. Blood 2003;102:2969–2975.

214. Towatari M, Iida H, Tanimoto M, Iwata H, Hamaguchi M, Saito H. Constitutive activation of mitogen-activated protein kinase pathway in acute leukemia cells. Leukemia 1997;11:479–484.

215. Kim S-C, Hahn J-S, Min Y-H, Yoo N-C, Ko Y-W, Lee W-J. Constitutive activation of extracellular signal-regulated kinase in human acute leukemias: combined role of activation of MEK, hyperexpression of extracellular signal-regulated kinase, and downregulation of a phosphatase, PAC1. Blood 1999;93:3893–3899.

216. O'Gorman DM, McKenna SL, McGahon AJ, Knox KA, Cotter TG. Sensitisation of HL60 human leukaemic cells to cytotoxic drug-induced apoptosis by inhibition of PI3-kinase survival signals. Leukemia 2000;14:602–611.

217. Xu Q, Simpson SE, Scialla TJ, Bagg A, Carroll M. Survival of acute myeloid leukemia cells requires PI3 kinase activation. Blood 2003;102:972–980.

218. Grandage VL, Gale RE, Linch DC, Khwaja A. PI3-kinase/Akt is constitutively active in primary acute myeloid leukaemia cells and regulates survival and chemoresistance via NF-kappaB, Mapkinase and p53 pathways. Leukemia 2005;19:586–594.

219. Andreeff M, Jiang S, Zhang X, et al. Expression of Bcl-2-related genes in normal and AML progenitors: changes induced by chemotherapy and retinoic acid. Leukemia 1999;13:1881–1892.

220. Zhao S, Konopleva M, Cabreira-Hansen M, et al. Inhibition of phosphatidylinositol 3-kinase dephospho-rylates BAD and promotes apoptosis in myeloid leukemias. Leukemia 2004;18:267–275.

221. Guzman ML, Neering SJ, Upchurch D, et al. Nuclear factor-kappaB is constitutively activated in primitive human acute myelogenous leukemia Cells. Blood 2001;98:2301–2307.

222. Birkenkamp KU, Geugien M, Schepers H, Westra J, Lemmink HH, Vellenga E. Constitutive NF-kappaB DNA-binding activity in AML is frequently mediated by a Ras/PI3-K/PKB-dependent pathway. Leukemia 2004;18:103–112.

223. Maniatis T. Catalysis by a multiprotein IkappaB kinase complex. Science 1997;278:818–819.

224. Baumgartner B, Weber M, Quirling M, et al. Increased IkappaB kinase activity is associated with activated NF-kappaB in acute myeloid blasts. Leukemia 2002;16:2062–2071.

225. Delwel R, Salem M, Pellens C, et al. Growth regulation of human acute myeloid leukemia: effects of five recombinant hematopoietic factors in a serum-free culture system. Blood 1988;72:1944–1949.

226. Zhang J, Li Y, Shen B. Up-regulation of XIAP by M-CSF is associated with resistance of myeloid leukemia cells to apoptosis. Leukemia 2002;16:2163–2165.

227. Carter BZ, Milella M, Tsao T, et al. Regulation and targeting of antiapoptotic XIAP in acute myeloid leukemia. Leukemia 2003;17:2081–2089.

228. Garrido SM, Appelbaum FR, Willman CL, Banker DE. Acute myeloid leukemia cells are protected from spontaneous and drug-induced apoptosis by direct contact with a human bone marrow stromal cell line (HS-5). Exp Hematol 2001;29:448–457.

229. Konopleva M, Konoplev S, Hu W, Zaritskey AY, Afanasiev BV, Andreeff M. Stromal cells prevent apoptosis of AML cells by up-regulation of anti-apoptotic proteins. Leukemia 2002;16:1713–1724.

230. Braess J, Schneiderat P, Schoch C, Fiegl M, Lorenz I, Hiddemann W. Functional analysis of apoptosis induction in acute myeloid leukaemia-relevance of karyotype and clinical treatment response. Br J Haematol 2004;126:338–347.

231. van Stijn A, Kok A, van der Pol MA, et al. A flow cytometric method to detect apoptosis-related protein expression in minimal residual disease in acute myeloid leukemia. Leukemia 2003;17:780–786.

232. van Stijn A, Feller N, Kok A, van der Pol MA, Ossenkoppele GJ, Schuurhuis GJ. Minimal residual disease in acute myeloid leukemia is predicted by an apoptosis-resistant protein profile at diagnosis. Clin Cancer Res 2005;11:2540–2546.

233. Carter BZ, Kornblau SM, Tsao T, et al. Caspase-independent cell death in AML: caspase inhibition in vitro with pan-caspase inhibitors or in vivo by XIAP or Survivin does not affect cell survival or prognosis. Blood 2003;102:4179–4186.

234. Garrido SM, Cooper JJ, Appelbaum FR, Willman CL, Kopecky K, Banker DE. Blasts from elderly acute myeloid leukemia patients are characterized by low levels of culture- and drug-induced apoptosis. Leuk Res 2001;25:23–32.

235. Suarez L, Vidriales MB, Moreno MJ, et al. Differences in anti-apoptotic and multidrug resistance phenotypes in elderly and young acute myeloid leukemia patients are related to the maturation of blast cells. Haematologica 2005;90:54–59.

236. Eischen CM, Kottke TJ, Martins LM, et al. Comparison of apoptosis in wild-type and Fas-resistant cells: chemotherapy-induced apoptosis is not dependent on Fas/Fas ligand interactions. Blood 1997;90:935–943.

237. Banerjee D. Genasense (Genta Inc). Curr Opin Invest Drugs 2001;2:574–580.

238. Dai G, Chan KK, Liu S, et al. Cellular uptake and intracellular levels of the bcl-2 antisense g3139 in cultured cells and treated patients with acute myeloid leukemia. Clin Cancer Res 2005;11:2998–3008.

239. Marcucci G, Byrd JC, Dai G, et al. Phase I and pharmacodynamic studies of G3139, a Bcl-2 antisense oligonucleotide, in combination chemotherapy in refractory or relapsed acute leukemia. Blood 2003;101:425–432.

240. Marcucci G, Stock W, Dai G, et al. Phase I study of oblimersen sodium, an antisense to Bcl-2, in untreated older patients with acute myeloid leukemia: pharmacokinetics, pharmacodynamics, and clinical activity. J Clin Oncol 2005;23:3404–3411.

241. Raffo A, Lai JC, Stein CA, et al. Antisense RNA down-regulation of bcl-2 expression in DU145 prostate cancer cells does not diminish the cytostatic effects of G3139 (Oblimersen). Clin Cancer Res 2004;10: 3195–3206.

242. Benimetskaya L, Wittenberger T, Stein CA, et al. Changes in gene expression induced by phosphorothioate oligodeoxynucleotides (including G3139) in PC3 prostate carcinoma cells are recapitulated at least in part by treatment with interferon-beta and -gamma. Clin Cancer Res 2004;10:3678–3688.

243. Bolanos-Meade J, Karp JE, Guo C, et al. Timed sequential therapy of acute myelogenous leukemia in adults: a phase II study of retinoids in combination with the sequential administration of cytosine arabinoside, idarubicin and etoposide. Leuk Res 2003;27:313–321.

244. Oltersdorf T, Elmore SW, Shoemaker AR, et al. An inhibitor of Bcl-2 family proteins induces regression of solid tumours. Nature 2005;435:677–681.

245. Kitada S, Leone M, Sareth S, Zhai D, Reed JC, Pellecchia M. Discovery, characterization, and structure-activity relationships studies of proapoptotic polyphenols targeting B-cell lymphocyte/leukemia-2 proteins. J Med Chem 2003;46:4259–4264.

246. Becattini B, Kitada S, Leone M, et al. Rational design and real time, in-cell detection of the proapoptotic activity of a novel compound targeting Bcl-X(L). Chem Biol 2004;11:389–395.

247. Oliver CL, Miranda MB, Shangary S, Land S, Wang S, Johnson DE. (−)-Gossypol acts directly on the mitochondria to overcome Bcl-2- and Bcl-X(L)-mediated apoptosis resistance. Mol Cancer Ther 2005;4:23–31.

248. Mohammad RM, Wang S, Aboukameel A, et al. Preclinical studies of a nonpeptidic small-molecule inhibitor of Bcl-2 and Bcl-X(L) [(−)-gossypol] against diffuse large cell lymphoma. Mol Cancer Ther 2005;4:13–21.

249. Cummings J, Ward TH, LaCasse E, et al. Validation of pharmacodynamic assays to evaluate the clinical efficacy of an antisense compound (AEG 35156) targeted to the X-linked inhibitor of apoptosis protein XIAP. Br J Cancer 2005;92:532–538.

250. McManus DC, Lefebvre CA, Cherton-Horvat G, et al. Loss of XIAP protein expression by RNAi and antisense approaches sensitizes cancer cells to functionally diverse chemotherapeutics. Oncogene 2004;23: 8105–8117.

251. Arnt CR, Kaufmann SH. The saintly side of Smac/DIABLO: giving anticancer drug-induced apoptosis a boost. Cell Death Diff 2003;10:1118–1120.

252. Schimmer AD. Inhibitor of apoptosis proteins: translating basic knowledge into clinical practice. Cancer Res 2004;64:7183–7190.

253. Guo F, Nimmanapalli R, Paranawithana S, et al. Ectopic overexpression of second mitochondria-derived activator of caspases (Smac/DIABLO) or cotreatment with N-terminus of Smac/DIABLO peptide potentiates epothilone B derivative-(BMS 247550) and apo-2L-TRAIL-induced apoptosis. Blood 2002;99: 3419–3426.

254. Li L, Thomas RM, Suzuki H, De Brabander JK, Wang X, Harran PG. A small molecule Smac mimic potentiates TRAIL- and TNFalpha-mediated cell death. Science 2004;305:1471–1474.

255. Oost TK, Sun C, Armstrong RC, et al. Discovery of potent antagonists of the antiapoptotic protein XIAP for the treatment of cancer. J Med Chem 2004;47:4417–4426.

256. Wu TY, Wagner KW, Bursulaya B, Schultz PG, Deveraux QL. Development and characterization of non-peptidic small molecule inhibitors of the XIAP/caspase-3 interaction. Chem Biol 2003;10:759–767.

257. Schimmer AD, Welsh K, Pinilla C, et al. Small-molecule antagonists of apoptosis suppressor XIAP exhibit broad antitumor activity. Cancer Cell 2004;5:25–35.

258. Carter BZ, Gronda M, Wang Z, et al. Small-molecule XIAP inhibitors derepress downstream effector caspases and induce apoptosis of acute myeloid leukemia cells. Blood 2005;105:4043–4050.

259. Gingras AC, Raught B, Sonenberg N. Regulation of translation initiation by FRAP/mTOR. Genes Dev 2001;15:807–826.

260. Bjornsti MA, Houghton PJ. The TOR pathway: a target for cancer therapy. Nat Rev Cancer 2004;4:335–348.

261. Wendel HG, De Stanchina E, Fridman JS, et al. Survival signalling by Akt and eIF4E in oncogenesis and cancer therapy. Nature 2004;428:332–337.

262. Wilhem SM, Carater C, Tang LJ, et al. BAY 43-9006 exhibits broad spectrum oral antitumor activity and targets the RAF/MEK/ERK pathway and receptor tyrosine kinases involved in tumor progression and angiogenesis. Cancer Res 2004;64:7099–7109.

263. Scheijen B, Ngo HT, Kang H, Griffin JD. FLT3 receptors with internal tandem duplications promote cell viability and proliferation by signaling through Foxo proteins. Oncogene 2004;23:3338–3349.

264. Kerr AH, James JA, Smith MA, Willson C, Court EL, Smith JG. An investigation of the MEK/ERK inhibitor U0126 in acute myeloid leukemia. Ann NY Acad Sci 2003;1010:86–89.

265. Shankar S, Srivastava RK. Enhancement of therapeutic potential of TRAIL by cancer chemotherapy and irradiation: mechanisms and clinical implications. Drug Resist Updat 2004;7:139–156.

266. Willis SN, Adams JM. Life in the balance: how BH3-only proteins induce apoptosis. Curr Opin Cell Biol 2005;17:617–625.

267. Smith BD, Levis M, Beran M, et al. Single-agent CEP-701, a novel FLT3 inhibitor, shows biologic and clinical activity in patients with relapsed or refractory acute myeloid leukemia. Blood 2004;103:3669–3676.

268. Giles FJ, Stopeck AT, Silverman LR, et al. SU5416, a small molecule tyrosine kinase receptor inhibitor, has biologic activity in patients with refractory acute myeloid leukemia or myelodysplastic syndromes. Blood 2003;102:795–801.

269. Fiedler W, Mesters R, Tinnefeld H, et al. A phase 2 clinical study of SU5416 in patients with refractory acute myeloid leukemia. Blood 2003;102:2763–2767.

270. O'Farrell AM, Foran JM, Fiedler W, et al. An innovative phase I clinical study demonstrates inhibition of FLT3 phosphorylation by SU11248 in acute myeloid leukemia patients. Clin Cancer Res 2003;9:5465–5476.

271. Fiedler W, Serve H, Dohner H, et al. A phase 1 study of SU11248 in the treatment of patients with refractory or resistant acute myeloid leukemia (AML) or not amenable to conventional therapy for the disease. Blood 2005;105:986–993.

272. Stone RM, De Angelo J, Galinsky I, et al. PKC 412 FLT3 inhibitor therapy in AML: results of a phase II trial. Ann Hematol 2004;83(suppl 1):S89–S90.

273. Kelley SK, Ashkenazi A. Targeting death receptors in cancer with Apo2L/TRAIL. Curr Opin Pharmacol 2004;4:333–339.

274. Witzig TE, Geyer SM, Ghobrial I, et al. Phase II trial of single-agent temsirolimus (CCI-779) for relapsed mantle cell lymphoma. J Clin Oncol 2005;23:5347–5356.

275. O'Gorman DM, McKenna SL, McGahon AJ, Knox KA, Cotter TG. Sensitization of HL60 human leukaemic cells to cytotoxic drug-induced apoptosis inhibition of PI3-kinase survival signals. Leukemia 2000;14:602–611.

276. Wright JJ, Zerivitz K, Gravell AE. Clinical trials referral resource. Current clinical trials of BAY 43-9006, Part 1. Oncology 2005;19:499–502.

277. Yu C, Bruzek LM, Meng XW, et al. The role of Mcl-1 downregulation in the proapoptotic activity of the multikinase inhibitor BAY 43-9006. Oncogene 2005;24:6861–6869.

278. O'Farrell AM, Yuen HA, Smolich B, et al. Effects of SU5416, a small molecule tyrosine kinase receptor inhibitor, on FLT3 expression and phosphorylation in patients with refractory acute myeloid leukemia. Leuk Res 2004;28:679–689.

7 Drug Resistance Transporters in AML

Douglas D. Ross

CONTENTS

Summary

Resistance to antineoplastic drugs is thought to be a major reason for failure to cure malignant diseases today. Multidrug resistance, defined as the development of resistance to a broad spectrum of antineoplastic agents following exposure to a single agent, can arise from a variety of mechanisms, among which is overexpression of members of the ATP-binding cassette (ABC) superfamily of transporter proteins. Notable among ABC transporters are those that cause multidrug resistance by effluxing anticancer agents from cells. P-glycoprotein (Pgp, product of the MDR1 gene and officially designated as ABCB1) and the multidrug resistance protein 1 (MRP1, or ABCC1) are the best studied in this context; however, other members of the MRP (ABCC) family and the recently discovered breast cancer resistance protein (BCRP, officially ABCG2) are also known to efflux anticancer drugs and to confer multidrug resistance to cancer cell lines. The recognition that a self-renewing stem cell compartment exists in AML and the expression of Pgp/ABCB1, BCRP/ABCG2, and perhaps other ABC transporters in these cells points to a need for future research on the contribution of these transporters to drug resistance in this target population.

1. TRANSPORTERS AS A CAUSE OF DRUG RESISTANCE IN LEUKEMIAS

Proteins involved with the intracellular transport of ions, xenobiotics, or bioorganic molecules comprise a large portion (15–25% by some estimates) of the human genome. This attests to the enormous importance these transporters have in the physiology of normal cells. It is therefore logical that the cancer genome may utilize a repertoire of transport proteins to adapt to the lethality of anticancer treatments. Acute myeloid leukemia (AML) is a chemotherapy-sensitive, potentially curable malignancy. However, approx 70% of AML cases will die from their disease, some as the result of primary drug resistance, but most as the result of acquired resistance to chemotherapy (1,2). In AML, a large body of research indicates that transport proteins do play a role in cellular resistance to antileukemic therapy; however, the full extent of this role is not fully unraveled. Furthermore, it is not yet understood how the interplay of transporter activity and drug resistance can be exploited for a therapeutic benefit. The majority of the research centers on resistance to multiple drugs that arises as a consequence of cellular expression members of the ATP-binding cassette (ABC) superfamily of transporter proteins, and this will be the focus of the review presented here.

From: *Contemporary Hematology: Acute Myelogenous Leukemia*
Edited by: J. E. Karp © Humana Press Inc., Totowa, NJ

It is important to note that resistance to drugs essential to AML therapy can arise as the result of alterations in transporters that are not ABC family members. For example, equilibrative nucleoside transporters facilitate nucleoside transport into and out of cells. Human equilibrative nucleoside transporter 1 (hENT1) transports ara-C into cells and, when extracellular ara-C is depleted, will transport intracellular ara-C back out of the cell. The consequence of the efflux role of hENT1 is probably overshadowed by intracellular trapping of ara-C by means of conversion to the triphosphate form. However, it has been shown that dipyridamole, an inhibitor of hENT1, can potentiate ara-C cytotoxicity by inhibiting drug efflux when given after exposure of HL-60 human AML cells to ara-C *(3)*. Despite this, hENT1 may play an important role in cellular accumulation of ara-C. A study of blast cells from 123 AML patients at time of diagnosis found that patients with blast cells deficient in hENT1 had a significantly shorter disease-free survival *(4)*.

1.1. ABC Transporters

The ABC transporter superfamily consists of 48 proteins distributed in seven subfamilies designated A through G. ABC transporters derive their name from their employment of the hydrolysis of ATP to shift drugs and xenobiotics unidirectionally out of cells. Hence, on a theoretical basis, cancer cellular overexpression of an ABC transporter can result in resistance to any anticancer drug that happens to be a substrate for that given transporter. This notion provided an explanation for the clinical phenomenon of multidrug resistance, where resistance to multiple agents accompanies recurrent cancer following initial successful treatment.

The ABC transporters most often associated with cancer multidrug resistance are ABCB1 (Pgp, or the product of the MDR1 gene), multidrug resistance protein (MRP) family members (ABCC subfamily), and ABCG2 (breast cancer resistance protein). However, members of the ABC superfamily other than ABCB1, ABCC1, and ABCG2 have recently been implicated as being capable of transporting clinically relevant antineoplastic drugs. For example, ABCB11, the bile salt transporter (BSEP), confers resistance to paclitaxel *(5)*. ABCB11/BSEP is expressed at high levels in liver tissue. Resistance to estramustine may be caused by ABCA2, a transporter normally involved in steroid transport, which is expressed in cytoplasmic endosomal/lysosomal vesicles *(6)*.

1.1.1. Pgp/MDR1/ABCB1

When one thinks of multidrug resistance, probably the first thing that comes to mind is P-glycoprotein (Pgp), the product of the multidrug resistance gene MDR1 *(7–9)*. In the nomenclature of the ABC transports, Pgp/MDR1 is designated ABCB1, or the first member of the B subfamily of the ABC superfamily. The MDR1 gene is located on chromosome 7. Pgp is an efflux transporter located in the plasma membrane, which effluxes xenobiotics, drugs, and certain physiological metabolites out of cells. Pgp was found to be responsible for efflux, and thus resistance, to multiple and often disparate classes of anticancer agents with very different chemical structures and mechanisms of action. These include some of the most active antineoplastic agents available today, such as etoposide, Vinca alkaloids, anthracyclines, and taxanes. Furthermore, laboratory selection of cancer cell lines with these drugs frequently led to the upregulation of Pgp. Hence, considerable excitement was engendered toward the notion that chemotherapeutic drug treatment resulted in Pgp upregulation in clinical cancers as an explanation of the phenomenon of clinical multidrug resistance. This excitement was heightened by the demonstration that a variety of pharmaceuticals could effectively inhibit Pgp drug efflux and could sensitize Pgp-expressing cancer cell lines to the cytotoxic effects of Pgp substrate drugs. To date, a number of very effective Pgp inhibitors are available for clinical use or are in clinical trials. Substrates and inhibitors for Pgp and other ABC transporters discussed in this chapter are displayed in Table 1.

A considerable body of literature supports the conclusion that the functional expression of Pgp/ABCG1 in blast cells from patients with AML predicts a poor outcome to treatment (e.g., refs. *10,11*). Furthermore, one study found that Pgp expression was greater in blast cells from older AML patients *(10)*, which led to the postulate that Pgp may contribute to the poorer response to treatment of AML in the elderly. Indeed, functional and physical expression of Pgp and MRP1 is observed in about 30% of *de novo* AML cases and may be of prognostic value *(12–14)*. Furthermore, expression of Pgp increases at time of disease relapse or in the presence of adverse prognostic factors or markers *(10,15–17)*. A number of inhibitors or blockers of Pgp-mediated drug efflux have been identified. Clinical trials with some of these agents have been conducted with mixed results. A CALGB trial of the Pgp inhibitor PSC-833 in combination with ara-C, etoposide, and daunorubicin therapy for *de novo* AML encountered excessive early mortality in the PSC-833 arm, but patients whose blast cells showed inhibition of drug efflux by PSC-833 in vitro had a longer disease-free survival if they were enrolled on the PSC-833 arm and worse outcomes if they were on the control arm *(18)*. A trial of PSC-833 in combination with mitoxantrone, etoposide, and cytarabine in relapsed or refractory AML and high-risk myelodysplastic syndrome revealed no benefit of the addition of PSC-833 *(19)*. However, a Southwest Oncology Group study of daunorubicin and ara-C induction and consolidation therapy with and without the Pgp inhibitor cyclosporin A resulted in prolonged duration of remission and improved overall survival in patients with poor-risk AML *(20)*. Despite these improvements, there was no improvement in the cure rate of AML as the result of Pgp inhibition, suggesting that other mechanisms of resistance, including transporter-based mechanisms *(10,12,13)*, may also be operative. Recently, it has been appreciated that cyclosporin A is a more broad-spectrum inhibitor of ABC transporters and may also inhibit MRP1/ABCC1 and BCRP/ABCG2, whereas PSC-833 inhibits only Pgp/ABCB1 *(21)*.

1.1.2. MRPs (ABCC FAMILY MEMBERS)

The second cancer multidrug resistance transporter to be identified is the multidrug resistance protein 1, or MRP1 *(22,23)*. MRP1 is the founding member of a series of related transporters within the C subfamily of the ABC superfamily *(24,25)*. Currently, the MRP family consists of nine distinct members; the first eight are currently associated with cancer drug resistance in laboratory models, but the clinical significance of MRP2-9 is currently under study. The chemotherapeutic drug substrate specificity of MRP1 overlaps considerably with that of Pgp/ABCB1, with the exception that paclitaxel and other taxanes are not substrates for MRP1 (Table 1). The substrate specificity of the other MRPs (MRP2-MRP9) broadens the classes of agents effluxed to include cisplatin, methotrexate, nucleosides (but not ara-C), nucleotides, fluoropyrimidines, and topoisomerase I inhibitors.

The importance of MRP transporters in conferring clinical drug resistance is somewhat unsettled at this time. Most clinical studies have focused on MRP1; hence more work is needed to determine the contributions of MRP2-MRP8 on clinical drug resistance. An early study using reverse transcription PCR suggested that MRP1 may have prognostic significance in AML *(26)*. Subsequent studies with monoclonal antibodies to MRP1 showed that MRP1 expression had no effect on remission induction rate, but may be associated with a shorter overall survival *(27)*; yet another study showed that the co-expression of MRP1 and Pgp/MDR1 adversely affected complete remission rate, but that neither MRP1 nor Pgp expression affected

Table 1
ABC Transporters Capable of Efflux of Chemotherapeutic Drugs

ABC family	Transporter	Substrate chemotherapeutic agents	Inhibitors
B	Pgp/MDR1/ ABCB1	Anthracyclines, etoposide, Vinca alkaloids, taxanes, imatinib	Cyclosporin A, verapamil, grapefruit juice, orange juice, PSC833, GF120918, VX-710, LY335979
	MDR2/ABCB4	Paclitaxel, vinblastine	—
	BSEP/ABCB11	Paclitaxel	—
C	MRP1/ABCC1	Anthracyclines, etoposide, methotrexate, Vinca alkaloids	Indomethacin, flavonoids, MK-571, cyclosporin A, VX-710
	MRP2/ABCC2	Cisplatin, doxorubicin, etoposide, methotrexate, mitoxantrone, Vinca alkaloids	Cyclosporin A, grapefruit juice, orange juice
	MRP3/ABCC3	Cisplatin, doxorubicin, etoposide, methotrexate, Vinca alkaloids	—
	MRP4/ABCC4	Methotrexate, thiopurines	—
	MRP5/ABCC5	6-Mercaptopurine, 6-thioguanine	—
	MRP6/ABCC6	Anthracyclines, etoposide, teniposide	—
	MRP7/ABCC10	Taxanes, Vinca alkaloids	—
	MRP8/ABCC11	Purine and pyrimidine nucleoside analogs	—
G	BCRP/ABCG2	Mitoxantrone, methotrexate (including polyglutamate forms), topotecan, SN-38, imatinib, flavopiridol	Fumitremorgin C, Ko-143, Iressa, imatinib, cyclosporin A, GF120918, novobiocin, VX-710, flavonoids, phytoestrogens, estrone, estradiol, benzimidazoles, nelfinavir, saquinavir, ritonavir

overall survival *(17)*. A study that used a functional assay to evaluate the activity of MRP1 in patient-derived AML blast cells found that MRP-activity-positive patients had a lower complete remission rate and shorter overall survival *(28)*. Because of the substrate specificity of some MRP family members, it is possible that these functional data reflect the activity of one or more MRP family members. Finally, a recent study of 331 adult AML patients revealed that MRP1 expression measured by reverse transcription polymerase chain reaction (PCR) was an independent predictor for disease-free survival *(11)*.

On the other hand, a number of studies of *de novo* or secondary AML indicate that MRP1 expression has no impact on treatment outcome, often using both protein and functional assays for MRP1 *(29–32)*. A study cited earlier from the Southwest Oncology Group reported that in a large series of adult AML patients, functional and protein expression of Pgp/MDR1 was a predictor of prognosis, but that MDR1 expression did not predict outcome *(10)*. Furthermore, MRP1 expression or function did not correlate with prognosis in myelodysplastic syndromes *(33)* or with emergence of minimal residual disease in AML *(34)*.

The MRP1 gene is located on chromosome 16. AML patients with an inverted 16 chromosome (inv[16]) are known to have a more favorable prognosis than other AML patients in general. In some (but not all) patients with inv(16), fluorescent *in situ* hybridization studies reveal that MRP1 is deleted, leading to the hypothesis that MRP1 loss may favorably affect clinical outcome *(35)*. A recent study of nine AML patients with inv(16) found no correlation between treatment outcome and deletion of MRP1; furthermore, the functional activity of MRP was maintained despite deletion or partial deletion of MRP1. This effect was attributed to possible upregulation of other MRP family genes *(36)*.

1.1.3. BCRP (ABCG2)

Accumulating evidence (e.g., ref. *12*) indicating that mechanisms of multidrug resistance other than Pgp and MRP1 occur in AML prompted a search for other transporter-based resistance mechanisms. A novel multidrug resistant human breast carcinoma cell line, MCF-7/AdrVp, which was selected with adriamycin in the presence of the Pgp inhibitor verapamil, display an ATP-dependent efflux of substrate anticancer drugs, but do not overexpress Pgp or MRP1 *(37)*. A novel ABC transporter was isolated from these breast cancer cells and was designated the breast cancer resistance protein, or BCRP *(38)*. BCRP is a member of the G subfamily of ABC transporters and is known officially as ABCG2 *(39)*. Transfection and enforced expression of BCRP in parental MCF-7 cells recapitulated the drug resistance phenotype of MCF-7/AdrVp cells, including resistance to adriamycin, doxorubicin, daunorubicin, and mitoxantrone *(38)*. Presently, the spectrum of antineoplastic drugs effluxed by BCRP also includes camptothecin-derived topoisomerase I inhibitors (topotecan, irinotecan, SN-38), methotrexate, and certain novel targeted therapeutic agents such as imatinib *(40)* and agents in clinical trials including quinazoline HER-tyrosine kinase inhibitors, flavopiridol, and benzoylphenylurea *(39)*.

Approximately 30% of AML cases express relatively high levels of BCRP mRNA using semi-quantitative reverse transcriptase (RT)-PCR methods, opening the possibility that BCRP expression in some patients might account for resistance to therapy *(41)*. Subsequently, a series of studies using real-time RT-PCR techniques suggested that BCRP expression correlated with poor outcome in AML: BCRP expression correlated with poor prognosis in childhood AML *(42)*, and in studies of 20 paired samples taken at diagnosis and at relapse, BCRP mRNA expression was found to increase in relapsed or refractory AML *(43)*. A study from our laboratory correlated BCRP mRNA measured by real-time RT-PCR with in vitro sensitivity to flavopiridol in blast cells from AML patients *(44)*.

Flow cytometric studies using BCRP protein or function as measures of expression, however, found low expression in the blast cell population overall, and that BCRP expression, when present, was confined to small subpopulations of blast cells with an immature phenotype *(45,46)*. The BCRP expressing immature subpopulations were often CD34$^+$ and CD38$^-$ and CD33$^-$, which are characteristics of the phenotype of the so-called leukemia stem cell, a self-renewing population described in more detail below. At first glance, these studies might suggest that BCRP expression in AML is inconsequential. However, if BCRP is expressed in the self-renewing leukemia stem cell population, chemoresistance governed by BCRP in this small yet highly consequential population of cells may be of great importance to the response of the disease to treatment. For example, leukemic stem cell populations as small as 1% or less of the total cell population may be sufficient to maintain self-renewal of the overall disease. In such a case, the levels of BCRP protein or function in the overall blast cell population might be low or undetectable, yet BCRP could contribute to poor response to treatment because of its leukemic stem cell protective effect. For treatment to be unsuccessful, the leukemia stem cell population need not expand at the time of relapse, but merely persist; perhaps this is why a study by van der Kolk et al. showed no consistent increase in BCRP expression or function at time of relapse in 20 paired samples of blast cells from AML patients, yet the predominant expression of BCRP was seen in CD34$^+$ subpopulations (46), both pretreatment and at relapse.

2. STEM CELL SURVIVAL: PRESENCE AND ROLE OF TRANSPORTERS

Normal hematopoietic stem cells (HSCs) have a capacity for self-renewal and can proliferate upon demand to give rise to the multiple lineages of blood cells. Some of the progeny of stem cells, termed progenitor cells, are capable of proliferation, but are not capable of self-renewal. The classical immunophenotype associated with HSCs is the expression of the CD34 surface antigen; however, recent evidence suggests that a more primitive, CD34$^-$ HSC exists (47). Such CD34$^-$ HSCs may be detected by their ability to exclude Hoechst dye (48–50) and are designated SP cells. Stem cells so identified appear as a "side population" (SP) upon flow-cytometric display of the red vs blue fluorescence of the Hoechst dye (Fig 1); SP cells constitute approx 0.03% of the cells in normal bone marrow (50). Recently it was discovered that BCRP/ABCG2 is expressed in SP cells and may be responsible, at least in part, for the SP phenotype, illustrated by the sorting experiments depicted in Fig. 1. Hoechst 33342 is a substrate for BCRP, and expression of BCRP in SP cells is thought to cause the low accumulation of the dye in these cells. Current thinking is that BCRP functions as a marker for the SP cell population but is not crucial for stem cell development. Expression of BCRP in stem cells probably serves to protect them from xenobiotics and a toxic environment.

Both human and mouse SP cells strongly express BCRP (49). In mouse models, upon differentiation to express CD34, SP cells show a marked downregulation of Bcrp1 (49). Hence the expression of BCRP in CD34$^+$ leukemic blast cells may represent an aberrant expression of this transporter compared to normal stem and progenitor cell counterparts. SP cells also express Pgp/ABCB1, which is also capable of transport of Hoechst 33342 dye; however, SP cells are present in normal numbers in Pgp-deficient (Mdr1a/1b$^{-/-}$) mice, suggesting that Pgp is not the major Hoechst transporter in mouse SP cells (49). In contrast, SP cells are markedly reduced in BCRP knockout mice (51).

Evidence is rapidly accumulating that cancers, similar to their normal tissue counterparts, possess a hierarchal organization of stem cells, progenitor cells, and more differentiated, nonproliferating progeny (52). In this hierarchical model, only the cancer stem cells have long-term repopulating ability and are responsible for sustaining tumor growth; more differentiated tumor progenitor cells, despite their ability to proliferate, ultimately are not capable of maintaining their numbers without input from the stem cell compartment and hence are irrelevant to the long-term growth and survival of the cancer. Hence, the ability to cure a given cancer may hinge on the ability of therapy to target the cancer stem cell. Compelling evidence for the existence of stem cells in AML derives from observations of the ability of blast cells from AML patients to engraft in NOD/SCID mice and produce leukemic cells virtually identical to those observed in the patient. Engraftment and initiation of leukemia by candidate human leukemic blast cell subpopulations in NOD/SCID mice is considered to be the definitive assay for self-renewal capacity and is measured by the quantification of human CD45$^+$ cells in the mouse bone marrow. When leukemia blast cell populations are subdivided by flow cytometric cell sorting, self-renewal capacity so measured resides mainly in certain CD34$^+$/CD38$^-$ subpopulations, and in leukemic SP cells (CD34$^{low/-}$, described below) (53,54).

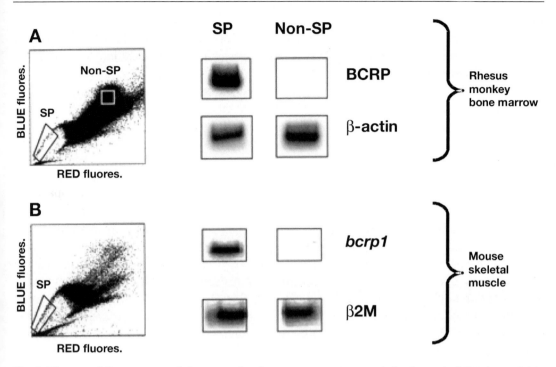

Fig. 1. Blue or red fluorescence of rhesus monkey bone marrow or mouse skeletal muscle following staining with Hoechst 33338 dye, analyzed by flow cytometry. The "side population" is identified by the rectangles marked "SP." The areas identified by the rectangles were sorted, then analyzed for human BCRP/ABCG2, mouse bcrp1/ABCG2, and human or mouse β-actin or β_2-microglobulin using reverse transcription polymerase chain reaction techniques. (From ref. *49*.)

2.1. SP Cells in Leukemias

A stem cell population with intrinsic capacity to efflux Hoechst 33342 dye, analogous to the side population that characterizes normal hematopoietic stem cells *(48)*, has been described recently in AML *(53)*. These AML SP cells all carried leukemia cytogenetic markers, effluxed mitoxantrone, had a CD34$^{low/-}$ immunophenotype, and were capable of engraftment and causing leukemia in NOD/SCID mice *(53)*. It is interesting that both normal and AML SP cells are CD34$^{low/-}$, suggesting that these cells may represent an even more immature phenotype than the CD34$^+$/CD38$^-$ cells that were found in earlier studies to be NOD/SCID-leukemia-initiating cells *(54)*. Unlike normal SP cells, which comprise, on average, 0.03% of bone marrow nucleated cells *(50)*, the percentage of SP cells in AML bone marrow ranged between 0.5 and 29.9% in one study *(55)*.

2.2. Chronic Myelogenous Leukemia, Imatinib, Stem Cells, and BCRP

Chronic myelogenous leukemia (CML) is a myeloproliferative disease that arises from a primitive hematopoietic cell transformed by Bcr-Abl, a chimeric protein formed as the result of the 9:22 translocation that produces the Philadelphia (Ph) chromosome *(56)*. Bcr-Abl is a functional tyrosine kinase that serves as the mitogenic driving force of the primitive Ph+ hematopoietic cells that are responsible for CML. The recent advent of imatinib (Gleevec, STI-571), a tyrosine kinase inhibitor that antagonizes Bcr-Abl, has revolutionized the treatment of chronic phase CML. Excluding bone marrow transplantation, imatinib is considered to be the single most effective agent used for the treatment of CML. Imatinib was recently shown to have a high-affinity interaction with BCRP *(40)* and to be a substrate for this transporter *(57)*. Cells selected for resistance to imatinib were found to upregulate BCRP and Pgp *(58)*.

Primitive Ph+ stem cells have been described in the chronic phase of CML that are $CD34^+$, but do not express CD38, CD45RA, or CD71 *(59)*. Such cells, like AML stem cells, are predominantly noncycling. Notably, Ph+, $CD34^+$ cells from chronic phase CML patients were found to be resistant to imatinib *(60)*. Remarkably, a recent paper found that Ph+, $CD34^+/CD38^+$ progenitor cells from chronic phase CML patients are capable of self-renewal and engraftment into NOD-SCID mice, unlike normal hematopoietic progenitor cells *(61)*. Hence, these CML cells with a progenitor cell phenotype ($CD34^+/CD38^+$) should probably be considered to be members of the CML stem cell population.

Although imatinib is presently the most effective agent available for the treatment of CML, molecular complete remissions, defined by negative PCR for Bcr-Abl, are rare, leading many to believe that because of the resistant self-renewing stem cells, imatinib treatment alone will not be curative for CML *(62)*. Currently, mechanisms of resistance to imatinib include mutations in Bcr-Abl and efflux transport by Pgp or BCRP *(63,64)*. Quiescent cells (eg., G_0) were at one time thought to be resistant to imatinib *(65)*; in fact, this was the resistance mechanism postulated for CML stem cells because they are in a quiescent state. However, a recent study demonstrated no correlation between proliferative status and the proapoptotic activity of imatinib in Bcr-Abl-expressing cells *(66)*.

Given the stem cell nature of CML, it is reasonable to hypothesize that Ph+ SP cells exist in CML and that these cells express BCRP and possibly Pgp. If this is true, then if BCRP and possibly Pgp is/are expressed in self-renewing CML stem cells, this expression may cause or contribute to imatinib resistance in the stem cells and failure to cure CML.

3. CONCLUSIONS

Resistance to antineoplastic therapy in AML likely arises from multiple mechanisms, including alterations in drug targets, alterations in susceptibility to various mechanisms of programmed cell death (described in Chapter 6), and cellular barriers that prevent drug from reaching or affecting its intracellular target. It is quite clear that many ABC transporters have the physical capacity to affect the latter mechanism based on work with cell lines in vitro demonstrating their capacity to efflux chemotherapeutic drugs from cells. Collectively, these transporters are capable of producing resistance to almost all antineoplastic agents available today. Clinical studies of the expression of these transporters in AML have largely focused on Pgp, MRP1, and BCRP/ABCG2. Although a number of studies relate the expression of these transporters to poor treatment outcome in AML, to date no single ABC transporter can be named a cause of failure to cure cases of AML. The expression of ABC transporters in normal HSCs and in their AML stem cell counterparts points to a need to understand further the role of these transporters in this potentially critical target population of self-renewing AML cells.

ACKNOWLEDGMENT

Dr. Ross is supported in part by a Department of Veterans Affairs Merit Review Grant.

REFERENCES

1. Mayer RJ, Davis RB, Schiffer CA, et al. 3rd Intensive postremission chemotherapy in adults with acute myeloid leukemia. Cancer and Leukemia Group B. N Engl J Med 1994;331:896–903.
2. Appelbaum FR, Kopecky KJ. Long-term survival after chemotherapy for acute myeloid leukemia: the experience of the Southwest Oncology Group. Cancer 1997;80:2199–2204.
3. Chan TC. Augmentation of 1-beta-D-arabinofuranosylcytosine cytotoxicity in human tumor cells by inhibiting drug efflux. Cancer Res 1989;49:2656–2660.
4. Galmarini CM, Thomas X, Calvo F, et al. In vivo mechanisms of resistance to cytarabine in acute myeloid leukaemia. Br J Haematol 2002;117:860–868.
5. Childs S, Yeh RL, Hui D, Ling V. Taxol resistance mediated by transfection of the liver-specific sister gene of P-glycoprotein. Cancer Res 1998;58:4160–4167.
6. Vulevic B, Chen Z, Boyd JT, et al. Cloning and characterization of human adenosine 5′-triphosphate-binding cassette, sub-family A, transporter 2 (ABCA2). Cancer Res 2001;61:3339–3347.
7. Juliano RL, Ling V. A surface glycoprotein modulating drug permeability in Chinese hamster ovary cell mutants. Biochim Biophys Acta 1976;455:152–162.
8. Ueda K, Cornwell MM, Gottesman MM, et al. The mdr1 gene, responsible for multidrug-resistance, codes for P-glycoprotein. Biochem Biophys Res Commun 1986;141:956–962.
9. Chen CJ, Chin JE, Ueda K, et al. Internal duplication and homology with bacterial transport proteins in the mdr1 (P-glycoprotein) gene from multidrug-resistant human cells. Cell 1986;47:381–389.
10. Leith CP, Kopecky KJ, Chen IM, et al. Frequency and clinical significance of the expression of the multidrug resistance proteins MDR1/P-glycoprotein, MRP1, and LRP in acute myeloid leukemia: a Southwest Oncology Group Study. Blood 1999;94:1086–1099.
11. Schaich M, Soucek S, Thiede C, Ehninger G, Illmer T. MDR1 and MRP1 gene expression are independent predictors for treatment outcome in adult acute myeloid leukaemia. Br J Haematol 2005;128:324–332.
12. Ross DD, Wooten PJ, Sridhara R, Ordonez JV, Lee EJ, Schiffer CA. Enhancement of daunorubicin accumulation, retention, and cytotoxicity by verapamil or cyclosporin A in blast cells from patients with previously untreated acute myeloid leukemia. Blood 1993;82:1288–1299.
13. Leith CP, Chen IM, Kopecky KJ, et al. Correlation of multidrug resistance (MDR1) protein expression with functional dye/drug efflux in acute myeloid leukemia by multiparameter flow cytometry: identification of discordant MDR-/efflux+ and MDR1+/efflux- cases. Blood 1995;86:2329–2342.
14. Ross DD. Novel mechanisms of drug resistance in leukemia. Leukemia 2000;14:467–473.
15. Legrand O, Simonin G, Perrot JY, Zittoun R, Marie JP. Pgp and MRP activities using calcein-AM are prognostic factors in adult acute myeloid leukemia patients. Blood 1998;91:4480–4488.
16. Legrand O, Simonin G, Beauchamp-Nicoud A, Zittoun R, Marie JP. Simultaneous activity of MRP1 and Pgp is correlated with in vitro resistance to daunorubicin and with in vivo resistance in adult acute myeloid leukemia. Blood 1999;94:1046–1056.
17. van der Kolk DM, de Vries EG, van Putten WJ, et al. P-glycoprotein and multidrug resistance protein activities in relation to treatment outcome in acute myeloid leukemia. Clin Cancer Res 2000;6:3205–3214.
18. Baer MR, George SL, Dodge RK, et al. A phase 3 study of the multidrug resistance modulator PSC-833 in previously untreated patients 60 years of age and older with acute myeloid leukemia: Cancer and Leukemia Group B Study 9720. Blood 2002;100:1224–1232.
19. Greenberg PL, Lee SJ, Advani R, et al. Mitoxantrone, etoposide, and cytarabine with or without valspodar in patients with relapsed or refractory acute myeloid leukemia and high-risk myelodysplastic syndrome: a phase III trial (E2995). J Clin Oncol 2004;22:1078–1086.
20. List AF, Kopecky KJ, Willman CL, et al. Benefit of cyclosporine modulation of drug resistance in patients with poor-risk acute myeloid leukemia: a Southwest Oncology Group study. Blood 2001;98:3212–3220.
21. Qadir M, O'Loughlin KL, Fricke SM, et al. Cyclosporin A is a broad-spectrum multidrug resistance modulator. Clin Cancer Res 2005;11:2320–2326.
22. Cole SP, Bhardwaj G, Gerlach JH, et al. Overexpression of a transporter gene in a multidrug-resistant human lung cancer cell line. Science 1992;258:1650–1654.
23. Kruh G, Chan A, Myers K, Gaughan K, Miki T, Aaronson SA. Expression complementary DNA library transfer establishes mrp as a multidrug resistance gene. Cancer Res 1994;54:1649–1652.
24. Borst P, Evers R, Kool M, Wijnholds J. A family of drug transporters: the multidrug resistance-associated proteins. J Natl Cancer Inst 2000;92:1295–1302.

25. Kruh GD, Belinsky MG. The MRP family of drug efflux pumps. Oncogene 2003;22:7537–7552.

26. Hart SM, Ganeshaguru K, Hoffbrand AV, Prentice HG, Mehta AB. Expression of the multidrug resistance-associated protein (MRP) in acute leukaemia. Leukemia 1994;8:2163–2168.

27. Filipits M, Stranzl T, Pohl G, et al. MRP expression in acute myeloid leukemia. An update. Adv Exp Med Biol 1999;457:141–150.

28. Laupeze B, Amiot L, Drenou B, et al. High multidrug resistance protein activity in acute myeloid leukaemias is associated with poor response to chemotherapy and reduced patient survival. Br J Haematol 2002;116: 834–838.

29. Filipits M, Suchomel RW, Zochbauer S, Brunner R, Lechner K, Pirker R. Multidrug resistance-associated protein in acute myeloid leukemia: no impact on treatment outcome. Clin Cancer Res 1997;3:1419–1425.

30. Borg AG, Burgess R, Green LM, Scheper RJ, Yin JA. Overexpression of lung-resistance protein and increased P-glycoprotein function in acute myeloid leukaemia cells predict a poor response to chemotherapy and reduced patient survival. Br J Haematol 1998;103:1083–1091.

31. van den Heuvel-Eibrink MM, Sonneveld P, Pieters R. The prognostic significance of membrane transport-associated multidrug resistance (MDR) proteins in leukemia. Int J Clin Pharmacol Ther 2000;38:94–110.

32. Tsimberidou AM, Paterakis G, Androutsos G, et al. Evaluation of the clinical relevance of the expression and function of P-glycoprotein, multidrug resistance protein and lung resistance protein in patients with primary acute myelogenous leukemia. Leuk Res 2002;26:143–154.

33. Poulain S, Lepelley P, Preudhomme C, et al. Expression of the multidrug resistance-associated protein in myelodysplastic syndromes. Br J Haematol 2000;110:591–598.

34. van der Pol MA, Broxterman HJ, Pater JM, et al. Function of the ABC transporters, P-glycoprotein, multidrug resistance protein and breast cancer resistance protein, in minimal residual disease in acute myeloid leukemia. Haematologica 2003;88:134–147.

35. Kuss BJ, Deeley RG, Cole SP, et al. Deletion of gene for multidrug resistance in acute myeloid leukaemia with inversion in chromosome 16: prognostic implications. Lancet 1994;343:1531–1534.

36. van Der Kolk DM, Vellenga E, van Der Veen AY, et al. Deletion of the multidrug resistance protein MRP1 gene in acute myeloid leukemia: the impact on MRP activity. Blood 2000;95:3514–3519.

37. Chen YN, Mickley LA, Schwartz AM, Acton EM, Hwang JL, Fojo AT. Characterization of adriamycin-resistant human breast cancer cells which display overexpression of a novel resistance-related membrane protein. J Biol Chem 1990;265:10,073–10,080.

38. Doyle LA, Yang W, Abruzzo LV, et al. A multidrug resistance transporter from human MCF-7 breast cancer cells. Proc Natl Acad Sci USA 1998;95:15,665–15,670.

39. Doyle LA, Ross DD. Multidrug resistance mediated by the breast cancer resistance protein BCRP (ABCG2). Oncogene 2003;22:7340–7358.

40. Ozvegy-Laczka C, Hegedus T, Varady G, et al. High-affinity interaction of tyrosine kinase inhibitors with the ABCG2 multidrug transporter. Mol Pharmacol 2004;65:1485–1495.

41. Ross DD, Karp JE, Chen TT, Doyle LA. Expression of breast cancer resistance protein in blast cells from patients with acute leukemia. Blood 2000;96:365–368.

42. Steinbach D, Sell W, Voigt A, Hermann J, Zintl F, Sauerbrey A. BCRP gene expression is associated with a poor response to remission induction therapy in childhood acute myeloid leukemia. Leukemia 2002;16:1443–1447.

43. van den Heuvel-Eibrink MM, Wiemer EA, Prins A, et al. Increased expression of the breast cancer resistance protein (BCRP) in relapsed or refractory acute myeloid leukemia (AML). Leukemia 2002;16:833–839.

44. Nakanishi T, Karp JE, Tan M, et al. Quantitative analysis of breast cancer resistance protein and cellular resistance to flavopiridol in acute leukemia patients. Clin Cancer Res 2003;9:3320–3328.

45. Abbott BL, Colapietro AM, Barnes Y, Marini F, Andreeff M, Sorrentino BP. Low levels of ABCG2 expression in adult AML blast samples. Blood 2002;100:4594–4601.

46. van der Kolk DM, Vellenga E, Scheffer GL, et al. Expression and activity of breast cancer resistance protein (BCRP) in de novo and relapsed acute myeloid leukemia. Blood 2002;99:3763–3770.

47. Osawa M, Hanada K, Hamada H, Nakauch, H. Long-term lymphohematopoietic reconstitution by a single CD34-low/negative hematopoietic stem cell. Science 1996;273:242–245.

48. Goodell MA, Brose K, Paradis G, Conner AS, Mulligan RC. Isolation and functional properties of murine hematopoietic stem cells that are replicating in vivo. J Exp Med 1996;183:1797–1806.

49. Zhou S, Schuetz JD, Bunting KD, et al. The ABC transporter Bcrp1/ABCG2 is expressed in a wide variety of stem cells and is a molecular determinant of the side-population phenotype. Nat Med 2001; 7:1028–1034.

50. Goodell MA, Rosenzweig M, Kim H, et al. Dye efflux studies suggest that hematopoietic stem cells expressing low or undetectable levels of CD34 antigen exist in multiple species. Nat Med 1997;3:1337–1345.

51. Krishnamurthy P, Ross DD, Nakanishi T, et al. The stem cell marker Bcrp/ABCG2 enhances hypoxic cell survival through interactions with heme. J Biol Chem 2004;279:24,218–24,225.

52. Reya T, Morrison SJ, Clarke MF, Weissman IL. Stem cells, cancer, and cancer stem cells. Nature 2001;414: 105–111.

53. Wulf GG, Wang RY, Kuehnle I, et al. A leukemic stem cell with intrinsic drug efflux capacity in acute myeloid leukemia. Blood 2001;98:1166–1173.

54. Blair A, Hogge DE, Sutherland HJ. Most acute myeloid leukemia progenitor cells with long-term proliferative ability in vitro and in vivo have the phenotype CD34(+)/CD71(−)/HLA-DR. Blood 1998;92:4325–4335.

55. Feuring-Buske M, Hogge DE. Hoechst 33342 efflux identifies a subpopulation of cytogenetically normal CD34(+)CD38(−) progenitor cells from patients with acute myeloid leukemia. Blood 2001;97:3882–3889.

56. Kalidas M, Kantarjian H, Talpaz M. Chronic myelogenous leukemia. JAMA 2001;286:895–898.

57. Burger H, Van Tol H, Boersma AW, et al. Imatinib mesylate (STI571) is a substrate for the BCRP/ABCG2 drug pump. Blood 2004;104:2940–2942.

58. Burger H, van Tol H, Boersma AW, et al. Imatinib mesylate (STI571) is a substrate for the breast cancer resistance protein (BCRP)/ABCG2 drug pump. Blood 2004;104:2940–2942.

59. Holyoake T, Jiang X, Eaves C, Eaves A. Isolation of a highly quiescent subpopulation of primitive leukemic cells in chronic myeloid leukemia. Blood 1999;94:2056–2064.

60. Graham SM, Jorgensen HG, Allan E, et al. Primitive, quiescent, Philadelphia-positive stem cells from patients with chronic myeloid leukemia are insensitive to STI571 in vitro. Blood 2002;99:319–325.

61. Jamieson CH, Ailles LE, Dylla SJ, et al. Granulocyte-macrophage progenitors as candidate leukemic stem cells in blast-crisis CML. N Engl J Med 2004;351:657–667.

62. Crossman LC, O'Brien SG. Imatinib therapy in chronic myeloid leukemia. Hematol Oncol Clin North Am 2004;18:605–617, viii.

63. Weisberg E, Griffin JD. Resistance to imatinib (Glivec): update on clinical mechanisms. Drug Resist Update 2003;6:231–238.

64. Illmer T, Schaich M, Platzbecker U, et al. P-glycoprotein-mediated drug efflux is a resistance mechanism of chronic myelogenous leukemia cells to treatment with imatinib mesylate. Leukemia 2004;18:401–408.

65. Knight GW, McLellan D. Use and limitations of imatinib mesylate (Glivec), a selective inhibitor of the tyrosine kinase Abl transcript in the treatment of chronic myeloid leukaemia. Br J Biomed Sci 2004;61:103–111.

66. La Rosee P, Shen L, Stoffregen EP, Deininger M, Druker BJ. No correlation between the proliferative status of Bcr-Abl positive cell lines and the proapoptotic activity of imatinib mesylate (Gleevec/Glivec). Hematol J 2003;4:413–419.

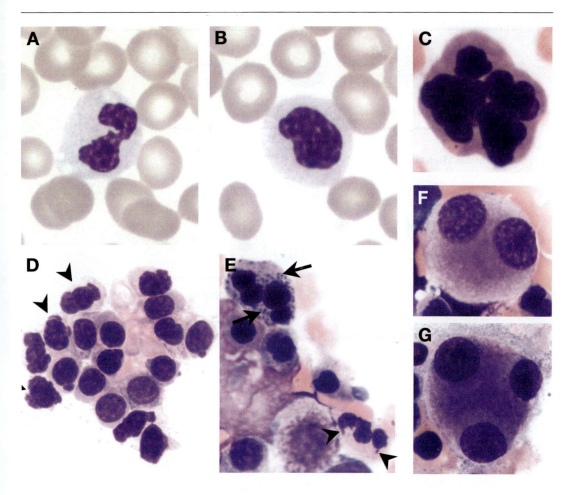

Color Plate 1. Fig. 4.1. *See* legend and discussion on p. 72.

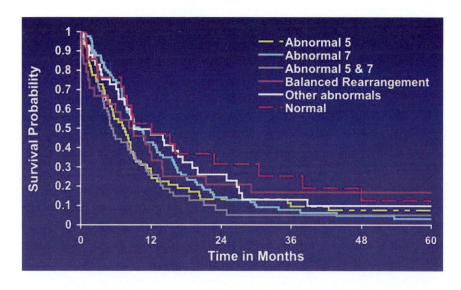

Color Plate 2. Fig. 4.3. *See* legend on p. 78 and discussion on p. 77.

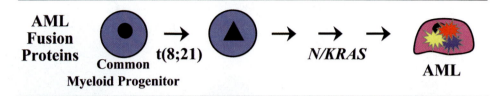

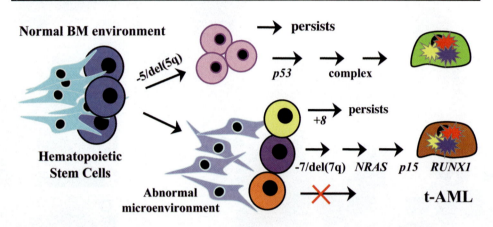

Color Plate 3. Fig. 4.4. *See* legend on p. 79 and discussion on p. 78.

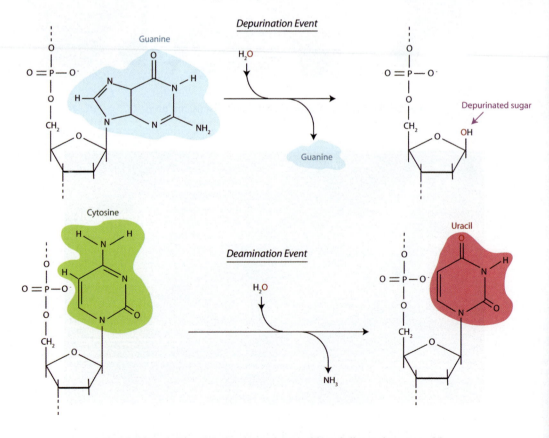

Color Plate 4. Fig. 5.1. *See* legend on p. 99 and discussion on p. 98.

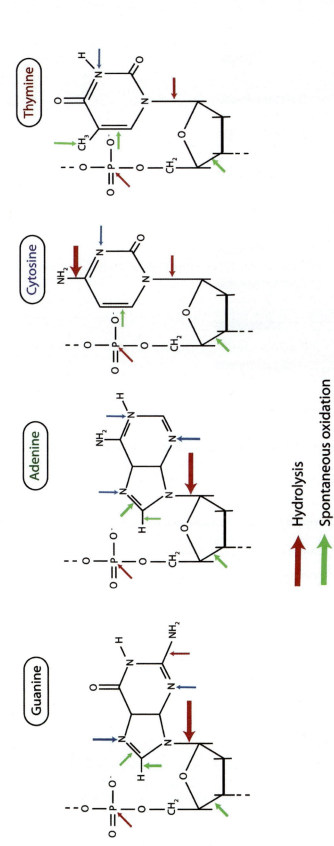

Color Plate 5. Fig. 5.2. *See* legend on p. 100 and discussion on p. 98.

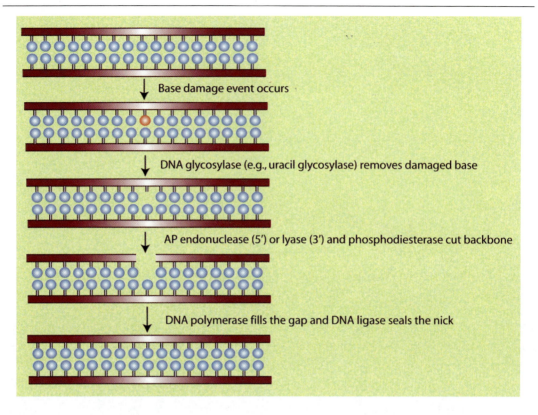

Color Plate 6. Fig. 5.3. *See* legend on p. 104 and discussion on p. 103.

*Please find Color Plate 7 on following page.

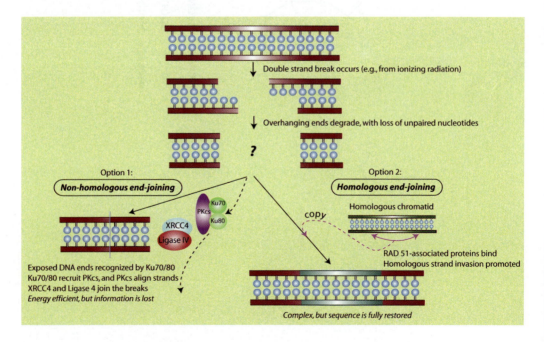

Color Plate 8. Fig. 5.5. *See* legend on p. 106 and discussion on p. 103.

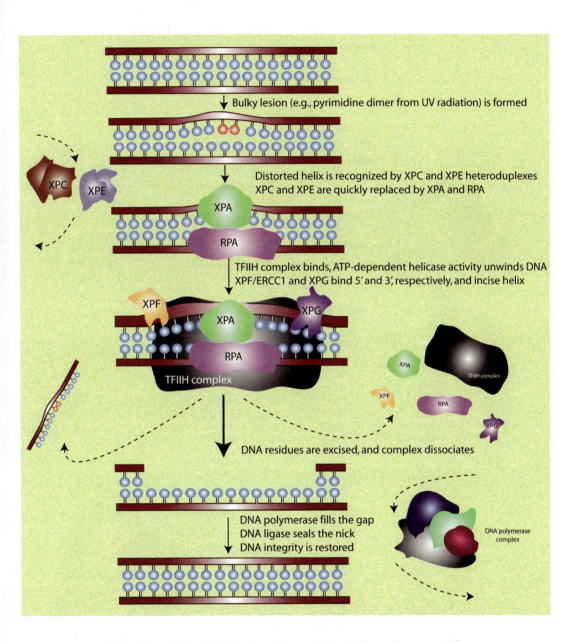

Color Plate 7. Fig. 5.4. *See* legend on p. 105 and discussion on p. 103.

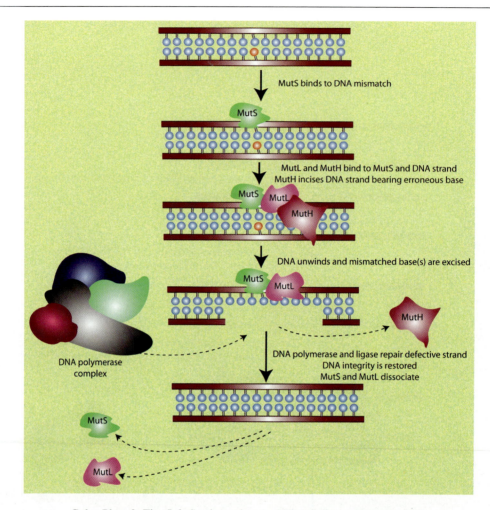

Color Plate 9. Fig. 5.6. *See* legend on p. 107 and discussion on p. 103.

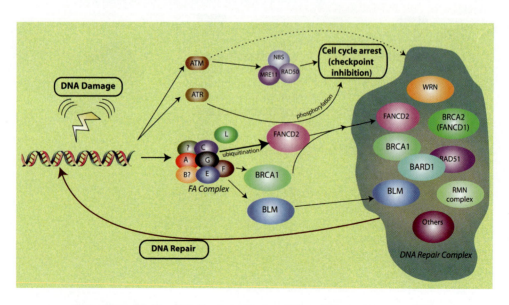

Color Plate 10. Fig. 5.7. *See* legend on p. 108 and discussion on p. 105.

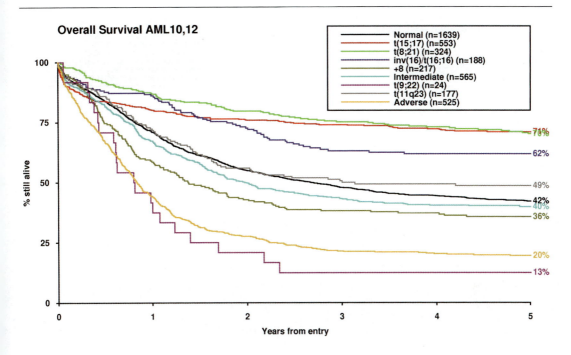

Color Plate 11. Fig. 8.1. *See* legend on p. 181 and discussion on p. 178.

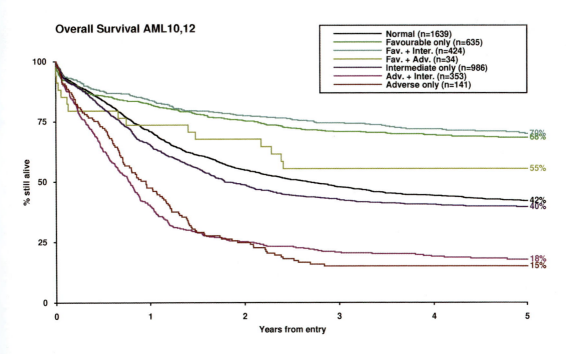

Color Plate 12. Fig. 8.2. *See* legend on p. 183 and discussion on p. 181.

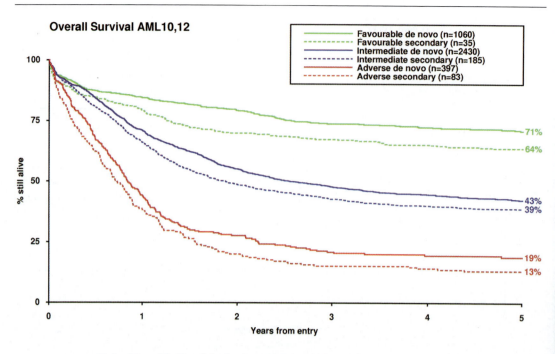

Color Plate 13. Fig. 8.3. *See* legend on p. 185 and discussion on p. 184.

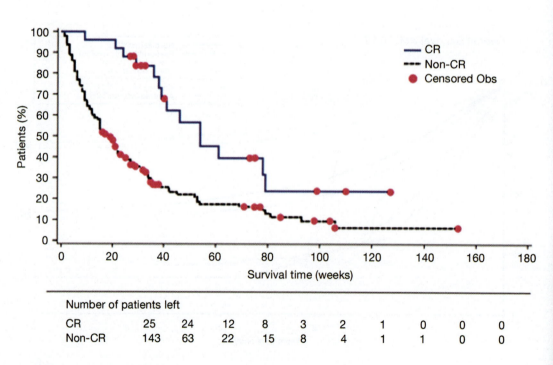

Color Plate 14. Fig. 12.4. *See* legend on p. 270 and discussion on p. 269.

III   TRANSLATING BIOLOGY INTO CLINICAL APPLICATION

8 Impact of Cytogenetics on Clinical Outcome in AML

David Grimwade

CONTENTS

Summary

Over the last three decades it has become clear that a significant proportion of cases of acute myeloid leukemia (AML) are characterized by at least one of a variety of recurrent chromosomal abnormalities. While there has been uncertainty as to which represent primary events in the pathogenesis of AML, those that provide critical second hits that are required for progression to full-blown leukemia or those that are merely markers of the leukemic process, it is nevertheless clear that diagnostic karyotype is a key determinant of outcome in this disease. Moreover, there is mounting evidence to support the notion that cytogenetic analysis can serve to identify biologically distinct subsets of AML that demand tailored therapeutic approaches. This underpins the trend toward more widespread adoption of routine cytogenetic and molecular analysis in the characterization of patients with a diagnosis of acute leukemia. A key challenge for the future is to use information gained from cytogenetic analyses in conjunction with molecular diagnostics and gene expression profiling to achieve greater consensus in risk group assignment of AML, which will provide a more reliable framework for determining the most appropriate treatment approach for individual patients with this disease.

Key Words: Cytogenetics; cryptic chromosomal rearrangements; fluorescence in situ hybridization; molecular screening in AML; risk stratification of AML; acquired uniparental disomy.

1. KARYOTYPIC FEATURES OF AML

AML is highly heterogeneous at the cytogenetic and molecular levels, with chromosomal breakpoint regions from more than 70 balanced reciprocal translocations having been cloned to date *(1)*. Although at first glance the number of genes disrupted in AML appears very daunting, common mechanistic themes in terms of the pathogenesis of the disease are beginning

From: *Contemporary Hematology: Acute Myelogenous Leukemia*
Edited by: J. E. Karp © Humana Press Inc., Totowa, NJ

to emerge. In particular, chromosomal translocations generate chimeric fusion proteins that mediate a block in differentiation through deregulation of transcription factors that play a key role in normal hematopoiesis. Notable examples include the t(8;21)(q22;q22) and inv(16) (p13q22)/t(16;16)(p13;q22), which disrupt genes encoding components of the heterodimeric core-binding factor (CBF) complex, with formation of *AML1-ETO* and *CBFB-MYH11* fusion genes, respectively. Similarly, chromosomal translocations involving 17q21, which typify acute promyelocytic leukemia (APL), disrupt the gene encoding RARα, which is implicated in myeloid differentiation, with PML being the most common fusion partner as a result of the t(15;17)(q22;q21). The *MLL* gene, which is located at 11q23, is also implicated in the pathogenesis of AML through partial tandem duplications (PTDs), which commonly occur in the context of trisomy 11, or as a promiscuous fusion partner as a result of chromosomal translocation. *MLL*-associated translocations are particularly prevalent in the pediatric age group, and to date more than 30 fusion partners of *MLL* have been identified; however, only a limited number are involved in the pathogenesis of AML in a significant number of patients (*see* Table 1). Other fusion genes arising as a result of rarer recurring chromosomal abnormalities occurring in AML are detailed in Table 1.

Overall, balanced reciprocal translocations are identified in over a third of AML cases arising in children and younger adults and are typically associated with *de novo* AML; however, a small proportion occur in therapy-related leukemias, particularly following exposure to drugs targeting DNA topoisomerase II. Interestingly, the nature of the prior drug exposure has a bearing on the molecular basis of therapy-related AML, with involvement of the *MLL* locus being linked with etoposide exposure, whereas therapy-related APL with t(15;17) most commonly arises following treatment with mitoxantrone or epirubicin *(2,3)*.

Population-based studies indicate that the incidence of AML with balanced translocations is relatively constant across all age groups. However, such abnormalities are relatively uncommon (accounting for <10% of cases) in AML presenting in older adults, in whom the disease is substantially more common and often characterized by a complex picture of chromosomal losses and gains *(4,5)*. This has led to the commonly held view that AML arising in older adults is biologically different from the disease associated with balanced translocations, reflecting an accumulation of multiple genetic lesions, more akin to secondary leukemias arising on a background of myelodysplasia, contributing to the relatively poor prognosis of AML in this age group.

2. PROGNOSTIC IMPACT OF KARYOTYPE IN AML

A large number of studies have established diagnostic karyotype as one of the most important determinants of outcome for patients with AML *(1)* (*see* Fig. 1; *see* Color Plate 11, following p. 174). As such, results of cytogenetic analysis are increasingly being used as a framework to determine treatment approach in children and younger adults with this disease.

2.1. Cytogenetic Abnormalities Predicting Relatively Favorable Outcome

In the majority of studies, t(15;17)(q22;q21), t(8;21)(q22;q22), and inv(16)(p13q22)/ t(16;16)(p13;q22) emerge as predicting the most favorable outcome (Table 2), and patients with such abnormalities are generally treated according to specific treatment protocols. In addition, the Southwest Oncology Group (SWOG) has traditionally included cases with deletions of 16q (del(16q)) within the favorable risk group alongside those with inv(16) and t(16;16) (Table 2). While the latter two abnormalities both generate the *CBFB-MYH11* fusion

Table 1
**Frequencies of Specific Cytogenetic Abnormalities According
to Analysis of a Series of 1584 Patients Treated in the MRC AML10 Trial**

Chromosomal aberrations associated with AML, grouped according to underlying molecular abnormality	Molecular consequence	Frequency in children and younger adults (0–55 years)	Clinical features
Core binding factor (CBF) gene rearrangement: *AML1 (CBFA2)* gene at 21q22 or *CBFB* gene at 16q22		**12%**	
t(3;21)(q26;q22)	*EAP/MDS1/ EVI1-AML1* fusion	Rare	
t(8;21)(q22;q22)	*AML1-ETO* fusion	8%	Significant proportion is classified as AML M2 and exhibit distinct morphological features
inv(16)(p13q22)/ t(16;16)(p13;q22)	*CBFB-MYH11* fusion	4%	Typically present as AML M4 with abnormal eosinophilic features (M4Eo)
t(16;21)(q24;q22)	*MTG16-AML1* fusion	Rare	
***RARA* gene rearrangement (17q12-21):**[a]		**12%**	**APL**
t(5;17)(q35;q12-21)	*NPM-RARA* fusion	Rare	ATRA sensitive
t(11;17)(q23;q21)	*PLZF-RARA* fusion	Rare	Distinct morphological features. ATRA and ATO resistant
t(15;17)(q22;q12-21)	*PML-RARA* fusion	12%	ATRA and ATO sensitive
***MLL* gene rearrangement (11q23):**[b]		**5%**	Associated with AML M4/M5
t(6;11)(q27;q23)	*AF6-MLL* fusion	<0.5%	
t(9;11)(p21-22;q23)	*AF9-MLL* fusion	1%	
t(10;11)(p11-13;q23)	*AF10-MLL* fusion	1%	
t(11;19)(q23;p13.3)	*MLL-ELL* fusion[b]	<0.5%	
Other		3%	
Involvement of zinc finger encoding genes by rearrangements of 3q: *EVI1* gene at 3q26 or *MDS/EVI1* homolog *MEL1* at 1p36			
inv(3)(q21q26)/ t(3;3)(q21;q26)	EVI1 overexpression	2%	Characteristic megakaryocyte morphology, can present with thrombocytosis

(Continued)

Table 1 (*Continued*)

Chromosomal aberrations associated with AML, grouped according to underlying molecular abnormality	*Molecular consequence*	*Frequency in children and younger adults (0–55 years)*	*Clinical features*
t(3;12)(q26;p13)	*MDS1/EVI1-TEL* fusion	<0.5%	
t(l;3)(p36;q21)	MEL1 overexpression	<0.5%	
Involvement of genes encoding factors involved in signal transduction:			
***ABL* at 9q34**			
t(9;22)(q34;q11)	*BCR-ABL* fusion	1%	
Nuclear pore component genes:			
***CAN (NUP214)* at 9q34, *NUP98* at 11p15**			
t(6;9)(p23;q34)	*DEK-CAN* fusion	1%	Associated with FAB type M2 and basophilia
t(11)(p15)	*NUP98* fusions	Rare	
Other genes encoding transcriptional regulators/chromatin modulators including:			
***MOZ* gene rearrangements at 8p11, *CBP* gene rearrangements at 16p13**			
t(l;22)(p13;q13)	*OTT-MAL* fusion	<0.5%	Associated with AML M7 in infants
inv(8)(p11q13)	*MOZ-TIF2* fusion	Rare	
t(8;16)(p11p13)	*MOZ-CBP* fusion	<0.5%	Associated with erythrophagocytosis
t(8;22)(p11;q13)	*MOZ-P300* fusion	Rare	
t(10;16)(q22;p13)	*MORF-CBP* fusion	Rare	
Ets family transcription factor genes:			
***TEL (ETV6)* gene rearrangements at 12p13, *ERG* gene rearrangement at 21q22**			
t(12)(p13)	*TEL (ETV6)* fusions	Rare	
t(16;21)(p11;q22)	*FUS-ERG* fusion	Rare	
Other recurrent translocations in AML:			
***NPM* on 5q35**			
t(3;5)(q25;q35)	*NPM-MLF1* fusion	<0.5%	

(*Continued*)

Table 1 (*Continued*)

AF10 on 10p12-p13			
t(10;11)(p12-p13; q14-q21)	*CALM-AF10* fusion	<0.5%	Associated with AMLM0

[a]*NuMA-RARA* and *STAT5b-RARA* associated with t(11;17)(q13;q21) and der(17) respectively, have been identified in only single patients with APL to date.

[b]More than 30 *MLL* fusion partners have been identified at the molecular level; only those lesions most commonly associated with AML are listed here. Three different *MLL* fusion partners have been identified in cases with t(11;19), with *ELL* being the commonest in AML. Cases listed as "Rare" were detected in ≤1 case in this series.

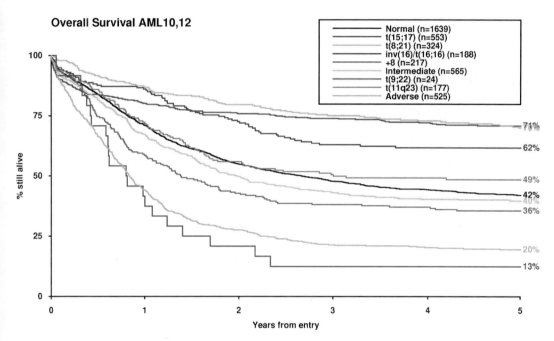

Fig. 1. (Color Plate 11, following p. 174) Overall survival of patients aged up to 60 years treated in UK Medical Research Council (MRC) AML10 and AML12 trials according to diagnostic karyotype. The t(15;17), t(8;21), inv(16)/t(16;16), t(11q23), and t(9;22) groups included cases in which other abnormalities were present. Outcome is shown for +8 as the sole abnormality. The Adverse category includes cases with abnormal 3q, −5, del(5q), −7 or complex karyotype (≥5 unrelated abnormalities) and lacking t(15;17), t(8;21), or inv(16)/t(16;16). All other abnormalities are included in the Intermediate category.

gene, cases with del(16q) are heterogeneous at the molecular level, and it seems sensible to exclude them from the favorable risk group unless an underlying *CBFB-MYH11* fusion is documented by fluorescence in situ hybridization or polymerase chain reaction (PCR).

There has been some debate as to whether additional cytogenetic abnormalities adversely affect the outcome of patients with t(15;17) and CBF leukemia. In APL, additional changes accompany the t(15;17) in approximately a third of cases, with trisomy 8 being the most common abnormality. Recent studies involving large cohorts of patients treated with all-*trans*-retinoic acid (ATRA) and anthracycline-based chemotherapy have indicated that additional cytogenetic abnormalities have no bearing on outcome (Fig. 2; *see* Color Plate 12, following p. 174). The t(8;21) is frequently associated with additional chromosomal abnormalities, with

Table 2
Variation in Cytogenetic Risk Group Classification Across Clinical Trial Groups

	MRC[a]	SWOG/ECOG[b]	CALGB[c]	GIMEMA/ AML10[d]	GERMAN AMLCG[e]
Favorable	t(15;17)	t(15;17)	t(15;17)	t(15;17)	t(15;17)
	t(8;21)	t(8;21)(lacking del(9q),	t(8;21)	t(8;21)	t(8;21)
	inv(16)/ t(16;16)	complex, i.e., ≥3 unrel abn) inv(16)/t(16;16)/ del(16q)	inv(16)/ t(16;16)	inv(16)/ t(16;16)	inv(16)/ t(16;16)
Intermediate	Normal	Normal	Normal	Normal	Normal
	Other non-complex	+6, +8, -Y, del(12p)	Other non-complex	−Y	Other non-complex
Adverse	abn(3q)	abn(3q),(9q), (11q),(21q),	inv(3)/t(3;3)	Other	inv(3)/t(3;3)
	−5/del(5q)	abn(17p)	−7		−5/del(5q)
	−7	−5/del(5q)	t(6;9)		−7/del(7q)
	Complex (≥5 unrel abn)	−7/del(7q)	t(6;11)		abn(11q23)
	(excluding those with favorable changes)	t(6;9) t(9;22) Complex (≥3 unrel abn)	t(11;19) +8 Complex (≥3 unrel abn) (excluding those with favorable changes)		del(12p) abn(17p)

[a]From ref. *11*.
[b]From ref. *8*.
[c]From ref. *42*.
[d]From ref. *43*.
[e]From ref. *41*.
Abbreviations: unrel abn, unrelated abnormality; abn, abnormal.

approximately half the cases featuring loss of a sex chromosome, which has no impact on outcome. An early report suggested that del(9q) adversely affects outcome in t(8;21)-associated AML *(6)*; however, it is likely that this was a chance finding reflecting small sample size and has not been borne out by subsequent larger studies. In accordance with cases with t(15;17) and t(8;21), no prognostic impact of additional abnormalities in the context of the inv(16), which is most commonly accompanied by trisomy 22, has been observed in the UK Medical Research Council (MRC) AML10 and AML12 trials (Fig. 2). This has led to the adoption of a hierarchical system of cytogenetic risk group classification whereby patients with t(15;17), t(8;21) or inv(16)/t(16;16) are assigned to the favorable risk group irrespective of the presence of additional cytogenetic abnormalities, including presence of abnormalities that in their own right would be thought to confer an adverse outcome (Figs. 1, 2; Table 2).

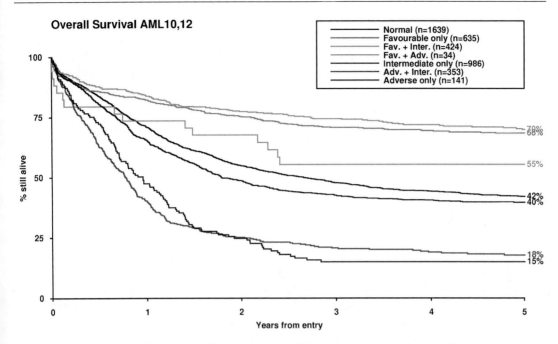

Fig. 2. (Color Plate 12, following p. 174) Impact of additional cytogenetic abnormalities on outcome in patients treated in UK Medical Research Council (MRC) AML10 and AML12 trials. Favorable (Fav): t(15;17), t(8;21), inv(16)/t(16;16). Adverse (Adv): abnormal 3q, −5, del(5q), −7, t(9;22), or complex karyotype (≥5 unrelated abnormalities). Intermediate (Inter): other abnormalities, not classified as favorable or adverse. Outcome of cases with normal karyotype is given for comparison.

2.2. Karyotypic Features Predicting Adverse Prognosis

In patients lacking a favorable cytogenetic marker or its molecular equivalent, a number of karyotypic abnormalities have been correlated with a poor response to initial therapy and significantly increased risk of relapse (Figs. 1, 2; Table 2). These include monosomies of chromosomes 5 and/or 7, deletion of the long arm of chromosome 5, and abnormalities of the long arm of chromosome 3, such as inv(3)(q21q26) and t(3;3)(q21;q26), which are associated with overexpression of the gene encoding the transcription factor EVI1, which is located at 3q26. The t(9;22)(q34;q11) leading to the BCR-ABL fusion is an uncommon abnormality in AML occurring in less than 1 % of cases, but is associated with an extremely poor outcome (Fig. 1). Most groups consider the t(6;9)(p23;q34), leading to the DEK-CAN fusion, as a poor prognostic indicator, particularly reflecting a high rate of relapse. In addition, AML with complex karyotype is assigned to the adverse risk group, although (as discussed later) there is currently no consensus as to how this group is most appropriately defined (Table 2). There is also some inconsistency in the risk-group assignment of cases with deletions involving the long arm of chromosome 7 (Table 2). This abnormality is commonly associated with other cytogenetic features conferring a poor prognosis, including loss of chromosome 5 material and complex karyotype.

Definitions of complex karyotype differ between groups, with the limit being set at three or five unrelated abnormalities. Evidence from the MRC trials data base suggests that patients with t(15;17), t(8;21), or inv(16)/t(16;16) are most appropriately assigned to the favorable risk group irrespective of karyotype complexity. Indeed, complex karyotype as defined by some groups is relatively common among patients with favorable risk lesions (e.g., t(8;21) accompanied by loss of sex chromosome and del(9q)) and, in the experience of the MRC, have a comparable outcome to other patients with the same primary abnormality, but with fewer secondary changes. While the presence of a favorable cytogenetic abnormality in the context of a very complex karyotype (defined as five or more abnormalities) is uncommon, evidence to date suggests that even these patients have a relatively favorable outcome. In practice, these distinctions are somewhat academic, because more reasoned decisions with respect to the most appropriate treatment approach in first complete remission (CR), including the role of transplantation, in such patients are likely to be reached using molecular monitoring for minimal residual disease (MRD) by quantitative PCR.

2.3. Karyotype Is an Independent Prognostic Factor in AML

In the hierarchical classification adopted in the MRC trials, AML patients with cytogenetic abnormalities not encompassed by favorable and adverse risk groups, including those with rare changes where limited sample sizes preclude reliable determination of the prognostic significance, are classified as standard risk along with those with normal karyotype. The MRC classification has subsequently been validated in independent data sets relating to trials conducted in children and younger adults by a number of groups, as well as in older adults (>55 years) (7–9). Cytogenetic risk group also retains its prognostic significance among patients with *de novo* and secondary AML, with a history of secondary leukemia predicting a poorer outcome within each respective risk group (*see* Fig. 3; *see* Color Plate 13, following p. 174). Moreover, diagnostic karyotype is a key predictor of outcome following bone marrow transplantation (BMT) in first CR (10,11).

3. DIAGNOSTIC KARYOTYPE IDENTIFIES BIOLOGICALLY DISTINCT SUBSETS OF AML

A key question is why diagnostic karyotype provides one of the strongest predictors of treatment outcome in AML. In a number of instances, cytogenetic analysis is almost certainly serving to identify the underlying molecular lesion that plays the primary role in initiating and determining the biological behavior of the leukemic clone. This is likely to be the case for balanced chromosomal rearrangements that generate chimeric oncoproteins; indeed, a number of such molecularly defined subsets of AML, including those with t(8;21)/AML1-ETO, inv(16)/CBFB-MYH11, and t(15;17)/PML-RARA, have been found to exhibit unique patterns of gene expression as determined by microarrays, which are apparent using unsupervised analytical approaches. One mechanism by which chimeric fusion proteins potentially contribute to leukemogenesis is by conferring self-renewal properties upon committed myeloid progenitors, as has recently been shown for the MOZ-TIF2 fusion (12). Indeed, immortalization of committed progenitors by leukemic oncoproteins could predispose to the acquisition of additional mutations that cooperate to give rise to full-blown leukemia. As such, a range of bone marrow progenitors could be potential targets for leukemic transformation, rather than just uncommitted multipotent progenitors, as was originally thought to be the case (13). This raises the possibility that the nature of the progenitor subject to leukemic transformation could be a key factor with a bearing upon treatment outcome, determining whether the leukemic clone can be successfully eliminated with conventional chemotherapy alone.

While balanced chromosomal rearrangements are directly related to disease pathogenesis and behavior through generation of chimeric oncoproteins (as discussed earlier) or gene

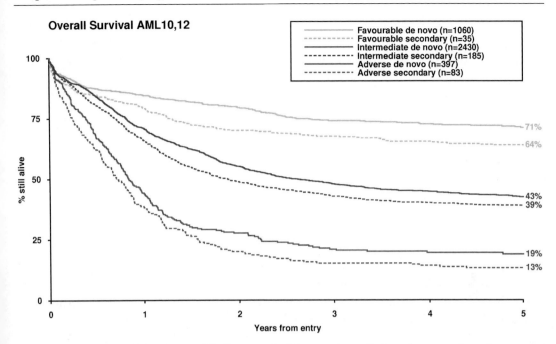

Fig. 3. (Color Plate 13, following p. 174) Cytogenetic risk group is predictive of outcome in patients treated in UK Medical Research Council (MRC) AML10 and AML12 trials with *de novo* and secondary AML. Favorable: t(15;17), t(8;21), inv(16)/ inv(16), alone or with other changes. Intermediate: normal karyotype and abnormalities not assigned to favorable or adverse groups. Adverse: abnormal 3q, −5, del(5q), −7, t(9;22), or complex karyotype (≥5 unrelated abnormalities) and lacking t(15;17), t(8;21), or inv(16)/t(16;16).

overexpression (e.g., EVI1), it has become apparent that gain or loss of particular chromosomes may provide a marker for underlying mutations within genes encoding transcription factors or chromatin modifiers that have been implicated in hematopoiesis. In some instances the mutation involves a gene on the chromosome subject to trisomy, with PTD of the *MLL* gene and mutation of *AML1* being correlated with +11 and +21, respectively *(14,15)*. The reasons for these associations are presently unclear, but it is possible that the process of chromosomal gain could potentially afford a selective advantage in the presence of the mutation. Recently, an association has been identified between mutation of the gene encoding the transcription factor CCAAT/enhancer-binding protein-α (CEBPA), which is located on chromosome 19, and deletions of the long arm of chromosome 9 *(16)*. The significance of this relationship is also currently obscure; however, it is interesting to note that, as discussed earlier, del(9q) is also a frequent secondary change in t(8;21)-associated AML and that CEBPA is a recognized target of the AML1-ETO fusion. This raises the possibility that del(9q) could occur through a common mechanism in these subsets of leukemia that is in some way related to abrogation of function of CEBPA. An alternative hypothesis is that disruption of CEBPA function coupled with the genetic events associated with del(9q) could cooperate in the process of leukemic transformation.

Investigation of cases of APL with cryptic formation of the *PML-RARA* fusion has revealed a similar spectrum of additional abnormalities to those with overt t(15;17), with +8 being the most common secondary change in both scenarios *(17)*. Overall, these data raise the possibility that leukemic oncoproteins may have a direct influence on the nature of secondary cytogenetic changes. Alternatively, particular secondary changes could arise through a common process of selection, providing the cooperating lesions required for leukemic transformation necessary to complement any given fusion protein. A further possibility is that the spectrum of observed secondary changes is a reflection of differences in the progenitor populations in which particular leukemias arise, with additional changes conferring characteristics that are required for leukemic transformation in any given population that are not provided by the chimeric oncoprotein itself in that particular cellular context.

The molecular events underlying cases of AML with miscellaneous numerical and structural cytogenetic abnormalities and those with adverse risk cytogenetics including loss of chromosomes 5 and 7 remain uncertain. However, it is possible that the heterogeneous pattern of chromosomal losses and gains observed in complex karyotypes reflects an underlying process of genomic instability that contributes to leukemogenesis.

While there is uncertainty as to which cytogenetic abnormalities represent primary events in the pathogenesis of AML, those that provide critical second hits required for progression to full-blown leukemia or those that are merely markers of the leukemic process, a number of lines of evidence support the notion that diagnostic karyotype identifies biologically distinct subsets of AML, which could have a bearing on the observed differences in response to therapy and outcome. In particular, AML blasts derived from cases with favorable, standard, and adverse risk karyotype have been found to exhibit different growth characteristics in semi-solid bone marrow cultures (18). Blasts with adverse karyotypic features show a greater propensity to autonomous growth, which is not a feature of cases with favorable cytogenetics (18). Karyotype has also been shown to influence engraftment characteristics of primary leukemic cells in NOD/SCID mice (13,19). Cells from adverse karyotype AML engraft to higher levels than those with favorable risk cytogenetics; moreover, high-level engraftment has been found to correlate with factor-independent growth in AML colony assays, which may reflect the potential for autocrine growth factor production (19). The NOD/SCID engraftment data could indicate that the relative proportion of leukemic stem cells differs according to cytogenetic risk group, being most prevalent in those with adverse karyotypic features. These data are also consistent with the hypothesis that leukemias with adverse cytogenetics arise in more primitive progenitors than those associated with favorable risk. Indeed this is in accordance with the recent observation that the BCR-ABL fusion cannot confer self-renewal properties upon committed myeloid progenitors, supporting the notion that the t(9;22), which predicts poor outcome in AML, arises in multipotent progenitors (12). The origin of the leukemic clone could have an important bearing upon treatment outcome, because involvement of multipotent progenitors could limit the capacity for normal hematopoietic repopulation after conventional chemotherapy. Moreover, primitive progenitors are characterized by expression of ABC transporters that render them potentially resistant to a number of chemotherapeutic agents.

4. IMPLICATIONS OF DIAGNOSTIC KARYOTYPE TO DETERMINE TREATMENT APPROACH

Conventional cytogenetics distinguishes a number of biologically distinct subsets of AML now being treated with specific treatment protocols. The management of APL with t(15;17) is based around use of ATRA and anthracycline-based chemotherapy regimens, with increasing use of arsenic trioxide. Treatment protocols for t(8;21) and inv(16)/t(16;16)-associated AML commonly involve high-dose cytosine arabinoside, based on a report of specific benefit from a Cancer and Leukemia Group B (CALGB) study (20). However, favorable outcomes have also been obtained for this subset of AML using regimens that do not include high-dose cytarabine; future studies will establish whether the CALGB data reflect a specific sensitivity of this subset of AML to cytarabine or are indicative of a more generalized sensitivity to chemotherapeutic agents.

The relatively favorable outcomes observed in patients with CBF leukemias treated with chemotherapy alone, and those with t(15;17)-associated APL treated with ATRA and chemotherapy combinations, have really called into question whether there is any role for transplantation in first CR for patients with favorable risk karyotype. Indeed, in the MRC AML10 and AML12 trials, any benefit in terms of reduction of relapse risk in this group was offset by transplant-related mortality such that there was no overall survival benefit for transplantation in first CR *(21,22)*. Although a benefit for transplant in first CR among patients with favorable karyotype has been suggested by the SWOG, this assertion was based on a comparison with good risk patients treated with chemotherapy alone, who actually fared more poorly than might have been expected (35% overall survival at 5 years) *(8)*. Therefore, routine use of transplantation in patients with favorable karyotype has now been abandoned by the majority of study groups; although some variation in practice still remains as a result of differences with respect to the precise definition of the good risk group (Table 2).

There has been a degree of inconsistency between different trial groups as to the cytogenetic abnormalities that are deemed to confer intermediate or adverse risk (Table 2), which most likely reflects problems associated with relatively small sample sizes, differences in median age of the study cohorts, and variation in therapy. However, it is important to realize that the distinction between intermediate and adverse risk groups is somewhat arbitrary and currently has little bearing on clinical management, given that evaluation of the role of transplantation in these groups remains a major focus of clinical trial activity. However, cytogenetic analysis may be helpful in identifying a group with extremely poor prognosis, with younger patients in this category typically being considered for allogeneic transplantation in first CR. This group of patients may also be considered candidates for more experimental treatment strategies; for example, although experience is limited, molecularly targeted therapies could potentially be of value in the management of *BCR-ABL*-associated AML. As far as older patients are concerned (>60 years), it is clear that presence of a complex karyotype is predictive of a dismal prognosis following intensive treatment associated with overall survival rates below 5% *(5,7)*, providing a rationale for adopting a nonintensive or palliative treatment approach to such patients.

5. LIMITATIONS OF CYTOGENETICS TO DETERMINE TREATMENT APPROACH IN AML

5.1. Classification of AML Cases With Cryptic Rearrangements

Although cytogenetic classification has provided a valuable framework on which to stratify treatment approach in AML, it has a number of limitations. In particular, conventional cytogenetic analysis does not firmly establish the fusion gene generated by any given translocation (e.g., t(10;11) can lead to *MLL-AF10* or *CALM-AF10* fusions depending upon chromosome 11 breakpoint location; *see* Table 1). Moreover, patients may be assigned to the incorrect risk group if purely based on the diagnostic karyotype, since approx 10% of cases with an underlying fusion gene associated with the good risk group lack the expected cytogenetic lesion because of unsuccessful cytogenetic analysis, variant translocations, or cryptic rearrangements *(17)*. Patients with morphological APL and an underlying *PML-RARA* fusion as determined by molecular methods, but lacking the classical t(15;17), have been shown to share the beneficial response to molecularly targeted therapies in the form of ATRA and arsenic trioxide and to have a favorable prognosis *(17,23)*. Therefore, it is assumed that patients with cryptic *AML1-ETO* or *CBFB-MYH11* gene fusions are biologically similar to those with cytogenetically apparent t(8;21) or inv(16)/t(16;16). In support of this notion, microarray analysis has shown that gene expression profiles of cases with cryptic rearrangements cluster with those cases with the overt respective cytogenetic lesion *(24,25)*. Therefore, patients with cryptic CBF leukemias represent a further group that could potentially be spared routine use of BMT in first CR. The identification of such patients supports routine molecular screening for CBF leukemias in AML, which also serves to identify additional patients who could be subject to MRD monitoring using a fusion gene marker.

5.2. Identification of Mutations by Molecular Screening With Implications for Prognosis and Novel Targeted Therapeutic Approaches

A further limitation as far as the use of karyotype for reliable risk stratification in AML is concerned is that it fails to take into account the prognostic and/or potential therapeutic impact of the growing number of cytogenetically cryptic mutations that have been implicated in the pathogenesis of the disease. In particular, recent studies have identified such mutations in a substantial proportion of patients with normal karyotype AML *(26–28)*. Indeed, approximately half of such cases have been shown to harbor mutations in the carboxy-terminus of the nucleolar phosphoprotein, nucleophosmin (NPM1); these lead to delocalization of the protein to the cytoplasm, which can be readily detected by immunostaining *(27)*. NPM1 mutation has been shown to correlate with M4/M5 FAB type, absent expression of CD34, and higher presenting leukocyte count. Another gene that is very frequently mutated in normal karyotype AML (~30%) is that encoding the Fms-like tyrosine kinase 3 (FLT3), with mutations leading to constitutive activation of the receptor. The most common type of mutation, found in approximately a quarter of cases, is an internal tandem duplication (ITD) of the juxtamembrane region. This is associated with higher presenting leukocyte count and provides an independent adverse prognostic indicator, predicting for an increased risk of relapse *(29)*. Interestingly, NPM1 mutation and FLT3-ITD commonly co-exist in normal karyotype AML, suggesting that they may cooperate in generating the leukemic phenotype; however, presence of FLT3-ITD appears to be the dominant factor in terms of predicting treatment outcome *(26,28)*. A less common form of FLT3 mutation (occurring in up to 10% of AML) involves the activation loop (tyrosine kinase domain, TKD); although, in contrast to FLT3-ITD, such mutations do not appear to affect prognosis. Other signal transduction molecules subject to activating mutations in AML, with potential implications for molecularly targeted therapy, include N- and K-RAS (~20%), c-KIT (~5%), and SHP-2 (~4%, encoded by *PTPN11* and associated with monosomy 7). In common with FLT3-TKD mutations, defects in RAS do not appear to affect prognosis *(30)*, whereas presence of KIT mutation in patients with CBF leukemia is correlated with higher presenting WBC and poorer prognosis *(31)*.

A number of genes encoding hematopoietic transcription factors have been shown to be mutated in AML. In the pediatric setting, GATA1 mutations have been specifically observed in the majority of myeloid proliferations arising on a background of Down syndrome, i.e., transient abnormal myelopoiesis (TAM) and acute megakaryoblastic leukemia, suggesting that gene deregulation associated with the constitutional trisomy 21 and somatically acquired mutation of GATA1 (leading to expression of a truncated form) cooperate in these processes.

In other age groups, the most common transcription factor gene subject to mutation is *CEBPA* (~10% of AML), which is associated with AML M2 morphology and normal or intermediate risk cytogenetic abnormalities (particularly del(9q), as discussed above). Interestingly, germline mutation of *CEBPA* has been identified in a kindred with familial AML, suggesting that in some instances deregulation of CEBPA may provide a primary lesion in leukemogenesis *(32).* The *AML1* gene, which was initially found to be mutated in the familial platelet disorder, a rare autosomal dominant condition characterized by progressive pancytopenia and dysplasia that ultimately progresses to AML, is also mutated in approx 3–5% of sporadic cases of AML, being particularly associated with FAB type M0 *(15).* As mentioned above, *AML1* mutations are frequently observed in the context of acquired +21, in which case they are commonly biallelic. Partial tandem duplication of the *MLL* gene is detected in approx 10% of AML, particularly those with normal karyotype or +11, and has been found to predict a poorer outcome *(33,34).*

Further insights into the pathogenesis of normal karyotype AML have been gained using single nucleotide polymorphism arrays, which have revealed acquired uniparental disomy (UPD) because of somatic recombination in approximately one-fifth of AML cases examined *(35).* Interestingly, the region of loss of heterozygosity on chromosome 19 included the *CEBPA* locus, which was subject to an apparently homozygous mutation *(35).* Subsequent studies have shown that similar mechanisms underlie homozygous mutation of *FLT3* in AML and *JAK2* in myeloproliferative disorders *(36)* and may very well be implicated in the generation of other biallelic mutations, e.g., involving *AML1.* Ongoing studies will establish whether other chromosomal regions subject to somatic recombination harbor mutations that contribute to the leukemic process.

It is now clear that a significant proportion of AML cases with apparently normal karyotype or miscellaneous cytogenetic abnormalities, which according to commonly applied cytogenetic classification systems would have been grouped together—classed as "standard risk," harbor cytogenetically cryptic mutations that have a significant impact upon disease characteristics, including response to therapy. Dissecting the biological and clinical significance of these findings is a major focus of current research, with recent studies suggesting that AML cases with mutation of NPM1 or CEBPA in the absence of FLT3 mutation represent novel subsets of AML with a relatively favorable prognosis and that such patients may not benefit from transplantation in first CR *(26,28,37,38).* Conversely, presence of MLL-PTD or FLT3-ITD has been shown to predict a poorer outcome *(34),* but it is not clear whether this can be improved by the use of BMT in first remission *(26,39).*

6. FUTURE PERSPECTIVE

Over the course of the next few years, it will be interesting to establish whether rarer recurring cytogenetically and molecularly defined entities have characteristic signatures on microarray analysis that would lend support to their recognition in future modifications to the World Health Organization classification for myeloid malignancies. However, although karyotype analysis has provided a valuable basis for determining treatment approach for patients with AML over the course of the last decade, it is clear that future risk-stratified protocols will need to take into account mutations identified by systematic molecular screening that predict outcome and in some instances define novel biological subsets of leukemia, which could potentially benefit from specific therapeutic approaches. It is also seems likely that experience gained through gene expression profiling will have an increasingly important bearing upon patient management, based upon improvements in disease classification and identification of pathways predicting likelihood of response to particular therapeutic agents. While conventional cytogenetics can provide an early indication of therapeutic response predicting likelihood of subsequent relapse *(40)*, MRD monitoring using more sensitive quantitative PCR and flow cytometric-based approaches seems set to play an increasingly important role in achieving greater individualization of antileukemic therapy. This should enable more informed decisions to be made with respect to the intensity of therapy in any given patient, permitting more informed decision making in the use of transplantation procedures in first complete remission.

ACKNOWLEDGMENTS

I am grateful to Robert Hills from the Clinical Trials Unit Birmingham for statistical analysis of MRC AML trials data (Figs. 1–3) and to the Leukaemia Research Fund of Great Britain for support for our research program. MRC trials databases are supported by Kay Kendall Leukaemia Fund and the Leukaemia Research Fund.

REFERENCES

1. Mrózek K, Heerema NA, Bloomfield CD. Cytogenetics in acute leukemia. Blood Rev 2004;18:115–136.
2. Beaumont M, Sanz M, Carli PM, et al. Therapy-related acute promyelocytic leukemia. J Clin Oncol 2003; 21:2123–2137.
3. Mistry AR, Felix CA, Whitmarsh RJ, et al. DNA topoisomerase II in therapy-related acute promyelocytic leukemia. N Engl J Med 2005;352:1529–1538.
4. Mauritzson N, Albin M, Rylander L, et al. Pooled analysis of clinical and cytogenetic features in treatment-related and *de novo* adult acute myeloid leukemia and myelodysplastic syndromes based on a consecutive series of 761 patients analyzed 1976–1993 and on 5098 unselected cases reported in the literature 1974–2001. Leukemia 2002;16:2366–2378.
5. Schoch C, Haferlach T, Haase D, et al. German AML Cooperative Group. Patients with *de novo* acute myeloid leukaemia and complex karyotype aberrations show a poor prognosis despite intensive treatment: a study of 90 patients. Br J Haematol 2001;112:118–126.
6. Schoch C, Haase D, Haferlach T, et al. Fifty-one patients with acute myeloid leukemia and translocation t(8;21)(q22;q22): an additional deletion in 9q is an adverse prognostic factor. Leukemia 1996;10:1288–1295.
7. Grimwade D, Walker H, Harrison G, et al. The predictive value of hierarchical cytogenetic classification in older adults with AML: analysis of 1,065 patients entered into the MRC AML11 trial. Blood 2001;98:1312–1320.
8. Slovak ML, Kopecky KJ, Cassileth PA, et al. Karyotypic analysis predicts outcome of preremission and postremission therapy in adult acute myeloid leukemia: a Southwest Oncology Group/Eastern Cooperative Oncology Group study. Blood 2000;96:4075–4083.
9. Visani G, Bernasconi P, Boni M, et al. The prognostic value of cytogenetics is reinforced by the kind of induction/consolidation therapy in influencing the outcome of acute myeloid leukemia—analysis of 848 patients. Leukemia 2001;15:903–909.
10. Ferrant A, Labopin M, Frassoni F, et al. Karyotype in acute myeloblastic leukemia: prognostic significance for bone marrow transplantation in first remission: A European Group for Blood and Marrow Transplantation study. Blood 1997;90:2931–2938.
11. Grimwade D, Walker H, Oliver F, et al. on behalf of the Medical Research Council Adult and Children's Leukaemia Working Parties. The importance of diagnostic cytogenetics on outcome in AML: analysis of 1,612 patients entered into the MRC AML10 trial. Blood 1998;92:2322–2333.
12. Huntly BJP, Shigematsu H, Deguchi K, et al. MOZ-TIF2, but not BCR-ABL, confers properties of leukemic stem cells to committed murine hematopoietic progenitors. Cancer Cell 2004;6:587–596.
13. Bonnet D, Dick JE. Human acute myeloid leukemia is organized as a hierarchy that originates from a primitive hematopoietic cell. Nature Med 1997;3:730–737.

14. Caligiuri M, Strout MP, Schichman SA, et al. Partial tandem duplication of ALL1 as a recurrent molecular defect in acute myeloid leukemia with trisomy 11. Cancer Res 1996;56:1418–1425.

15. Preudhomme C, Warot-Loze D, Roumier C, et al. High incidence of biallelic point mutations in the Runt domain of the AML1/PEBP2αB gene in M0 acute myeloid leukemia and in myeloid malignancies with acquired trsomy 21. Blood 2000;96:2862–2869.

16. Fröhling S, Schlenk RF, Krauter J, et al. Acute myeloid leukemia with deletion 9q within a noncomplex karyotype is associated with CEBPA loss-of-function mutations. Genes Chromosomes and Cancer 2005; 42:427–432.

17. Grimwade D, Biondi A, Mozziconacci M-J, et al. Characterization of acute promyelocytic leukemia cases lacking the classical t(15;17): results of the European working party. Blood 2000;96:1297–1308.

18. Öhler L, Berer A, Aletaha D, et al. Cytogenetic risk groups in acute myeloblastic leukaemia differ greatly in their semi-solid colony growth. Br J Haematol 2001;113:120–125.

19. Ailles LE, Gerhard B, Kawagoe H, Hogge DE. Growth characteristics of acute myelogenous leukemia progenitors that initiate malignant hematopoiesis in nonobese diabetic/severe combined immunodeficient mice. Blood 1999;94:1761–1772.

20. Bloomfield CD, Lawrence D, Byrd JC, et al. Frequency of prolonged remission duration after high-dose cytarabine intensification in acute myeloid leukemia varies by cytogenetic subtype. Cancer Res 1998;58: 4173–4179.

21. Burnett AK, Goldstone AH, Stevens RM, et al. Randomised comparison of addition of autologous bone-marrow transplantation to intensive chemotherapy for acute myeloid leukaemia in first remission: results of MRC AML 10 trial. Lancet 1998;351:700–708.

22. Burnett AK, Wheatley K, Goldstone AH, et al. Medical Research Council Adult and Paediatric Working Parties. The value of allogeneic bone marrow transplant in patients with acute myeloid leukaemia at differing risk of relapse: results of the UK MRC AML10 trial. Br J Haematol 2002;118:385–400.

23. Burnett AK, Grimwade D, Solomon E, Wheatley K, Goldstone AH. Presenting white blood cell count and kinetics of molecular remission predict prognosis in acute promyelocytic leukemia treated with all-*trans* retinoic acid: result of the randomized MRC trial. Blood 1999;93:4131–4143.

24. Haferlach T, Kohlmann A, Schnittger S, et al. Global approach to the diagnosis of leukemia using gene expression profiling. Blood 2005;106:1189–1198.

25. Valk PJM, Verhaak RGW, Beijen MA, et al. Prognostically useful gene-expression profiles in acute myeloid leukemia. N Engl J Med 2004;350:1617–1628.

26. Döhner K, Schlenk RF, Habdank M, et al. Mutant *nucleophosmin* (*NPM1*) predicts favorable prognosis in younger adults with acute myeloid leukemia and normal cytogenetics – interaction with other gene mutations. Blood 2005;106:3740–3746.

27. Falini B, Mecucci C, Tiacci E, et al. Cytoplasmic nucleophosmin in acute myelogenous leukemia with a normal karyotype. N Engl J Med 2005;352:254–266.

28. Schnittger S, Schoch C, Kern W, et al. Nucleophosmin gene mutations are predictors of favorable prognosis in acute myelogenous leukemia with a normal karyotype. Blood 2005;106:3733–3739.

29. Kottaridis PD, Gale RE, Linch DC. FLT3 mutations and leukaemia. Br J Haematol 2003;122:523–538.

30. Bowen DT, Frew ME, Hills R, et al. RAS mutation in acute myeloid leukemia is associated with distinct cytogenetic subgroups but does not influence outcome in patients <60 years. Blood 2005;106:2113–2119.

31. Reilly JT. Pathogenesis of acute myeloid leukaemia and inv(16)(p13q22): a paradigm for understanding leukaemogenesis? Br J Haematol 2005;128:18–34.

32. Sith ML, Cavenagh JD, Lister TA, Fitzgibbon J. Mutation of *CEBPA* in familial acute myeloid leukemia. New Engl J Med 2004;351:2403–2407.

33. Döhner K, Tobis K, Ulrich R, et al. Prognostic significance of partial tandem duplications of the *MLL* gene in adult patients 16 to 60 years old with acute myeloid leukemia and normal cytogenetics: a study of the Acute Myeloid Leukemia Study Group Ulm. J Clin Oncol 2002;20:3254–3261.

34. Schnittger S, Kinkelin U, Schoch C, et al. Screening for MLL tandem duplication in 387 unselected patients with AML identify a prognostically unfavorable subset of AML. Leukemia 2000;14:796–804.

35. Raghavan M, Lillington DM, Skoulakis S, et al. Genome-wide single nucleotide polymorphism analysis reveals frequent partial uniparental disomy due to somatic recombination in acute myeloid leukemia. Cancer Res 2005;65:375–378.

36. Kralovics R, Passamonti F, Buser AS, et al. A gain-of-function mutation of JAK2 in myeloproliferative disorders. New England Journal of Medicine 2005;352:1779–1790.

37. Fröhling S, Schlenk RF, Stolze I, et al. *CEBPA* mutations in younger adults with acute myeloid leukemia and normal cytogenetics: prognostic relevance and analysis of cooperating mutations. J Clin Oncol 2004;22:624–633.
38. Preudhomme C, Sagot C, Boissel N, et al. ALFA Group. Favorable prognostic significance of *CEBPA* mutations in patients with de novo acute myeloid leukemia: A study from the Acute Leukemia French Association (ALFA). Blood 2002;100:2717–2723.
39. Gale RE, Hills R, Kottaridis PD, et al. No evidence that FLT3 status should be considered as an indicator for transplantation in acute myeloid leukemia (AML): an analysis of 1135 patients excluding acute promyelocytic leukemia from the UK MRC AML10 and 12 trials. Blood, 2005;106:3658–3665.
40. Marcucci G, Mrózek K, Ruppert AS, et al. Abnormal cytogenetics at date of morphologic complete remission predicts short overall and disease-free survival, and higher relapse rate in adult acute myeloid leukemia: results from Cancer and Leukemia Group B Study 8461. J Clin Oncol 2004;22:2410–2418.
41. Schoch C, Schnittger S, Klaus M, Kern W, Hiddemann W, Haferlach T. AML with 11q23/*MLL* abnormalities as defined by the WHO classification: incidence, partner chromosomes, FAB subtype, age distribution, and prognostic impact in an unselected series of 1897 cytogenetically analyzed AML cases. Blood 2003;102: 2395–2402.
42. Byrd JC, Mrózek K, Dodge RK, et al. Pretreatment cytogenetic abnormalities are predictive of induction success, cumulative incidence of relapse, and overall survival in adult patients with de novo acute myeloid leukemia: results from Cancer and Leukemia Group B (CALGB 8461) Blood 2002;100:4325–4336.
43. Suciu S, Mandelli F, de Witte T, et al. EORTC and GIMEMA Leukemia Groups. Allogeneic compared with autologous stem cell transplantation in the treatment of patients younger than 46 years with acute myeloid leukemia (AML) in first complete remission (CR1): an intention-to-treat analysis of the EORTC/GIMEMA AML-10 trial. Blood 2003;102:1232–1240.

9 APL: A Classic Tale of Bench to Bedside

Olga Frankfurt, LoAnn C. Peterson,
Robert Gallagher, and Martin S. Tallman

CONTENTS

Summary

Acute promyelocytic leukemia (APL), a distinct subtype of acute myeloid leukemia (AML), is characterized by a unique molecular aberration, the presence of circulating promyelocytes, and, frequently, a life-threatening coagulopathy. The outcome of the patients with APL has improved dramatically over the last 40 years. Discovery that in APL the (15;17) translocation is associated with rearrangement and fusion of retinoic acid receptor-α (RARα) and promyelocytic leukemia (PML) genes and the clinical observation that APL is uniquely sensitive to *all-trans*-retinoic acid (ATRA) provided a foundation for the further breakthroughs in understanding the mechanism of the disease. Development of sophisticated molecular techniques led to improved diagnosis and monitoring of patients with APL and provides an invaluable tool in guiding therapy. Multiple clinical trials have explored the optimal doses, schedules, and duration of chemo- and targeted therapy, with the goals of minimizing toxicity without sacrificing the outstanding outcomes now readily achieved in most patients. In this chapter we have summarized the basic mechanisms implicated in the pathogenesis of APL as well as the targeted therapeutic strategies that transformed APL from one of the most lethal acute leukemias to one that is highly curable.

Key Words: Acute promyelocytic leukemia; PML-RARα; coagulopathy; *all-trans*-retinoic acid; arsenic trioxide; retinoic acid syndrome.

1. INTRODUCTION

The outcome of acute promyelocytic leukemia (APL), designated M3 by the French–American–British (FAB) classification, has evolved during the last 40 years from one of the most fatal leukemias to one that is highly curable. Insights into its genetic and biological

From: *Contemporary Hematology: Acute Myelogenous Leukemia*
Edited by: J. E. Karp © Humana Press Inc., Totowa, NJ

mechanisms, as well as the development of specific and effective therapeutic strategies, have made APL a compelling and inspiring example of the potential of modern molecular medicine to conquer human malignancy.

APL was first described in 1957 by Hillestad, who reported three patients presenting with a hemorrhagic diathesis, hypofibrinogenemia, and typical morphology of hypergranular APL *(1)*. Bernard and colleagues subsequently provided a detailed description of the disease based on the evaluation of 20 patients and, a decade later, were the first to point out the peculiar sensitivity of APL to daunorubicin *(2,3)*.

Two important discoveries provide a foundation for the vast body of knowledge available today addressing the pathogenesis, targeted therapy, and resistance to treatment in APL. The first one, began with the discovery in the mid-1970s that APL is consistently associated with a balanced reciprocal translocation between the long arms of chromosomes 15 and 17 *(4)*. The second finding stemmed from the observation that APL cells possess a unique property of undergoing terminal differentiation upon exposure in tissue culture to supraphysiological concentrations of *all-trans*-retinoic acid (ATRA) *(5)*. The clinical relevance of the in vitro findings became apparent when Chinese investigators showed that ATRA therapy resulted in significant number of complete, albeit relatively short-lived, remissions in APL patients *(6)*. The seminal discovery that the t(15;17) translocation consistently produces a rearrangement of the retinoic acid receptor-α (RARα) gene on chromosome 17q11-21 unified these two lines of investigation *(7–9)*. Subsequently, the fusion partner of the RARα gene from chromosome 15 was identified and initially called myl, but then renamed PML (promyelocytic leukemia) *(10–12)*. Therefore, the two hybrid gene products that result from the reciprocal t(15;17) translocation in APL are PML-RARα and RARα-PML. Subsequently, four alternative fusion gene partners of RARα, generically referred as X-RARα, have been identified, each one of which is associated with unique chromosomal translocation (Table 1) *(10,13–17)*. All of the fusion proteins include the same portion of RAR-α, highlighting its central role in the pathogenesis of APL and response to ATRA.

2. MOLECULAR CHARACTERISTICS OF APL

2.1. Retinoids and Retinoid Receptors

ATRA, a naturally occurring derivative of vitamin A, exhibits profound antiproliferative and pro-differentiating effects on a variety of tumor cells in vivo and in vitro by modulating gene transcription *(18–22)*. Cellular retinoic acid-binding protein-II (CRABP-II) appears to function as a carrier of bound ATRA from the cytoplasm to the nuclear RARs, with which it can interact directly, and is believed to facilitate the formation of the RAR-RA complex *(23,24)*.

RARs belong to the steroid/thyroid hormone receptor gene superfamily, which encodes proteins that acts as ligand-dependent regulators of gene transcription *(25)*. RAR protein contains two essential domains: a DNA-binding domain (DBD) at a NH_2 terminus and a ligand-binding domain (LBD) at the COOH terminus. The DBD of the RARs includes two characteristic zinc finger motifs, which recognize retinoic acid response elements (RAREs) in the promoter region of ATRA-responsive genes.

Two groups of RARs have been identified: retinoid receptors (RAR types α, β, γ), activated by ATRA and its natural isomer 9-cis-retinoic acid, and rexinoid receptors (RXR types α, β, γ), activated by 9-*cis*-retinoic acid only *(18,19,26)*. These receptor subtypes may form either homodimers (RXR-RXR) or heterodimers (RAR-RXR), which bind to the RARE elements

Table 1
Alternative RARα Fusion Genes

Fusion gene (ref.)	Karyotype	Frequency	Reciprocal product	Response to ATRA
PML-RARα (10–12,251,252)	t(15;17)(q22;q11-21)	>99%	Yes (75%)	Yes
PLZF-RARα (13)	t(11;17)(q23; q11-21)	~20 cases	Yes	No
NPM-RARα (14)	t(5;17)(q32; q11-21)	3 cases	Yes	Yes
NuMA-RARα (15)	t(11;17)(q13; q11-21)	1 case	No	Yes
STAT5b-RARα (16,17)	t(17;17)(q11-21;q11-21)	2 cases	No	No

RARα, retinoid acid receptor α; PML, promyelocytic leukemia; PLZF, promyelocytic leukemia zinc finger; NPM, nucleophosmin; NuMA, nuclear mitotic apparatus; STAT5b, signal transduction and transcription factor 5b.

to initiate transcription of the genes essential for cell growth and differentiation. RXRs are also capable of forming heterodimers with other nuclear receptors, such as thyroid hormone receptors, the vitamin D_3 receptor, and the peroxisome proliferator-activated receptors (PRARs) (19,26).

In the absence of ligand binding, the RAR/RAX heterodimer acts as a transcriptional repressor by recruiting histone deacetylases (HDACs), nuclear co-repressor molecules, such as N-CoR (nuclear receptor co-repressors) or SMRT (silencing mediator of retinoid and thyroid receptors), and Sin 3A or Sin 3B. This protein complex produces histone deacetylation and chromatin condensation, events that silence gene transcription (22,26). Binding of the RA results in allosteric changes in the LBD of the receptor, leading to the dissociation of the co-repressor complex, recruitment of histone acetyl transferase (HAT) co-activators, and chromatin decondensation, causing transcriptional activation (22,26). Co-activator molecules recruited in the RAR complexes exert regulatory effects on the retinoid-mediated gene transcription via inducing transactivation of the activator function-2 (AF-2) domain of the retinoid receptors. Some of the identified nuclear receptors co-activators include NcoA-1/SRC-1, CBP/p300, p/CIP, and ACTR. These complexes possess intrinsic HAT activity, which can cause relaxation of condensed chromatin, allowing DNA accessibility to the basal transcriptional machinery in the promoters of the RA-dependent genes (19,26).

In addition to DNA-binding and ligand-binding domains, designated C and E regions, respectively, there are three other subregions of RARα. The A region, which constitutes the amino-terminus of the RARα-X fusion proteins, has autonomous, ligand-independent transcriptional activation function (AF-1), regulated by a specific serine residue (27). The D region, located at the carboxy-terminus, serves a "hinge" function important for the RAR-RXR heterodimer formation on RARE and contains Co-R Box, essential for interaction with co-repressor proteins (28). The function of the F-region, unique to RARs, is unknown.

RARα is preferentially expressed in the cells of myeloid lineage and plays a major role in the induction of the RA effects on myelopoesis (29). When a mutant RARα protein with a defective LBD is expressed in FDCP mix A4 murine multipotent hematopoietic cell line, the cells fail to differentiate into mature granulocytes or macrophages (30). Similarly, a RA-resistant HL-60 cell variant expresses a mutant form of RARα, which appears to be responsible for RA insensitivity, since re-expression of wild-type RARα in these cells restores normal RA-mediated cell differentiation (31).

2.2. Structure and Function of PML

The PML gene, originally characterized in APL patients, exhibits tumor suppressor characteristics *(10)*. The PML protein mediates growth inhibitory and pro-apoptotic effects and is expressed at low levels in a wide variety of cell types *(32–34)*. In hematopoietic cells, the PML is expressed at highest levels in the immature myeloid cells, where it appears to be important for terminal differentiation.

The PML protein consists of a distinct cystein/histidine-rich zinc finger domain termed the RING domain, followed by two additional cysteine/histidine clusters (B-boxes), and α-helical coiled-coil motif (collectively referred to as the RBCC domain) *(34,35)*. The RBCC domain does not possess DNA-binding capacity and is believed to mediate PML multimerization, PML-NB localization, and PML-RAR heteromerization via protein–protein interactions *(34)*. PML has a characteristic cellular localization in the nucleus, where it is associated with organelles called nuclear bodies (NBs)—also referred to as promyelocytic oncogenic domains (PODs), Kremer bodies, or nuclear domain 10 (ND10)—that form part of the nuclear matrix *(36–38)*. These NBs are discrete speckled subnuclear structures, where PML complexes with other proteins, such as SUMO-1, Sp 100, Sp 140, CBP, DAXX, p53, and Rb *(32,39,40)*. It is well established that the normal structure of PML-NB is disrupted in PML$^{-/-}$ primary cells and in APL blasts and that after ATRA or arsenic trioxide (ATO)-induced remission, the normal appearance of the PML-nuclear bodies is restored *(39,41,42)*. PML is critical for the formation and stability of the NB, it turn implying that the function of multiple NB components may be impaired in the APL blasts or in cells lacking PML *(43)*. It is possible that abnormal redistribution of PML-NBs may play a role in the pathogenesis of APL, although the finding that disruption of PML-NB structure does not occur in all of the APL subtypes argues against this *(18,21,44,45)*.

Several findings support the role of PML as a tumor suppressor gene *(33,34)*. PML inactivation promotes a marked survival and proliferative advantage to cells of various histological origins *(33,41)* and impairs cellular senescence in response to oncogenic stimuli *(46,47)*. Additionally, PML inactivation impairs cellular differentiation by differentiating agents such as ATRA and vitamin D *(48,49)*. Conversely, overexpression of PML gene by transfection in a variety of cell lines, including the APL cell line NB4, results in potent growth inhibition *(50–52)*. PML exhibits antitumor effects by regulation of Fas- and caspase-dependent apoptosis. Its function appears essential for the induction of apoptosis in response to tumor necrosis factor (TNF)-α, ceramide, and interferon (IFN), because PML inactivation results in protection from the aforementioned apoptotic stimuli *(33)*. The Fas-mediated pathway has been demonstrated to involve the recruitment to NBs and binding to PML of the chromatin binding protein Daxx, an important mediator of Fas-induced apoptosis *(39,53)*. In the absence of PML, Daxx acquires a dispersed nuclear pattern, and activation-induced cell death of splenocytes is profoundly impaired. Furthermore, PML inactivation results in the complete abrogation of the Daxx pro-apoptotic activity. In APL cells Daxx is delocalized from NBs; however, upon treatment with ATRA it returns to PML-NBs, suggesting that PML and Daxx cooperate in a NB-dependent p53-independent pathway for apoptosis *(53)*. PML can also act as a positive regulator of p53-dependent apoptotic pathway via physical interaction with p53 in vivo and in vitro, and it is required for proper acetylation of p53 upon γ-irradiation *(41)*. In PML$^{-/-}$ thymocytes, p53-dependent DNA damage-induced apoptosis, p53 DNA-binding ability, and the induction of p53 target genes such as BAX are impaired upon γ-irradiation *(41)*.

A biological effect of PML is at least partially related to its function as a transcriptional cofactor. There is no evidence that PML interacts directly with DNA, and the interaction is likely to occur via binding to recruited proteins that have direct or indirect transcriptional repressor and activator activities *(46,54–56)*. The net biological effect appears to be primarily inhibitory, since PML-mediated activation of retinoid receptors, p53, and GATA-2 all result in decreased cell proliferation *(48)*.

PML-RARα transgenic mice with an inactivating mutation in the RARα region develop leukemia whereas RARα transgenic mice with the same mutation do not, suggesting that the PML domain plays an essential role in the PML-RARα leukemogenesis *(57)*.

2.3. Structure, Expression, and Role of PML-RARα in Leukemogenesis

In APL, the PML-RARα gene is created by the fusion of the PML gene on chromosome 15 with a break in one of the three breakpoint cluster regions (bcr) and the RARα gene on chromosome 17 with a break in randomly distributed sites throughout the second intron *(58)* (Fig. 1). Three isoforms of PML-RARα fusion transcripts have been described *(59,60)*. The long (L) isoform results from a genomic break (bcr1) in PML intron 6, whereas the short (S) isoform is a consequence of a breakpoint (bcr3) in PML intron 3. The S transcript lacks two major structural motifs: a serine/proline-rich region with several potential phosphorylation sites and nuclear localization sequence (NLS), both encoded by the PML exon 6 *(60)*. In a small subset of APL patients, the breakpoint (bcr2) occurs in or near the 3′-end of PML exon 6 (or, rarely, in PML exon 5), causing the deletion of variable amounts of coding sequence and expressing a variable (V) isoform of PML-RARα fusion transcript *(61)*. Frequently, a variable number of nucleotides derived from RARα intron 2 is incorporated in the PML-RARα V isoform transcript, preserving the translational open reading frame (ORF) *(61)*. Among 221 patents with PML-RARα-positive APL entered in the first North American Intergroup Trial (I0129), the frequency of the L-, S-, and V-form fusion proteins were 55, 37, and 8%, respectively *(58)*.

The t(15;17) chromosomal translocation occurs in almost 99% of cases of APL and results in the generation of PML-RARα and RARα-PML gene fusion transcripts, which encode PML-RARα and RARα-PML chimeric proteins, respectively *(22,45)*. The PML-RARα transcript and fusion protein are detected in essentially all of the APL patients, whereas RARα-PML transcript is detected in approx 75% of APL cases *(22,45,62)*. In other far less common translocations seen in APL, the RARα gene is fused with either the promyelocytic leukemia zinc finger (PLZF) gene on chromosome 11, the nuclear mitotic apparatus (NUMA) gene on chromosome 5, the nucleophosmin gene on chromosome 11, or the signal transducer and activator of transcription (STAT5B) gene on chromosome 17 *(22,45,62)*. It appears that APL patients with PLZF-RARα and STAT5B-RARα fusion genes have the poorest outcome because of a resistance to chemotherapy and unresponsiveness to differentiation by ATRA *(22,45,62)*.

The PML-RARα chimeric protein has oncogenic properties both in vivo and in vitro. Transfection experiments demonstrate that the introduction of the PML-RARα fusion protein into U937 cell line *(63)* and into primary human hematopoietic progenitor cells *(64)* results in a ATRA-responsive promyelocytic differentiation block. However, introduction of a variant form PML-RARα with mutation within the co-repressor binding AF-2 domain does not result in leukemic transformation, underscoring the importance of co-repressor proteins in the APL leukemogenesis *(64)*.

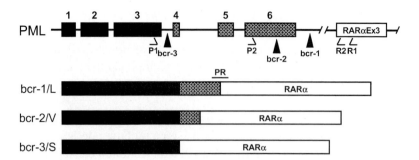

Fig. 1. Schematic representation of promyelocytic leukemia (PML) breaksites and PML-RARα fusion mRNAs. The three PML breakpoint cluster regions (bcr-1, -2, -3) are indicated by vertical arrowheads, and the resultant L, V, and S PML-RARα isoforms are diagrammed. PML exons are indicated by numbered, shaded rectangles. The positions of primers used to amplify PML-RARα mRNA are indicated below their respective exons. (From ref. *61*.)

Transgenic mouse experiments also support the pathogenic role of PML-RARα in APL *(44,49,65–67)*. Ten to 30% of PML-RARα transgenic mice developed APL-like syndrome, manifested by leukocytosis, anemia, thrombocytopenia, and extensive infiltration of the bone marrow and spleen by leukemic blasts Treatment with ATRA induced differentiation of the leukemic blast and resulted in hematological remission *(44,49)*. However, PLZF-RARα transgenic mice were resistant, mimicking ATRA resistance observed in human APL patients bearing the t(11;17) translocation *(44,49)*. Those experiments demonstrated a long latency (6–12 months) and variable rates of induction of leukemia, suggesting that other somatic alterations are required for leukemia to develop. Consistent with this hypothesis, retroviral transduction of a FLT3 internal tandem duplication (ITD) mutation into the bone marrow of the PML-RARα transgenic mice resulted in the evolution of APL with a short-latency phenotype and complete penetrance *(68,69)*. It has also been suggested that RARα-PML, which by itself is incapable of inducing APL, may enhance the oncogenic potential of PML-RARα and accelerate the development of leukemia *(49,70)*. However, the above-mentioned observation was based on utilization of the S isoform of RARα-PML with the L isoform PML-RARα transgene, casting doubt on this interaction under natural conditions.

Although extensive studies have established the leukemogenic potential of PML-RARα, the precise mechanism of its action remains to be fully elucidated. One of the means by which PML-RARα transforms cells involves a dominant-negative "silencing" effect on the action of RAR-RXR heterodimers *(44)*. PML-RARα exhibits the same affinity for RA as normal RARα, and it can form a complex with RARα that binds to a RARE via the binding domain of RARα. This property allows PML-RARα to sequester RXR from the RAR-RXR heterodimer, ultimately resulting in the dominant-negative silencing of RARE-dependent gene transcription *(18,21,22,44,62)*. This dominant negative activity of the fusion protein on PML is crucial for APL leukemogenesis, since a dominant negative RARα mutant that is unable to interfere with PML function fails to induce leukemia *(57,71–73)*. By exhibiting a dominant-negative effect on PML activities, the PML-RARα fusion protein in hematopoietic progenitor cells renders them resistant to Fas-, TNF-, and IFN-dependent apoptosis *(33,74)*.

The dominant negative effect of PML-RARα is compounded by its ability to recruit abnormal quantities of tightly bound co-repressor proteins to RARE-regulated gene promoters *(64,75,76)*. This occurs primarily via binding of the co-repressor complex to the LBD of the RARα-region of the PML-RARα, which maintains genes required for terminal neutrophilic differentiation in a transcriptionally inactive state, at least partly due to associated histone deacetylase (HDAC) activity. It has been postulated that HDAC-nuclear co-repressor-dependent gene silencing is responsible for the maturation arrest seen in APL and that high pharmacological doses of ATRA are needed to dissociate HDAC-co-repressor complex from PML-RARα and to reverse transcriptional silencing *(18,21,22,26,44)*. In the subset of APL with the t(11;17) translocation resulting in the PLZF-RARα gene product, the fusion protein binds to the HDAC–co-repressor complex via both the RARα and PLZF moieties. Consequently, ATRA is not sufficient to induce dissociation of the complex from the basal transcriptional machinery, explaining the resistance of this APL subtype to differentiating effect of RA *(18,21,22,26,44)*. Not surprisingly, HDAC inhibitors such as trichostatin A could overcome the transcriptional repressive activity of PML-RARα and PLZF-RARα as wells as unresponsiveness of PLZF-RARα leukemic cells to ATRA *(21,77,78)*.

Recently, Gurrieri and colleagues described truncating mutations in the PML allele *not* involved in the PML-RARα translocation in two APL cases characterized by an aggressive course: ATRA resistance and poor clinical outcome *(79)*. In model systems, truncated PML was no longer concentrated in the nucleus (in PML-NBs), but instead displayed an aberrant cytoplasmic localization pattern, where it was unable to exert nuclear and NB-dependent function attributed to PML *(80)*. Because PML is reduced to heterozygosity in APL as a consequence of the t(15;17) translocation, the truncating mutation in the other PML allele results in its complete inactivation. This loss of PML function was associated with a decreased response in vitro of the leukemic blasts to ATRA and would in turn confer a proliferative and survival advantage based on experimental system data *(79,80)*.

Another potential mechanism by which PML-RARα may mediate leukemogenesis via inhibition of the normal PML function relates to the recently described interaction of PML with the Jak-Stat pathway. It was demonstrated that normal PML interacts with Stat3 protein via its B-box and carboxy-terminus region and that it exhibits negative regulatory effects on Stat3 activation by inhibiting its ligand-dependent DNA-binding capacity *(72)*. In cells expressing PML-RARα, there is a dissociation of Stat3 from PML despite the fact that PML-RARα does not interact directly with Stat3. Such dissociation leads to enhancement of Stat3 transcriptional activity and promotes Stat3 anti-apoptotic responses *(72)*.

PML-RARα leukemic cells from murine models display numerous recurrent chromosomal abnormalities, suggesting that PML-RARα may favor the accumulation of these genetic lesions by rendering cells genomically unstable *(81)*. Indeed, a number of proteins involved in maintenance of genomic stability, including the Bloom syndrome DNA helicase (BLM), whose absence from the cells is associated with a high level of sister-chromatid exchange (SCE) and cancer predisposition, accumulate in the PML-NB *(82–84)*. In APL cells carrying PML-RARα oncoprotein, both PML and BLM are delocalized from the NB into microspeckled nuclear regions *(40)*. In PML$^{-/-}$ cells BLM fails to accumulate in the NB and the frequency of SCE is greatly augmented, suggesting that the PML-dependent localization of BLM in the PML-NB is required for its normal function *(40)*. Thus, PML-RARα could favor genomic instability and the accumulation of additional genetic events that might participate in the leukemogenic process.

The identification of gene products regulated by the RARα is of importance since it is likely that some of them are mediators of the antileukemic effect of ATRA. In a recent study, 169 genes were found to be modulated by ATRA treatment of the NB-4 APL cell line *(85)*. ATRA treatment resulted in the expression upregulation of 100 genes, whereas transcription of 69 genes was diminished. Among the genes found to be induced by ATRA were the transcription factors CCAAT/enhancer-binding protein (c/EBPε) and Hox A1, the cell cycle inhibitor p21^{WAF} and GADD153, the anti-apoptotic protein Bcl-2-related(A1) and DAD-1, and the granulocyte differentiation markers CD11b and CD18 *(85)*. Some of the target proteins whose gene expression was inhibited by ATRA were c-MYC, NF-κB, and GATA2, all known transcription factors that can mediate cell signals that promote cell growth *(85)*. However, the temporal and the cause-and-effect relationship between changes in PML-RARα and these gene-modulation events remain to be determined.

2.4. Role of PML-RARα in the Response to Therapy

The generation of PML-RARα is a key oncogenic event upon which the leukemic cells depend in order to proliferate and thrive, even if additional genetic events coexist with it in the leukemic blasts *(86)*. This observation has important therapeutic implications in that agents that directly target the activity and stability of the PML-RARα fusion protein may be effective in t(15;17) APL. Indeed, both ATRA and ATO have the common property of inducing proteolytic degradation of the PML-RARα fusion transcript in NB4 APL cells, including ATRA-resistant cell lines, and in fresh APL cells *(77,87–91)*. One explanation for the therapeutic effect of these agents is that by removing the dominant negative effect of PML-RARα, they allow normal RARα and PML, produced by the nontranslocated gene loci, to re-establish physiological pathways leading to the terminal granulocytic differentiation and apoptosis *(87,92,93)*. However, the experimental evidence suggests that the underlying molecular mechanisms are not only more complex, but also significantly different for the two agents. After exposure to ATRA, an initial reduction in the expression level of the L-isoform of PML-RARα is noted within 1 hour *(94)*. Greater reduction occurs at 6–12 hours and is accompanied by the appearance of a proteolytic fragment, dPML-RARα, between 12 and 48 hours *(87,90,94)*. After 48 hours, continuing proteolysis results in the virtual disappearance of PML-RARα and dPML-RARα *(94,95)*. During that time, the RARα protein level is reduced, the RARα mRNA level is unchanged or increased, and PML-RARα mRNA level is unchanged *(94,95)*.

Response to ATO is different from that following ATRA exposure in several respects: it occurs more rapidly (6–12 hours), it is not associated with the generation of a proteolytic fragment, and it is associated with the more rapid reformation of PML-NB. Several cellular and molecular studies have shown that ATO targets PML-RARα via induction of a rapid SUMO (small ubiquitin-related modifier)-1-mediated degradation of the PML moiety of the fusion protein *(91)*. However, other studies show that recruitment of hypersumoylated PML to NB after ATO exposure produced protein stabilization rather than degradation *(96)*. Although ATO treatment induces increased sumoylation of PML and restoration of NBs in APL cells, the molecular basis of this process remains to be clarified *(91,97)*. Arsenic can activate several signaling pathways, including extracellular-signal-regulated protein kinases (ERKs), c-Jun N-terminal kinases (JNKs), and p38 kinase pathways *(98)*. In NB4 cells, ATO induces apoptosis and differentiation via MAP kinase signaling and phosphorylation of the important PML-RARα co-repressor, SMRT. This leads to the dissociation of SMRT from its nuclear receptor partners, RARα and PML-RARα, and to a release form the dominant-negative effect of transcriptional repression *(99,100)*.

ATO induces partial differentiation and apoptosis of APL cells in a dose-dependent manner. In NB4 cells, at low concentration (<0.5 μM) ATO exhibits a modest differentiation effect, whereas at high concentrations (>1 μM) it produces apoptosis *(77,101)*. In ATO-treated patients, signs of both apoptosis and partial differentiation of APL cells can be detected in the bone marrow after 2–3 weeks of therapy *(101,102)*. Additionally, at certain concentrations (1–5 μM), ATO can cause apoptosis in many other types of neoplastic hematopoietic cells, including non-APL myeloid leukemias, acute lymphoblastic leukemia, and multiple myeloma *(89,103)*.

Both caspase activation and direct proteasome targeting have been implicated in the degradation on PML-RARα, although neither is sufficient for complete degradation *(87,92, 94,104)*. The primary site for caspase proteolysis resides in PML exon 6 of PML-RARα *(94,104)*. The S-form of the PML-RARα lacks PML exon 6 and is modestly resistant to ATRA-induced proteolysis *(60)*. The proteasome-mediated degradation of PML-RARα and RARα primarily depends on the binding of SUG-1 in the AF2 transactivation domain of RARα to the 19S proteasome *(94)*.

2.5. The Alternative Translocations and Fusion Partners in APL

In APL, four other RARα fusion gene partners have been described: PLZF *(13)*, NPM (NucleoPhosMin) *(14)*, NuMa (nuclear mitotic apparatus) *(15)*, and STAT5b (signal transduction and transcription factor 5b) *(16)* (Table 1). Although the number of APL patients with these alternative gene translocations is small, it appears that the novel fusion partners may confer different clinical and biological characteristic. In all cases, the coding exons for the B to F regions of RARα are fused to a 5′ segment of the alternative fusion gene.

2.5.1. PLZF-RARα APL

Acute leukemia with the t(11;17) translocation expressing the PLZF-RARα fusion gene was first described by Chen and colleagues in 1993 (13). It occurs in 0.5–1% of APL patients and has been associated with unfavorable clinical outcome and poor response to ATRA and ATO therapy in vivo and in vitro *(13,105–108)*. At the molecular level, the t(11:17) involves the PLZF gene on chromosome 11, and the RARα gene on chromosome 17, resulting in two hybrid RARα-PLZF and PLZF-RARα genes. PLZF protein is a transcriptional repressor and in its wild-type form acts as a powerful growth suppressor of myeloid cells *(44)*. Both chimeric RARα-PLZF and PLZF-RARα proteins have been shown to produce an APL-like syndrome in transgenic mice *(49)*.

ATRA and ATO do not induce remission in PLZF-RARα APL. Yet each has been shown to induce the degradation of PLZF-RARα, both in vivo and in vitro, suggesting that the maintenance of the leukemic phenotype does not depend entirely on the continuous presence of the chimeric oncoprotein. However, undetectable amounts of PLZF-RARα may be sufficient to exert leukemogenic effect, or additional genetic events may render PLZF-RARα redundant for maintenance of malignant phenotype, or PLZF-RARα may affect transcription though epigenetic mechanisms. Aberrant transcriptional regulation would be, therefore, maintained throughout cell replication even in the absence of the PLZF-RARα oncoprotein *(86)*. This is supported by the finding that PLZF-RARα can directly interact via PLZF with nuclear co-repressors and NCoR/SMRT-Sin3A-histone deacetylase, leading to chromatin remodeling *(21,77,78,109)*. Methylation has been associated with epigenetic transcriptional inactivation and cancer pathogenesis *(110)*. A link between gene methylation and histone deacetylation has been established by protein MeCP2, which binds mSin-3/NCor/SMRT-Sin3A-histone deacetylases complex to methylate cytosines *(111)*.

ATRA insensitivity may be due to the amino-terminal structure of PLZF, called the POZ- (Poxvirus and Zinc finger) or BTB- (broad complex-tramtrac-Bric-a-brac) domain *(44,112)*. This amino-terminal domain can bind the same nuclear co-repressor protein as RARα, but in a non-ATRA-dependent manner *(21,77,109,112)*. Thus, ATRA therapy of PLZF-RARα APL may lead to displacement of the co-repressor from the RARα-binding site and perhaps even to the recruitment of co-activator proteins, but it is unable to displace the co-repressors from the POZ domain. A number of other molecular mechanisms may contribute to the ATRA insensitivity, such as the sequestration of RXR, loss of association of PLZF-RARα with a carboxy-situated binding component, possibly PML, and the limited positive transactivation activity of PLZF-RARα on RARE-regulated genes *(44,113–115)*. The differentiation block imposed by PLZF-RARα can be at least partially overcome by treatment with HDAC inhibitors which bypass the blocked RAR pathway *(77,109,116)*.

2.5.2. OTHER FUSION GENES

Like PML and PLZF, NPM is a complex multifunctional nuclear matrix phosphoprotein, localized to the nucleolus, which plays an important role in ribosomal RNA assembly *(44)*. It has been reported to have chaperoning functions and nuclease activity and may play a role in regulation of centrosomal duplication *(117)*. NPM level may play a regulatory role in cell growth and differentiation via binding to the transcription factor Yin Yang 1 and IFN response factor-1. Formation of NMP-RARα homo- or oligomers likely results in displacement of normal NPM from its nucleolar location to a disperse nuclear pattern characteristic for NPM-RARα APL *(118)*. NPM-RARα is also able to displace PLZF, but not PML, from its normal nuclear distribution *(118)*. NPM-RARα APL cells behave similarly to PML-RARα in their positive differentiation response to ATRA and in the failure of the NPM moiety to bind co-repressors *(119,20)*. NPM-RARα-RXR heterodimers bind DNA 10-fold more avidly than NPM-RARα homodimers, suggesting that RXR sequestration may play a particularly important role in this type of APL *(119)*. Limited information is available regarding the function and clinical relevance of NuMa-RARα and STAT5b-RARα fusion genes *(15–17)*. The NuMa-RARα contains the N-terminal 1883 amino acids of NuMA, which encode domains responsible for NuMA nuclear reassembly, oligomerization, and spindle association function *(121)*. NuMA-RARα APL described in a 6-month-old boy had an undetectable reciprocal RARα-NuMA mRNA level and was ATRA sensitive *(15)*.

The first case of STAT5b-RARα APL was described in a 67-year-old patient with ATRA-resistant leukemia *(16)*. Immunophenotypically, the second patient, who was 57 years old at diagnosis, had all the features of APL (CD11a⁻, CD18-, CD34⁻, HLA-DR⁻, except weakly CD133⁺). The break/fusion point of the STAT5b gene, as determined by the sequence analysis of the STAT5b-RARα mRNA, was the same in both cases *(17)*. According to Dong and colleagues, STAT5b-RARα has overall similar DNA-binding preferences to PML-RARα, although it binds weakly to RARE-p21-WAF *(122)*. While PML-RARα and PLZF-RARα are able to form both single and multimeric heterodimers with RXRα, STAT5b-RARα is able to form only single RXRα heterodimer. The significance of STAT5b-RARα insensitivity to ATRA-induced degradation is unclear, since PLZF-RARα is sensitive to ATRA-induced degradation, yet results in ATRA-resistant disease. It has been postulated that persistent interaction of STAT5b-RARα with nuclear receptor transcriptional repressor complex corepressor (CoR) in the presence of pharmacological levels of ATRA may contribute to ATRA unresponsiveness *(16)*.

3. EPIDEMIOLOGY

APL accounts for 10–15% of cases of adult AML. The median age at diagnosis among patients with APL (40 years) is considerably lower than that of patients with other AML

Table 2
Putative Adverse Prognostic Factors in APL

Clinical features

Age (>50–60) *(130,253)*

Male gender *(130,134)*

Laboratory findings

High leukocyte count (>10 × 10^9/L) *(131,134)*

Platelet count (<40 × 10^9/L) *(131)*

Coagulopathy at diagnosis *(254)*

Persistent minimal residual disease *(255)*

CD56 expression *(256,257)*

CD34 expression *(258,259)*

Multidrug resistance (MDR) gene expression *(259)*

FLT3 gene mutation *(134)*

PML-RARα fusion at PML bcr3 *(255)*

Aberrant p15 promoter hypermethylation *(260)*

HLA-B13 *(151)*

subtypes (70 years). There appears to be no increase in the incidence of APL with increasing age *(123,124)* and no difference in the incidence of APL between the sexes *(125)*. Patients of Hispanic heritage seem to have an increased incidence of APL compared to other ethnic groups with 20–30% of Hispanic patients with AML having the M3 subtype *(126,127)*. Some epidemiological studies have implicated electromagnetic fields and radon exposure in the etiology of APL *(124)*. Of interest, elevated body mass index (BMI) was associated with the diagnosis of APL among patients with AML ($p = 0.0003$) *(126)*.

4. PROGNOSTIC FACTORS IN APL

It is essential to identify patients at high risk of relapse in APL, because they may potentially benefit from high-dose therapy and hematopoietic stem cell transplantation (SCT) or novel agents (Table 2).

4.1. Clinical and Laboratory Parameters

The presenting white blood cell count (WBC) has been the most significant prognostic factor in APL patients treated with the combination of ATRA and chemotherapy *(128–130)*. Based on the PETHEMA and GIMEMA experience, Sanz and colleagues have identified initial WBC and platelet counts as the only prognostically significant risk factors *(131)* (Fig. 2). Patients with a low risk of relapse presented with WBC <10,000/μL and platelets > 40,000/μL, intermediate risk if WBC <10,000/μL and platelets <40,000/μL, or high risk if WBC >10,000/μL and platelets <40,000/μL.

Older age and male gender appear to be unfavorable prognostic factors in newly diagnosed APL *(130,132–135)* (Fig. 3).

4.2. PML-RARα Isoforms

Although a less favorable outcome associated with the short PML-RARα fusion transcripts has been reported in some studies *(136)*, most have failed to show a significant difference *(58)*. In a recent study conducted by Gupta and colleagues, the short isoform was associated with

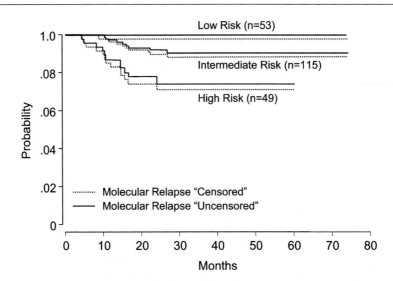

Fig. 2. Kaplan-Meier product-limit estimate of RFS according to the risk groups defined by the predictive model.

elevated WBC and significantly decreased relapse-free survival (RFS), although it had no effect on rate of molecular complete remission (CR) and overall survival (OS) *(129)*.

4.3. CD56 Expression

Expression of CD56, which reflects the neural crest adhesion molecule and is possibly involved in trafficking of the leukemia cells, was suggested to be an unfavorable prognostic factor, associated with the leukemogenic mutation at the primitive hematopoietic progenitor cell level, short remission duration, and increased risk of extramedullary relapse after ATRA and chemotherapy *(137)*. However, more recent data failed to demonstrate an unfavorable prognostic value of CD56 expression *(138)*.

4.4. Secondary Chromosomal Abnormalities

Additional chromosomal abnormalities do not appear to influence the outcome in patients with APL treated with a combination of chemotherapy and ATRA *(139–142)*. In 292 patients with APL treated with ATRA and chemotherapy, 26% had additional chromosomal abnormalities, with trisomy 8 being the most frequent secondary change (46% of the cases with secondary change), followed by chromosomes 17, 9, and 7. No significant differences were observed with regard to age, sex, presenting WBC, percent of circulating blasts, platelet count, fibrinogen level, and incidence of hypogranular variants between patients with and without additional rearrangements. Follow-up at 2 years failed to show a significant difference between the groups with regard to CR, event-free survival (EFS), rate of relapse, and OS *(139)*. Although several small studies suggested that additional chromosomal aberrations may render patients less sensitive to ATRA and negatively influence CR and early death rates *(143,144)*, a retrospective analysis of 418 patients with *de novo* APL enrolled in two consecutive PETHEMA trials (APL96 and APL99) showed no clinical, biological, morphological, immunophenotypic, or molecular differences between the patients with t(15;17) translocation alone and the group of patients with additional chromosomal abnormalities *(142)*.

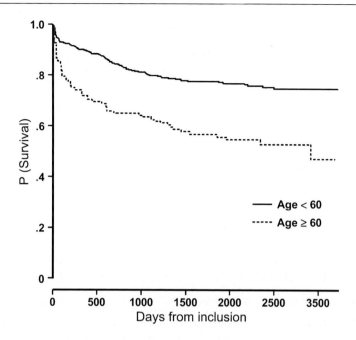

Fig. 3. Overall survival according to age of patients with acute promyelocytic leukemia. The estimated 4-year survival was 57.8% in patients older than 60 years compared to 78% in younger adults ($p < 0.0001$). (From ref. *135*.)

4.5. Internal Tandem Duplication of the FLT3

It has been suggested that FLT-3 aberrations, in the form of internal tandem duplication (ITD) or mutation at the activation loop position 835 (D835), may be associated with worse outcome in APL, although data are not conclusive *(134)*. In several small studies FLT-3 ITD (20–38%) and D835 (7.8–18.7%) had no significant influence on OS, CR, or DFS, although ITDs were associated with the PML breakpoint at bcr3 and hypogranular morphology *(145–147)*. However, in 90 APL patients from Italy treated with ATRA and idarubicin, the FLT-3 ITDs were associated with elevated WBC, hypogranular morphology, PML breakpoint at bcr3, and an inferior DFS due to increased rate of relapse *(148)*. In other recent studies, FLT-3 mutations were a significant unfavorable prognostic factor because of the association with high WBC and increased rate of death during induction *(134,149)*. Based on the analysis of the 119 APL patients enrolled in the two consecutive APL-93 and APL-2000 trials, FLT3-ITD and FLT3- D835 mutations were associated with high WBC, bcr3, and V/S PML RARα isoforms. Although rates of CR, induction mortality, death in CR, as well as cumulative incidence of relapse were not affected by FLT3 mutations, there was a trend for the shorter overall survival in FLT3-ITD patients ($p = 0.09$) because of poor postrelapse survival ($p = 0.02$) *(150)*. The above finding suggests that underlying genetic instability in APL patients with FLT3-ITD leads to acquisition of additional unknown poor-prognostic gene mutations at relapse.

A study of 102 patients with APL treated with ATRA and idarubicin (AIDA protocol) found a statistically significant association between HLA-B13 and risk of relapse by univariate and multivariate analysis *(151)*.

5. THERAPY

5.1. Immediate Supportive Care

Once a diagnosis of APL is suspected by clinical and morphological evaluation, it should be managed as a medical emergency because of the high rate of spontaneous and potentially fatal hemorrhage. Supportive measures to reverse the coagulopathy must be instituted promptly and include aggressive platelet, fresh frozen plasma, and fibrinogen transfusions. A fibrinogen level of 100–150 mg/dL and platelets level of $30–50 \times 10^9$/L should be maintained until disappearance of all the clinical and laboratory features of coagulopathy (152). Because of the significant improvement of the coagulopathy with ATRA (153), ATRA therapy in combination with supportive care should be initiated as soon as diagnosis is suspected, even prior to the genetic confirmation of APL.

5.2. Induction

Based on the cumulative experience of multiple cooperative groups, induction therapy should consist of ATRA and anthracycline-based chemotherapy (20,133,154).

5.2.1. THE ROLE OF CYTARABINE IN INDUCTION

The role of cytarabine in the induction regimen for APL remains controversial. Two retrospective analyses failed to show a difference in the rate of CR among patients treated with daunorubicin alone or in combination with cytarabine (155,156). In the pre-ATRA era, the investigators from the GIMEMA group conducted a prospective randomized trial showing a CR of 76.3% in patients receiving single-agent idarubicin (60 mg/m^2), compared to 66.6% in patients receiving combination of idarubicin (48 mg/m^2) and cytarabine (157). A 7-year follow-up showed a 35% EFS in a single-agent idarubicin arm compare to 23% in a combination arm ($p = 0.035$). To confirm the hypothesis that anthracycline alone may be as effective as anthracycline–cytarabine combination, Fenaux and colleagues randomized newly diagnosed APL patients with WBC <10,000/mm^3 and age <60 years to two groups that differ only in the lack of cytarabine in induction and consolidation regimens. CR of 98% and one early death were noted in a combination group as compared to 92% CR, three early deaths, and two cases of resistant disease in the group that did not receive cytarabine. The 2-year incidence of relapse, EFS, and OS was 3.8% vs 11.9% ($p = 0.021$), 93.6% vs 83.4% ($p = 0.019$), and 97.4% vs 89.9% ($p = 0.085$) in groups with and without cytarabine, respectively. Based on these results, the authors could not recommend the omission of cytarabine from the therapy of newly diagnosed APL in patients with WBC <10,000/mm^3 and younger than 60 years (158).

5.2.2. COMBINING ATRA WITH CHEMOTHERAPY FOR INDUCTION

A dramatic response to therapy with oral ATRA in APL patients was originally reported in 1988 by the Shanghai group and subsequently confirmed by others (6,159,160). Despite the initial impressive results, remission induced by ATRA alone was short-lived, prompting the addition of conventional chemotherapy (161).

In a pilot study by Fenaux and colleagues, out of 26 APL patients treated with ATRA until CR and followed by three courses of daunorubicin and cytarabine, 96% (25/26) achieved a CR compare to 76% in the historical controls treated with chemotherapy alone (162). At 4 years, EFS (62% vs 28%), disease-free interval (DFI) (70% vs 42%), and OS (77% vs 40%) were significantly better after a combination of ATRA and chemotherapy. The European APL and the North American Intergroup trials compared ATRA to daunorubicin plus cytarabine (163) (Table 3). In both studies the CR rates and early death rates were not statistically

Table 3
Prospective Randomized Trials of ATRA With/Without Chemotherapy in APL

Trial (ref.)	Induction	No. of patients	CR (%)	ED (%)	DFS/EFS, 2–3 years (%)
APL91 (163)	ATRA (+chemo)	54	97	9	79
	Chemotherapy	47	81	8	50
North American	ATRA	172	72	11	69
Intergroup (164)	Chemo	174	69	14	29
APL93 (133)	ATRA→chemo	109	95	8	75
	ATRA + chemo	99	94	7	86
MRC (168)	ATRA (5d)→chemo	119	70	23	59
	ATRA + chemo	120	87	12	78

CR, complete response; ED, early death; DFS, disease-free survival; EFS, event-free survival; ATRA, *all-trans*-retinoic acid; chemo, chemotherapy; MRC, Medical Research Council.

different, but the DFS at 2–3 years was better for ATRA-treated patients (130,164). A phase III prospective randomized trial conducted by the European APL group showed that concurrent-administration ATRA and chemotherapy resulted in a better outcome than sequential treatment (133). The EFS at 2 years was 84% in the concurrent arm, and 77% is sequential. This difference was attributable to a significantly lower risk of relapse at 2 years: 6% vs 16% in the concurrent and the sequential arms, respectively ($p = 0.004$) (133).

5.2.3. Gemtuzumab Ozogamicin

Considering the high rate of CD33 expression in APL, Estey and colleagues evaluated the role of a potent cytotoxic agent gemtuzumab ozogamicin (GO; Mylotarg TM), an anti-CD33 monoclonal antibody conjugated with calicheamicin, in the induction regimen (165). Nineteen patients with newly diagnosed APL were treated with ATRA in combination with GO (three patients required an addition of IDA because of elevated WBC). The CR rate in patients who received ATRA and GO was 88% (14/16). Although the CR rate appeared comparable to ATRA and chemotherapy combination, randomized data are essential to establish the role of GO in the induction regimen of patients with APL.

GO is also highly effective as a single agent for the therapy of the patients with molecularly relapsed APL, including those with advanced disease. Of 16 patients with APL relapsed at molecular level (8 in 1st relapse, 5 in 2nd, 2 in 3rd, and 1 in 4th) and treated with GO, 9 out of 11 achieved a molecular remission (MR) after the two doses and 13 out of 13 after the third dose. Of the 3 remaining patients, 1 achieved MR after the first dose and received no further therapy because of hepatotoxicity and 2 patients suffered disease progression during therapy with GO (166).

Takeshita and colleagues evaluated the role of GO in the APL cells resistant to ATRA and ATO and determined that gemtuzumab is effective against ATO- and ATRA-resistant APL cells that do not express P-glycoprotein. These investigators also established that the mechanism of resistance to GO was not related to the mechanism of resistance to ATRA and ATO in APL cells (167).

5.3. Postremission Therapy

5.3.1. Consolidation Therapy in APL

The benefits of consolidation chemotherapy in APL have been investigated in a number of clinical trials, showing molecular remissions in more than 90% of the patients receiving two to three cycles of postremission therapy, irrespective of the type of drug combined with anthracyclines during consolidation *(168–170)*. The goal of consolidation therapy in APL is to eradicate the leukemic clone, as determined by a negative polymerase chain reaction (PCR), as this has been convincingly correlated with improved outcome in several clinical trials *(168–170)*. Moreover, failure to achieve a PCR-negative state at the end of consolidation warrants initiation of salvage therapy *(171,172)*. Although a consensus regarding the crucial role of anthracyclines in APL consolidation has been reached and most investigators utilize two to three cycles of consolidation therapy, the optimal number of cycles remains to be determined.

The question as to whether cytarabine is necessary during consolidation remains a matter of debate. The results of the several trials utilizing standard and high-dose cytarabine (1–3 g/m^2) in consolidation suggest that the dose of cytarabine may not be important *(128,132,133, 164,173)*. Furthermore, other studies suggest that cytarabine may not be needed.

In a prospective nonrandomized study by the PETHEMA group, cytarabine was omitted from the induction and consolidations regimens *(169)*. All patients received anthracycline monotherapy as consolidation, with patients in the intermediate- and high-risk categories receiving a combination of higher dose of anthracycline and ATRA. The DFS and OS at 3 years were 90% and 85%, respectively.

The APL 2000 trial addressed the role of cytarabine in consolidation by randomizing low-risk patients (age < 60 years, WBC <10,000/mm^3) between a standard group A (treated with ATRA, DNR 60 mg/m^2/d × 3 days, and cytarabine 200 mg/m^2/d × 7 days for induction, the same chemotherapy for the first consolidation, DNR 45 mg/m^2/d × 3 days and cytarabine 1 g/m^2/d × 4 days for the second consolidation, and maintenance with ATRA 15 days every 3 months, 6MP, and MTX for 2 years) and group B, who received the same treatment, but without cytarabine. In group A 98% (79/80) of patients achieved a CR with one early death as compared to 94% (82/87) CR, three ED, and two resistant leukemia in group B. The 2-year incidences of relapse, EFS, and OS were 3.8% vs 11.9% ($p = 0.021$), 93.6% vs 83.4% ($p = 0.019$), and 97.4% vs 89.9% ($p = 0.085$) in groups A and B, respectively *(158)*. The results of this study do not support the omission of cytarabine, at least with the lower dose of anthracycline (495 mg/m^2), in consolidation chemotherapy of newly diagnosed APL patients.

5.3.2. MAINTENANCE THERAPY IN APL

Several clinical trials convincingly demonstrated the benefits of maintenance therapy in patients with APL *(155,174,175)* (Table 4; Fig. 4). Based on the results of the European APL93 study, combination of ATRA, methotrexate, and 6-MP resulted in the lowest relapse rate compared to the single-agent ATRA or chemotherapy groups and proved particularly effective for patients with elevated WBC count at presentation *(133)*. However, more recent studies failed to show the benefit of maintenance therapy in APL patients who achieved a PCR-negative status after the third consolidation *(176)*.

Maintenance therapy remains a subject of investigation with respect to optimal schedule, dose, and targeted patient population.

6. RETINOID ACID TOXICITY

6.1. Retinoic Acid Syndrome

Retinoic acid syndrome (RAS), the most life-threatening toxicity of ATRA, is manifested by unexplained fever, weight gain, respiratory distress with or without radiographic evidence

Table 4
Maintenance Therapy in APL

Trial (ref.)	Maintenance	n	Relapse rate
North American	ATRA	94	32
Intergroup *(130)*	Observation	105	57
APL 93 *(133)*	ATRA	63	20
	ATRA + chemo	64	9
	Chemo	63	22
	Observation	67	32
PETHEMA *(169)*	ATRA + chemo	123	5

of interstitial infiltrates, pericardial and pleural effusions, periodic hypotension, and acute renal failure *(177)*. RAS usually occurs between the second day and the third week of ATRA therapy, with an incidence of 5–27% and mortality (of those who develop RAS) of 5–29% *(133,136,178–181)*. Although earlier data suggested that baseline leukocytosis, rapidly rising WBC count, and expression of CD13 on APL blasts might predispose to the development of RAS *(182)*, subsequent studies failed to identify risk factors for the development of RAS in APL patients treated with ATRA *(58,136,181,183)*. Retrospective analysis of the small number of patients suggested that the development of the RAS may predispose to the extramedullary relapse, particularly in the CNS *(184–187)*.

6.1.1. PREVENTION OF RAS

The early addition of chemotherapy to ATRA is believed to decrease the incidence of the RAS *(168,178)*. Although there are anecdotal data showing decreased incidence of RAS and mortality compared to historic controls with the prophylactic administration of corticosteroids *(179)*, there are no prospective randomized data to confirm such a benefit of corticosteroids *(188)*.

At the earliest onset of symptoms suggestive of RAS, therapy with 10 mg of dexamethasone every 12 hours should be instituted. If the symptoms are mild, ATRA may be continued concomitantly with steroids under careful observation. However, if the symptoms are severe or fail to respond to steroid therapy, ATRA should be temporary discontinued *(183)*. RAS rarely occurs in patients receiving ATRA as postremission therapy *(183)*.

6.1.2. PATHOGENESIS OF RAS

The pathogenesis of RAS has not been clearly delineated. The constellation of histological findings such as edema, hemorrhage, fibrinous exudates, and leukocytes infiltration likely results from microvascular damage and is frequently seen in a variety of conditions , including trauma, sepsis, and acute respiratory distress syndrome.

There is evidence that cathepsin G, a serine protease known to enhance capillary permeability, is stimulated in patients treated with ATRA *(189)*. ATRA also is known to increase expression of LFA-1 and other cellular adhesion molecules on the surface of APL cells, resulting in increased binding to adhesion molecules on the epithelium *(190,191)*. Hematopoietic growth factors, such as interleukin (IL)-1β, TNF-α, and IL-6, known to promote leukocyte activation, may play a role in the clinical feature of hypotension and pulmonary infiltrates.

6.2. Other ATRA Toxicities

Other complications of ATRA therapy are less severe and include musculoskeletal pain, myositis, xerostomia, elevation of liver enzymes, hypertriglyceridemia, thrombocytosis, and

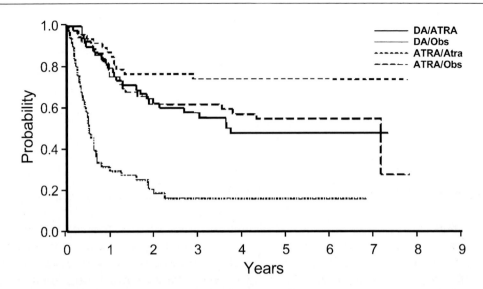

Fig. 4. Kaplan-Meier estimates of disease-free survival based on both the induction and maintenance randomizations. (From ref. *130.*)

skin rash, occasionally evolving into erythema nodosum *(183,192–196)*. Pseudotumor cerebri *(197)*, Sweet's syndrome *(198–200)*, hemophagocytic syndrome *(201)*, and a case of scrotal ulceration have been described *(202)*. Additionally, serious thrombotic complications, such as myocardial and splenic infarctions, cerebral thrombosis, and pulmonary emboli in the setting of thrombocytopenia have been reported *(203–205)*.

7. PROGNOSTIC SIGNIFICANCE OF MINIMAL RESIDUAL DISEASE

In recent years, a number of studies have highlighted the importance of PML-RARα detection by reverse transcriptase (RT)-PCR in the diagnosis and management of patients with APL *(172, 206–208)*. A positive PML-RARα test after consolidation reliably predicts subsequent hematological relapse, whereas repeatedly negative results are associated with long-term survival in the majority of patients. In the prospective study by the Diverio and colleagues, 163 patients with newly diagnosed APL received an induction and consolidation with a combination of ATRA and chemotherapy *(172)*. All of the patients achieved a CR as determined by RT-PCR after completion of consolidation therapy. RT-PCR assay for PML-RARα was conducted at regular pre-established time points from CR after consolidation. Of 21 patients who became PCR positive thereafter, 20 experienced hematological relapse at a median time of 3 months (range 1–14 months) from the first PCR-positive result. Of 142 patients who remained persistently PCR negative in more than two tests after consolidation, only 8 had hematological relapse, making the estimated risk of relapse at 3 years 10%. Patients who become PCR positive can be salvaged prior to development of the overt disease, and this approach may result in an improved outcome compared to delaying treatment until morphological appearance of the disease. A reasonable schedule for testing is to obtain at least two successive marrow samples at the end of consolidation, then every 3 months for the first 2 years of CR, then every 6 months for the next 2–3 years. With contemporary therapeutic strategies, this schedule may be most applicable to patients with high risk disease.

Approximately 50% of patients in CR after induction therapy are PCR positive, even if low-sensitivity methods are used. Several clinical trials (e.g., MCR, North American

Intergroup, GIMEMA, and PETHEMA) have failed to find correlation between post-induction PCR status and patient outcome. Hence, there is no indication to either increase the treatment intensity or change therapy for patients who test PCR positive prior to consolidation. Additionally, it remains to be determined from prospective analyses whether quantitative measurements of the level of PML-RARa by real-time RT-PCR in bone marrow or peripheral blood samples will provide even greater prognostic accuracy than nonquantitative, low-sensitivity RT-PCR methods *(170,209)*.

8. THE ROLE OF ARSENIC TRIOXIDE IN APL

Approximately 10–30% of patients treated with the combination of ATRA and chemotherapy eventually relapse *(164,168,180,210)*. Although second remissions are common, particularly if the last exposure to ATRA occurred more than 6–12 months prior to relapse, they are not durable. Investigators from China were the first to report that an herbal mixture containing arsenic induces CR in patients with relapsed and refractory as well as newly diagnosed APL *(211–213)* (Table 4). Since 1996, a large number of studies demonstrated 85–90% ATO-induced CR rates in patients with newly diagnosed and relapsed APL *(214)* (Table 5).

8.1. ATO in Untreated APL

A summary of data from the Harbin Medical University shows a CR rate of 88% in untreated APL patients, similar to that of the patients with relapsed and refractory disease *(215)*. Studies from India and Iran reported similar findings as well as a high rate of molecular remission and absence of drug resistance in patients treated with the single agent ATO *(216,217)*. The postremission therapy used in those patients was not uniform, with some receiving ATO alone and some treated with additional chemotherapy.

Using ATO for induction, consolidation, and maintenance, George and colleagues demonstrated a 95% hematological remission in 58 patients with newly diagnosed APL who were unable to receive ATRA-based therapy *(218)*. At a median follow-up of 23 months, 4 patients (8.6%) relapsed (although 3 achieved a second remission with a combination of ATO and ATRA), and 45 (77.5%) were alive and in molecular remission with a leukemia-free survival of 91.3% *(218)*. In another recent study, 73 patients with newly diagnosed APL were treated with ATO induction and consolidation *(219)*. Complete remissions were achieved in 66 patients (90.4%), and early death occurred in 7 patients primarily from APL maturation syndrome. Fourteen relapses were observed at 17 +/− 12.7 months of follow-up, although 11 achieved a second CR after retreatment with ATO. One and 2/3-year survival were 86% and 84%, respectively *(219)*.

Although ATO therapy results in high rates of remission and appears to be an acceptable first-line intervention in APL, without randomized data, it is uncertain if such an approach results in higher cure rates than that achieved by standard therapy with ATRA and chemotherapy combination *(212,215)*.

8.2. ATO in Relapsed APL

In the United States, trials of ATO in patients with relapsed APL replicated the Chinese experience, showing hematological and molecular CR rates of 85–91% and 72–78%, respectively *(102,220,276)*. The 2-year RFS and OS estimates for combined trials were 49% and 63%, respectively, indicating an impressive survival rate induced by ATO in patients with refractory or relapsed APL *(221)* (Fig. 5). The therapeutic efficacy of ATO has been further

Table 5
Arsenic Trioxide in APL

Study (ref.)	Year	Arsenic compound	Disease status	Number	CR (%)
Sun *(261)*	1992	Ailin-1	*De novo* and relapsed	32	65.6
Zhang *(262)*	1996	ATO	*De novo*	30	73.3
			Relapsed	42	52
Chen	1996	ATO	Relapsed	16	93.7
Soignet *(102)*	1998	ATO	Relapsed/Refractory	12	92
Niu *(212)*	1999	ATO	Relapsed	47	85
			De novo	11	72.7
Zhang *(215)*	1999	ATO	*De novo* Relapsed/Refractory	242	75
Camacho *(235)*	2000	ATO	Relapsed/Refractory	26	88
Soignet *(220)*	2001	ATO	Relapsed/Refractory	40	85
Shalabi *(222)*	2001	ATO	Relapsed/Refractory	57	74
Lazo *(223)*	2003	ATO	Relapsed	12	100

confirmed by the studies from the National Cancer Insitute and MD Anderson Cancer Center *(222,223)* (Table 4). It appears that in relapsed APL patients, ATO therapy leads to high CR rates, high molecular remission rates, is associated with infrequent drug resistance even when anthracyclines, ATRA, and SCT fail, and is associated with mild and reversible adverse reactions. Additionally, because ATO as a single agent is able to induce high CR rates in this patient population, chemotherapy may be omitted, allowing for a less toxic approach.

According to several studies from China, the use of ATO maintenance therapy for varying durations resulted in prolonged remissions in the number of patients *(212,215)*. For example, in a study by Au and colleagues, at a median follow-up of 15 months, relapse rate was 12.5% in maintenance group vs 58.8% without ATO maintenance ($p = 0.003$) *(224)*.

8.3. ATO to Induce a Second Complete Remission Prior to HSCT

The role of hematopoietic stem cell transplantation (HSCT) as a consolidation strategy in relapsed APL patients after ATO-induced CR has been addressed in several small studies *(225,226)*. In the US multicenter trial, 18 patients underwent SCT after ATO therapy. At the time of transplantation 14 patients were in CR (11 allogeneic, 3 autologous), whereas 4 patients relapsed after the last ATO treatment (3 allogeneic and 1 autologous). All 4 patients who underwent auto-SCT and 10 of 14 patients treated with allo-SCT were alive at 3 years follow-up (first half of 2002) *(225)*.

Although further randomized prospective studies are required to fully establish the role of ATO in the transplantation setting, it appears to be an effective and relatively nontoxic agent able to induce CR prior to transplantation. Patients who achieve CR with ATO are likely to be in better condition at the time of transplantation, which may translate into reduced transplantation-related morbidity and mortality.

8.4. ATO and ATRA Combination Therapy

Based on the above-mentioned clinical trials as well as extensive safety analysis, ATO was approved by the U.S. Food and Drug Administration in September 2000 for the induction and consolidation therapy of patients with t(15;17) APL who are refractory to, or have relapsed after, retinoid and anthracycline therapy.

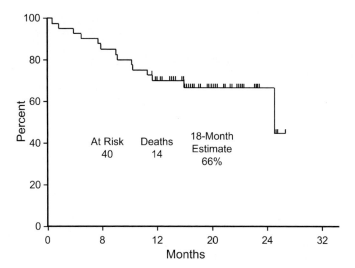

Fig. 5. Kaplan-Meier overall survival curve of patients with relapsed acute promyelocytic leukemia treated with arsenic trioxide. (From ref. *220.*)

Because ATRA and ATO degrade PML-RARα via different pathways and appear to have synergistic effects in vivo and in vitro studies, it has been postulated that the combination of these two drugs may result in improved outcome in APL patients. To address this hypothesis, Shen and colleagues randomized 61 patients with newly diagnosed APL to three treatment groups: ATRA at 25 mg/m^2/day until CR, ATO at 0.16 mg/kg/day until CR, or a combination of ATRA and As$_2$O$_3$ at the above-mentioned doses *(227)*. After achieving a CR, all three groups received the same three consecutive consolidation chemotherapy regimens. Maintenance treatments were different among the three groups: ATRA-only group was given ATRA, 6-MP, or MTX; ATO-only group was treated with As$_2$O$_3$, 6-MP, or MTX; and combination group was given ATRA, arsenic, and MTX or 6-MP. Although the CR rates were similar in all three groups (>90%), the time to achieve CR was the shortest in the combination arm. Earlier platelet recovery also was noted in the combination arm. The disease burden as reflected by fold change in PML-RARα transcripts at CR decreased more significantly in the combination arm compared to ATRA or arsenic alone groups (p <0.01); this difference also persisted at consolidation (p <0.05). Importantly, all 20 cases treated with the combination of ATO and ATRA remained in CR, while 7 of 37 cases treated with monotherapy relapsed after a follow-up of 8–30 months (median 18 months) (Fig. 6). The synergism of ATRA and ATO in apoptosis and degradation of PML-RARα oncoprotein provide a plausible explanation for the superior efficacy of combination therapy.

Estey and colleagues also demonstrated that 28 of 32 (88%) patients with untreated APL achieved a CR with an ATRA/ATO combination, maintained with the same drugs without chemotherapy *(228,229)*. Although several patients required GO for elevated WBC and in five patients GO was substituted for ATO because of cardiac toxicity, the results compared favorably with those for the patients treated with ATRA and idarubicin at the same institution *(228,229)*.

Additional ongoing trials are exploring the combination of ATO with ATRA, HuM195, and reduced doses of idarubicin in patients with newly diagnosed APL *(221)*.

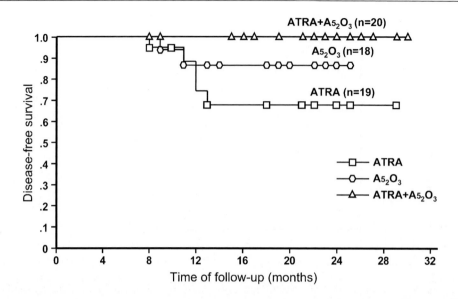

Fig. 6. Kaplan-Meier disease-free survival curves. The relative risk (RR) of the single-agent groups is significantly higher than that of the *all-trans*-retinoic acid (ATRA) + arsenic trioxide (ATO) combination group ($p = 0.0202$, Fisher's exact test). When patients from the two monotherapy groups are put together, the RR is also statistically higher than that of the combination group ($p = 0.038$). (From ref. *227.*)

8.5. Mechanisms of Action of ATO

The mechanisms behind the efficacy of arsenic therapy in APL are not entirely understood. They are believed to involve apoptosis induction at relatively high concentrations ($0.5–2 \times 10^{-6} M$) as well as partial cellular differentiation at low concentrations ($0.1–0.5 \times 10^{-6} M$), via degradation of the PML-RARα *(88,97,102,230)*.

Studies of APL-derived cell lines and transgenic mice carrying the PML-RARα fusion proteins indicate that arsenic trioxide induces degradation of both the chimeric PML-RARα and native PML from the nuclei of malignant cells, allowing partial differentiation of the leukemic population to proceed *(97)*. ATO may induce apoptosis of APL cells independently of the expression of PML-RARα fusion protein by indirectly impairing H_2O_2 catabolism, which leads to a decrease in mitochondrial membrane potential, release of cytochrome c, and activation and upregulation of caspases 1, 2, 3, and 8 *(102,103,231,232)*. Other suggested mechanisms include downregulation of bcl-2 expression and modulation of the intracellular content of reduced glutathione *(233,234)*.

8.6. ATO-Associated Toxicity

The most significant toxicities of arsenic include hyperleukocytosis, APL differentiation syndrome, and ventricular arrhythmia as a result of prolongation of QT interval *(235,236)*.

8.6.1. Hyperleukocytosis and APL Differentiation Syndrome

Hyperleukocytosis, similar to that observed in patients treated with ATRA, occurs in nearly 50% of patients receiving ATO therapy *(235)*. Typically, the WBC reaches its peak 20 days after the beginning of therapy and resolves, on average, 10.5 days thereafter. ATO therapy may be continued, presuming patients are monitored closely for the development of the cardiopulmonary symptoms.

At the earliest signs of the APL differentiation syndrome, which develops in about 20–30% patients with hyperleukocytosis, dexamethasone therapy should be instituted *(152,237)*. As symptoms improve, dexamethasone may be tapered and discontinued. If the patient has persistent leukocytosis despite resolution of the syndrome, it may be prudent to continue dexamethasone until WBC decreases to <10,000/μL. Additional cytotoxic therapy does not appear to be required *(152)*.

8.6.2. CARDIAC AND OTHER TOXICITIES

ATO therapy has been associated with serious cardiac toxicity, such as delayed cardiac repolarization, manifesting by QT prolongation, ventricular premature contractions, development of torsades de pointes, and several episodes of sudden death *(238–240)*. However, close cardiac monitoring, maintaining QT interval < 460 ms and potassium and magnesium levels >4.0 mEq/L and 2.0 mg/dL, respectively, allows for safe administration of ATO in patients with APL *(152,241,242)*.

It has been suggested that ATO increases the cardiac calcium current and reduces the surface expression of the cardiac potassium channel human ether-a-go-go-related gene (hERG), causing QT prolongation and torsades *(243)*.

Alopecia, hepatotoxicity, peripheral neuropathy, acute renal failure, and neuromuscular degenerative changes have been reported in APL patients treated with ATO *(212,220,223, 227,236,244)*.

9. HEMATOPOIETIC STEM CELL TRANSPLANTATION IN APL

Considering the excellent outcome of the combination of ATRA and chemotherapy in patients with APL, HSCT is not indicated in the first CR. Most studies of HSCT in the CR2 were performed prior to the introduction of arsenic, and since many patients with relapsed and refractory disease may be treated successfully with ATO without introducing transplantation-related toxicity, the optimal timing for transplantation is unclear. Data from the European Bone Marrow Transplant Registry collected in the pre-ATRA era demonstrated a leukemia-free survival (LFS) of 48% for auto-HSCT and 42% for allo-HSCT conducted in CR1, with treatment-related mortality (TRM) of 19% and 42%, respectively. Patients who received transplantation in CR2 had a LFS of 32% for auto-HSCT and 22% for allo-HSCT, with TRM of 23% and 41%, respectively *(245)*.

To address the role of HSCT in the CR2 after the re-induction with a combination of ATRA and chemotherapy, de Botton and colleagues retrospectively analyzed an outcome of auto- and allo-HSCT in 73 patients *(246)*. Seven-year RFS, EFS, and OS in the auto-HSCT group were 79.4%, 60.6%, and 59.8%, respectively, with TRM of 6%. In the auto-HSCT group, out of 28 PCR-negative, 2 PCR-positive, and 20 PCR-undetermined patients prior to the transplantation, 3 (11%), 1, and 6 (30%) relapsed, respectively. Patients in molecular remission at the time of stem cell harvest had a 7-year RFS, EFS, and OS of 87.3%, 76.5%, and 75%, respectively, as compared with 69.8%, 49.2%, and 51.1% in PCR-positive patients. These results confirm the existing data demonstrating that molecular remission prior to Auto-HSCT, as determined by RT-PCR, is an important predictor of a favorable outcome *(247,248)*. Thus, auto-HSCT appears to be an important approach in the management of patients in the CR2, with low TRM and prolonged remission in 60% of the patients. In the allo-HSCT group, 7-year RFS, EFS, and OS were 92.3%, 52.2%, and 51.8%, respectively, with 39% TRM. OS was significantly better in the auto-HSCT group than in the allo-HSCT group ($p = 0.04$), whereas RFS and EFS did not differ significantly ($p = 0.19$ and $p = 0.11$, respectively). In the allo-HSCT group, out of 6 PCR-positive patients prior to transplant, only one relapsed, suggesting the effectiveness of allo-HSCT in this group of patients and confirming the results of a prior series showing two of six relapses in RT-PCR positive patients prior to allo-HSCT (249). Although postinduction therapy was not randomized in this study, the relapse rate appeared higher (39%) among patients who did not undergo auto- or allo-HSCT in CR2.

Based on the available data, autologous (PCR-negative) or allogeneic (PCR-positive) HSCT may be indicated in APL patients in second remission. Although the results of auto-HSCT appear superior to those of allogeneic HSCT, it is important to remember that the data are retrospective. Patients undergoing allo-HSCT had more high-risk features (e.g., higher WBC, shorter duration of first CR, greater incidence of CR positivity) and sustained more TRM. Successful outcome of matched unrelated donor (MUD) transplant after ATO consolidation in patient with ATRA and CT refractory APL has been reported (250).

10. CONCLUSIONS

The therapy for APL has changed significantly over the last 40 years and continues to evolve. Current therapeutic strategies consisting of ATRA and anthracycline-based chemotherapy result in prolonged DFS and a potential cure for more than 80% of patients. Early recognition of therapy-related complications and advances in supportive care undoubtedly contribute to improved survival. The ability to monitor minimal residual disease provides additional information crucial for clinical decision making. Current research efforts attempt to further delineate the role of cytarabine in induction and consolidation regimens and focus on the risk-adapted strategies to reduce treatment-related toxicity. The roles of ATO and GO are being explored in the setting of persistent minimal residual disease, HSCT, as part of the first-line regimen, and in high-risk patients. Novel therapeutic agents such as histone deacetylase inhibitors and histone methyltransferase inhibitors, which target chromatin modifications, as well as FLT-3 kinase inhibitors and p38 MAP-kinase inhibitors, are being evaluated in the laboratory and may be the focus of future clinical trials.

REFERENCES

1. Hillestad LK. Acute promyelocytic leukemia. Acta Med Scand 1957;159(3):189–194.
2. Bernard J, Mathe G, Boulay J, Ceoard B, Chome J. [Acute promyelocytic leukemia: a study made on 20 cases.]. Schweiz Med Wochenschr 1959;89:604–608.
3. Bernard J, Weil M, Boiron M, Jacquillat C, Flandrin G, Gemon MF. Acute promyelocytic leukemia: results of treatment by daunorubicin. Blood 1973;41(4):489–496.
4. Rowley JD, Golomb HM, Dougherty C. 15/17 translocation, a consistent chromosomal change in acute promyelocytic leukaemia. Lancet 1977;1(8010):549–550.
5. Breitman TR, Collins SJ, Keene BR. Terminal differentiation of human promyelocytic leukemic cells in primary culture in response to retinoic acid. Blood 1981;57(6):1000–1004.
6. Huang ME, Ye YC, Chen SR, et al. Use of all-trans retinoic acid in the treatment of acute promyelocytic leukemia. Blood 1988;72(2):567–572.
7. Borrow J, Goddard AD, Sheer D, Solomon E. Molecular analysis of acute promyelocytic leukemia breakpoint cluster region on chromosome 17. Science 1990;249(4976):1577–1580.

8. de The H, Chomienne C, Lanotte M, Degos L, Dejean A. The t(15;17) translocation of acute promyelocytic leukaemia fuses the retinoic acid receptor alpha gene to a novel transcribed locus. Nature 1990;347(6293): 558–561.

9. Longo L, Pandolfi PP, Biondi A, et al. Rearrangements and aberrant expression of the retinoic acid receptor alpha gene in acute promyelocytic leukemias. J Exp Med 1990;172(6):1571–1575.

10. de The H, Lavau C, Marchio A, Chomienne C, Degos L, Dejean A. The PML-RAR alpha fusion mRNA generated by the t(15;17) translocation in acute promyelocytic leukemia encodes a functionally altered RAR. Cell 1991;66(4):675–684.

11. Kakizuka A, Miller WH, Jr., Umesono K, et al. Chromosomal translocation t(15;17) in human acute promyelocytic leukemia fuses RAR alpha with a novel putative transcription factor, PML. Cell 1991;66(4):663–674.

12. Pandolfi PP, Grignani F, Alcalay M, et al. Structure and origin of the acute promyelocytic leukemia myl/RAR alpha cDNA and characterization of its retinoid-binding and transactivation properties. Oncogene 1991;6(7):1285–1292.

13. Chen Z, Brand NJ, Chen A, et al. Fusion between a novel Kruppel-like zinc finger gene and the retinoic acid receptor-alpha locus due to a variant t(11;17) translocation associated with acute promyelocytic leukaemia. EMBO J 1993;12(3):1161–1167.

14. Redner RL, Rush EA, Faas S, Rudert WA, Corey SJ. The t(5;17) variant of acute promyelocytic leukemia expresses a nucleophosmin-retinoic acid receptor fusion. Blood 1996;87(3):882–886.

15. Wells RA, Catzavelos C, Kamel-Reid S. Fusion of retinoic acid receptor alpha to NuMA, the nuclear mitotic apparatus protein, by a variant translocation in acute promyelocytic leukaemia. Nat Genet 1997;17(1): 109–113.

16. Arnould C, Philippe C, Bourdon V, Gr goire MJ, Berger R, Jonveaux P. The signal transducer and activator of transcription STAT5b gene is a new partner of retinoic acid receptor alpha in acute promyelocytic-like leukaemia. Hum Mol Genet 1999;8(9):1741–1749.

17. Gallagher R, Mark S, Paietta E, et al. Identification of a second Acute Promyelocytic Leukemia (APL) Patient with the STAT5b-RARalpha Fusion Gene among PML-RARalpha-Negative Eastern Cooperative Oncology Group (ECOG) APL protocol Registrants. Blood 2004;104(11):3005.

18. Altucci L, Gronemeyer H. The promise of retinoids to fight against cancer. Nat Rev Cancer 2001;1(3): 181–193.

19. Mangelsdorf DJ, Thummel C, Beato M, et al. The nuclear receptor superfamily: the second decade. Cell 1995;83(6):835–839.

20. Tallman MS, Nabhan C, Feusner JH, Rowe JM. Acute promyelocytic leukemia: evolving therapeutic strategies. Blood 2002;99(3):759–767.

21. He LZ, Guidez F, Triboli C, et al. Distinct interactions of PML-RARalpha and PLZF-RARalpha with co-repressors determine differential responses to RA in APL. Nat Genet 1998;18(2):126–135.

22. Pandolfi PP. Oncogenes and tumor suppressors in the molecular pathogenesis of acute promyelocytic leukemia. Hum Mol Genet 2001;10(7):769–775.

23. Dong D, Ruuska SE, Levinthal DJ, Noy N. Distinct roles for cellular retinoic acid-binding proteins I and II in regulating signaling by retinoic acid. J Biol Chem 1999;274(34):23,695–23,698.

24. Zhou D, Hallam SJ, Lee SJ, Wiernik PH, Tallman MS, Gallagher RE. Constitutive expression of cellular retinoic acid binding protein II and lack of correlation with sensitivity to all-trans retinoic acid in acute promyelocytic leukemia cells. Cancer Res 1998;58(24):5770–5776.

25. Chambon P. A decade of molecular biology of retinoic acid receptors. FASEB J 1996;10(9):940–954.

26. Glass CK, Rosenfeld MG. The coregulator exchange in transcriptional functions of nuclear receptors. Genes Dev 2000;14(2):121–141.

27. Rochette-Egly C, Adam S, Rossignol M, Egly JM, Chambon P. Stimulation of RAR alpha activation function AF-1 through binding to the general transcription factor TFIIH and phosphorylation by CDK7. Cell 1997;90(1):97–107.

28. Kurokawa R, Soderstrom M, Horlein A, et al. Polarity-specific activities of retinoic acid receptors determined by a co-repressor. Nature 1995;377(6548):451–454.

29. Zhu J, Heyworth CM, Glasow A, et al. Lineage restriction of the RARalpha gene expression in myeloid differentiation. Blood 2001;98(8):2563–2567.

30. Tsai S, Bartelmez S, Heyman R, Damm K, Evans R, Collins SJ. A mutated retinoic acid receptor-alpha exhibiting dominant-negative activity alters the lineage development of a multipotent hematopoietic cell line. Genes Dev 1992;6(12A):2258–2269.

31. Collins SJ, Robertson KA, Mueller L. Retinoic acid-induced granulocytic differentiation of HL-60 myeloid leukemia cells is mediated directly through the retinoic acid receptor (RAR-alpha). Mol Cell Biol 1990;10(5):2154–2163.
32. Strudwick S, Borden KL. Finding a role for PML in APL pathogenesis: a critical assessment of potential PML activities. Leukemia 2002;16(10):1906–1917.
33. Wang ZG, Ruggero D, Ronchetti S, et al. PML is essential for multiple apoptotic pathways. Nat Genet 1998;20(3):266–272.
34. Salomoni P, Pandolfi PP. The role of PML in tumor suppression. Cell 2002;108(2):165–170.
35. Borden KL, Boddy MN, Lally J, et al. The solution structure of the RING finger domain from the acute promyelocytic leukaemia proto-oncoprotein PML. EMBO J 1995;14(7):1532–1541.
36. Chang KS, Fan YH, Andreeff M, Liu J, Mu ZM. The PML gene encodes a phosphoprotein associated with the nuclear matrix. Blood 1995;85(12):3646–3653.
37. Weis K, Rambaud S, Lavau C, et al. Retinoic acid regulates aberrant nuclear localization of PML-RAR alpha in acute promyelocytic leukemia cells. Cell 1994;76(2):345–356.
38. Jensen K, Shiels C, Freemont PS. PML protein isoforms and the RBCC/TRIM motif. Oncogene 2001;20(49)(October 29):7223–7233.
39. Zhong S, Muller S, Ronchetti S, Freemont PS, Dejean A, Pandolfi PP. Role of SUMO-1-modified PML in nuclear body formation. Blood 2000;95(9):2748–2752.
40. Zhong S, Hu P, Ye TZ, Stan R, Ellis NA, Pandolfi PP. A role for PML and the nuclear body in genomic stability. Oncogene 1999;18(56):7941–7947.
41. Guo A, Salomoni P, Luo J, et al. The function of PML in p53-dependent apoptosis. Nat Cell Biol 2000; 2(10):730–736.
42. Bachleitner-Hofmann T, Kees M, Gisslinger H. Arsenic trioxide: acute promyelocytic leukemia and beyond. Leuk Lymphoma 2002;43(8):1535–1540.
43. Grignani F, Testa U, Rogaia D, et al. Effects on differentiation by the promyelocytic leukemia PML/RARalpha protein depend on the fusion of the PML protein dimerization and RARalpha DNA binding domains. EMBO J 1996;15(18):4949–4958.
44. Melnick A, Licht JD. Deconstructing a disease: RARalpha, its fusion partners, and their roles in the pathogenesis of acute promyelocytic leukemia. Blood 1999;93(10):3167–3215.
45. Ruthardt M, Testa U, Nervi C, et al. Opposite effects of the acute promyelocytic leukemia PML-retinoic acid receptor alpha (RAR alpha) and PLZF-RAR alpha fusion proteins on retinoic acid signalling. Mol Cell Biol 1997;17(8):4859–4869.
46. Pearson M, Carbone R, Sebastiani C, et al. PML regulates p53 acetylation and premature senescence induced by oncogenic Ras. Nature 2000;406(6792):207–210.
47. Ferbeyre G, de Stanchina E, Querido E, Baptiste N, Prives C, Lowe SW. PML is induced by oncogenic ras and promotes premature senescence. Genes Dev 2000;14(16):2015–2027.
48. Zhong S, Delva L, Rachez C, et al. A RA-dependent, tumour-growth suppressive transcription complex is the target of the PML-RARalpha and T18 oncoproteins. Nat Genet 1999;23(3):287–295.
49. Rego EM, Pandolfi PP. Analysis of the molecular genetics of acute promyelocytic leukemia in mouse models. Semin Hematol 2001;38(1):54–70.
50. Koken MH, Linares-Cruz G, Quignon F, et al. The PML growth-suppressor has an altered expression in human oncogenesis. Oncogene 1995;10(7):1315–1324.
51. Mu ZM, Chin KV, Liu JH, Lozano G, Chang KS. PML, a growth suppressor disrupted in acute promyelocytic leukemia. Mol Cell Biol 1994;14(10):6858–6867.
52. Ahn MJ, Nason-Burchenal K, Moasser MM, Dmitrovsky E. Growth suppression of acute promyelocytic leukemia cells having increased expression of the non-rearranged alleles: RAR alpha or PML. Oncogene 1995;10(12):2307–2314.
53. Zhong S, Salomoni P, Ronchetti S, Guo A, Ruggero D, Pandolfi PP. Promyelocytic leukemia protein (PML) and Daxx participate in a novel nuclear pathway for apoptosis. J Exp Med 2000;191(4):631–640.
54. Vallian S, Chin KV, Chang KS. The promyelocytic leukemia protein interacts with Sp1 and inhibits its transactivation of the epidermal growth factor receptor promoter. Mol Cell Biol 1998;18(12):7147–7156.
55. Doucas V, Tini M, Egan DA, Evans RM. Modulation of CREB binding protein function by the promyelocytic (PML) oncoprotein suggests a role for nuclear bodies in hormone signaling. Proc Natl Acad Sci USA 1999;96(6):2627–2632.

56. Tsuzuki S, Towatari M, Saito H, Enver T. Potentiation of GATA-2 activity through interactions with the promyelocytic leukemia protein (PML) and the t(15;17)-generated PML-retinoic acid receptor alpha oncoprotein. Mol Cell Biol 2000;20(17):6276–6286.

57. Kogan SC, Hong SH, Shultz DB, Privalsky ML, Bishop JM. Leukemia initiated by PMLRARalpha: the PML domain plays a critical role while retinoic acid-mediated transactivation is dispensable. Blood 2000;95(5):1541–1550.

58. Gallagher RE, Willman CL, Slack JL, et al. Association of PML-RAR alpha fusion mRNA type with pretreatment hematologic characteristics but not treatment outcome in acute promyelocytic leukemia: an intergroup molecular study. Blood 1997;90(4):1656–1663.

59. Grignani F, Fagioli M, Alcalay M, et al. Acute promyelocytic leukemia: from genetics to treatment. Blood 1994;83(10).

60. Slack JL, Yu M. Constitutive expression of the promyelocytic leukemia-associated oncogene PML-RARalpha in TF1 cells: isoform-specific and retinoic acid-dependent effects on growth, bcl-2 expression, and apoptosis. Blood 1998;91(9):3347–3356.

61. Slack JL, Willman CL, Andersen JW, et al. Molecular analysis and clinical outcome of adult APL patients with the type V PML-RARalpha isoform: results from intergroup protocol 0129. Blood 2000;95(2):398–403.

62. Parrado A, Chomienne C, Padua RA. Retinoic acid receptor alpha (RAralpha) Mutations in Human Leukemia. Leuk Lymphoma 2000;39(3-4):271–282.

63. Testa U, Grignani F, Barberi T, et al. PML/RAR alpha+ U937 mutant and NB4 cell lines: retinoic acid restores the monocytic differentiation response to vitamin D3. Cancer Res 1994;54(16):4508–4515.

64. Grignani F, Valtieri M, Gabbianelli M, et al. PML/RAR alpha fusion protein expression in normal human hematopoietic progenitors dictates myeloid commitment and the promyelocytic phenotype. Blood 2000; 96(4):1531–1537.

65. Brown D, Kogan S, Lagasse E, et al. A PMLRARalpha transgene initiates murine acute promyelocytic leukemia. Proc Natl Acad Sci USA 1997;94(6):2551–2556.

66. Grisolano JL, Wesselschmidt RL, Pelicci PG, Ley TJ. Altered myeloid development and acute leukemia in transgenic mice expressing PML-RAR alpha under control of cathepsin G regulatory sequences. Blood 1997;89(2):376–387.

67. He LZ, Tribioli C, Rivi R, et al. Acute leukemia with promyelocytic features in PML/RARalpha transgenic mice. Proc Natl Acad Sci USA 1997;94(10):5302–5307.

68. Schnittger S, Schoch C, Dugas M, et al. Analysis of FLT3 length mutations in 1003 patients with acute myeloid leukemia: correlation to cytogenetics, FAB subtype, and prognosis in the AMLCG study and usefulness as a marker for the detection of minimal residual disease. Blood 2002;100(1):59–66.

69. Kelly LM, Kutok JL, Williams IR, et al. PML/RARalpha and FLT3-ITD induce an APL-like disease in a mouse model. Proc Natl Acad Sci USA 2002;99(12):8283–8288.

70. Pollock JL, Westervelt P, Kurichety AK, Pelicci PG, Grisolano JL, Ley TJ. A bcr-3 isoform of RARalpha-PML potentiates the development of PML-RARalpha-driven acute promyelocytic leukemia. Proc Natl Acad Sci USA 1999;96(26):15,103–15,108.

71. de The H. Altered retinoic acid receptors. FASEB J 1996;10(9):955–960.

72. Kawasaki A, Matsumura I, Kataoka Y, Takigawa E, Nakajima K, Kanakura Y. Opposing effects of PML and PML/RAR alpha on STAT3 activity. Blood 2003;101(9):3668–3673.

73. Pandolfi PP. In vivo analysis of the molecular genetics of acute promyelocytic leukemia. Oncogene 2001;20(40):5726–5735.

74. Grignani F, Ferrucci PF, Testa U, et al. The acute promyelocytic leukemia-specific PML-RAR alpha fusion protein inhibits differentiation and promotes survival of myeloid precursor cells. Cell 1993;74(3):423–431.

75. Lin RJ, Evans RM. Acquisition of oncogenic potential by RAR chimeras in acute promyelocytic leukemia through formation of homodimers. Mol Cell 2000;5(5):821–830.

76. Minucci S, Maccarana M, Cioce M, et al. Oligomerization of RAR and AML1 transcription factors as a novel mechanism of oncogenic activation. Mol Cell 2000;5(5):811–820.

77. Lin RJ, Nagy L, Inoue S, Shao W, Miller WH, Jr., Evans RM. Role of the histone deacetylase complex in acute promyelocytic leukaemia. Nature 1998;391(6669):811–814.

78. Grignani F, De Matteis S, Nervi C, et al. Fusion proteins of the retinoic acid receptor-alpha recruit histone deacetylase in promyelocytic leukaemia. Nature 1998;391(6669):815–818.

79. Gurrieri C, Nafa K, Merghoub T, et al. Mutations of the PML tumor suppressor gene in acute promyelocytic leukemia. Blood 2004;103(6):2358–2362.

80. Zhong S, Salomoni P, Pandolfi PP. The transcriptional role of PML and the nuclear body. Nat Cell Biol 2000;2(5):E85–E90.

81. Zimonjic DB, Pollock JL, Westervelt P, Popescu NC, Ley TJ. Acquired, nonrandom chromosomal abnormalities associated with the development of acute promyelocytic leukemia in transgenic mice. Proc Natl Acad Sci USA 2000;97(24):13,306–13,311.

82. Ellis NA, Groden J, Ye TZ, et al. The Bloom's syndrome gene product is homologous to RecQ helicases. Cell 1995;83(4):655–666.

83. Lombard DB, Guarente L. Nijmegen breakage syndrome disease protein and MRE11 at PML nuclear bodies and meiotic telomeres. Cancer Res 2000;60(9):2331–2334.

84. Johnson FB, Lombard DB, Neff NF, et al. Association of the Bloom syndrome protein with topoisomerase IIIalpha in somatic and meiotic cells. Cancer Res 2000;60(5):1162–1167.

85. Liu TX, Zhang JW, Tao J, et al. Gene expression networks underlying retinoic acid-induced differentiation of acute promyelocytic leukemia cells. Blood 2000;96(4):1496–1504.

86. Rego EM, He LZ, Warrell RP, Jr., Wang ZG, Pandolfi PP. Retinoic acid (RA) and As2O3 treatment in transgenic models of acute promyelocytic leukemia (APL) unravel the distinct nature of the leukemogenic process induced by the PML-RARalpha and PLZF-RARalpha oncoproteins. Proc Natl Acad Sci USA 2000;97(18):10,173–10,178.

87. Yoshida H, Kitamura K, Tanaka K, et al. Accelerated degradation of PML-retinoic acid receptor alpha (PML-RARA) oncoprotein by all-trans-retinoic acid in acute promyelocytic leukemia: possible role of the proteasome pathway. Cancer Res 1996;56(13):2945–2948.

88. Chen GQ, Zhu J, Shi XG, et al. In vitro studies on cellular and molecular mechanisms of arsenic trioxide (As2O3) in the treatment of acute promyelocytic leukemia: As2O3 induces NB4 cell apoptosis with downregulation of Bcl-2 expression and modulation of PML-RAR alpha/PML proteins. Blood 1996;88(3):1052–1061.

89. Zhu XH, Shen YL, Jing YK, et al. Apoptosis and growth inhibition in malignant lymphocytes after treatment with arsenic trioxide at clinically achievable concentrations. J Natl Cancer Inst 1999;91(9):772–778.

90. Jing Y, Wang L, Xia L, et al. Combined effect of all-trans retinoic acid and arsenic trioxide in acute promyelocytic leukemia cells in vitro and in vivo. Blood 2001;97(1):264–269.

91. Muller S, Matunis MJ, Dejean A. Conjugation with the ubiquitin-related modifier SUMO-1 regulates the partitioning of PML within the nucleus. EMBO J 1998;17(1):61–70.

92. Raelson JV, Nervi C, Rosenauer A, et al. The PML/RAR alpha oncoprotein is a direct molecular target of retinoic acid in acute promyelocytic leukemia cells. Blood 1996;88(8):2826–2832.

93. Chen G, Shen Z, Zhu AP. [Pharmacokinetics and efficacy of low-dose all-trans retinoic acid in the treatment of acute promyelocytic leukemia]. Zhonghua Nei Ke Za Zhi 1997;36(5):295–299.

94. Zhu J, Gianni M, Kopf E, et al. Retinoic acid induces proteasome-dependent degradation of retinoic acid receptor alpha (RARalpha) and oncogenic RARalpha fusion proteins. Proc Natl Acad Sci USA 1999;96(26):14,807–14,812.

95. Duprez E, Lillehaug JR, Naoe T, Lanotte M. cAMP signalling is decisive for recovery of nuclear bodies (PODs) during maturation of RA-resistant t(15;17) promyelocytic leukemia NB4 cells expressing PML-RAR alpha. Oncogene 1996;12(11):2451–2459.

96. Sternsdorf T, Puccetti E, Jensen K, et al. PIC-1/SUMO-1-modified PML-retinoic acid receptor alpha mediates arsenic trioxide-induced apoptosis in acute promyelocytic leukemia. Mol Cell Biol 1999;19(7):5170–5178.

97. Zhu J, Koken MH, Quignon F, et al. Arsenic-induced PML targeting onto nuclear bodies: implications for the treatment of acute promyelocytic leukemia. Proc Natl Acad Sci USA 1997;94(8):3978–3983.

98. Bode AM, Dong Z. The paradox of arsenic: molecular mechanisms of cell transformation and chemotherapeutic effects. Crit Rev Oncol Hematol 2002;42(1):5–24.

99. Hong SH, Yang Z, Privalsky ML. Arsenic trioxide is a potent inhibitor of the interaction of SMRT corepressor with Its transcription factor partners, including the PML-retinoic acid receptor alpha oncoprotein found in human acute promyelocytic leukemia. Mol Cell Biol 2001;21(21):7172–7182.

100. Hayakawa F, Privalsky ML. Phosphorylation of PML by mitogen-activated protein kinases plays a key role in arsenic trioxide-mediated apoptosis. Cancer Cell 2004;5(4):389–401.

101. Chen GQ, Shi XG, Tang W, et al. Use of arsenic trioxide (As2O3) in the treatment of acute promyelocytic leukemia (APL): I. As2O3 exerts dose-dependent dual effects on APL cells. Blood 1997;89(9):3345–3353.

102. Soignet SL, Maslak P, Wang ZG, et al. Complete remission after treatment of acute promyelocytic leukemia with arsenic trioxide. N Engl J Med 1998;339(19):1341–1348.

103. Wang ZG, Rivi R, Delva L, et al. Arsenic trioxide and melarsoprol induce programmed cell death in myeloid leukemia cell lines and function in a PML and PML-RARalpha independent manner. Blood 1998;92(5):1497–1504.

104. Nervi C, Ferrara FF, Fanelli M, et al. Caspases mediate retinoic acid-induced degradation of the acute promyelocytic leukemia PML/RARalpha fusion protein. Blood 1998;92(7):2244–2251.

105. Licht JD, Chomienne C, Goy A, et al. Clinical and molecular characterization of a rare syndrome of acute promyelocytic leukemia associated with translocation (11;17). Blood 1995;85(4):1083–1094.

106. Sainty D, Liso V, Cantu-Rajnoldi A, et al. A new morphologic classification system for acute promyelocytic leukemia distinguishes cases with underlying PLZF/RARA gene rearrangements. Group Francais de Cytogenetique Hematologique, UK Cancer Cytogenetics Group and BIOMED 1 European Coomunity-Concerted Acion "Molecular Cytogenetic Diagnosis in Haematological Malignancies. Blood 2000;96(4): 1287–1296.

107. Grimwade D, Gorman P, Duprez E, et al. Characterization of cryptic rearrangements and variant translocations in acute promyelocytic leukemia. Blood 1997;90(12):4876–4885.

108. Bennett JM, Catovsky D, Daniel MT, et al. Hypergranular promyelocytic leukemia: correlation between morphology and chromosomal translocations including t(15;17) and t(11;17). Leukemia 2000;14(7): 1197–1200.

109. Guidez F, Ivins S, Zhu J, Soderstrom M, Waxman S, Zelent A. Reduced retinoic acid-sensitivities of nuclear receptor corepressor binding to PML- and PLZF-RARalpha underlie molecular pathogenesis and treatment of acute promyelocytic leukemia. Blood 1998;91(8):2634–2642.

110. Baylin SB, Herman JG, Graff JR, Vertino PM, Issa JP. Alterations in DNA methylation: a fundamental aspect of neoplasia. Adv Cancer Res 1998;72:141–196.

111. Nan X, Ng HH, Johnson CA, et al. Transcriptional repression by the methyl-CpG-binding protein MeCP2 involves a histone deacetylase complex. Nature 1998;393(6683):386–389.

112. Melnick A, Carlile G, Ahmad KF, et al. Critical residues within the BTB domain of PLZF and Bcl-6 modulate interaction with corepressors. Mol Cell Biol 2002;22(6):1804–1818.

113. Licht JD, Shaknovich R, English MA, et al. Reduced and altered DNA-binding and transcriptional properties of the PLZF-retinoic acid receptor-alpha chimera generated in t(11;17)-associated acute promyelocytic leukemia. Oncogene 1996;12(2):323–336.

114. Dong S, Zhu J, Reid A, et al. Amino-terminal protein-protein interaction motif (POZ-domain) is responsible for activities of the promyelocytic leukemia zinc finger-retinoic acid receptor-alpha fusion protein. Proc Natl Acad Sci USA 1996;93(8):3624–3629.

115. Koken MH, Reid A, Quignon F, et al. Leukemia-associated retinoic acid receptor alpha fusion partners, PML and PLZF, heterodimerize and colocalize to nuclear bodies. Proc Natl Acad Sci USA 1997;94(19):10,255–10,260.

116. Petti MC, Fazi F, Gentile M, et al. Complete remission through blast cell differentiation in PLZF/RARalpha-positive acute promyelocytic leukemia: in vitro and in vivo studies. Blood 2002;100(3): 1065–1067.

117. Okuda M, Horn HF, Hoffmann IA, Snyder JD, Bove KE, Fukasawa K. Nucleophosmin/B23 is a target of CDK2/cyclin E in centrosome duplication. Cell 2000;103:127–140.

118. Hummel JL, Wells RA, Dube ID, Licht JD, Kamel-Reid S. Deregulation of NPM and PLZF in a variant t(5;17) case of acute promyelocytic leukemia. Oncogene 1999;18(3):633–641.

119. Redner RL, Chen JD, Rush EA, Li H, Pollock SL. The t(5;17) acute promyelocytic leukemia fusion protein NPM-RAR interacts with co-repressor and co-activator proteins and exhibits both positive and negative transcriptional properties. Blood 2000;95(8):2683–2690.

120. Redner RL, Corey SJ, Rush EA. Differentiation of t(5;17) variant acute promyelocytic leukemic blasts by all-trans retinoic acid. Leukemia 1997;11(7):1014–1016.

121. Redner RL. Variations on a theme:the alternate translocations in APL. Leukemia 2002;16(10):1927–1932.

122. Dong D, Tweardy DJ. Interactions of STAT5b-RARalpha, a novel acute promyelocytic leukemia fusion protein, with retinoic acid receptor and STAT3 signaling pathways. Blood 2002;99(8):2637–2646.

123. Vickers M, Jackson G, Taylor P. The incidence of acute promyelocytic leukemia appears constant over most of a human lifespan, implying only one rate limiting mutation. Leukemia 2000;14(4):722–726.

124. Pulsoni A, Stazi A, Cotichini R, et al. Acute promyelocytic leukaemia: epidemiology and risk factors. A report of the GIMEMA Italian archive of adult acute leukaemia. GIMEMA Cooperative Group. Eur J Haematol 1998;61(5):327–332.

125. Mele A, Stazi MA, Pulsoni A, et al. Epidemiology of acute promyelocytic leukemia. Haematologica 1995;80(5):405–408.

126. Estey E, Thall P, Kantarjian H, Pierce S, Kornblau S, Keating M. Association between increased body mass index and a diagnosis of acute promyelocytic leukemia in patients with acute myeloid leukemia. Leukemia 1997;11(10):1661–1664.

127. Douer D, Preston-Martin S, Chang E, Nichols PW, Watkins KJ, Levine AM. High frequency of acute promyelocytic leukemia among Latinos with acute myeloid leukemia. Blood 1996;87(1):308–313.

128. Burnett AK, Grimwade D, Solomon E, Wheatley K, Goldstone AH. Presenting white blood cell count and kinetics of molecular remission predict prognosis in acute promyelocytic leukemia treated with all-trans retinoic acid: result of the Randomized MRC Trial. Blood 1999;93(12):4131–4143.

129. Gupta V, Yib QL, Brandwein J, et al. Clinico-biological features and prognostic significance of PML/RARalpha isoforms in adult patients with acute promyelocytic leukemia treated with all trans retinoic acid (ATRA) and chemotherapy. Leuk Lymphoma 2004;45(3):469–480.

130. Tallman MS, Andersen JW, Schiffer CA, et al. All-trans retinoic acid in acute promyelocytic leukemia: long-term outcome and prognostic factor analysis from the North American Intergroup protocol. Blood 2002;100(13):4298–4302.

131. Sanz MA, Lo Coco F, Martin G, et al. Definition of relapse risk and role of nonanthracycline drugs for consolidation in patients with acute promyelocytic leukemia: a joint study of the PETHEMA and GIMEMA cooperative groups. Blood 2000;96(4):1247–1253.

132. Asou N, Adachi K, Tamura J, et al. Analysis of prognostic factors in newly diagnosed acute promyelocytic leukemia treated with all-trans retinoic acid and chemotherapy. Japan Adult Leukemia Study Group. J Clin Oncol 1998;16(1):78–85.

133. Fenaux P, Chastang C, Chevret S, et al. A randomized comparison of all transretinoic acid (ATRA) followed by chemotherapy and ATRA plus chemotherapy and the role of maintenance therapy in newly diagnosed acute promyelocytic leukemia. The European APL Group. Blood 1999;94(4):1192–1200.

134. Au WY, Fung A, Chim CS, et al. FLT-3 aberrations in acute promyelocytic leukaemia: clinicopathological associations and prognostic impact. Br J Haematol 2004;125(4):463–469.

135. Ades L, Chevret S, De Botton S, et al. Outcome of acute promyelocytic leukemia treated with all trans retinoic acid and chemotherapy in elderly patients: the European group experience. Leukemia 2005;19(2):230–233.

136. Vahdat L, Maslak P, Miller WH, Jr., et al. Early mortality and the retinoic acid syndrome in acute promyelocytic leukemia: impact of leukocytosis, low-dose chemotherapy, PMN/RAR-alpha isoform, and CD13 expression in patients treated with all-trans retinoic acid. Blood 1994;84(11):3843–3849.

137. Ferrara F, Morabito F, Martino B, et al. CD56 expression is an indicator of poor clinical outcome in patients with acute promyelocytic leukemia treated with simultaneous all-trans-retinoic acid and chemotherapy. J Clin Oncol 2000;18(6):1295–1300.

138. Montesinos P, De la Serna J, Vellenga E. Clinical features and outcome of patients with acute promyelocytic leukemiapresenting CD56 antigen expression treated with PETHEMA LPA99 trial. Haematologica Reports 2005;1:C20.

139. De Botton S, Chevret S, Sanz M, et al. Additional chromosomal abnormalities in patients with acute promyelocytic leukaemia (APL) do not confer poor prognosis: results of APL 93 trial. Br J Haematol 2000;111(3):801–806.

140. Grimwade D, Walker H, Oliver F, et al. The importance of diagnostic cytogenetics on outcome in AML: analysis of 1,612 patients entered into the MRC AML 10 trial. The Medical Research Council Adult and Children's Leukaemia Working Parties. Blood 1998;92(7):2322–2333.

141. Schoch C, Haase D, Haferlach T, et al. Incidence and implication of additional chromosome aberrations in acute promyelocytic leukaemia with translocation t(15;17)(q22;q21): a report on 50 patients. Br J Haematol 1996;94(3):493–500.

142. Cervera JM, G; Hernandez, J; et al. Additional chromosome abnormalities have no prognostic value in acute promyelocytic leukemia patients treated with simultaneous ATRA and anthracycline-based chemotherapy: an update of the APL96 and APL99 pethema protocols. Blood 2004;104(11):2019.

143. Pantic M, Novak A, Marisavljevic D, et al. Additional chromosome aberrations in acute promyelocytic leukemia: characteristics and prognostic influence. Med Oncol 2000;17(4):307–313.

144. Xu L, Zhao WL, Xiong SM, et al. Molecular cytogenetic characterization and clinical relevance of additional, complex and/or variant chromosome abnormalities in acute promyelocytic leukemia. Leukemia 2001;15(9):1359–1368.

145. Kiyoi H, Naoe T, Yokota S, et al. Internal tandem duplication of FLT3 associated with leukocytosis in acute promyelocytic leukemia. Leukemia Study Group of the Ministry of Health and Welfare (Kohseisho). Leukemia 1997;11(9):1447–1452.

146. Kainz B, Heintel D, Marculescu R, et al. Variable prognostic value of FLT3 internal tandem duplications in patients with de novo AML and a normal karyotype, t(15;17), t(8;21) or inv(16). Hematol J 2002;3(6):283–289.

147. Shih LY, Kuo MC, Liang DC, et al. Internal tandem duplication and Asp835 mutations of the FMS-like tyrosine kinase 3 (FLT3) gene in acute promyelocytic leukemia. Cancer 2003;98(6):1206–1216.

148. Noguera NI, Breccia M, Divona M, et al. Alterations of the FLT3 gene in acute promyelocytic leukemia: association with diagnostic characteristics and analysis of clinical outcome in patients treated with the Italian AIDA protocol. Leukemia 2002;16(11):2185–2189.

149. Grimwade D, Gale RE, Hills R, et al. The relationship between FLT3 mutation status, biological characteristics and outcome in patients with acute promyelocytic leukemia. Blood 2003;102:334.

150. Callens C, Chevret S, Cayuela JM, et al. Prognostic implication of FLT3 and Ras gene mutations in patients with acute promyelocytic leukemia (APL): a retrospective study from the European APL Group. Leukemia 2005;Jul 19(17):1153–1160.

151. Bolognesi E, Cimino G, Diverio D, et al. HLA class I in acute promyelocytic leukemia (APL): possible correlation with clinical outcome. Leukemia 2000;14(3):393–398.

152. Sanz MA, Tallman MS, Lo-Coco F. Tricks of the trade for the appropriate management of newly diagnosed acute promyelocytic leukemia. Blood 2005;105(8):3019–3025.

153. Barbui T, Finazzi G, Falanga A. The impact of all-trans-retinoic acid on the coagulopathy of acute promyelocytic leukemia. Blood 1998;91(9):3093–3102.

154. Ohno R, Asou N, Ohnishi K. Treatment of acute promyelocytic leukemia: strategy toward further increase of cure rate. Leukemia 2003;17(8):1454–1463.

155. Marty M, Ganem G, Fischer J, et al. [Acute promyelocytic leukemia: retrospective study of 119 patients treated with daunorubicin]. Nouv Rev Fr Hematol 1984;26(6):371–378.

156. Petti MC, Avvisati G, Amadori S, et al. Acute promyelocytic leukemia: clinical aspects and results of treatment in 62 patients. Haematologica 1987;72(2):151–155.

157. Avvisati G, Petti MC, Lo-Coco F, et al. Induction therapy with idarubicin alone significantly influences event-free survival duration in patients with newly diagnosed hypergranular acute promyelocytic leukemia: final results of the GIMEMA randomized study LAP 0389 with 7 years of minimal follow-up. Blood 2002;100(9):3141–3146.

158. Ades L, Raffoux, E, Chevret S, et al. Is ARAC required in the treatment of newly diagnosed APL? Results of a randomised trial (APL 2000). Blood 2004;104(11):391.

159. Castaigne S, Chomienne C, Daniel MT, et al. All-trans retinoic acid as a differentiation therapy for acute promyelocytic leukemia. I. Clinical results. Blood 1990;76(9):1704–1709.

160. Warrell RP, Jr., Frankel SR, Miller WH, Jr., et al. Differentiation therapy of acute promyelocytic leukemia with tretinoin (all-trans-retinoic acid). N Engl J Med 1991;324(20):1385–1393.

161. Chen ZX, Xue YQ, Zhang R, et al. A clinical and experimental study on all-trans retinoic acid-treated acute promyelocytic leukemia patients. Blood 1991;78(6):1413–1419.

162. Fenaux P, Castaigne S, Dombret H, et al. All-transretinoic acid followed by intensive chemotherapy gives a high complete remission rate and may prolong remissions in newly diagnosed acute promyelocytic leukemia: a pilot study on 26 cases. Blood 1992;80(9):2176–2181.

163. Fenaux P, Le Deley MC, Castaigne S, et al. Effect of all transretinoic acid in newly diagnosed acute promyelocytic leukemia. Results of a multicenter randomized trial. European APL 91 Group. Blood 1993; 82(11):3241–3249.

164. Tallman MS, Andersen JW, Schiffer CA, et al. All-trans-retinoic acid in acute promyelocytic leukemia. N Engl J Med 1997;337(15):1021–1028.

165. Estey EH, Giles FJ, Beran M, et al. Experience with gemtuzumab ozogamycin ("mylotarg") and all-trans retinoic acid in untreated acute promyelocytic leukemia. Blood 2002;99(11):4222–4224.

166. Lo-Coco F, Cimino G, Breccia M, et al. Gemtuzumab ozogamicin (Mylotarg) as a single agent for molecularly relapsed acute promyelocytic leukemia. Blood 2004;104(7):1995–1999.

167. Takeshita A, Shinjo K, Naito K, et al. Efficacy of gemtuzumab ozogamicin on ATRA- and arsenic-resistant acute promyelocytic leukemia (APL) cells. Leukemia 2005;Aug 19(8):1306–1311.

168. Mandelli F, Diverio D, Avvisati G, et al. Molecular remission in PML/RAR alpha-positive acute promyelocytic leukemia by combined all-trans retinoic acid and idarubicin (AIDA) therapy. Gruppo Italiano-Malattie

Ematologiche Maligne dell'Adulto and Associazione Italiana di Ematologia ed Oncologia Pediatrica Cooperative Groups. Blood 1997;90(3):1014–1021.

169. Sanz MA, Martin G, Rayon C, et al. A modified AIDA protocol with anthracycline-based consolidation results in high antileukemic efficacy and reduced toxicity in newly diagnosed PML/RARalpha-positive acute promyelocytic leukemia. PETHEMA group. Blood 1999;94(9):3015–3021.

170. Gallagher RE, Yeap BY, Bi W, et al. Quantitative real-time RT-PCR analysis of PML-RAR alpha mRNA in acute promyelocytic leukemia: assessment of prognostic significance in adult patients from intergroup protocol 0129. Blood 2003;101(7):2521–2528.

171. Lo-Coco F, Breccia M, Diverio D. The importance of molecular monitoring in acute promyelocytic leukaemia. Best Pract Res Clin Haematol 2003;16(3):503–520.

172. Diverio D, Rossi V, Avvisati G, et al. Early detection of relapse by prospective reverse transcriptase-polymerase chain reaction analysis of the PML/RARalpha fusion gene in patients with acute promyelocytic leukemia enrolled in the GIMEMA-AIEOP multicenter "AIDA" trial. GIMEMA-AIEOP Multicenter "AIDA" Trial. Blood 1998;92(3):784–789.

173. Lengfelder E, Reichert A, Schoch C, et al. Double induction strategy including high dose cytarabine in combination with all-trans retinoic acid: effects in patients with newly diagnosed acute promyelocytic leukemia. German AML Cooperative Group. Leukemia 2000;14(8):1362–1370.

174. Kantarjian HM, Keating MJ, Walters RS, Smith TL, McCredie KB, Freireich EJ. Role of maintenance chemotherapy in acute promyelocytic leukemia. Cancer 1987;59(7):1258–1263.

175. Fenaux P, Degos L. Treatment of acute promyelocytic leukemia with all-trans retinoic acid. Leuk Res 1991;15(8):655–657.

176. Avvisati G, Petti M, Lo Coco F, Testi A, Fazi P. AIDA:The Italian Way of Treating Acute Promyelocytic Leukemia (APL), Final Act. Blood 2003;102(11):142a.

177. Frankel SR, Eardley A, Heller G, et al. All-trans retinoic acid for acute promyelocytic leukemia. Results of the New York Study. Ann Intern Med 1994;120(4):278–286.

178. De Botton S, Dombret H, Sanz M, et al. Incidence, clinical features, and outcome of all trans-retinoic acid syndrome in 413 cases of newly diagnosed acute promyelocytic leukemia. The European APL Group. Blood 1998;92(8):2712–2718.

179. Wiley JS, Firkin FC. Reduction of pulmonary toxicity by prednisolone prophylaxis during all-trans retinoic acid treatment of acute promyelocytic leukemia. Australian Leukaemia Study Group. Leukemia 1995;9(5):774–778.

180. Avvisati G, Lo Coco F, Diverio D, et al. AIDA (all-trans retinoic acid + idarubicin) in newly diagnosed acute promyelocytic leukemia: a Gruppo Italiano Malattie Ematologiche Maligne dell'Adulto (GIMEMA) pilot study. Blood 1996;88(4):1390–1398.

181. Santos FL, Dore AI, Lima AS, et al. [Hematological features and expression profile of myeloid antigens of acute promyelocytic leukemia patients: analysis of prognostic factors for development of the retinoic acid syndrome]. Rev Assoc Med Bras 2004;50(3):286–292.

182. Fenaux P, Castaigne S, Chomienne C, Dombret H, Degos L. All trans retinoic acid treatment for patients with acute promyelocytic leukemia. Leukemia 1992;6 (suppl 1):64–66.

183. Tallman MS, Andersen JW, Schiffer CA, et al. Clinical description of 44 patients with acute promyelocytic leukemia who developed the retinoic acid syndrome. Blood 2000;95(1):90–95.

184. Ko BS, Tang JL, Chen YC, et al. Extramedullary relapse after all-trans retinoic acid treatment in acute promyelocytic leukemia—the occurrence of retinoic acid syndrome is a risk factor. Leukemia 1999;13(9):1406–1408.

185. Weiss MA, Warrell RP, Jr. Two cases of extramedullary acute promyelocytic leukemia. Cytogenetics, molecular biology, and phenotypic and clinical studies. Cancer 1994;74(7):1882–1886.

186. Evans GD, Grimwade DJ. Extramedullary disease in acute promyelocytic leukemia. Leuk Lymphoma 1999;33(3–4):219–229.

187. Liso V, Specchia G, Pogliani EM, et al. Extramedullary involvement in patients with acute promyelocytic leukemia: a report of seven cases. Cancer 1998;83(8):1522–1528.

188. Sanz MA, Martin G, Gonzalez M, et al. Risk-adapted treatment of acute promyelocytic leukemia with all-trans-retinoic acid and anthracycline monochemotherapy: a multicenter study by the PETHEMA group. Blood 2004;103(4):1237–1243.

189. Seale J, Delva L, Renesto P, et al. All-trans retinoic acid rapidly decreases cathepsin G synthesis and mRNA expression in acute promyelocytic leukemia. Leukemia 1996;10(1):95–101.

190. Larson RS, Brown DC, Sklar LA. Retinoic acid induces aggregation of the acute promyelocytic leukemia cell line NB-4 by utilization of LFA-1 and ICAM-2. Blood 1997;90(7):2747–2756.

191. Brown DC, Tsuji H, Larson RS. All-trans retinoic acid regulates adhesion mechanism and transmigration of the acute promyelocytic leukaemia cell line NB-4 under physiologic flow. Br J Haematol 1999; 107(1):86–98.

192. Hakimian D, Tallman MS, Zugerman C, Caro WA. Erythema nodosum associated with all-trans-retinoic acid in the treatment of acute promyelocytic leukemia. Leukemia 1993;7(5):758–759.

193. Losada R, Espinosa E, Hernandez C, Dorticos E, Hernandez P. Thrombocytosis in patients with acute promyelocytic leukaemia during all-trans retinoic acid treatment. Br J Haematol 1996;95(4):704–705.

194. Martinez-Chamorro C, Martinez E, Gil-Fernandez JJ, Alonso A, Escudero A, Fernandez-Ranada JM. ATRA-induced myositis in induction therapy of acute promyelocytic leukemia. Haematologica 2002;87(2):ECR08.

195. Miranda N, Oliveira P, Frade MJ, Melo J, Marques MS, Parreira A. Myositis with tretinoin. Lancet 1994;344(8929):1096.

196. Fabbiano F, Magrin S, Cangialosi C, Felice R, Mirto S, Pitrolo F. All-trans retinoic acid induced cardiac and skeletal myositis in induction therapy of acute promyelocytic leukaemia. Br J Haematol 2005;129(3): 444–445.

197. Colucciello M. Pseudotumor cerebri induced by all-trans retinoic acid treatment of acute promyelocytic leukemia. Arch Ophthalmol 2003;121(7):1064–1065.

198. Shirono K, Kiyofuji C, Tsuda H. Sweet's syndrome in a patient with acute promyelocytic leukemia during treatment with all-trans retinoic acid. Int J Hematol 1995;62(3):183–187.

199. Christ E, Linka A, Jacky E, Speich R, Marincek B, Schaffner A. Sweet's syndrome involoving the musculo-skeletal system during treatment of promyelocytic leukemia with all-trans retinoic acid. Leukemia 1996;10(4):731–734.

200. Park CJ, Bae YD, Choi JY, et al. Sweet's syndrome during the treatment of acute promyelocytic leukemia with all-trans retinoic acid. Korean J Intern Med 2001;16(3):218–221.

201. Garcia-Suarez J, Banas H, Krsnik I, De Miguel D, Reyes E, Burgaleta C. Hemophagocytic syndrome associated with retinoic acid syndrome in acute promyelocytic leukemia. Am J Hematol 2004;76(2):172–175.

202. Mourad YA, Jabr F, Salem Z. Scrotal ulceration induced by all-trans retinoic acid in a patient with acute promyelocytic leukemia. Int J Dermatol 2005;44(1):68–69.

203. Goldschmidt N, Gural A, Ben Yehuda D. Extensive splenic infarction, deep vein thrombosis and pulmonary emboli complicating induction therapy with all-trans-retinoic acid (ATRA) for acute promyelocytic leukemia. Leuk Lymphoma 2003;44(8):1433–1437.

204. Torromeo C, Latagliata R, Avvisati G, Petti MC, Mandelli F. Intraventricular thrombosis during all-trans retinoic acid treatment in acute promyelocytic leukemia. Leukemia 2001;15(8):1311–1313.

205. Falanga A, Marchetti M, Barbui T. All-trans-retinoic acid and bleeding/thrombosis. Pathophysiol Haemost Thromb 2003;33 (suppl 1):19–21.

206. Lo Coco F, Diverio D, Falini B, Biondi A, Nervi C, Pelicci PG. Genetic diagnosis and molecular monitoring in the management of acute promyelocytic leukemia. Blood 1999;94(1):12–22.

207. Miller WH, Jr., Kakizuka A, Frankel SR, et al. Reverse transcription polymerase chain reaction for the rearranged retinoic acid receptor alpha clarifies diagnosis and detects minimal residual disease in acute promyelocytic leukemia. Proc Natl Acad Sci USA 1992;89(7):2694–2698.

208. Grimwade D. The pathogenesis of acute promyelocytic leukaemia: evaluation of the role of molecular diagnosis and monitoring in the management of the disease. Br J Haematol 1999;106(3):591–613.

209. Schnittger S, Weisser M, Schoch C, Hiddemann W, Haferlach T, Kern W. New score predicting for prognosis in PML-RARA+, AML1-ETO+, or CBFBMYH11+ acute myeloid leukemia based on quantification of fusion transcripts. Blood 2003;102(8):2746–2755.

210. Wang Z, Sun G, Shen Z, Chen S, Chen Z. Differentiation therapy for acute promyelocytic leukemia with all-trans retinoic acid: 10-year experience of its clinical application. Chin Med J (Engl) 1999;112(11): 963–967.

211. Sun GL, Ouyang RR, Chen SJ, et al. Treatment of acute promyelocytic leukemia with all-trans retinoic acid. A five-year experience. Chin Med J (Engl) 1993;106(10):743–748.

212. Niu C, Yan H, Yu T, et al. Studies on treatment of acute promyelocytic leukemia with arsenic trioxide: remission induction, follow-up, and molecular monitoring in 11 newly diagnosed and 47 relapsed acute promyelocytic leukemia patients. Blood 1999;94(10):3315–3324.

213. Shen ZX, Chen GQ, Ni JH, et al. Use of arsenic trioxide (As2O3) in the treatment of acute promyelocytic leukemia (APL): II. Clinical efficacy and pharmacokinetics in relapsed patients. Blood 1997;89(9): 3354–3360.
214. Wang ZY. Ham-Wasserman lecture: treatment of acute leukemia by inducing differentiation and apoptosis. Hematology (Am Soc Hematol Educ Program) 2003:1–13.
215. Zhang P. The use of arsenic trioxide (As2O3) in the treatment of acute promyelocytic leukemia. J Biol Regul Homeost Agents 1999;13(4):195–200.
216. Mathews V, Balasubramanian P, Shaji RV, George B, Chandy M, Srivastava A. Arsenic trioxide in the treatment of newly diagnosed acute promyelocytic leukemia: a single center experience. Am J Hematol 2002;70(4):292–299.
217. Ghavamzadeh AA, Aghdami M. Treatment of new cases of acute promyelocytic leukemia by arsenic trioxide. In: Am Soc Clin Oncol 39th Annual Meeting, May 31– June 3, 2003; Chicago, IL, 2003.
218. George BM, Vishwabanadhya A. Arsenic trioxide (As_2O_3) in the treatment of patients with newly diagnosed acute promyelocytic leukemia (APML)—toxicity and outcome. Blood 2004;104(11):889.
219. Ghavamzadeh AA, Hamidlah G, et al. Treatment of new cases of acute promyelocytic leukemia by arsenic trioxide. Blood 2004;104(11):396.
220. Soignet SL, Frankel SR, Douer D, et al. United States multicenter study of arsenic trioxide in relapsed acute promyelocytic leukemia. J Clin Oncol 2001;19(18):3852–3860.
221. Dombret H, Fenaux P, Soignet SL, Tallman MS. Established practice in the treatment of patients with acute promyleocytic leukemia and the introduction of arsenic trioxide as a novel therapy. Semin Hematol 2002;39(2 suppl 1):8–13.
222. Shalabi AF, Cheson BD. Arsenic trioxide in relpased or refractory acute promyelocytic leukemia: An NCI special exception (compassionate use) program. Blood 2001;98:596a.
223. Lazo G, Kantarjian H, Estey E, Thomas D, O'Brien S, Cortes J. Use of arsenic trioxide (As_2O_3) in the treatment of patients with acute promyelocytic leukemia: the M. D. Anderson experience. Cancer 2003;97(9): 2218–2224.
224. Au WYC, Lie AK, at al. Teatment of relapsed acute promyelocytic leukemia by arsenic-based strategies without hematopoietic stem cell transplantation in Hong Kong: a seven-year experince. Blood 2004; 104(11):395.
225. Douer D, Hu W, Giralt S, Lill M, DiPersio J. Arsenic trioxide (trisenox) therapy for acute promyelocytic leukemia in the setting of hematopoietic stem cell transplantation. Oncologist 2003;8(2):132–140.
226. Leoni F, Gianfaldoni G, Annunziata M, et al. Arsenic trioxide therapy for relapsed acute promyelocytic leukemia: a bridge to transplantation. Haematologica 2002;87(5):485–489.
227. Shen ZX, Shi ZZ, Fang J, et al. All-trans retinoic acid/As_2O_3 combination yields a high quality remission and survival in newly diagnosed acute promyelocytic leukemia. Proc Natl Acad Sci USA 2004;101(15): 5328–5335.
228. Estey EF, Giles F. All-trans retinoic acid (ATRA) +arsenic trioxide (ATO) to minimize or eliminate chemotherapy in untreated APL. Blood 2003;102:618a–619a.
229. Estey EG-M, Ferrajoli A, et al. Use of all-transretinoic acid (ATRA) + arsenic trioxide (ATO) to eliminate or minimize use of dhemotherapy (CT) in untreated acute promyelocytic leukemia. Blood 2004; 104(11):393.
230. Shao W, Fanelli M, Ferrara FF, et al. Arsenic trioxide as an inducer of apoptosis and loss of PML/RAR alpha protein in acute promyelocytic leukemia cells. J Natl Cancer Inst 1998;90(2):124–133.
231. Jing Y, Dai J, Chalmers-Redman RM, Tatton WG, Waxman S. Arsenic trioxide selectively induces acute promyelocytic leukemia cell apoptosis via a hydrogen peroxide-dependent pathway. Blood 1999;94(6): 2102–2111.
232. Kitamura K, Minami Y, Yamamoto K, et al. Involvement of CD95-independent caspase 8 activation in arsenic trioxide-induced apoptosis. Leukemia 2000;14(10):1743–1750.
233. Dai J, Weinberg RS, Waxman S, Jing Y. Malignant cells can be sensitized to undergo growth inhibition and apoptosis by arsenic trioxide through modulation of the glutathione redox system. Blood 1999;93(1): 268–277.
234. Davison K, Cote S, Mader S, Miller WH. Glutathione depletion overcomes resistance to arsenic trioxide in arsenic-resistant cell lines. Leukemia 2003;17(5):931–940.
235. Camacho LH, Soignet SL, Chanel S, et al. Leukocytosis and the retinoic acid syndrome in patients with acute promyelocytic leukemia treated with arsenic trioxide. J Clin Oncol 2000;18(13):2620–2625.

236. Che-Pin L, Huang MJ, Chang IY, Lin WY, Sheu YT. Retinoic acid syndrome induced by arsenic trioxide in treating recurrent all-trans retinoic acid resistant acute promyelocytic leukemia. Leuk Lymphoma 2000; 38(1–2):195–198.
237. Douer DT, MS. Arsenic trioxide: new clinical experience with an old medication in hematologic malignancies. J Clin Oncol 2005;23:2396–2410.
238. Ohnishi K, Yoshida H, Shigeno K, et al. Prolongation of the QT interval and ventricular tachycardia in patients treated with arsenic trioxide for acute promyelocytic leukemia. Ann Intern Med 2000;133(11): 881–885.
239. Unnikrishnan D, Dutcher JP, Varshneya N, et al. Torsades de pointes in 3 patients with leukemia treated with arsenic trioxide. Blood 2001;97(5):1514–1516.
240. Westervelt P, Brown RA, Adkins DR, et al. Sudden death among patients with acute promyelocytic leukemia treated with arsenic trioxide. Blood 2001;98(2):266–271.
241. Barbey JT, Pezzullo JC, Soignet SL. Effect of arsenic trioxide on QT interval in patients with advanced malignancies. J Clin Oncol 2003;21(19):3609–3615.
242. Singer JK, B; Frank K. Safety experience with Trisenox (arsenic trioxide). Blood 2003;102:509b.
243. Ficker E, Kuryshev YA, Dennis AT, et al. Mechanisms of arsenic-induced prolongation of cardiac repolarization. Mol Pharmacol 2004;66(1):33–44.
244. Huang SY, Chang CS, Tang JL, et al. Acute and chronic arsenic poisoning associated with treatment of acute promyelocytic leukaemia. Br J Haematol 1998;103(4):1092–1095.
245. Mandelli F, Labopin M, Granena A, et al. European survey of bone marrow transplantation in acute promyelocytic leukemia (M3). Working Party on Acute Leukemia of the European Cooperative Group for Bone Marrow Transplantation (EMBT). Bone Marrow Transplant 1994;14(2):293–298.
246. de Botton S, Fawaz A, Chevret S, et al. Autologous and allogeneic stem-cell transplantation as salvage treatment of acute promyelocytic leukemia initially treated with all-trans-retinoic acid: a retrospective analysis of the European acute promyelocytic leukemia group. J Clin Oncol 2005;23(1):120–126.
247. Meloni G, Diverio D, Vignetti M, et al. Autologous bone marrow transplantation for acute promyelocytic leukemia in second remission: prognostic relevance of pretransplant minimal residual disease assessment by reverse-transcription polymerase chain reaction of the PML/RAR alpha fusion gene. Blood 1997;90(3):1321–1315.
248. Ferrara F, Palmieri S, Annunziata M, Pocali B, Viola A, Pane F. Prolonged molecular remission after autologous stem cell transplantation in relapsed acute promyelocytic leukemia. Haematologica 2004;89(5): 621–622.
249. Lo-Coco F, Romano A, Mengarelli A, et al. Allogeneic stem cell transplantation for advanced acute promyelocytic leukemia: results in patients treated in second molecular remission or with molecularly persistent disease. Leukemia 2003;17(10):1930–1933.
250. Iguchi T, Yokoyama K, Miyamoto K, et al. [Successful bone marrow transplantation with a matched unrelated donor in an acute promyelocytic leukemia patient after reinduction therapy with arsenic trioxide]. Rinsho Ketsueki 2004;45(1):75–77.
251. Borrow J, Goddard AD, Gibbons B, et al. Diagnosis of acute promyelocytic leukaemia by RT-PCR: detection of PML-RARA and RARA-PML fusion transcripts. Br J Haematol 1992;82(3):529–540.
252. Alcalay M, Zangrilli D, Fagioli M, et al. Expression pattern of the RAR alpha-PML fusion gene in acute promyelocytic leukemia. Proc Natl Acad Sci USA 1992;89(11):4840–4844.
253. Asou N, Adachi K, Tamura U, et al. Analysis of prognostic factors in newly diagnosed patients with acute promyelocytic leukemia: the APL92 study of the Japan Adult Leukemia Study Group (JALSG). Cancer Chemother Pharmacol 2001;48 (suppl 1):S65–S71.
254. Sanz MA, Jarque I, Martin G, et al. Acute promyelocytic leukemia. Therapy results and prognostic factors. Cancer 1988;61(1):7–13.
255. Jurcic JG, Nimer SD, Scheinberg DA, DeBlasio T, Warrell RP, Jr., Miller WH, Jr. Prognostic significance of minimal residual disease detection and PML/RAR-alpha isoform type: long-term follow-up in acute promyelocytic leukemia. Blood 2001;98(9):2651–2656.
256. Murray CK, Estey E, Paietta E, et al. CD56 expression in acute promyelocytic leukemia: a possible indicator of poor treatment outcome? J Clin Oncol 1999;17(1):293–297.
257. Ito S, Ishida Y, Oyake T, et al. Clinical and biological significance of CD56 antigen expression in acute promyelocytic leukemia. Leuk Lymphoma 2004;45(9):1783–1789.
258. Lee JJ, Cho D, Chung IJ, et al. CD34 expression is associated with poor clinical outcome in patients with acute promyelocytic leukemia. Am J Hematol 2003;73(3):149–153.

259. Candoni A, Damiani D, Michelutti A, et al. Clinical characteristics, prognostic factors and multidrug-resistance related protein expression in 36 adult patients with acute promyelocytic leukemia. Eur J Haematol 2003;71(1):1–8.
260. Chim CS, Wong SY, Kwong YL. Aberrant gene promoter methylation in acute promyelocytic leukaemia: profile and prognostic significance. Br J Haematol 2003;122(4):571–578.
261. Sun HD, Ma L, Hu XC, Zhang TD. AiLin I treated 32 cases of acute promyelocytic leukemia. Chin J Integrat Chin West Med 1992;12:170–171.
262. Zhang P, Wang SY, Hu XH. Arsenic trioxide treated 72 cases of acute promyelocytic leukemia. Chin J Hematol 1996;17:58–62.

IV   MOLECULAR THERAPEUTICS OF AML: SELECTED TARGETED APPROACHES

10 Emerging Therapeutics for AML

Edward A. Sausville

CONTENTS

INTRODUCTION
PRECLINICAL STUDIES
COMBINATIONS IN PRECLINICAL STUDY
RECENT CLINICAL TRIALS
CONCLUSIONS
REFERENCES

Summary

Emerging therapeutics for acute myeloid leukemia (AML) have evolved from disparate sources. In addition to oncogene, epigenetic, or cytokine pathway-directed therapies (discussed in other chapters), recent research has defined an eclectic collection of novel opportunities in leukemia treatment. These derive variously from natural products, including aplidine and triterpenoids; synthetic chemicals such as adaphostin; and biologicals such as antibody-directed therapeutics. This chapter will endeavor to summarize the state of preclinical and clinical development of these treatments and to define emerging trends in leukemia directed developmental therapeutics. Strategies to modulate resistance, either intrinsic or acquired, are of continued importance; however, strategies to evoke leukemic cell "stress" by perturbing signaling pathways are of great interest to explore further. Likely progress in the latter goal will be achieved by defining combinations of novel targeted agents. These are envisioned to allow modulation of cytotoxicity evoked not only by classical agents, but also by affecting critical pathways activated during leukemogenesis to sustain the leukemic cell's survival. These approaches will, it is hoped, augment the success of, or provide totally new, strategies to achieve response and improve survival of patients with AML.

Key Words: New agents; targeted therapy; vaccines; VEGF signaling; adaphostin; triterpenoids.

1. INTRODUCTION

Acute myeloid leukemia (AML) presents both an enormous set of opportunities as well as challenges. For developers of novel drugs, AML, like other hematological neoplasms, offers the intellectual and practical satisfaction of allowing very readily the opportunity to assess the ability of a novel treatment to affect its intended target and therefore of providing "real-time" feedback to the development process. However, AML is clearly a heterogeneous collection of diseases for which gene-based classifications are potentially possible *(1,2)*, but where for the most part the promise of biological guidance in the design and selection of therapy has yet to reach clinical practice. AML treatment utilizes standard approaches that are the same in many of their particulars now as they were 20 years ago, with the promise of ultimate curative value in at best 40% of patients in "average prognosis" groups. At worst,

From: *Contemporary Hematology: Acute Myelogenous Leukemia*
Edited by: J. E. Karp © Humana Press Inc., Totowa, NJ

for certain subtypes curative potential is far less frequent, because patients with unfavorable cytogenetics including many elderly patients possess either intrinsically resistant disease to the lynchpin agents of current therapy or have medical impediments to the successful completion of such regimens. The noteworthy counterexample that stands in contrast to these concerns is the continuing success of building retinoids into the up-front and maintenance therapy of acute promyelocytic leukemia *(3)*. Nonetheless, the achievement of cures in any fraction of patients with AML is a major achievement, and current regimens, despite their limitations, are the considered result of painstaking clinical research over the past 50 years.

The goal of this chapter is to consider a range of current therapeutic agents and strategies that are very early in their potential development or application to AML. Other chapters will consider more focused approaches, including cytokines, FLT3 and farnesyl transferase inhibitors, epigenetic modulation (including DNA methyltransferase inhibitors and histone deacetylase inhibitors) and differentiation-based strategies.

A conceptual framework that may be useful in considering further opportunities departs from the proposal of Gilliland and colleagues that a "successful" leukemic state in AML (in terms of causing clinically dire disease for a patient) arises from that patient's dominant malignant clone containing certain combinations of genetic lesions that block differentiation along normal hematopoietic precursor pathways, as well as those that activate proliferation pathways by, for example, certain tyrosine kinases, as exemplified by flt3 *(4)*. In addition, the successful AML cell will adopt one or more anti-apoptotic strategies, including bcl2 family members and other anti-anti-apoptotic, pro-survival molecules *(5,6)*. Included as contributing to such influences are more general, poorly understood "cell stress buffers," which defend against redox, unfolded protein, DNA damage, and mitotic spindle lesions. Their characterization in AML, as in other tumor types, remains at an early stage, and these could be the basis of therapeutic strategies in their own right.

One thesis to consider in developing novel therapeutic approaches to AML is that the genetic lesions now defined by cytogenetic approaches may suggest particular targets for drug-discovery campaigns, while the regulators of cell stress pathways may provide a basis of increasing susceptibility to pro-apoptotic signals. These cell stress-related systems could take advantage of the transient function of the normal progeny of myeloid differentiation in challenging environments, such as the sites of inflammatory lesions, where the cells must survive in hypoxic, poorly perfused, and pathogen-rich states, and then die with the successful completion of their task in defending the organism. By this reasoning, understanding in a more refined way how myeloid cell stress is modulated in relation to activation of growth-regulatory pathways might suggest novel therapeutic strategies. Implicit in this reasoning is the need for combinations of agents. One member of a useful combination of this type would affect a survival or proliferation signal, and another would modulate the cellular stress emerging from the signaling-directed agent's activity. This theme has emerged in several recent preclinical studies to be discussed here and is poised to enter into clinical studies as well.

2. PRECLINICAL STUDIES

2.1. Novel Cytotoxics

2.1.1. CDK INHIBITORS

Flavopiridol is a semi-synthetic flavonoid originally of interest as an inhibitor of cyclin-dependent kinases *(7)*. More recent studies have defined that in addition to regulating progression through the cell cycle, CDK family members also encompass activities regulating transcription as well as secretory cell and neuronal function *(8)*, an outcome that has complicated the clinical development of CDK inhibitors. Nonetheless, older preclinical data emphasized the potential capacity of this agent to affect AML cells in in vitro and in vivo models *(9)*. A property particularly relevant to AML treatment is the recently defined capacity of flavopiridol to cause evidence of mitochondrial dysfunction and induction of apoptosis in AML cells in combination with phorbol 12-myristate,13-acetate *(10)*, even in the presence of cells engineered to express bcl2. Because flavopiridol enhanced the dephosphorylation of the phospho-RB tumor suppressor protein, flavopiridol's capacity to downmodulate CDK activity may have contributed to this outcome. Alternatively, an entirely novel flavopiridol target may be relevant to this effect. Subsequent studies have confirmed an influence of flavopiridol on the mitochondrial pathway of apoptosis. Specifically, flavopiridol- mediated induction of apoptosis in U937 cells was not influenced by expression of bcl2 full-length protein (in contrast to cytosine-arabinoside-induced lethality), while surprisingly the same cells expressing a bcl2-loop deleted (residues 32–80) protein were resistant to flavopiridol-mediated apoptosis, and inhibitors of caspase 8 activation did not attenuate flavopiridol-mediated apoptosis *(11)*.

Nakanishi et al. evaluated cells isolated from patients with AML for sensitivity to flavopiridol and observed little correlation of flavopiridol sensitivity to expression of the multidrug-resistance protein PGP(mdr-1). In contrast, the breast cancer resistance protein (BCRP) mRNA expression correlated with cellular viability to a fixed concentration of flavopiridol *(12)*.

The recent recognition from clinical studies in chronic lymphocytic leukemia that "hybrid" bolus/infusion schedules of administration of flavopiridol *(13)* may have value in maximizing responses calls for an evaluation of these schedules in AML also, as well as a definition of whether transcriptional effects on cell survival genes or cell cycle regulatory endpoints are most important in mediating cell killing by "pan CDK inhibitors." The evaluation of other CDK inhibitors including such clinically available molecules as R-Roscovitine and BMS-387032 in AML preclinical models or in patients has not been completed.

2.1.2. ADAPHOSTIN

AG957 is a tyrphostin originally found to have anti p210[bcr/abl] activity in vitro *(14)* and in living cells *(15)*. In addition, it clearly modulates tyrosine kinase signaling in non-chronic myeloid leukemia cells *(16)*. Adaphostin is a derivative of the tyrphostin AG957 with improved pharmacokinetic features *(17)*. Svingen and colleagues demonstrated that in addition to direct inhibition of p210[bcr/abl], adaphostin in living cells shared with AG957 the capacity to downregulate the expression of native p210[bcr/abl] *(18)*. Chandra and colleagues recently demonstrated that in a variety of cells including isolates from patients with AML, adaphostin in addition caused intracellular peroxide production, DNA strand breaks, and evidence of activation of p53 damage response pathways in p53 wild-type cells *(19)*. These studies raise the possibility that in addition to modulation of tyrosine kinase signaling, adaphostin can modulate redox susceptibility in hematopoietic cells including AML-derived blasts. Yu and colleagues amplified these findings by confirming the capacity of adaphostin to diminish signaling downstream of tyrosine kinases including MEK, ERK1/2, and Akt in cells of both myeloid (U937) and lymphoid (Jurkat) lineages, as well of antioxidants to attenuate adaphostin-mediated toxicity *(20)*. In addition, this study provided evidence that activation of MEK, raf, and akt signaling in adaphostin-exposed cells could also attenuate drug-induced apoptosis, but did not block adaphostin-mediated generation of reactive oxygen species. These studies clearly demonstrate that both signaling and redox-related effects are attributable to adapostin.

Monks et al. very recently *(21)* have provided one potential basis for adaphostin-mediated generation of redox active species by demonstrating that adaphostin could alter intracellular labile Fe homeostasis. This would potentially provide a source of radical generation by, for example, Fenton reaction-derived H_2O_2, O_2^-, and $\cdot OH$ species. The source of the released Fe was not clear and remains to be defined, as does the relevance of this mechanism to adaphostin cytotoxicity in a broader range of cell types. Of interest, therefore, is the possibility that adaphostin has the dual capacity to modulate signaling of cell survival pathways while serving as a source of cell-damaging free radical intermediates.

2.1.3. RAPAMYCIN

Great interest has recently focused on the mammalian target of rapamycin (mTOR) as a mediator of signaling downstream of the Akt proto-oncogene, which mediates enhanced translational capacity of cancer cells. Recher and colleagues have documented *(22)* that rapamycin caused prominent diminution of the clonogenic capacity of AML cells obtained from patients in comparison to its effects on normal hematopoietic precursors, with evidence of downmodulation of phosphorylation of the mTOR targets 4EBP1 and p70S6K. In selected cell lines there was block in G0 or G1. Preliminary evidence of clinical benefit in relapsed and refractory acute myeloid leukemia patients was also noted.

2.1.4. NOVEL TRITERPENOIDS

Sporn and colleagues introduced the novel triterpenoid 2-cyano-3,12-dioxooleana-1,9,-dien-28-oic acid (CDDO) and its methyl ester as a modulator of a variety of signal transduction pathways in human leukemia cells, including nuclear factor (NF)κB and sustained activation of the c-Jun N-terminal kinase, with prominent induction of apoptosis induced in every leukemia cell line tested including those with overexpression of pro-survival bcl family members *(23)*. Reed et al. confirmed prominent induction of apoptosis by these compounds in AML cells and in addition demonstrated prominent activation of caspase 8, potentially by downregulating FLIP, an endogenous caspase 8 inhibitor *(24)*.

A basis for mechanistic pleiotropy for CDDO and its derivatives was suggested by the studies of Kufe et al. *(25)*, which documented that CDDO increased reactive oxygen intermediates with prominent diminution of glutathione, a feature shared by CDDO's methyl and imidazolide esters. Apoptosis was diminished by addition of *N*-acetylcysteine or glutathione, further implicating the capacity to alter redox status as a prominent mechanistic feature of the drugs. Further confirming the potential import of redox regulation in triterpenoid action, Konopleva et al. *(26)* have recently demonstrated a capacity of CDDO to directly release cytochrome c from isolated mitochondria, raising the possibility that the compound has a unique ability to affect a mitochondrial target directly.

A plethora of other phenomena have been associated with CDDO action in leukemia as well as other cell types, including suppression of ERK signaling with p38 stress kinase activation *(27)*; downregulation of PML/RARα in the NB4 APL cell line as well as in primary APL isolates, with sensitization to arsenic trioxide-related apoptosis *(28)*; modulation of peroxisome proliferator-activated receptor(PPAR)-γ-signaling and heme oxygenase-1, Nrf2/ARE *(29,30)*; as well as inappropriate elevations of Ca^{2+}, albeit the latter effect was in epithelial cells *(31)*. A unifying mechanism to explicate the phenomena associated with CDDO and its derivatives is currently not available. Since the compound is an α, β unsaturated ketone, the possibility exists that a central feature of its action could be alkylation by the drug of thiols. These thiol moieties could either be small redox buffers, such as glutathione, or thiols in a variety of target proteins, depending on the affinity of the drug for the region of the target protein bearing the thiol. The resulting cellular dysfunction may then vary depending on the pathway affected as well as activation of proteolytic mechanisms to degrade the damaged proteins. Whether triterpenoids will have a therapeutic index in human subjects will be of interest, but the ultimate basis for their value may lie at least in part in the relative susceptibility of leukemic cells to redox stress.

2.1.5. 2-METHOXYESTRADIOL

This metabolite of estrogen was found to have anti-angiogenic and antiproliferative properties and has been demonstrated to bind to the colchicine site of tubulin in a way that differs from other known antimicrotubule agents *(32,33)*. Gao et al. have recently demonstrated that in U937 cells 2-methoxyestradiol was able to activate an apoptotic pathway in a way that was attenuated by activation of the Akt pathway and by redox scavengers, including catalase and a superoxide dismutase mimetic *(34)*. A model for 2-methoxyestradiol action was proposed that may be distinct for leukemia cells in that primary oxidative rather than tubulin-mediated damage is proposed, initiating the apoptotic pathway. This would be an important correlate of clinical trials that are now possible with this compound.

2.1.6. APLIDINE

This is a most interesting novel marine natural product that demonstrated preclinical activity in acute lymphoid blasts in a way that is thought to be somewhat sparing of normal myelopoeisis. The compound, a depsipeptide, also displayed potent capacity to inhibit proliferation of AML-derived cell lines under conditions where it also appeared to decrease elaboration of vascular endothelial growth factor (VEGF) *(35)*. These preclinical results clearly support the entry of the molecule, which is in phase II studies in solid tumors, into human studies in patients with AML.

2.2. Novel Biologics

2.2.1. ANTI-CD33

Anti-CD33-directed therapies continue to dominate the field of emerging biological approaches to treat AML. Interestingly, Balanian and Ball *(36)* found that unconjugated anti- CD33 itself amplified cytosine arabinoside- and idarubicin-mediated diminution of primary AML isolate proliferation and clonogenicity, but not the effects evoked by bryostatin or VP16-213, a property recently explored in a phase III trial to be described below.

A targeted effect utilizing an anti-CD33 directed antibody is the basis for the clinically approved gemtuzumab ozogamicin (GO; Mylotarg®) *(37)*. This drug utilizes a humanized anti-CD33 antibody to deliver the extremely potent ene-diyne antibiotic calicheamicin to cells expressing the CD33 determinant. However, certain infrequently observed but medically troublesome toxicities with this agent, including hepatic vein thrombosis *(38)*, argue for continuing consideration of alternate toxicity-conveying elements utilizing the anti-CD33 delivery strategy. Marks et al. *(39)* describe the creation of an antibody–amphipathic peptide construct, which did kill one of three AML cell lines. Because the antibody–peptide conjugate must be properly internalized, a basis for resistance clearly exists and optimally some ability to define the capacity for internalization should be developed to optimize this strategy.

2.2.2. CYTOKINES

AML cells express receptors for a variety of cytokines including colony-stimulating factors, interleukins, fibroblast growth factors (FGFs), and VEGF. Recent preclinical studies have been summarized showing that downstream signaling pathways activated by these receptors through Raf/MEK/ERK and PI3 kinase pathways may be suitable for the development of novel therapeutic strategies *(40)*.

VEGF in particular has emerged as a key mediator in pathways participating in an "autocrine" loop in AML cells, in particular through the VEGF receptor 2(VEGF-R2 or KDR). This pathway operates both through external stimulation, as an anti-VEGF antibody was capable of blocking NFκB activation, and intracellular pathways, as an intracellularly acting inhibitor of KDR function prominently inhibited the operation of both the PI3 kinase and MAP kinase pathways, with inception of apoptosis *(41)*. Interestingly, the anti-VEGF antibody alone had little effect on cell survival, emphasizing the importance of the internal pathway.

Another important receptor present in a subset of leukemia cells is the FLT3 receptor, discussed elsewhere in this volume. Of interest here is the demonstration that FLT3 activated by mutations in the juxtamembrane domain activated the transcription of distinct gene subsets, distinct from gene sets found in AML cells with wild-type or N-ras point mutants *(42)*. Discriminating genes included genes prominently involved in cell cycle control, gene transcription, and signal transduction. This emphasizes the potential for selection of drug targets based on the expression patterns of genes and perhaps ultimately the selection of patients for treatment using these approaches. Likewise, basic FGF was found to be expressed by immunohistochemistry in bone marrow biopsies from AML patients *(43)*. AML cell lines in the same study exposed to FGF had augmented colony formation that is blocked by an anti-FGF antibody. Lacking at present, however, is a clear perception of the "heirarchy" of growth factor control of AML cell proliferation. The possibility exists that truly valuable agents in AML would be agents that act across the targets of several signaling systems or combined agents directed at respective "most important" signaling systems.

3. COMBINATIONS IN PRECLINICAL STUDY

A key concept guiding the evolution of current regimens to treat AML was the value of combinations of agents as a basis for therapeutic success. In the currently widely used cytotoxic regimens, combinations evolved driven in many cases by pharmacological considerations related to what toxicities were tolerable in given dosing regimens. The advent of so-called molecularly targeted cancer therapeutics allows the concept of drug treatments tailored to disrupt pathways important in maintaining a "successful" cancer cell *(44,45)*, including uncontrolled proliferation, disordered cell death regulation, and loss of tumor suppressor mechanisms (all of which could be construed as being targeted by "conventional cytotoxics") as well as the more recently recognized capacity of tumor cells to acquire the capacity to divide indefinitely and activate altered stroma functions including invasion and angiogenesis. The interesting possibility in considering strategies for AML "regimen building" is the possibility that cytotoxic chemotherapy could be regarded as either a perturbation of proliferation or as an activator of cell stress response pathways. These pathways in turn become targets for drug development in an effort to augment cell stress. This is combination therapy with a new twist, driven not solely by pharmacological opportunity, but rather by a consideration of the biological function of cellular pathways responding to stress. Several recent studies have considered different strategies to address these goals.

3.1. Protein Kinase Modulation

Grant and colleagues *(46)* have demonstrated that modulators of protein kinase C (PKC), including bryostatin (which transiently activates and then downregulates PKC) and the PKC inhibitors staurosporine and 7-hydroxystaurosporine (UCN-01), could sensitize cells made resistant to ara-C by overexpression of bcl2. This was manifest by increased apoptosis as well as colony-forming assays. These workers also demonstrated that PKC-dependent pathways influenced AML cell response to flavopiridol. One aspect contributing to bryostatin's enhancement of flavopiridol-mediated apoptosis was postulated to be through upregulation of signaling through the tumor necrosis factor (TNF)-α pathway *(47)*, as the combination of bryostatin and flavopiridol evoked increased release of TNF-α. Apoptosis was retarded by expression of a TNF receptor-dominant negative death domain. Interestingly, the pro-survival molecule mcl-1 was downregulated, likely reflecting flavopiridol's inhibition of mcl1 mRNA synthesis thorough effects on the transcription-related CDK family members *(8)*. Flavopiridol was also demonstrated to augment induction of apoptosis and downegulation of mcl-1, activation of JNK kinase, and diminished expression of p21$^{WAF1/CIP1}$ in the setting of con-comitant proteosome inhibition in another study *(48)*. A mechanism causing these latter effects was proposed to be the diminished DNA binding of NFκB in the setting of cell cycle blockade and transcriptional modulation induced by flavopiridol. Thus, flavopiridol interaction with the therapeutic effect of the proteosome inhibitor could occur through CDK-related effects (augmentation of cell cycle block; decrease of mcl1), as well as through a kinase target to be defined (affecting NFκB).

UCN-01 (7-hydroxystaurosporine) is a protein kinase inhibitor with three principal sets of potent (IC$_{50}$ <50 n*M*) activities. It inhibits PKCs of the α,β,γ-classes, with less potent (5- to 10-fold) activity against PKCs δ and ε, and is without activity against PKCζ *(49)*. It was sub-sequently recognized to be a potent inhibitor of the DNA damage-activated checkpoint kinase chk1 *(50,51)*, with some evidence of ability to modulate chk2 under certain conditions *(52)*. Most recently, Tsuruo et al. have demonstrated UCN-01 as capable of modulating akt signal-ing through its capacity for inhibition of the phospatidylinositide-dependent kinase (PDK)1 *(53)*. The latter activity is thought to contribute substantially to the clinically observed but manageable toxicity of hyperglycemia *(54,55)*. Although UCN-01 has been incompletely evaluated in AML as a single agent, substantial preclinical studies would support its further evaluation, particularly in combination with agents modulating other proliferation pathways.

In U937 cells, UCN-01 alone caused evidence of cell cycle arrest, with paradoxical activation of MEK/ERK signaling and activation of the c-Jun N terminal kinase activity *(56)*. In combination with farnesyl transferase inhibitors, UCN-01 caused noteworthy apoptosis, evidenced by prominent mitochondrial dysfunction. Which of the kinases sensitive to UCN-01 was most responsible for this outcome was not clear, although protection from apoptosis by transfection of a constitutively activated, myristoylated akt but not MEK did call attention to the PDK1-related pathways *(57)*.

If akt-related signaling is of great importance in AML, a possibility well supported by the observations of Andreef, Carroll, and colleagues in freshly isolated leukemic cells *(58,59)*, then targeting of cells with UCN-01 (to modulate PDK signaling) and rapamycin (to modulate mTOR activation) might be of value. This is supported by marked synergism of UCN-01 and rapamycin *(60)* in inducing apoptosis in U937 cells, although in these studies co-administration of constitutively activated MEK and of inhibitors of JNK activation also somewhat attenuated the effect of the combination.

Other studies with UCN-01 in AML cells have focused on its ability to modulate sensitivity to cytotoxic agents, presumptively by its prominent capacity to modulate PKC or chk kinase function. Shao et al. *(61)* demonstrated that in HL60 AML cells, as expected, UCN-01 inhi-bited PKCs β and δ with little effect on PKCζ. PKCα was also inhibited shortly after addition, but its activity increased as cells went into apoptosis, a finding enhanced by co-administration of camptothecin and etoposide and attributed to PKCα's hyperphosphorylation. Alteration of PKC activities was proposed to emanate in part from activation of apoptosis-related caspases. Plunkett et al. *(62)* took a somewhat different tack, using low, cytostatic concentrations of fludarabine to arrest AML cells in S phase, with increased Tyr 15 phosphorylation of CDK2 suggesting the primary mediation of the effect by inhibition of chk1/cdc25 phosphatase DNA damage response pathway. Immunocomplex coprecipitation studies supoprted this idea by demonstrating complexes containing CDK2, CDC25A, and Chk1. Subsequent addition of UCN-01 to the fludarabine-arrested cells demonstrated prominent exit from S phase, loss of CDK2 Tyr 15 phosphorylation, and increase of cdc25 phosphatase A activity. These results strongly support the idea of further clinical pursuit in AML of activity-modulating strategies employing UCN-01 with S-phase checkpoint-activating strategies. The fact that UCN-01 actually should not be thought of as working only through PKC was called to the fore by recent studies of Grant et al. *(63)* demonstrating that co-administration of the PKC modulator bisindolylmaleimide could reverse bryostatin-mediated potentiation of ara-C toxicity, but not that invoked by UCN-01. Modulation, however, of the mitochondrial pathway of apoptosis appeared to attenuate UCN-01/araC toxicity but not that of bryostatin/ara C, concordant with this group's prior observations *(46)*.

3.2. Heat Shock Protein (hsp)90 Modulators

Heat shock proteins have been increasingly recognized as mediating crucial aspects of the folding and proper intracellular location of an increasing list of proteins. Hsp90 is a key regulator of the folding state of such "client" proteins as tyrosine kinase receptors, cell cycle checkpoint modulators (such as chk1), and steroid hormone receptors *(64)*. Because survival of cells exposed to nucleoside analogs is clearly influenced by the intactness of the chk1 pathway, it became of interest to define the effect of modulators of hsp90 such as the clinically available 17-allylamino,17-demethoxygeldanamycin (17-AAG). Mesa et al. *(65)* demonstrated that low concentrations of ara-C could activate chk1, with S-phase slowing. Concomitant treatment with clinically achievable concentrations of 17-AAG greatly decreased colony formation by AML cells. This effect was mimicked by si-RNA-mediated depletion of chk-1, but not by disruption of signaling through PI-3K. These results support clinical studies of combinations of ara-C and hsp90 modulators in AML.

3.3. Histone Deacetylase Inhibitors

Histone deacetylase inhibitors (HDACI)s have been proposed as major therapeutic opportunities owing to their ability to relieve repression of aberrant transcription in cancer cells, particularly AML *(66,67)*. Several aspects of HDACI pharmacology and clinical staudies are described elsewhere in this volume. One major pathway modulated by HDACIs in AML cells is through NFκB. Both of the HDACIs MS-275 and suberoylanilide hydroxamic acid (SAHA) caused hyperacetylation and nuclear translocation of RelA/p65 and activation of genes governed by NFκB. Pharmacological inhibitors or genetic strategies to modulate NFκB markedly potentiated apoptosis induced by HDACIs, the latter occurring in the face of increased reactive oxygen species and activation of JNK *(68)*. Modulation of NFκB-regulated pathways would be expected to act as a potentiator of apoptosis relevant to drugs affecting several other pathways. Indeed, minimally toxic concentrations of fludarabine are potentiated by MS-275 with augmented activation of mitochondrial injury pathways, but without change in fludarabine triphosphate formation or incorporation of enhanced fludarabine into DNA *(69)*.

Perifosine is an alkylphospholipid recently recognized as clearly affecting akt signaling *(70)*. HDAC inhibitors co-administered with perifosine to myeloid and lymphoid leukemia cell lines caused enhanced apoptosis, evidence of caspase 3 and 8 activation, and inactivation of ERK1/2 and Akt. Because apoptosis was partially blocked by constitutively active, myristoylated Akt, as well as by expressed activated MEK signaling, modulation of signaling through both pathways could plausibly be related to the combined action of these agents *(71)*.

Bhalla and colleagues recently demonstrated that certain HDACIs were also capable of inducing not only acetylation of histones, but also Hsp90, with modulation of Hsp90 function in a way that mimicked direct modulators of Hsp90 function *(72)*. Whether this implies a second way to modulate Hsp90 function that is truly distinct from those afforded by the geldanamycins or related molecules will be of interest to explore clinically.

4. RECENT CLINICAL TRIALS

Addition of new agents to "standard" induction regimens is a time-honored approach to constructing new regimens for AML. For example, cladribine has been added in the salvage setting to ara-C and mitoxantrone with granulocyte colony-stimulating factor (G-CSF) to form the CLAG-M regimen. In 43 patients (25 primary resistant and 18 relapsed), complete response (CR) was obtained in 49% of patients, with 69% of those disease-free at 1 year *(73)*. Although the authors felt cladribine definitely added value to the regimen, comparative trials would be needed to assess its real contribution.

While these types of studies may define ultimately valuable additions to the AML therapeutic armamentarium, other novel clinical strategies in AML would derive from the preclinical studies described above, with attempts to modulate the key molecules in specific pathways known to be important in leukemogenesis. The following trials are but the vanguard of this latter type, hoping to manipulate pathways sustaining the viability of the malignant cell as targets for intervention.

4.1. Small Molecules

4.1.1. ANGIOGENESIS MODULATORS

The VEGF-R antagonist SU5416 was studied in a cohort of 43 patients with refractory AML or elderly patients not judged to be medically fit for intensive induction chemotherapy. One patient had a morphological CR of 2 months' duration, while seven patients had a greater than 50% reduction in blasts for 1–5 months. A trend toward better response in patients with high levels of VEGF by polymerase chain reaction was observed *(74)*. Because of preliminary evidence of efficacy in myelodysplastic syndromes, thalidomide was studied at 200–400 mg per day in a phase I/II study, and partial responses (PRs; decrease in blast cell marrow infiltration by at least 50% for 1 month) were observed in four patients, with an additional CR of greater than 20 months *(75)*. These results collectively argue for continued evaluation of "anti-angiogenic" strategies, but caution must be exercised in inferring the mechanism causing these responses. As discussed above and elsewhere in this volume, the VEGF signaling axis apparently functions as a survival factor for hematopoietic neoplasm cells *per se*, and therefore SU5416 may be acting on the neoplastic cell compartment and not on marrow vasculature. Likewise, thalidomide is known to be metabolized into a host of electrophilic metabolites, some of which have the potential to function as alkylating agents.

Attempting to capitalize on VEGF both as a survival factor and as a pro-angiogenic cytokine, Karp et al. *(76)* added the anti-VEGF monoclonal antibody bevacizumab (10 mg/kg on day 8) after attempted reinduction therapy with "timed sequential therapy" including ara-C (2 g/M^2 over 72 hours on day 1) and mitoxantrone 40 mg/M^2 beginning on day 4 in patients with refractory or relapsed AML. Overall response was 48% in 48 patients, with CR in 33. Eighteen patients went on to receive at least one consolidation treatment, and 5 went on to allogeneic transplant. Patients with a CR had a median disease-free survival of 16 months and overall survival of 7 months. The serum concentration of VEGF was modulated in the majority of patients. Toxicities were within what would be expected in this population, with 6% suffering decreased ejection fraction, cerebrovascular bleed in 4%, and 15% mortality.

4.1.2. RESISTANCE MODULATORS

Preclinical evidence has suggested that the proteosome inhibitor bortezomib can potentiate the actions of anthracyclines. Therefore, Orlowski et al. conducted a dose-finding study of bortezomib when given with pegylated liposomal doxorubicin in patients with relapsed and refractory hematopoetic malignancies, including AML, in which there were two PRs to a regimen of 1.3 and 30 mg/M^2 of bortezomib and liposomal doxorubicin, respectively *(77)*. Grade 3 and 4 toxicities in at least 10% of patients included cytopenias, pneumonia, and peripheral neuropathy.

Classical multidrug resistance mediated by the P-glycoprotein remains an attractive yet unfulfilled target in AML. Zosuquidar trihydrochloride (Z.3HCL) was studied in a dose-finding study with daunorubicin and ara-C in 16 previously untreated patients. Eleven patients achieved a CR and one a PR, comparable to expected outcomes from induction chemotherapy *(78)*. Z.3HCL rapidly inhibited rhodamine 123 efflux in $CD56^+$ cells in 16/16 patients and in 6/10 $CD33^+$ cells. Evidence of a decrease in doxorubicin's IC_{50} for AML cells from Z.3HCL-treated patients was evident.

As outlined previously, abundant evidence of resistance modulation by PKC- interactive agents exists. Bryostatin-1, a transient PKC activator, but long-term PKC downregulator, was co-administered in a dose-finding trial with high-dose ara-C (1.5 g/M^2 q 12 h × 4 doses). The bryostatin 1 maximal tolerated dose was 50 μg/M^2, with dose-limiting toxicity principally related to myalgia. Four of 23 patients achieved CR. There was variable success in modulating PKC, with increases in two, decreases in four, and no change in three of the nine patients in which it was assayed *(79)*.

Retinoic acid is known to act as a differentiation agent for certain leukemia cells. In an exploratory trial designed to evaluate the impact of *all-trans*-retinoic acid (ATRA) on the tolerance of standard AML regimens, Bassan et al. administered 25 mg/M^2 on days 1–14 and 45 mg/M^2 on days 15–28 of two standard courses of idarubicin, ara-C, etoposide, and G-CSF followed by up to three courses of cytarabine plus G-CSF *(80)*. Nineteen patients treated with this regimen were compared to 29 comparable cases without ATRA. Headache with high-dose ara-C was noted. There was not a noteworthy difference in complete remission rate, disease-free survival, or overall survival at 3 years comparing the two experiences. ATRA added in vitro to the leukemic blasts did not exhibit an inhibitory or pro-apoptotic effect.

A well-understood basis for resistance to chemotherapeutic agents in a wide variety of neoplasms extends from the action of bcl2-related family members *(81)*. Oblimersen sodium is an antisense oligonucleotide developed against the bcl2 molecule itself. A phase I study of oblimersen was undertaken added to continuous infusion ara-C and two dose levels of doxorubicin in primary or secondary AML in patients who were ≥60 years of age, followed by consolidation with oblimersen plus high-dose ara-C *(82)*. Of 29 patients treated, 14 had CR, with persistence to 12 months in about 50%. No dose-limiting side effects of the oblimersen were encountered, and modulation of bcl2 mRNA was actually seen in leukemic blasts after the 72–hour infusion of oblimersen. These results point to the potential value of anti-bcl2 therapy, but a comparative trial would be necessary to reach a definitive conclusion as to the value of this approach. An additional issue is the recent recognition that oblimersen contains a "CpG" motif capable of activating innate immunity through interaction with Toll-like receptors *(83)*, adducing the possibility of this additional mechanism for oblimersen's effect.

4.2. Biologics

4.2.1. LINTUZUMAB

This unconjugated, humanized monoclonal antibody directed to the CD33 determinant was studied in a phase III trial where 191 patients with relapsed or refractory AML were randomly assigned to either mitoxantrone, etoposide, and ara-C (MEC) chemotherapy with or without lintuzumab 12 mg/M^2. The drug was well tolerated, with only infusion-related toxicity and no exacerbation of expected adverse events related to chemotherapy. There was no difference in CR rate or overall median survival (156 days) between the two groups *(84)*.

4.2.2. GEMTUZUMAB OZOGAMICIN

This antibody conjugate of an anti-CD33 humanized antibody with the DNA-damaging agent calicheamicin was approved for use in elderly patients with AML who are not viewed as medically fit for induction chemotherapy *(37)*. Its potential movement to other regimens was considered in a phase II trial *(85)* where it was administered in sequence with conventional chemotherapy to a population of elderly AML patients. Eligible patients between 61 and 75 years of age received GO on days 1 and 15, followed by one course of mitoxantrone, ara-C, and etoposide, without further planned treatment for complete responders. Of 57 evaluable patients, 38 completed the entire sequence, and the CR rate was 35% (CR with incomplete platelet recovery of 19%). Treatment-related mortality or resistant disease was 14% and 30%, respectively. Myelosuppression and liver toxicity were the main adverse events in both segments. This study is of interest because of the possibility of a reduced intensity of treatment with chemotherapy compared to standard approaches, yet with preservation of a meaningful response rate, compared to standard induction and consolidation AML in a similar population. On the other hand, the clear superiority to treatment of an analogous population with GO alone would need to be established in a *bona fide* randomized approach, as Nabhan et al. have reported of 12 patients treated solely with GO a response of 27% with a median duration of 7.6 months *(86)*.

A phase I trial of GO in pediatric patients has recently been reported by Arceci et al. *(87)*. GO was well tolerated at 6 mg/M^2 for two doses, with dose-limiting toxicities of veno-occlusive disease (VOD) at 9 mg/M^2. Of 13 patients receiving hematopoietic stem cell transplantation within 4 months of completing GO, 40% developed VOD. Overall, of 29 patients treated with GO, 28% achieved overall remission. These results were interpreted by the investigators as a basis for further study in combination with standard induction therapy for AML in children.

4.2.3. VACCINE STRATEGIES

The Wilms' tumor gene is overexpressed in leukemia and MDS patient samples. Wu et al. *(88)* demonstrated the existence of IgG subclass spectrum of expression of IgGs 1, 2, and 3 subclasses suggested Th1-type immune activation in patients with leukemia and MDS as compared to normal volunteers and compared to the incidence of Th2-type immune activation in the same patient population. These results were taken to imply the potential value of stimulating further Th1-based immune responses against leukemia cells as a therapeutic strategy.

5. CONCLUSIONS

This overview gives some idea of the emerging approaches to define new agents suitable for evaluation in AML. A consistent theme in these approaches is that a continuing refinement of our understanding of the biology of AML is providing targets whose basis for enthusiasm is their ability to cause stress of the tumor cell's homeostatic pathways in a way that increases susceptibility to apoptosis. Classical DNA-directed therapeutics such as ara-C, doxorubicin, mitoxantrone, and the like were used clinically before being recognized as being modulators of DNA damage response-induced signaling as well as conveying DNA damage *per se*. Selection of agents to modulate the stress response pathway without conveying DNA damage are now of interest to consider. The resistance mechanisms utilized by AML cells, including drug efflux pumps and bcl2 family member expression, also remain incompletely exploited but certainly are ripe for clinical investigation.

While cytokine and oncogene receptor-related therapeutic manipulation exemplified by flt3 activation are considered in other chapters in this volume, such growth factor-related signaling systems including raf, MAP kinase, and akt activation remain important contributors to cellular stress adaptation, the successful manipulation of which will offer analogous clinical trial opportunities. Additional cell stress mechanisms such as unfolded protein checkpoints, redox balance, and metabolic susceptibility (e.g., fatty acid synthesis and glucose metabolism) can now also begin to be considered as target areas for new therapy discovery and development.

The challenge in AML therapeutics is clear. Conventional approaches have "maxed out" survival at about 30–40%, considering all prognostic groups together. The tools of modern cancer cell biology have defined a range of potential therapeutic targets for clinical investigators to consider and in which industry could invest discovery and development resources. AML, by virtue of its ready accessibility to query in the malignant compartment, will ideally spur pilot phase efforts that will quickly allow an assessment of best available strategies for more widespread development that will have a positive impact on patient outcome. This is particularly true for the increasing problem of AML in the elderly population, for whom the conversion of AML to a more chronic phase capable of coexistence with a patient's physiological state remains a potentially useful outcome of several of the more current strategies.

REFERENCES

 1. Golub TR. Genomic approaches to the pathogenesis of hematologic malignancy. Curr Opin Hematol 2001;8:252–261.
 2. Gutierrez NC, Lopez Perez R, Hernandez JM, et al. Gene expression profile reveals deregulation of genes with relevant functions in the different subclasses of acute myeloid leukemia. Leukemia 2005;19:402–409.
 3. Tallman MS. Acute promyelocytic leukemia as a paradigm for targeted therapy. Semin Hematol 2004; 41(2 suppl 4):27–32.
 4. Sternberg DW, Gilliland DG. The role of signal transducer and activator of transcription factors in leukemogenesis. J Clin Oncol 2004;22:361–371.
 5. Konopleva M, Zhao S, Hu W, et al. The anti-apoptotic genes bcl-x(L) and bcl-2 are over expressed and contribute to chemoresistance of non-proliferating leukaemic CD 34+ cells. Br J Hematol 2002;18:521–534.

6. Invernizzi R, Travaglino E, Lunghi M, et al. Survivin expression in acute leukemias and myelodysplastic syndromes. Leuk Lymphoma 2004;45:2229–2237.

7. Shapiro GI. Preclinical and clinical development of the cyclin depenent kinase inhibitor flavopiridol. Clin Cancer Res 2004;10:4270s–4275s.

8. Sausville EA. Complexities in the development of cyclin-dependent kinase inhibitor drugs.Trends Mol Med 2002;8(4 suppl):S32–S37.

9. Arguello F, Alexander M, Sterry JA, et al. Flavopiridol induces apoptosis of normal lymphoid cells, causes immunosuppression, and has potent antitumor activity in vivo against human leukemia and lymphoma xenografts. Blood 1998;91:2482–2490.

10. Cartee L, Wang Z, Decker RH, et al. The cyclin-dependent kinase inhibitor (CDKI) flavopiridol disrupts phorbol 12-myristate 13-acetate- induced differentiation and CDK1 expression while enhancing apoptosis in human myeloid leukemia cells. Cancer Res 2001;61:2583–2591.

11. Decker RH, Wang S, Dai Y, Dent P, Grant S. Loss of bcl-2 phosphorylation loop domain is required to protect human myeloid leukemia cells from flavopiridol-mediated mitochondrial damage and apoptosis. Cancer Biol Ther 2002;1:136–144.

12. Nakanishi T, Karp JE, Tan M, et al. Quantitative analysis of breast cancer resistance; protein and cellular resistance to flavopiridol in acute leukemia patients. Clin Cancer Res 2003;9:3320–3328.

13. Byrd JC, Peterson BL, Gabrilove J, et al. Cancer and Leukemia Group B. Treatment of relapsed chronic lymphocytic leukemia by 72-hour continuous infusion or 1-hour bolus infusion of flavopiridol: results from Cancer and Leukemia Group B study 19805. Clin Cancer Res 2005;11:4176–4181.

14. Kaur G, Gazit A, Levitzki A, Stowe E, Cooney DA, Sausville EA. Tyrphostin induced growth inhibition: correlation with effect on p210bcr-abl autokinase activity in K562 chronic myelogenous leukemia. Anticancer Drugs 1994;5:213–222.

15. Kaur G, Sausville EA. Altered physical state of p210bcr-abl in tyrphostin AG957-treated K562 cells. Anticancer Drugs 1996;7:815–824.

16. Losiewicz MD, Kaaur G, Sausville EA. Different early effects of tyrphostin AG957 and geldanamycins on mitogen-activated protein kinase and p120cbl phosphorylation in anti CD-3-stimulated T-lymphoblasts. Biochem Pharmacol 1999;57:281–289.

17. Kaur G, Narayanan VL, Risbood PA, et al. Synthesis, structure-activity relationship, and p210(bcr-abl) protein tyrosine kinase activity of novel AG 957 analogs. Bioorg Med Chem 2005;13:1749–1761.

18. Svingen PA, Tefferi A, Kottke TJ, et al. Effects of the bcr/abl kinase inhibitors AG957 and NSC 680410 on chronic myelogenous leukemia cells in vitro. Clin Cancer Res 2000;6:237–249.

19. Chandra J, Hackbarth J, Le S, et al. Involvement of reactive oxygen species in adaphostin-induced cytotoxicity in human leukemia cells. Blood 2003;102:4512–4519.

20. Yu C, Rahmani M, Alemenara J, Sausville EA, Dent P, Grant S. Induction of apoptosis in human leukemia cells by the tyrosine kinase inhibitor adaphostin proceeds though a RAF-1/MEK/ERK and AKT-dependent process. Oncogene 2004;23:1364–1376.

21. Hose C, Kaur G, Sausville EA, Monks A. Transcriptional profiling identifies altered intracellular labile iron homeostasis as a contributing factor to the toxicity of adaphostin: decreased VEGF secretion is independent of HIF-1 regulation. Clin Cancer Res 2005;11:6370–6381.

22. Recher C, Beyne-Rauzy O, Demur C, et al. Antileukemic activity of rapamycin in acute myeloid leukemia. Blood 2005;105:2527–2534.

23. Stadheim TA, Suh N, Ganju N, Sporn MB, Eastman A. The novel triterpenoid 2-cyano-3,12-dioxoooleana-1,9-dien-28-oic acid (CDDO) potently enhances apoptosis induced by tumor necrosis factor in human leukemia cells. J Biol Chem 2002;277:16,448–16,455.

24. Suh WS, Kim YS, Schimmer AD, et al. Synthetic triterpenoids activate a pathway for apoptosis in AML cells involving downregulation of FLIP and sensitization to TRAIL. Leukemia 2003;17:2122–2129.

25. Ikeda T, Sporn M, Honda T, Gribble GW, Kufe D. The novel triterpenoid CDDO and its derivatives induce apoptosis by disruption of intracellular redox balance. Cancer Res 2003;63:5551–5558.

26. Konopleva M, Tsao T, Estrov Z, et al. The synthetic triterpenoid 2-cyano, 3,12-dioxoooleana-1,9-dien-28-oic acid induces caspase-dependent and independent apoptosis in acute myelogenous leukemia. Cancer Res 2004;64:7927–7935.

27. Konopleva M, Contractor R, Kurinna SM, Chen W, Andreef M, Ruvolo PP. The novel triterpenoid CDDO-Me suppresses MAPK pathways and promotes p38 activation in acute myeloid leukemia cells. Leukemia 2005; 19:1350–1354.

28. Ikeda T, Kimura F, Nakata Y, et al. Triterpenoid CDDO-Im downregulates PML/RARα. Cell Death Differ 2005;12:523–531.
29. Mix KS, Coon CI, Rosen ED, Suh N, Sporn MB, Brinckerhoff CE. Peroxisome proliferator activated receptor-gamma independent repression of collagenase gene expression by 2-cyano, 3,12-dioxooleana-1,9-dien-28-oic acid and prostaglandin 15-deoxy-delta(12,14) J2: role for SMAD signaling. Mol Pharmacol 2004;65:309–318.
30. Liby K, Hock T, Yore MM, et al. The synthetic triterpenoids, CDDO and CDDO-imidazolide, are potent inducers of heme oxygenase-1 and Nrf2/ARE signaling. Cancer Res 2005;65:4789–4798.
31. Hail N Jr, Konopleva M, Sporn M, Lotan R, Andreeff M. Evidence supporting a role for calcium in apoptosis induction by the synthetic triterpenoid 2-cyano, 3,12-dioxooleana-1,9-dien-28-oic acid (CDDO) J Biol Chem 2004;279:11,179–11,187.
32. Lakhani NJ, Sarkar, MA, Venitz J, Figg WD. 2-Methoxyestradiol, a promising anticancer agent. Pharmacotherapy 2003;23:165–172.
33. D'Amato RJ, Lin CM, Flynn E, Folkman J, Hamel, E. 2-Methoxyestradiol, an endogenous mammalian metabolite, inhibits tubulin polymerization by interacting at the colchicine site. Proc Natl Acad Sci USA 1994;91:3964–3968.
34. Gao N, Rahmani M, Dent P, Grant S. 2-Methoxyestradiol-induced apoptosis in human leukemia cells proceeds through a reactive oxygen species and Akt-dependent process. Oncogene 2005;24:3797–3809.
35. Biscardi M, Caporale R, Balestri F, Gavazzi S, Jimeno J, Grossi A. AEGF inhibition and cytotoxic effect of aplidin in leukemia cell lines and cells from acute myeloid leukemia. Ann Oncol 2005;16:1667–1674.
36. Balanian L, Ball ED. Anti-CD33 monoclonal antibodies enhance the cytotoxic effects of cytosine arabinoside and idarubicin on acute myeloid leukemia cells through similarities in their signaling pathways. Exp Hematol 2005;33:199–211.
37. Linenberger ML. CD33-directed therapy with gemtuzumab ozogamicin in acute myeloid leukemia: progress in understanding cytotoxicity and potential mechanisms of drug resistance.Leukemia 2005;19:176–182.
38. Nabhan C, Rundhagen L, Jatoi M, et al. Gemtuzumab ozogamicin (MylotargTM) is infrequently associated with sinusoidal obstructive syndrome/veno-occlusive disease. Ann Oncol 2004;15:1231–1236
39. Marks AJ, Cooper MS, Anderson RJ, et al. Selective apoptotic killing of malignant hemopoetic cells by antibody-targeted delivery of an amphipathic peptide. Cancer Res 2005;65:2373–2377.
40. Chang F, Steelman LS, Lee JT, et al. Signal transduction mediated by the ras/raf/mek/erk pathway from cytokine receptors to transcription factors: potential targeting for therapeutic intervention. Leukemia 2003;17:1263–1293.
41. Santos SC, Dias S. Internal and external autocrine VEGF/KDR loops regulate survival of subsets of acute leukemia through distinct signaling pathways. Blood 2004;103:3883–3889.
42. Neben K, Schnittger S, Brors B, et al. Distinct gene expression patterns associated with FLT3-and NRAS-activating mutations in acute myeloid leukemia with normal karyotype. Oncogene 2005;24:1580–1588.
43. Bieker R, Padro T, Kramer J, et al. Overexpression of basic fibroblast growth factor and autocrine stimulation in acute myeloid leukemia. Cancer Res 2003;63:7241–7246.
44. Decker S, Sausville EA. Pre-clinical modeling of combination treatments: fantasy or requirement. Ann NY Acad Sci 2005;1059:61–69.
45. Hanahan D, Weinberg RA. The hallmarks of cancer. Cell 2000;100:57–70.
46. Wang S, Vrana JA, Bartimole TM, et al. Agents that down-regulate or inhibit protein kinase C circumvent resistance to 1-beta-D-arabinofuranosylcytosine-induced apoptosis in human leukemia cells that overexpress bcl-2. Mol Pharmacol 1997;52:1000–1009.
47. Cartee L, Maggio SC, Smith R, Sankala HM, Dent P, Grant S. Protein kinase C-dependent activation of the tumor necrosis factor receptor-mediated extrinsic death pathway underlies enhanced apoptosis in human myeloid leukemia cells exposed to bryostatin-1 and flavopiridol. Mol Cancer Ther 2003;2:83–93.
48. Dai Y, Rahmani M, Grant S. Proteasome inhibitors potentiate leukemic cell apoptosis induced by the cyclin-dependent kinase inhibitor flavopiridol through a SAPK/JNK-and NF-kappaB-dependent process. Oncogene 2003;22:7108–7122.
49. Seynaeve CM, Kazianetz MG, Blumberg PM, Sausville EA., Worland PJ. Differential inhibition of protein kinase C isozymes by UCN-01, a staurosporine analogue. Mol Pharmacol 1994;45:1207–1214.
50. Graves PR, Yu L, Schwarz JK, et al. The Chk1 protein kinase and the Cdc25C regulatory pathways are targets of the anticancer agent UCN-01. J Biol Chem 2000;275:5600–5605.
51. Busby EC, Leistritz DF, Abraham RT, Karnitz LM, Sarkaria JN. The radiosensitizing agent 7-hydroxystaurosporine (UCN-01) inhibits the DNA damage checkpoint kinase hChk1. Cancer Res 2000;60:2108–2112.

52. Yu Q, La Rose J, Zhang H, Takemura H, Kohn KW, Pommier Y. UCN-01 inhibits p53 up-regulation and abrogates gamma-radiation-induced G(2)-M checkpoint independently of p53 by targeting both of the checkpoint kinases, Chk2 and Chk1. Cancer Res 2002;62:5743–5748.

53. Sato S, Fujita N, Tsuruo T. Interference with PDK1-Akt survival signaling pathway by UCN-01 (7-hydroxystaurosporine). Oncogene 2002;21:1727–1738.

54. Sausville EA, Arbuck SG, Messmann R, et al. Phase I trial of 72-hour continuous infusion UCN-01 in patients with refractory neoplasms. J Clin Oncol 2001;19:2319–2333.

55. Kondapaka SB, Zarnowski M, Yver DR, Sausville EA, Cushman SW. 7-hydroxystaurosporine (UCN-01) inhibition of Akt Thr308 but not Ser473 phosphorylation: a basis for decreased insulin-stimulated glucose transport. Clin Cancer Res 2004;10:7192–7198.

56. Dai Y, Yu C, Singh V, et al. Pharmacological inhibitors of the mitogen-activated protein kinase (MAPK) kinase/MAPK cascade interact synergistically with UCN-01 to induce mitochondrial dysfunction and apoptosis in human leukemia cells. Cancer Res 2001;61:5106–5115.

57. Dai Y, Rahmani M, Pei XY, et al. Farnesyltransferase inhibitors interact synergistically with the CHk1 inhibitor UCN-01 to induce apoptosis in human leukemia cells through interruption of both Akt and MED/ERK pathways and activation of SEK1/JNK. Blood 2005;105:1706–1716.

58. Xu Q, Simpson SE, Scialla TJ, Bagg A, Carroll M. Survival of acute myeloid leukemia cells requires PI3 kinase activation. Blood 2003;102:972–980.

59 Zhao S, Konopleva M, Cabreira-Hansen M, et al. Inhibition of phosphatidylinositol 3-kinase dephosphorylates BAD and promotes apoptosis in myeloid leukemias Leukemia 2004;18:267–275.

60. Hahn M, Li W, Yu C, Rahmani M, Dent P, Grant S. Rapamycin and UCN-01 synergistically induce apoposis in human leukemia cells through a process that is regulated by the raf-1/mek/erk, akt, and jnk signal transduction pathways. Mol Cancer Ther 2005;4:457–470.

61. Shao RG, Cao CX, Pommier Y. Activation of PKCalpha downstream from caspases during apoptosis induced by 7-hydroxystaurosporine or the topoisomerase inhibitors, camptothecin and etoposide, in human myeloid leukemia HL60 cells. J Biol Chem 1997;272:31,321–31,325.

62. Sampath D, Shi Z, Plunkett W. Inhibition of cyclin dependent kinase 2 by the chk1-cdc25A pathway during the S-phase checkpoint activated by fludarabine: dysregulation by 7-hydroxystaurosporine. Mol Pharmacol 2002;62:680–688.

63. Wang S, Wang Z, Grant S. Bryostatin 1 and UCN-01 potentiate 1-beta-D-arabinofuranosylcytosine-induced apoptosis in human myeloid leukemia cells through disparate mechanisms Mol Pharmacol 2003;63:232–242.

64. Isaacs JS, Xu W, Neckers L. Heat shock protein 90 as a molecular target for cancer therapeutics. Cancer Cell 2003;3:213–217.

65. Mesa RA, Loegering D, Powell HL, et al. Heat shock protein 90 inhibition sensitizes acute myelogenous leukemia cells to cytarabine. Blood 2005;106:318–327.

66. Melnick AM, Adelson K, Licht JD. The theoretical basis of transcriptional therapy of cancer: can it be put into practice? J Clin Oncol 2005;23:3957–3970.

67. Bhalla K. Epigenetic and chromatin modifiers as targeted therapy of hematologic malignancies. J Clin Oncol 2005;23:3971–3993.

68. Dai Y, Rahmani M, Dent P, Grant S. Blockade of histone deacetylase inhibitor-induced RelA/p65 acetylation and NF-{kappa}B activation potentiates apoptosis in leukemia cells through a process mediated by oxidative damage, XIAP downregulation, and c-Jun N-terminal kinase 1 activation. Mol Cell Biol 2005;25: 5429–5444.

69. Maggio SC, Rosato RR, Kramer LB, et al. The histone deacetylase inhibitor MS-275 interacts synergistically with fludarabine to induce apoptosis in human leukemia cells. Cancer Res 2004;64:2590–2600.

70. Kondapacka SB, Singh SS, Dasmahapatra GP, Sausville E, Roy KK. Perifosine, a novel alkylphospholipid, inhibits protein kinase B activation. Mol Cancer Ther 2003;2:1093–1103.

71. Rahmani M, Reese E, Dai Y, et al. Coadministration of histone deacetylase inhibitors and perifosine synergistically induces apoptosis in human leukemia cells through Akt and ERK1/2 inactivation and the generation of ceramide and reactive oxygen species. Cancer Res 2005;65:2422–2432.

72. Bali P, Pranpat M, Bradner J, et al. Inhibition of histone deacetylase 6 acetylates and disrupts the chaperone function of heat shock protein 90: a novel basis for antileukemia activity of histone deacetylase inhibitors. J Biol Chem 2005;280:26,729–26,734.

73. Wrzesien-Kus A, Robak T, Wierzbowska A, et al. A multicenter, open, non-comparative, Phase II study of the combination of cladribine (2-chlorodeoxyadenosine), cytarabine, granulocyte colony-stimulating factor

and mitoxantrone as induction therapy in refractory acute myeloid leukemia: a report of the Polish adult leukemia group. Ann Hematol 2005;84:557–564.

74. Fiedler W, Mesters R, Tinnefeld H, et al. A phase 2 clinical study of SU5416 in patients with refractory acute myeloid leukemia. Blood 2003;102:2763–2767.

75. Steins MB, Bieker R, Padro T, et al. Thalidomide for the treatment of acute myeloid leukemia. Leuk Lymphoma 2003;44:1489–1493.

76. Karp JE, Gojo I, Pili R, et al. Targeting vascular endothelial growth factor for relapsed and refractory adult acute myelogenous leukemias: therapy with sequential 1-beta-d-arabinofuranosylcytosine, mitoxantrone, and bevacizumab. Clin Cancer Res 2004;10:3577–3585.

77. Orlowski RZ, Voorhees PM, Garcia RA, et al. Phase 1 trial of the proteasome inhibitor bortezomib and pegylated liposomal doxorubicin in patients with advanced hematologic malignancies. Blood 2004;105:3058–3065.

78. Gerrard G, Payne E, Baker RJ, et al. Clinical effects and P-glycoprotein inhibition in patients with acute myeloid leukemia treated with zosuquidar trihydrochloride, daunorubicin, and cytarabine. Haematologica 2004;89:782–790.

79. Cragg LH, Andreeff M, Feldman E, et al. Phase I trial and correlative laboratory studies of bryostatin 1 (NSC 339555) and high-dose 1-B-D-arabinofuranosylcytosine in patients with refractory acute leukemia. Clin Cancer Res 2002;8:2123–2133.

80. Bassan R, Chiodini B, Lerede T, et al. Prolonged administration of all-trans retinoic acid in combination with intensive chemotherapy and G-CSF for adult acute myelogenous leukemia: single-center pilot study in different risk groups. Hematol J 2002;3:193–200.

81. Deng X, Kornblau, SM, Ruvolo, PP, May, WS, Jr. Regulation of Bcl2 phosphorylation and potential significance for leukemic cell chemoresistance. J Natl Cancer Inst Monogr 2001;28:30–37.

82. Marcucci G, Stock W, Dai G, et al. Phase I study of oblimersen sodium, an antisense to bcl2, in untreated older patients with acute myeloid leukemia: pharmacokinetics, pharmacodynamics, and clinical activity. J Clin Oncol 2005;23:3404–3411.

83. Wang H, Rayburn E, Zhang R. Synthetic oligodeoxynucleotides containing deoxycytidyl-deoxyguanosine dinucleotides (CpG ODNs) and modified analogs as novel anticancer therapeutics. Curr Pharm Des 2005;11: 2889–2907.

84. Feldman EJ, Brandwein J, Stone R, et al. Phase III randomized multicenter study of a humanized anti-CD33 monoclonal antibody, lintuzumab, in combination with chemotherapy, versus chemotherapy alone in patients with refractory or first-relapsed acute myeloid leukemia. J Clin Oncol 2005;23:4110–4116.

85. Amadori S, Suciu S, Willemze R, et al. De Witte EORTC leukemia group; GIMEMA leukemia group. Sequential administration of gemtuzumab ozogamicin and conventional chemotherapy as first line therapy in elderly patients with acute myeloid leukemia: a phase II study (AML-15) of the EORTC and GIMEMA leukemia groups. Haematologica 2004;89:950–956.

86. Nabhan C, Rundhaugen LM, Riley MB, et al. Phase II pilot trial of gemtuzumab ozogamicin (GO) as first line therapy in acute myeloid leukemia patients age 65 or older. Leuk Res 2005;29:53–57.

87. Arceci RJ, Sande J, Lange B, et al. Safety and efficacy of gemtuzumab ozogamicin (Mylotarg®) in pediatric patients with advanced CD33-positive acute myeloid leukemia. Blood 2005;106:1183–1188.

88. Wu F, Oka Y, Tsuboi A, et al. Th1-biased humoral immune responses against Wilms tumor gene WT1 product in the patients with hematopoietic malignancies. Leukemia 2005;19:268–274.

11 FLT3: A Prototype Receptor Tyrosine Kinase Target in AML

Mark Levis

CONTENTS

Summary

The receptor tyrosine kinase FLT3 is an important regulatory molecule in hematopoiesis and is expressed on the blasts in most cases of acute leukemia. Activating mutations of this receptor are present in roughly 30% of acute myeloid leukemia (AML) patients and are associated with a distinctly worse clinical outcome. Efforts to target this mutation and improve outcomes in this subgroup of AML patients have led to the investigation of several novel small-molecule FLT3 tyrosine kinase inhibitors. These compounds derive from a wide variety of chemical classes and differ significantly in both their potency and selectivity. This review summarizes the data validating FLT3 as a therapeutic target in AML and reviews the results of preliminary clinical trials using these agents for the treatment of AML patients harboring FLT3 mutations.

Key Words: Kinase; FLT3; AML; prognosis; inhibitor; stem cell.

1. INTRODUCTION

Constitutively activated tyrosine kinases have been investigated by scientists and clinicians alike for their role in the pathogenesis of cancer. The fact that these oncogene products play

From: *Contemporary Hematology: Acute Myelogenous Leukemia*
Edited by: J. E. Karp © Humana Press Inc., Totowa, NJ

such a role is no longer subject to debate. Still being debated is how effectively these enzymes can be targeted and whether or not such targeting can have a meaningful impact in the treatment of the disease. Tyrosine kinases seem be particularly important in the pathogenesis of hematological malignancies, especially myeloid leukemias. Starting with the recognition that the product of the Philadelphia chromosome (BCR/ABL) is an activated tyrosine kinase, to the recent discovery of a PDGFRα fusion protein in hypereosinophilic syndrome (HES) and eosinophilic leukemia and a gain of function mutation of Janus kinase 2 (JAK2), mutation-activated kinases continue to be identified as causative factors in hematopoietic disorders *(1–5)*. The first successful clinical use of a small molecule kinase inhibitor was, in fact, in the treatment of chronic myelogenous leukemia (CML) *(6)*.

The receptor tyrosine kinase FLT3 (FMS-like tyrosine kinase-3) is a relatively recent addition to the list of kinases implicated in leukemogenesis. This chapter will review the data implicating FLT3 in the pathogenesis of acute myeloid leukemia (AML), evaluate the credentials of this enzyme as a therapeutic target, and summarize the recent efforts to incorporate small-molecule FLT3 inhibitors into AML therapy.

2. WHAT MAKES A GOOD THERAPEUTIC TARGET?

Which kinases shoule one target for leukemia therapy? Presumably, the focus should be on those kinases that are essential in generating or maintaining the transformed state. BCR/ABL, the *sine qua non* of CML, is an example of such a kinase. Other choices are less obvious, however, which is not surprising given that malignant transformation is probably a multistep process, with many aberrant proteins playing a role *(7)*. Nonetheless, some guiding principles can be used to establish the credentials of a kinase as a suitable target for therapy. First, the highest priority targets should probably be kinases that have increased activity through some form of mutation. The precedence for this approach actually comes both from experience in solid tumors as well as in leukemia. CML, of course, is practically defined by the presence of the constitutively activated BCR-ABL kinase. Activating mutations of JAK2 have now been found in a majority of cases of the Philadelphia chromosome negative myeloproliferative diseases *(3–5)*. Gastrointestinal stromal tumors (GIST) likewise are characterized by activated KIT, and thus have a high response rate to KIT inhibition *(8)*. More subtle examples exist, however. For example, only a small fraction of lung cancer patients respond to treatment with a small molecule inhibitor of the epidermal growth factor receptor (EGFR). These patients, however, typically harbor activating mutations of EGFR *(9)*. Breast cancer patients whose tumors have HER2 amplification represent the only subset of patients to derive clinical benefit from the antibody targeting this kinase, trastuzumab *(10,11)*.

Cytogenetic analysis, performed on virtually all clinical cases of leukemia, facilitated the relatively early discovery of fusion oncoproteins such as BCR/ABL (a product of the 9;21 translocation in CML) or TEL-PDGFR (caused by the 5;12 translocation occasionally seen in chronic myelomonocytic leukemia) *(12–14)*. Nonetheless, translocations (at least those that are apparent with clinical cytogenetic analysis) cause only a fraction of the known kinase-activating mutations associated with cancer. Other types of constitutive activating mutations are less easily identified, because there are remarkably diverse means of abnormally upregulating the activity of a kinase. The receptor tyrosine kinases offer a useful illustration of this point.

A receptor tyrosine kinase (Fig. 1) typically consists of an extracellular ligand-binding domain, a transmembrane domain, and, intracellularly, a juxtamembrane domain and a kinase domain containing the ATP-binding pocket *(15)*. Upon the binding of ligand, the receptors

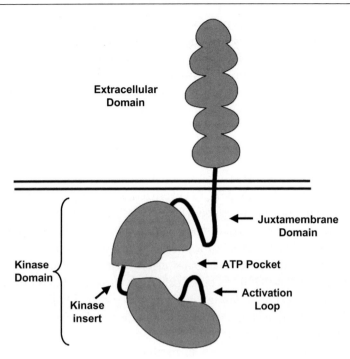

Fig. 1. Simplified diagram of the FLT3 receptor in monomeric form. The juxtamembrane domain and the activation loop both act as structural regulatory elements for access to the ATP-substrate binding pocket.

dimerize and undergo autophosphorylation, a covalent modification that stimulates the activity of the kinase domain. The activated receptor then transduces its signals via transfer of phosphate from ATP to tyrosine residues on various downstream proteins. For many cell surface receptors, the juxtamembrane domain serves as a negative regulatory domain, inhibiting the activity of the kinase domain until ligand binding occurs *(16)*.

Abnormal activation of these receptors can occur in a variety of ways. Perhaps the simplest is through overexpression of the wild-type receptor. This can occur via gene amplification, or possibly through epigenetic alterations affecting transcription, translation, or perhaps even receptor turnover. A classic example of this type of gene amplification is found with the epidermal growth factor family of receptors in solid tumors, most notably c-erb-B in breast cancer *(10)*. Point mutations localized to the so-called activation loop of the kinase domain can constitutively activate a receptor by shifting the ATP-binding pocket to a more open, accessible conformation. Such kinase domain mutations have been identified in KIT, MET, FLT3, and PDGFRα, all associated with malignancy *(17–20)*. Crystal structure analyses of the EphB2 receptor and of the FLT3 receptor suggest that mutations within the juxtamembrane region disrupt the inhibitory influence this domain exerts over the kinase domain *(21,22)*. Point mutations, deletions, insertions, and internal tandem duplications have all been found in the juxtamembrane domain of the KIT receptor in GISTs, all associated with constitutively phosphorylated receptor *(23)*. Likewise, internal tandem duplications of the FLT3 gene (FLT3/ITD mutations) constitutively activate FLT3 and are one of the most common molecular abnormalities found in AML *(24,25)*. Finally, activating mutations can be found within the extracellular domain. Some of these mutations in the KIT receptor in GIST appear to activate the receptor by promoting dimerization via an abnormal disulfide bond *(26)*. For other mutations in the extracellular domain, the mechanism of constitutive activation is unclear *(27)*.

Adding to the complexity of this situation is the likelihood that a given kinase inhibitor will be effective against only a subset of the mutations affecting a particular kinase. In particular, a number of small molecule kinase inhibitors appear to be ineffective against the kinase domain mutations. For example, imatinib has little effect on the activity of some of the less frequent KIT kinase domain mutations that occur in GIST, and AG1296, a tyrphostin, is ineffective against the analogous mutations in the FLT3 receptor *(28,29)*.

3. THE FLT3 RECEPTOR

Human FLT3 was cloned a decade ago by two independent groups *(30,31)*. It contains 993 amino acids and, on electrophoretic gels, is visualized as a doublet corresponding to 130 and 160 kDa (the larger being the mature, glycosylated form). It has an extracellular ligand-binding region with five immunoglobulin-like domains and a single transmembrane domain (Fig. 1). The cytoplasmic portion is comprised of a juxtamembrane domain followed by the tyrosine kinase domain, which is interrupted by a kinase insert domain. These structural features allow FLT3 to be grouped with the PDGF receptor subfamily (so-called class III) of receptor tyrosine kinases *(15)*. It is closest in homology to KIT and the two PDGF receptors and has lesser homology with the members of the nerve growth factor (NGF/TRK) and the vascular endothelial growth factor receptor subfamilies.

The juxtamembrane domain of FLT3 is of particular interest because of its negative regulatory influence on the tyrosine kinase activity of the receptor. Upon binding FLT3 ligand (FL), wild-type FLT3 dimerizes and undergoes a conformational change. This causes the so-called activation loop, localized to the N-terminal kinase domain, to assume an open conformation and allow ATP access to the ATP-binding pocket. Upon ligand-induced dimerization, FLT3 undergoes autophosphorylation and transduces signals promoting cell growth and inhibiting apoptosis through pathways linked to cytoplasmic proteins such as Ras-GAP, PLC-β, STAT5, and ERK1/2 *(32–38)*.

FL is expressed in virtually all cell types thus far examined *(39,40)*. In contrast, FLT3 has a fairly narrow range of cell expression, being localized primarily to hematopoietic and neural tissues, which presumably confines its functions to these cell types *(31)*. In bone marrow, FLT3 is expressed the CD34$^+$ fraction of hematopoietic cells, and in a smaller fraction of CD34$^-$ cells destined to become dendritic cells *(41)*. Recent evidence implicates it in "lymphoid-primed" hematopoietic precursors *(42)*. FLT3 is clearly an important receptor in hematopoietic development. Its ligand acts in synergy with other cytokines to promote hematopoietic precursor expansion, and targeted disruption of either FLT3 or FL in mice leads to a reduction in hematopoietic precursors (although such disruption is nonlethal) *(43–50)*.

4. FLT3 AS A THERAPEUTIC TARGET IN LEUKEMIA

In 1996, internal tandem duplication mutations of FLT3 (FLT3/ITD mutations) localized to the juxtamembrane domain were discovered in a significant fraction of AML cases *(51)*. Cases harboring these mutations were noted to have a worse clinical outcome than those lacking a mutation. Subsequently, point mutations at aspartate 835 (D835, within the activation loop), analogous to previously described mutations in the KIT gene, were found in 7% of cases *(19,52)*. Both types of mutations constitutively activate FLT3 *(19,53,54)*. The FLT3/ITD mutations presumably destabilize the negative regulatory function of the juxtamembrane domain. The D835 mutations, meanwhile, are precisely analogous to point mutations that have been well characterized for other receptors *(17,55,56)*. These mutations, localized to the kinase domain, shift the so-called activation loop to an open configuration. Following these initial observations, dozens of studies comprising the results of screening more than 5000 adult and pediatric AML samples have been published *(57–69)*. From these studies, FLT3/ITD mutations can be estimated to occur in 22.9% of *de novo* AML (i.e., AML not arising from pre-existing myelodysplasia), and their presence clearly confers a worse prognosis *(25)*. D835 mutations occur in 7% of cases, with a less certain clinical impact.

The signaling properties of a FLT3 receptor with an ITD mutation differ from those of the wild-type receptor in a manner that clearly contributes to the process of leukemogenesis. STAT5 and FOXO transcription factors are abnormally activated in response to FLT3/ITD, but not FLT3 wild-type, signaling *(70–73)*. Microarray studies have identified upregulation of the Pim-1 and Pim-2 proto-oncogenes, as well as interaction with the Wnt signaling pathway, in FLT3/ITD leukemia cells *(70,74,75)*. Finally, c/EBPα, a transcription factor involved in myeloid differentiation, is downregulated by the mutant receptors, indicative of the differentiation block that so characterizes leukemia cells *(70,76)*. This downregulation is possibly mediated by RGS2 *(72)*.

Overall, FLT3 mutations now represent one of the most common molecular abnormalities in AML, and the large body of data regarding the incidence and prognostic impact of FLT3 mutations establishes this receptor as a worthy therapeutic target.

5. FLT3 LEUKEMIA: CLINICAL CHARACTERISTICS

The only test currently available to confirm the presence of a FLT3 mutation in AML is polymerase chain reaction (PCR) based *(51,77)*. With regard to the FLT3/ITD mutations, however, there are a number of consistent clinical features that offer clues to their presence. Patients harboring FLT3/ITD mutations tend to present with leukocytosis and a packed bone marrow, features consistent with a highly proliferative disease. The blasts tend to have monocytic features, and cytogenetics are most commonly normal—with two exceptions. The most prominent exception is the case of acute promyelocytic leukemia (APL), in which over one-third of cases harbor a FTL3/ITD mutation. While these cases tend to be the microgranular variants, thus far there has been no evidence for an adverse prognosis associated with the mutations in M3 AML *(78–82)*. Another interesting exception to the normal cytogenetics rule is the association of FLT3/ITD mutations with 6;9 translocations (which are known to carry an adverse prognosis) *(67,83)*. The general consensus is that FLT3/ITD mutations do not affect the likelihood of achieving a complete remission, but rather increase the likelihood of relapse. However, the data upon which this conclusion is based consist of outcomes derived from clinical trials of AML, almost all of which were testing induction regimens more intensive than the traditional "7+3." It is entirely possible that intensity of therapy can impact the remission rate with this AML subtype. Further studies will be required to clarify this issue.

6. FLT3 MUTATIONS AND LEUKEMIA STEM CELLS

For AML, it is reasonable to speculate that the malignant transforming event occurs in a primitive hematopoietic stem cell and that relapsing or refractory disease occurs because of the persistence of these leukemia stem cells following initial therapy. These difficult-to-isolate leukemia stem cells have been best studied using the NOD/SCID mouse model, in which human leukemia cells expressing CD34 (a stem cell marker) but lacking CD38 (a lineage commitment marker) have been shown to contain the so-called leukemia-initiating population, a population capable of self-renewal *(84,85)*. In this regard, FLT3 appears to play a prominent role in stem cell biology, where its expression is first detected on short-term ("low-quality") stem cells, and recent work implicates this receptor as a marker for commitment to a nonerythroid nonmegakaryocytic lineage. Wild-type FLT3 is expressed on the leukemic blasts in the majority of cases of acute leukemia, and the expression is no longer tightly coupled to CD34 expression *(86–90)*. A reasonable supposition, therefore, is that the FLT3/ITD mutations occur within the leukemia stem cell population. In support of this is the recent finding that the mutations are present in $CD34^+/CD38^-$ NOD/SCID leukemia-initiating cells *(91)*.

Two clinical observations, however, offer perhaps the best glimpse of the role these mutations may play in leukemogenesis. The first observation is that the ratio of FLT3 mutant to wild-type DNA may vary among patients and may serve as a predictor for clinical outcome, with patients whose AML cells are homozygous for mutant alleles having the most dismal outcomes *(62)*. Along these lines, the FLT3 mutant-to-wild-type ratio may vary from the time of diagnosis to the time of relapse *(92–95)*. In occasional cases, mutations present at diagnosis (typically those with low mutant-to-wild-type ratios) were lost at relapse. Alternately, in other patients mutations only appeared at relapse. In most cases, however, the mutant allele was present at diagnosis and the mutant-to-wild-type ratio increased at relapse. This suggests that the pool of leukemia stem cells is heterogeneous in nature (supported by recent data using the NOD/SCID model) *(96)* and that in most cases the FLT3 mutations may provide a selective advantage to the stem cell clones that harbor them.

7. FLT3 INHIBITORS

Imatinib mesylate (Gleevec; Norvartis), a small-molecule inhibitor of BCR-ABL, KIT, and PDGF-Rα/β, has been shown to have remarkable clinical efficacy in CML, GIST, and HES *(2,6,8,97)*. These successes, combined with the credentials of FLT3 as a potential target for therapy, have spurred widespread interest in the development of FLT3 inhibitors for the treatment of acute leukemia. Thus far, at least 17 different compounds, derived from five unique chemical classes, have been introduced into the literature with this purpose *(98)*.

Several different small-molecule kinase inhibitors with activity against FLT3 have now been tested in clinical trials (Table 1). The FLT3 inhibitors characterized to date are heterocyclic compounds that either act as ATP competitors or structurally resemble the intermediary complex of a tyrosine covalently bound to ATP. Crystal structure data from other drug–receptor combinations, as well as from studies of the FLT3 receptor, allow some speculation about the structure–activity relationships of these inhibitors *(99–101)*. While most of them likely fit into the ATP-binding pocket of FLT3, the exact mechanism probably varies from inhibitor to inhibitor. For example, some compounds may bind via an induced-fit mechanism (as is seen with staurosporine binding to CSK), while others might bind in a lock-and-key manner (such as imatinib binding to ABL). Adding to this potential variation, FLT3 inhibitors may bind to the active, inactive, or transitional state of FLT3. The selectivity of an inhibitor for FLT3 may be greatly influenced by a single amino acid change. For example, FLT3 is normally insensitive to inhibition by imatinib mesylate (IC_{50} >3 µM). Substitution of Phe-691 with threonine renders the receptor susceptible to the drug (IC_{50} 0.1–0.3 µM) *(100)*. Recently, FLT3 inhibitors were found to have variable potency against different activating mutations *(29)*. This is perhaps not a surprising finding, because FLT3 activating mutations all likely have direct influence over the ATP-binding pocket where the inhibitors bind.

Table 1
FLT3 Inhibitors Previously or Currently Being Studied in Clinical Trials

Compound	Chemical class	Status
SU5416	3-Substituted indolinone	Phase 3
SU11248	3-Substituted indolinone	Phase 2
CEP-701	Indolocarbazole	Phase 2
PKC412	Indolocarbazole	Phase 2
MLN518	Quinazoline	Phase 2
CHIR-258	Benzimidalzole-quinolinone	Phase 1

Activating mutations of FLT3 occur in up to 30% of AML, and AML samples harboring these mutations consistently respond in vitro more dramatically than wild-type samples to FLT3 inhibition *(102–104)*. A recent report examined the level of FLT3 transcripts in primary AML samples using quantitative PCR and concluded that overexpression of wild-type FLT3 was associated with a poor prognosis and that such cases may potentially respond clinically to FLT3 inhibitors *(105)*.

8. SU5416

This intravenously administered indolinone with activity against FLT3 and the VEGF receptor family has been studied clinically as a single agent in two phase 2 studies in AML *(106,107)*. In one study 43 AML patients who either had refractory disease or were too elderly for conventional therapy were treated twice weekly in 4-week cycles *(106)*. One patient achieved a reduction in bone marrow blasts to less than 5% (but did not recover neutrophils or platelets), and 7 obtained a 50% or greater reduction in bone marrow or peripheral blasts. The reported response rate was therefore 19%, with responses lasting 1–5 months. Although they observed an association between blast VEGF RNA expression and response, they did not assess the in vivo phosphorylation status of either FLT3 or the VEGF receptors in the study population. None of the responding patients harbored FLT3/ITD mutations. It is difficult, therefore, to draw any meaningful conclusions from this particular trial, largely because it is not clear if the targets (FLT3 or VEGF receptors) were affected. In the second trial of 33 AML patients and 22 MDS patients, there were 3 partial responses and 1 hematological improvement *(107)*. No information obtained on the in vivo activity of the targeted receptors. Nonetheless, in an elegant follow-up study of these patients, the same group demonstrated in vivo inhibition of FLT3 phosphorylation immediately after drug infusion *(108)*. SU5416, however, has a relatively short half-life, and only sustained inhibition of FLT3 is predicted to result in leukemia cell death. Thus it was not surprising that correlative studies from this trial demonstrated short-lived inhibition of FLT3 autophosphorylation lasting only a few hours after dosing. The important conclusion from this follow-up work was that the major limitation of SU5416 appeared to be pharmacokinetic, not pharmacodynamic.

9. SU11248

Another indolinone, SU11248 has been touted as a "multitargeted" inhibitor. It is orally available, more potent in vitro than SU5416, and inhibits a rather broad range of receptor tyrosine kinases, including FLT3, the VEGF receptors, KIT, and the PDGF receptors *(98)*.

Perhaps not surprisingly, this reduction in selectivity may have resulted in an increase in toxicity. In a phase 1 study, 29 patients received a single dose, in escalating fashion, of SU11248 *(109)*. The primary endpoint of the study was the all-important one: confirmation of target inhibition. This data was then followed up with a more traditional phase I study in which 16 AML patients, including 4 with FLT3 mutations, were treated in prolonged fashion *(110)*. Six patients had transient reductions in peripheral and bone marrow blasts, including all 4 patients with FLT3 mutations. While inhibition of FLT3 phosphorylation (and appropriate downstream targets) was achieved with the higher dose levels, it became apparent that the drug would not be tolerated in sustained fashion because of toxicity that likely relates to the larger number of cellular targets inhibited by SU11248. In another recent report, SU11248 was demonstrated to have synergistic effects in vitro when combined with cytarabine and daunorubicin, with clinical trials of this approach being designed for future testing *(111)*.

10. CEP-701

This indolocarbazole derivative was initially introduced as an inhibitor of TrkA for possible use in prostate cancer *(112)* but was recognized subsequently as a potent FLT3 inhibitor *(103)*. A clinical laboratory correlative phase 1/2 trial in relapsed or refractory AML patients with FLT3 mutations was initiated *(113)*. The correlative assays from this trial revealed that if a patient had leukemic blasts that died when exposed to CEP-701 in vitro, and if that patient achieved a level of CEP-701 in plasma sufficient to significantly inhibit FLT3 autophosphorylation in sustained fashion, then a clinical response was observed. Five out of 14 patients showed a response, typically with reductions in peripheral blasts. One patient achieved a decrease in marrow blasts to less than 5% for 3 months.

Finally, data from a recent report of in vitro studies combining CEP-701 with chemotherapy have provided the basis for a recently launched, multicenter clinical trial *(114)*. The data suggest that pretreatment of AML cells with CEP-701 causes a cell cycle arrest, blunting the effects of chemotherapy. Synergistic effects were seen when CEP-701 was administered immediately following chemotherapy, and a phase 2 trial of chemotherapy followed by CEP-701 is being conducted in adults with AML harboring FLT3 mutations in first relapse.

11. PKC412

PKC412, another indolocarbazole derivative, was originally investigated as a protein kinase C inhibitor (hence, PKC). It was then recognized as a potent FLT3 inhibitor and tested in a phase 2 trial of AML patients, again using a relapsed or refractory group that harbored FLT3 mutations *(115,116)*. Twenty patients were treated with a fixed dosing schedule of 75 mg orally three times daily, and 14 of these showed a clinical response, primarily in peripheral blast reduction. Six patients achieved a greater than 50% reduction in bone marrow blast count, and 3 achieved less than 5% blasts. Responses correlated with in vivo FLT3 inhibition. Currently, PKC412 is being tested in combination with conventional chemotherapy as part of induction therapy for newly diagnosed AML patients *(117)*.

12. MLN518

This compound, previously known as CT53518, inhibits FLT3, KIT, and PDGFRβ with a similar potency *(118,119)*. Preliminary results of a phase 2 trial in FLT3/ITD AML showed a reduction in peripheral blasts in 6 of 18 patients, similar to other FLT3 inhibitors *(120)*. Of note, this inhibitor has little effect on FLT3 kinase domain point mutants and therefore may be somewhat more limited in scope of efficacy *(121)*.

13. CHIR-258

CHIR-258 is a recently introduced multitargeted compound with potent in vitro efficacy against FLT3, KIT, VEGFR1-3, PDGFR, and fibroblast growth factor receptor *(122)*. Phase 1 data are not yet available.

14. OTHER ISSUES SURROUNDING FLT3 INHIBITORS

Myelosuppression (beyond that normally seen in AML) has not thus far been a major toxicity observed in the FLT3 inhibitor trials, although this has been a concern in planning trials combining the inhibitors with chemotherapy. MLN518 was tested in colony-forming assays of normal and leukemic human bone marrow samples as well as in a murine bone marrow transplant model *(123)*. MLN518 had no significant effects on the growth of normal hematopoietic progenitors and had only minimal effects on recovery from chemotherapy-induced myelosuppression.

15. RESISTANCE TO FLT3 INHIBITORS

Resistance to imatinib is now a well-described phenomenon in CML *(124)*, so investigators have quickly moved to identify mutations in FLT3 that confer resistance to the various inhibitors in development *(121,125,126)*. Point mutations in the ATP-binding pocket and the activation loop of the kinase domain have been generated that display varying degrees of resistance to different FLT3 inhibitors. The potential clinical significance of these mutations is as yet unclear. For all FLT3 inhibitors thus far studied in clinical trials, resistance to mono-therapy with the inhibitor has emerged relatively rapidly, but few data are available as to the exact mechanism of resistance. With the indolocarbazoles (CEP-701 and PKC412), loss of response has been related to inadequate plasma drug levels, i.e., pharmacokinetic causes. Out of eight patients treated with CEP-701, two had blasts that were resistant to the drug in vitro prior to any therapy, suggesting that even sustained, effective FLT3 inhibition will be ineffective for some FLT3/ITD AML patients.

16. CONCLUSIONS

Since their discovery nearly a decade ago, FLT3 mutations have come to define an important new subset of AML, much like the 15;17 translocation defines APL. Unlike APL, FLT3 AML has a rather grim prognosis with currently available therapy. It is important to remember, however, that prior to the introduction of *all-trans*-retinoic acid (ATRA) to target this molecular defect, APL was likewise a poor-risk disease. Hence, there is great hope that targeting FLT3 will likewise convert FLT3 AML into one of the more curable leukemias. The consensus from the initial clinical trials is that monotherapy with small-molecule FLT3 inhibitors can lead to significant but nonsustained clinical effects in relapsed AML patients harboring activating mutations. Extending the analogy further, APL is not generally curable with ATRA alone. FLT3 inhibitors are more likely to be useful either in some form of combination with conventional chemotherapy or as maintenance therapy after remission has been achieved.

REFERENCES

1. Ben-Neriah Y, Daley GQ, Mes-Masson AM, Witte ON, Baltimore D. The chronic myelogenous leukemia-specific P210 protein is the product of the bcr/abl hybrid gene. Science 1986;233(4760):212–214.
2. Cools J, DeAngelo DJ, Gotlib J, et al. A tyrosine kinase created by fusion of the PDGFRA and FIP1L1 genes as a therapeutic target of imatinib in idiopathic hypereosinophilic syndrome. N Engl J Med 2003;348(13): 1201–1214.
3. Kralovics R, Passamonti F, Buser AS, et al. A gain-of-function mutation of JAK2 in myeloproliferative disorders. N Engl J Med 2005;352(17):1779–1790.
4. Levine RL, Wadleigh M, Cools J, et al. Activating mutation in the tyrosine kinase JAK2 in polycythemia vera, essential thrombocythemia, and myeloid metaplasia with myelofibrosis. Cancer Cell 2005;7(4):387–397.
5. James C, Ugo V, Le Couedic JP, et al. A unique clonal JAK2 mutation leading to constitutive signalling causes polycythaemia vera. Nature 2005;434(7037):1144–1148.
6. Druker BJ, Talpaz M, Resta DJ, et al. Efficacy and safety of a specific inhibitor of the BCR-ABL tyrosine kinase in chronic myeloid leukemia. N Engl J Med 2001;344(14):1031–1037.
7. Vogelstein B, Kinzler KW. The multistep nature of cancer. Trends Genet 1993;9(4):138–141.
8. Demetri GD, von Mehren M, Blanke CD, et al. Efficacy and safety of imatinib mesylate in advanced gastrointestinal stromal tumors. N Engl J Med 2002;347(7):472–480.
9. Lynch TJ, Bell DW, Sordella R, et al. Activating mutations in the epidermal growth factor receptor underlying responsiveness of non-small-cell lung cancer to gefitinib. N Engl J Med 2004;350(21):2129–2139.
10. Slamon DJ, Clark GM, Wong SG, Levin WJ, Ullrich A, McGuire WL. Human breast cancer: correlation of relapse and survival with amplification of the HER-2/neu oncogene. Science 1987;235(4785):177–182.
11. Hortobagyi GN. Overview of treatment results with trastuzumab (Herceptin) in metastatic breast cancer. Semin Oncol 2001;28(6 suppl 18):43–47.
12. Nowell P, Hungerford D. Chromosome Studies on Normal and Leukemic Human Leukocytes. J Natl Cancer Inst 1960;25:85–109.
13. Rowley JD. Letter: A new consistent chromosomal abnormality in chronic myelogenous leukaemia identified by quinacrine fluorescence and Giemsa staining. Nature 1973;243(5405):290–293.
14. Golub TR, Barker GF, Lovett M, Gilliland DG. Fusion of PDGF receptor beta to a novel ets-like gene, tel, in chronic myelomonocytic leukemia with t(5;12) chromosomal translocation. Cell 1994;77(2):307–316.
15. van der Geer P, Hunter T, Lindberg RA. Receptor protein-tyrosine kinases and their signal transduction pathways. Annu Rev Cell Biol 1994;10:251–337.
16. Hubbard SR. Theme and variations: juxtamembrane regulation of receptor protein kinases. Mol Cell 2001; 8(3):481–482.
17. Jeffers M, Schmidt L, Nakaigawa N, et al. Activating mutations for the met tyrosine kinase receptor in human cancer. Proc Natl Acad Sci USA 1997;94(21):11,445–11,450.
18. Furitsu T, Tsujimura T, Tono T, et al. Identification of mutations in the coding sequence of the proto-oncogene c-kit in a human mast cell leukemia cell line causing ligand-independent activation of c-kit product. J Clin Invest 1993;92(4):1736–1744.
19. Yamamoto Y, Kiyoi H, Nakano Y, et al. Activating mutation of D835 within the activation loop of FLT3 in human hematologic malignancies. Blood 2001;97(8):2434–2439.
20. Hirota S, Ohashi A, Nishida T, et al. Gain-of-function mutations of platelet-derived growth factor receptor alpha gene in gastrointestinal stromal tumors. Gastroenterology 2003;125(3):660–667.
21. Wybenga-Groot LE, Baskin B, Ong SH, Tong J, Pawson T, Sicheri F. Structural basis for autoinhibition of the Ephb2 receptor tyrosine kinase by the unphosphorylated juxtamembrane region. Cell 2001;106(6): 745–757.
22. Griffith J, Black J, Faerman C, et al. The structural basis for autoinhibition of FLT3 by the juxtamembrane domain. Mol Cell 2004;13(2):169–178.
23. Antonescu CR, Sommer G, Sarran L, et al. Association of KIT exon 9 mutations with nongastric primary site and aggressive behavior: KIT mutation analysis and Clinical correlates of 120 gastrointestinal stromal tumors. Clin Cancer Res 2003;9(9):3329–3337.

24. Gilliland DG, Griffin JD. The roles of FLT3 in hematopoiesis and leukemia. Blood 2002;100(5): 1532–1542.

25. Levis M, Small D. FLT3: ITDoes matter in leukemia. Leukemia 2003;17(9):1738–1752.

26. Santoro M, Carlomagno F, Romano A, et al. Activation of RET as a dominant transforming gene by germline mutations of MEN2A and MEN2B. Science 1995;267(5196):381–383.

27. Lux ML, Rubin BP, Biase TL, et al. KIT extracellular and kinase domain mutations in gastrointestinal stromal tumors. Am J Pathol 2000;156(3):791–795.

28. Frost MJ, Ferrao PT, Hughes TP, Ashman LK. Juxtamembrane mutant V560GKit is more sensitive to Imatinib (STI571) compared with wild-type c-kit whereas the kinase domain mutant D816VKit is resistant. Mol Cancer Ther 2002;1(12):1115–1124.

29. Grundler R, Thiede C, Miething C, Steudel C, Peschel C, Duyster J. Sensitivity toward tyrosine kinase inhibitors varies between different activating mutations of the FLT3 receptor. Blood 2003;102(2):646–651.

30. Rosnet O, Schiff C, Pebusque MJ, et al. Human FLT3/FLK2 gene: cDNA cloning and expression in hemato-poietic cells. Blood 1993;82(4):1110–1119.

31. Small D, Levenstein M, Kim E, et al. STK-1, the human homolog of Flk-2/Flt-3, is selectively expressed in CD34+ human bone marrow cells and is involved in the proliferation of early progenitor/stem cells. Proc Natl Acad Sci USA 1994;91(2):459–463.

32. Dosil M, Wang S, Lemischka IR. Mitogenic signalling and substrate specificity of the Flk2/Flt3 receptor tyrosine kinase in fibroblasts and interleukin 3-dependent hematopoietic cells. Mol Cell Biol 1993;13(10): 6572–6585.

33. Rosnet O, Buhring HJ, deLapeyriere O, et al. Expression and signal transduction of the FLT3 tyrosine kinase receptor. Acta Haematol 1996;95(3–4):218–223.

34. Lavagna-Sevenier C, Marchetto S, Birnbaum D, Rosnet O. FLT3 signaling in hematopoietic cells involves CBL, SHC and an unknown P115 as prominent tyrosine-phosphorylated substrates. Leukemia 1998;12(3): 301–310.

35. Lavagna-Sevenier C, Marchetto S, Birnbaum D, Rosnet O. The CBL-related protein CBLB participates in FLT3 and interleukin-7 receptor signal transduction in pro-B cells. J Biol Chem 1998;273(24):14,962–14,967.

36. Zhang S, Mantel C, Broxmeyer HE. Flt3 signaling involves tyrosyl-phosphorylation of SHP-2 and SHIP and their association with Grb2 and Shc in Baf3/Flt3 cells. J Leukoc Biol 1999;65(3):372–380.

37. Marchetto S, Fournier E, Beslu N, et al. SHC and SHIP phosphorylation and interaction in response to activation of the FLT3 receptor. Leukemia 1999;13(9):1374–1382.

38. Zhang S, Fukuda S, Lee Y, et al. Essential role of signal transducer and activator of transcription (Stat)5a but not Stat5b for Flt3-dependent signaling. J Exp Med 2000;192(5):719–728.

39. Hannum C, Culpepper J, Campbell D, et al. Ligand for FLT3/FLK2 receptor tyrosine kinase regulates growth of haematopoietic stem cells and is encoded by variant RNAs. Nature 1994;368(6472):643–648.

40. Lyman SD, James L, Johnson L, et al. Cloning of the human homologue of the murine flt3 ligand: a growth factor for early hematopoietic progenitor cells. Blood 1994;83(10):2795–2801.

41. Gotze KS, Ramirez M, Tabor K, Small D, Matthews W, Civin CI. Flt3high and Flt3low CD34+ progenitor cells isolated from human bone marrow are functionally distinct. Blood 1998;91(6):1947–1958.

42. Adolfsson J, Mansson R, Buza-Vidas N, et al. Identification of flt3(+) lympho-myeloid stem cells lacking erythro-megakaryocytic potential a revised road map for adult blood lineage commitment. Cell 2005; 121(2):295–306.

43. Mackarehtschian K, Hardin JD, Moore KA, Boast S, Goff SP, Lemischka IR. Targeted disruption of the flk2/flt3 gene leads to deficiencies in primitive hematopoietic progenitors. Immunity 1995;3(1):147–161.

44. McKenna HJ, Stocking KL, Miller RE, et al. Mice lacking flt3 ligand have deficient hematopoiesis affecting hematopoietic progenitor cells, dendritic cells, and natural killer cells. Blood 2000;95(11):3489–3497.

45. Ray RJ, Paige CJ, Furlonger C, Lyman SD, Rottapel R. Flt3 ligand supports the differentiation of early B cell progenitors in the presence of interleukin-11 and interleukin-7. Eur J Immunol 1996;26(7):1504–1510.

46. Veiby OP, Jacobsen FW, Cui L, Lyman SD, Jacobsen SE. The flt3 ligand promotes the survival of primitive hemopoietic progenitor cells with myeloid as well as B lymphoid potential. Suppression of apoptosis and counteraction by TNF-alpha and TGF-beta. J Immunol 1996;157(7):2953–2960.

47. Broxmeyer HE, Lu L, Cooper S, Ruggieri L, Li ZH, Lyman SD. Flt3 ligand stimulates/costimulates the growth of myeloid stem/progenitor cells. Exp Hematol 1995;23(10):1121–1129.

48. Hirayama F, Lyman SD, Clark SC, Ogawa M. The flt3 ligand supports proliferation of lymphohematopoietic progenitors and early B-lymphoid progenitors. Blood 1995;85(7):1762–1768.

49. Nicholls SE, Winter S, Mottram R, Miyan JA, Whetton AD. Flt3 ligand can promote survival and macrophage development without proliferation in myeloid progenitor cells. Exp Hematol 1999;27(4):663–672.

50. Sitnicka E, Buza-Vidas N, Larsson S, Nygren JM, Liuba K, Jacobsen SE. Human CD34+ hematopoietic stem cells capable of multilineage engrafting NOD/SCID mice express flt3: distinct flt3 and c-kit expression and response patterns on mouse and candidate human hematopoietic stem cells. Blood 2003;102(3):881–886.

51. Nakao M, Yokota S, Iwai T, et al. Internal tandem duplication of the flt3 gene found in acute myeloid leukemia. Leukemia 1996;10(12):1911–1918.

52. Abu-Duhier FM, Goodeve AC, Wilson GA, Care RS, Peake IR, Reilly JT. Identification of novel FLT-3 Asp835 mutations in adult acute myeloid leukaemia. Br J Haematol 2001;113(4):983–988.

53. Kiyoi H, Towatari M, Yokota S, et al. Internal tandem duplication of the FLT3 gene is a novel modality of elongation mutation which causes constitutive activation of the product. Leukemia 1998;12(9):1333–1337.

54. Kiyoi H, Ohno R, Ueda R, Saito H, Naoe T. Mechanism of constitutive activation of FLT3 with internal tandem duplication in the juxtamembrane domain. Oncogene 2002;21(16):2555–2563.

55. Nagata H, Worobec AS, Oh CK, et al. Identification of a point mutation in the catalytic domain of the proto-oncogene c-kit in peripheral blood mononuclear cells of patients who have mastocytosis with an associated hematologic disorder. Proc Natl Acad Sci USA 1995;92(23):10,560–10,564.

56. Till JH, Ablooglu AJ, Frankel M, Bishop SM, Kohanski RA, Hubbard SR. Crystallographic and solution studies of an activation loop mutant of the insulin receptor tyrosine kinase: insights into kinase mechanism. J Biol Chem 2001;276(13):10,049–10,055.

57. Kiyoi H, Naoe T, Nakano Y, et al. Prognostic implication of FLT3 and N-RAS gene mutations in acute myeloid leukemia. Blood 1999;93(9):3074–3080.

58. Rombouts WJ, Blokland I, Lowenberg B, Ploemacher RE. Biological characteristics and prognosis of adult acute myeloid leukemia with internal tandem duplications in the Flt3 gene. Leukemia 2000;14(4):675–683.

59. Abu-Duhier FM, Goodeve AC, Wilson GA, et al. FLT3 internal tandem duplication mutations in adult acute myeloid leukaemia define a high-risk group. Br J Haematol 2000;111(1):190–195.

60. Stirewalt DL, Kopecky KJ, Meshinchi S, et al. FLT3, RAS, and TP53 mutations in elderly patients with acute myeloid leukemia. Blood 2001;97(11):3589–3595.

61. Kottaridis PD, Gale RE, Frew ME, et al. The presence of a FLT3 internal tandem duplication in patients with acute myeloid leukemia (AML) adds important prognostic information to cytogenetic risk group and response to the first cycle of chemotherapy: analysis of 854 patients from the United Kingdom Medical Research Council AML 10 and 12 trials. Blood 2001;98(6):1752–1759.

62. Whitman SP, Archer KJ, Feng L, et al. Absence of the wild-type allele predicts poor prognosis in adult de novo acute myeloid leukemia with normal cytogenetics and the internal tandem duplication of FLT3: a cancer and leukemia group B study. Cancer Res 2001;61(19):7233–7239.

63. Iwai T, Yokota S, Nakao M, et al. Internal tandem duplication of the FLT3 gene and clinical evaluation in childhood acute myeloid leukemia. The Children's Cancer and Leukemia Study Group, Japan. Leukemia 1999; 13(1):38–43.

64. Xu F, Taki T, Yang HW, et al. Tandem duplication of the FLT3 gene is found in acute lymphoblastic leukaemia as well as acute myeloid leukaemia but not in myelodysplastic syndrome or juvenile chronic myelogenous leukaemia in children. Br J Haematol 1999;105(1):155–162.

65. Kondo M, Horibe K, Takahashi Y, et al. Prognostic value of internal tandem duplication of the FLT3 gene in childhood acute myelogenous leukemia. Med Pediatr Oncol 1999;33(6):525–529.

66. Meshinchi S, Woods WG, Stirewalt DL, et al. Prevalence and prognostic significance of Flt3 internal tandem duplication in pediatric acute myeloid leukemia. Blood 2001;97(1):89–94.

67. Thiede C, Steudel C, Mohr B, et al. Analysis of FLT3-activating mutations in 979 patients with acute myelogenous leukemia: association with FAB subtypes and identification of subgroups with poor prognosis. Blood 2002;99(12):4326–4335.

68. Schnittger S, Schoch C, Dugas M, et al. Analysis of FLT3 length mutations in 1003 patients with acute myeloid leukemia: correlation to cytogenetics, FAB subtype, and prognosis in the AMLCG study and usefulness as a marker for the detection of minimal residual disease. Blood 2002;100(1):59–66.

69. Boissel N, Cayuela JM, Preudhomme C, et al. Prognostic significance of FLT3 internal tandem repeat in patients with de novo acute myeloid leukemia treated with reinforced courses of chemotherapy. Leukemia 2002;16(9):1699–1704.

70. Mizuki M, Fenski R, Halfter H, et al. Flt3 mutations from patients with acute myeloid leukemia induce transformation of 32D cells mediated by the Ras and STAT5 pathways. Blood 2000;96(12):3907–3914.

71. Mizuki M, Schwable J, Steur C, et al. Suppression of myeloid transcription factors and induction of STAT response genes by AML-specific Flt3 mutations. Blood 2003;101(8):3164–3173.

72. Scheijen B, Ngo HT, Kang H, Griffin JD. FLT3 receptors with internal tandem duplications promote cell viability and proliferation by signaling through Foxo proteins. Oncogene 2004;23(19):3338–3349.

73. Choudhary C, Schwable J, Brandts C, et al. AML-associated Flt3 kinase domain mutations show signal transduction differences in comparison to Flt3 ITD mutations. Blood 2005.

74. Kim KT, Baird K, Ahn JY, et al. Pim-1 is up-regulated by constitutively activated FLT3 and plays a role in FLT3-mediated cell survival. Blood 2005;105(4):1759–1767.

75. Tickenbrock L, Schwable J, Wiedehage M, et al. Flt3 tandem duplication mutations cooperate with Wnt signaling in leukemic signal transduction. Blood 2005;105(9):3699–3706.

76. Zheng R, Friedman AD, Levis M, Li L, Weir EG, Small D. Internal tandem duplication mutation of FLT3 blocks myeloid differentiation through suppression of C/EBP{alpha} expression. Blood 2004;103(5): 1883–1890.

77. Murphy KM, Levis M, Hafez MJ, et al. Detection of FLT3 Internal Tandem Duplication and D835 Mutations by a Multiplex Polymerase Chain Reaction and Capillary Electrophoresis Assay. J Mol Diagn 2003;5(2):96–102.

78. Kiyoi H, Naoe T, Yokota S, et al. Internal tandem duplication of FLT3 associated with leukocytosis in acute promyelocytic leukemia. Leukemia Study Group of the Ministry of Health and Welfare (Kohseisho). Leukemia 1997;11(9):1447–1452.

79. Arrigoni P, Beretta C, Silvestri D, et al. FLT3 internal tandem duplication in childhood acute myeloid leukaemia: association with hyperleucocytosis in acute promyelocytic leukaemia. Br J Haematol 2003; 120(1):89–92.

80. Noguera NI, Breccia M, Divona M, et al. Alterations of the FLT3 gene in acute promyelocytic leukemia: association with diagnostic characteristics and analysis of clinical outcome in patients treated with the Italian AIDA protocol. Leukemia 2002;16(11):2185–2189.

81. Shih LY, Kuo MC, Liang DC, et al. Internal tandem duplication and Asp835 mutations of the FMS-like tyrosine kinase 3 (FLT3) gene in acute promyelocytic leukemia. Cancer 2003;98(6):1206–1216.

82. Schlenk RF, Germing U, Hartmann F, et al. High-dose cytarabine and mitoxantrone in consolidation therapy for acute promyelocytic leukemia. Leukemia 2005.

83. Oyarzo MP, Lin P, Glassman A, Bueso-Ramos CE, Luthra R, Medeiros LJ. Acute myeloid leukemia with t(6;9)(p23;q34) is associated with dysplasia and a high frequency of flt3 gene mutations. Am J Clin Pathol 2004;122(3):348–358.

84. Blair A, Hogge DE, Sutherland HJ. Most acute myeloid leukemia progenitor cells with long-term proliferative ability in vitro and in vivo have the phenotype CD34(+)/CD71(-)/HLA-DR. Blood 1998;92(11): 4325–4335.

85. Bonnet D, Dick JE. Human acute myeloid leukemia is organized as a hierarchy that originates from a primitive hematopoietic cell. Nat Med 1997;3(7):730–737.

86. Meierhoff G, Dehmel U, Gruss HJ, et al. Expression of FLT3 receptor and FLT3-ligand in human leukemia-lymphoma cell lines. Leukemia 1995;9(8):1368–1372.

87. Drexler HG. Expression of FLT3 receptor and response to FLT3 ligand by leukemic cells. Leukemia 1996;10(4):588–599.

88. Carow CE, Levenstein M, Kaufmann SH, et al. Expression of the hematopoietic growth factor receptor FLT3 (STK-1/Flk2) in human leukemias. Blood 1996;87(3):1089–1096.

89. Birg F, Courcoul M, Rosnet O, et al. Expression of the FMS/KIT-like gene FLT3 in human acute leukemias of the myeloid and lymphoid lineages. Blood 1992;80(10):2584–2593.

90. Rosnet O, Buhring HJ, Marchetto S, et al. Human FLT3/FLK2 receptor tyrosine kinase is expressed at the surface of normal and malignant hematopoietic cells. Leukemia 1996;10(2):238–248.

91. Levis M, Murphy KM, Pham R, et al. Internal tandem duplications of the FLT3 gene are present in leukemia stem cells. Blood 2005.

92. Nakano Y, Kiyoi H, Miyawaki S, et al. Molecular evolution of acute myeloid leukemia in relapse: unstable N-ras and FLT3 genes compared with p53 gene. Br J Haematol 1999;104(4):659–664.

93. Kottaridis PD, Gale RE, Langabeer SE, Frew ME, Bowen DT, Linch DC. Studies of FLT3 mutations in paired presentation and relapse samples from patients with acute myeloid leukemia: implications for the role of FLT3 mutations in leukemogenesis, minimal residual disease detection, and possible therapy with FLT3 inhibitors. Blood 2002;100(7):2393–2398.

94. Shih LY, Huang CF, Wu JH, et al. Internal tandem duplication of FLT3 in relapsed acute myeloid leukemia: a comparative analysis of bone marrow samples from 108 adult patients at diagnosis and relapse. Blood 2002;100(7):2387–2392.

95. Tiesmeier J, Muller-Tidow C, Westermann A, et al. Evolution of FLT3-ITD and D835 activating point mutations in relapsing acute myeloid leukemia and response to salvage therapy. Leuk Res 2004;28(10):1069–1074.

96. Hope KJ, Jin L, Dick JE. Acute myeloid leukemia originates from a hierarchy of leukemic stem cell classes that differ in self-renewal capacity. Nat Immunol 2004;5(7):738–743.

97. Druker BJ, Sawyers CL, Kantarjian H, et al. Activity of a specific inhibitor of the BCR-ABL tyrosine kinase in the blast crisis of chronic myeloid leukemia and acute lymphoblastic leukemia with the Philadelphia chromosome. N Engl J Med 2001;344(14):1038–1042.

98. Levis M, Small D. Small molecule FLT3 tyrosine kinase inhibitors. Curr Pharm Des 2004;10(11): 1183–1193.

99. Lamers MB, Antson AA, Hubbard RE, Scott RK, Williams DH. Structure of the protein tyrosine kinase domain of C-terminal Src kinase (CSK) in complex with staurosporine. J Mol Biol 1999;285(2):713–725.

100. Bohmer FD, Karagyozov L, Uecker A, et al. A single amino acid exchange inverts susceptibility of related receptor tyrosine kinases for the ATP site inhibitor STI-571. J Biol Chem 2003;278(7):5148–5155.

101. Nagar B, Bornmann WG, Pellicena P, et al. Crystal structures of the kinase domain of c-Abl in complex with the small molecule inhibitors PD173955 and imatinib (STI-571). Cancer Res 2002;62(15):4236–4243.

102. Levis M, Tse KF, Smith BD, Garrett E, Small D. A FLT3 tyrosine kinase inhibitor is selectively cytotoxic to acute myeloid leukemia blasts harboring FLT3 internal tandem duplication mutations. Blood 2001;98(3): 885–887.

103. Levis M, Allebach J, Tse KF, et al. A FLT3-targeted tyrosine kinase inhibitor is cytotoxic to leukemia cells in vitro and in vivo. Blood 2002;99(11):3885–3891.

104. Brown P, Meshinchi S, Levis M, et al. Pediatric AML primary samples with FLT3/ITD mutations are preferentially killed by FLT3 inhibition. Blood 2004;104(6):1841–1849.

105. Ozeki K, Kiyoi H, Hirose Y, et al. Biologic and clinical significance of the FLT3 transcript level in acute myeloid leukemia. Blood 2004;103(5):1901–1908.

106. Fiedler W, Mesters R, Tinnefeld H, et al. A phase II clinical study of SU5416 in patients with refractory acute myeloid leukemia. Blood 2003.

107. Giles FJ, Cooper MA, Silverman L, et al. Phase II study of SU5416—a small-molecule, vascular endothelial growth factor tyrosine-kinase receptor inhibitor—in patients with refractory myeloproliferative diseases. Cancer 2003;97(8):1920–1928.

108. O'Farrell AM, Yuen HA, Smolich B, et al. Effects of SU5416, a small molecule tyrosine kinase receptor inhibitor, on FLT3 expression and phosphorylation in patients with refractory acute myeloid leukemia. Leuk Res 2004;28(7):679–689.

109. O'Farrell AM, Foran JM, Fiedler W, et al. An innovative phase I clinical study demonstrates inhibition of FLT3 phosphorylation by SU11248 in acute myeloid leukemia patients. Clin Cancer Res 2003;9(15): 5465–5476.

110. Fiedler W, Serve H, Dohner H, et al. A phase 1 study of SU11248 in the treatment of patients with refractory or resistant acute myeloid leukemia (AML) or not amenable to conventional therapy for the disease. Blood 2005;105(3):986–993.

111. Yee KW, Schittenhelm M, O'Farrell AM, et al. Synergistic effect of SU11248 with cytarabine or daunorubicin on FLT3 ITD-positive leukemic cells. Blood 2004;104(13):4202–4209.

112. George DJ, Dionne CA, Jani J, et al. Sustained in vivo regression of Dunning H rat prostate cancers treated with combinations of androgen ablation and Trk tyrosine kinase inhibitors, CEP-751 (KT-6587) or CEP-701 (KT-5555). Cancer Res 1999;59(10):2395–2401.

113. Smith BD, Levis M, Beran M, et al. Single-agent CEP-701, a novel FLT3 inhibitor, shows biologic and clinical activity in patients with relapsed or refractory acute myeloid leukemia. Blood 2004;103(10): 3669–3676.

114. Levis M, Pham R, Smith BD, Small D. In vitro studies of a FLT3 inhibitor combined with chemotherapy: sequence of administration is important to achieve synergistic cytotoxic effects. Blood 2004;104(4):1145–1150.

115. Weisberg E, Boulton C, Kelly LM, et al. Inhibition of mutant FLT3 receptors in leukemia cells by the small molecule tyrosine kinase inhibitor PKC412. Cancer Cell 2002;1(5):433–443.

116. Stone RM, DeAngelo DJ, Klimek V, et al. Patients with acute myeloid leukemia and an activating mutation in FLT3 respond to a small-molecule FLT3 tyrosine kinase inhibitor, PKC412. Blood 2005;105(1):54–60.

117. Giles F, Schiffer C, Kantarjian H, et al. Phase 1 study of PKC412, an oral FLT3 kinase inhibitor, in sequential and xoncomitant xombinations with daunorubicin and cytarabine (DA) induction and high-dose cytarabine (HDAra-C) consolidation in newly diagnosed patients with AML. Blood 2004;104:262a.

118. Kelly LM, Yu JC, Boulton CL, et al. CT53518, a novel selective FLT3 antagonist for the treatment of acute myelogenous leukemia (AML). Cancer Cell 2002;1(5):421–432.

119. Pandey A, Volkots DL, Seroogy JM, et al. Identification of orally active, potent, and selective 4-piper-azinylquinazolines as antagonists of the platelet-derived growth factor receptor tyrosine kinase family. J Med Chem 2002;45(17):3772–3793.

120. De Angelo D, Stone R, Heaney M, et al. Phase II evaluation of the tyrosine kinase inhibitor MLN518 in patients with acute myeloid leukemia (AML) bearing a FLT3 internal tandem duplication (ITD) mutation. Blood 2004;104(11):496a.

121. Clark JJ, Cools J, Curley DP, et al. Variable sensitivity of FLT3 activation loop mutations to the small mole-cule tyrosine kinase inhibitor MLN518. Blood 2004;104(9):2867–2872.

122. Trudel S, Li ZH, Wei E, et al. CHIR-258, a novel, multitargeted tyrosine kinase inhibitor for the potential treatment of t(4;14) multiple myeloma. Blood 2005;105(7):2941–2948.

123. Griswold IJ, Shen LJ, La Rosee P, et al. Effects of MLN518, a dual FLT3 and KIT inhibitor, on normal and malignant hematopoiesis. Blood 2004;104(9):2912–2918.

124. Shah NP, Nicoll JM, Nagar B, et al. Multiple BCR-ABL kinase domain mutations confer polyclonal resist-ance to the tyrosine kinase inhibitor imatinib (STI571) in chronic phase and blast crisis chronic myeloid leukemia. Cancer Cell 2002;2(2):117–125.

125. Bagrintseva K, Schwab R, Kohl TM, et al. Mutations in the tyrosine kinase domain of FLT3 define a new molecular mechanism of acquired drug resistance to PTK inhibitors in FLT3-ITD-transformed hematopoietic cells. Blood 2004;103(6):2266–2275.

126. Cools J, Mentens N, Furet P, et al. Prediction of resistance to small molecule FLT3 inhibitors: implications for molecularly targeted therapy of acute leukemia. Cancer Res 2004;64(18):6385–6389.

12 Farnesyl Transferase Inhibitors in the Therapy of AML

Jeffrey E. Lancet

CONTENTS

Summary

Farnesyl transferase inhibitors (FTIs) are signal transduction inhibitors that impede critical cell growth and survival signals. Clinical studies in elderly adults with acute myeloid leukemia (AML), particularly AML evolving from myelodysplastic syndromes, demonstrate modest but definite and reproducible clinical activity that is associated with prolongation of survival. FTI therapy is accompanied by a relatively low toxicity profile, thereby providing an important alternative to traditional cytotoxic approaches for elderly patients who are not likely to tolerate or even benefit from aggressive chemotherapy. One rationale upon which the clinical testing of FTIs in myeloid malignancies was based was the ability of FTIs to interrupt the farnesylation of oncogenic Ras proteins and the significant incidence of activating *ras* gene mutations in hematological malignancies. Provocatively, responses appear to be independent of *ras* mutations. Current studies continue to define the determinants of FTI antitumor activity and resistance. Preliminary microarray data suggest that FTIs modulate the activities of genetic networks involved in cell cycle progression, apoptosis, cell adhesion and cytoskeletal organization, and immune reactivity. The full development of FTIs in the therapeutic armamentarium for hematological malignancies will require the design and testing of rational combinations of cytotoxic, biological, and immunomodulatory agents in the laboratory and the clinic.

Key Words: Farnesylation; farnesyltransferase inhibition; signal transduction.

1. INTRODUCTION

An improved understanding of basic mechanisms in leukemia biology has driven the development of novel and targeted therapies in acute myeloid leukemia (AML). In recent years small molecule inhibitors have been developed for targets including FLT-3, vascular endothelial growth factor (VEGF), c-kit, histone deacetylases, DNA methyltransferases, and farnesyltransferase (FTase). These and other targets are discussed throughout this book in the contexts of pathogenesis and molecular therapeutics.

From: *Contemporary Hematology: Acute Myelogenous Leukemia*
Edited by: J. E. Karp © Humana Press Inc., Totowa, NJ

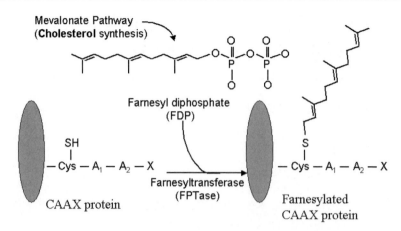

Fig. 1. Farnesylation reaction: FPTase transfers a fernasyl group onto the cysteine terminal portion of a substrate protein, such as Ras. (Adapted from ref. *2*.)

Farnesyl transferase inhibitors (FTIs) are a new class of signal transduction inhibitor that inhibit critical growth and survival signals. These agents potently and selectively inhibit intracellular FTase, an enzyme that catalyzes the transfer of a lipid farnesyl moiety to the cysteine terminal residue of a substrate protein (Fig. 1) *(1)*. Several intracellular proteins serve as substrates for prenylation via FTase, including Ras, Rho-B, Rac, and Lamin proteins *(2)*. Disrupting the normal prenylation process of these substrate proteins may thereby inhibit cellular events that are governed by them.

To date, several classes of FTIs have been developed *(3)*. Farnesyl diphosphate (FDP) analogs represent one class of FTIs. A second class of FTIs, known as peptidomimetics, compete with the terminal cysteine portion (C-A-A-X) of Ras and related proteins for FTase. A third class of FTIs is the bisubstrate analogs, which incorporate the structural motifs of both FTase and the C-A-A-X tetrapeptide. Nonpeptidomimetic inhibitors of FTase, identified from random screening of compound libraries, comprise a fourth class of FTIs. Collectively, the FTI subtypes share an ability to potently and selectively inhibit farnesylation; however, it appears likely that individual classes of FTIs, and perhaps the individual compounds within each class, ultimately display dissimilar functional activity within specific cancer types.

In the clinical arena, several FTIs have been developed (Fig. 2). Tipifarnib (Zarnestra®, R115777, Johnson & Johnson PRD), an orally bioavailable nonpeptidomimetic inhibitor, is the most developed compound in AML. Lonafarnib (Sarasar®, SCH66336, Schering-Plough Pharmaceuticals) and BMS-214662 (Bristol-Myers Squibb) are other FTIs that are undergoing development in hematological malignancies, including AML.

2. TARGETS FOR FTIS

The putative targets of FTIs are farnesylated proteins, several of which have important implications in the governance of intracellular events pertaining to proliferation and survival (Table 1).

2.1. Ras

The Ras family of oncoproteins, which guides a crucial network of signal transduction pathways that affects cellular proliferation, survival, and differentiation, was the principal

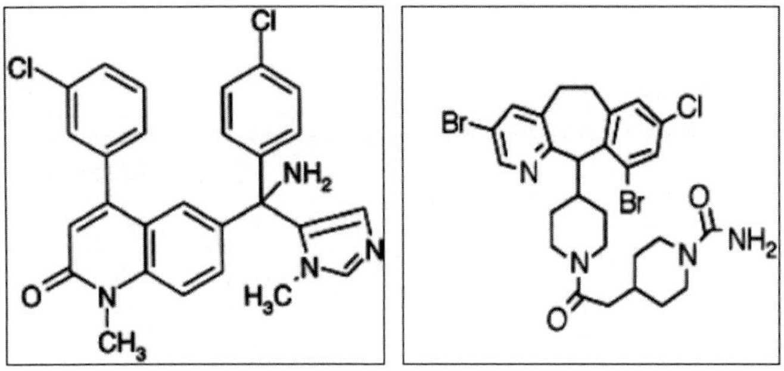

Tipifarnib (R115777)   Lonafarnib (SCH66336)

Fig. 2. Biochemical structures of farnesyltransferase inhibitors in clinical testing.

Table 1
Selected Intracellular Proteins Undergoing Farnesylation

Proteins	Cell structure/function
Res (H-, K-, N-)	Signal transduction
RHO (B, E)	Cytoskeletal organization, adhesion
Lamins (A, B)	Nuclear membrane structure
HDJ-2	Chaperone protein
Centromeric (CENPs)	Centromere–microtubule interaction proteins

target for which FTIs were initially developed (Fig. 3) *(2,4,5)*. The posttranslational modification of Ras involves its isoprenylation within the cytosol, at which point it is then enabled to migrate to the cell membrane, where it can activate downstream signaling events *(1,6)*. While membrane bound, Ras alternates between an active GTP-bound form and an inactive GDP-bound form, an equilibrium regulated by surface proteins such as SOS (a guanine nucleotide exchange factor), and GTPase activating protein (GAP) *(4)*. When mutated, Ras may fail to interact appropriately with its negative regulators, thereby leading to its constitutive activation in the GTP-bound form *(5)*.

The relatively high rate of mutated or activated *ras* in AML justifies its applicability as a relevant therapeutic target. Mutations of the N-*ras* oncogene, for example, occur in up to 48% of cases, although there is considerable variation in these rates amongpublished series *(7–12)*. Excessive signaling through Ras may occur independent of an activating mutation. One conceivable mechanism might involve an imbalance or excess of membrane-associated regulatory proteins that positively regulate Ras function. Indeed, one such recently discovered protein, RasGRP4, appears to be preferentially expressed in myeloid cells, including AML cell lines *(13)*. Similarly, disrupting the Grb-2/SOS complex, a key guanine nucleotide exchange factor that positively regulates Ras, greatly inhibits both Ras mediated cell proliferation in both BCR-ABL cell lines and freshly isolated chronic myeloid leukemia (CML) blasts *(14)*. Abnormal signaling upstream from Ras may represent a second putative mechanism through which unmutated Ras may be overactivated. With regard once again to the BCR-ABL model of leukemogenesis, introduction of dominant negative (inactive) *ras* into BCR-ABL transfected hematopoietic or fibroblast cells results in a complete blockage of malignant transformation *(15)*. Internal tandem duplication of the *FLT-3* gene, a common event in AML, may also mediate increased Ras activity via upstream mechanisms, in that transfection with a dominant-negative form of Ras inhibits colony formation in cells containing the *FLT-3* ITD

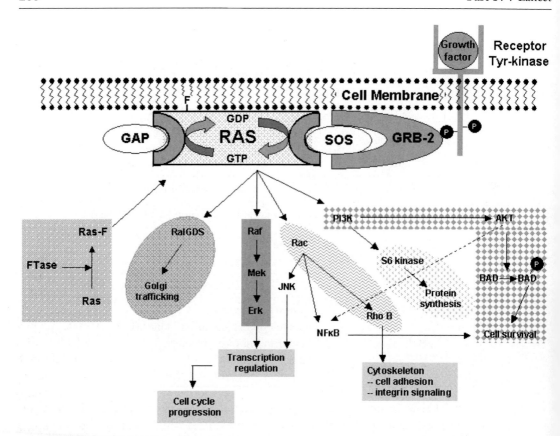

Fig. 3. Ras-mediated signaling. Posttranslationally farnesylated Ras localizes to the cell membrane, where it interacts with the regulatory factors GAP and SOS. In its activated GTP-bound form, Ras is capable of various kinase pathways that ultimately govern cellular proliferation and survival.

mutation *(16)*. Collectively, these observations suggest that inhibition of posttranslationally modified Ras via compounds such as FTIs is a viable therapeutic strategy in AML. It is important to recognize, however, that the precise level of Ras activity within a cell likely has important consequences on proliferation and survival, such that perturbation of this activity may not correlate directly with growth or survival inhibition. An excellent illustration of this assertion can be found in recent study wherein transduced human hematopoietic cells with a high level of H-Ras activity were found to be relatively nonproliferative and well differentiated. Moderate inhibition of Ras activity via FTI exposure resulted in increased proliferation and an elevated frequency of blast-like progenitors with enhanced self-renewal capacity, suggesting that the amplitude of Ras pathway signaling is a determinant of myeloid cell fate and that only moderate Ras activity within primitive hematopoietic cells may trigger leukemic growth and phenotype *(17)*. As such, therapeutic approaches to Ras inhibition should certainly be undertaken with caution.

Downstream effectors of Ras may also play relevant roles in leukemogenesis. Two such signaling cascades include the Raf-MEK mitogen-associated protein kinase (MAPK) pathway and the phosphatidylinositol-3-kinase (PI3K)/protein kinase B (PKB, AKT) pathway. Raf is a serine-threonine protein kinase that binds Ras *(18–20)*, after which it initiates a downstream cascade of phosphorylation, ultimately resulting in MAPK phosphorylation *(21–23)*. MAPK then localizes to the nucleus, where it activates transcription factors that govern cellular proliferation and apoptosis *(24–26)*. In the case of PI3K/AKT, Ras first interacts directly with the PI3K catalytic subunit to phosphorylate and activate the pivotal "second messenger" serine-threonine kinase AKT *(27–29)*. AKT then phosphorylates substrates involved in cell proliferation and survival following DNA damage or other cellular stresses.

Both the Raf-Mek-MAPK and the PI3K/AKT pathways appear to be germane to the regulation of leukemogenesis. For instance, constitutively activated mutant Raf can abrogate growth factor dependency in hematopoietic cells *(30)*, and pharmacological or antisense inhibition of MEK function can block Ras- or Raf-mediated transformation and cytokine-stimulated growth *(31)*. MAPK itself may be overexpressed or constitutively activated in hematopoietic malignancies, including AML. Constitutive activation of MAPK in clinical AML marrow samples, as determined by immunoblot and in vitro kinase analyses, has been demonstrated in a high proportion of AML cases at baseline *(32–34)*. Elevated baseline expression of phospho-MAPK may also adversely affect survival *(33)*.

The importance of PI3K/AKT signaling in cancers, including leukemia, can be demonstrated through several preclinical models. One in vitro model examining BCR-ABL-mediated leukemogenesis showed that intact PI3K-AKT signaling is essential for transformation and colony growth *(35)*. In another model, Ras mutants incapable of activating the Raf-MEK-ERK pathway were still able to inhibit apoptosis in interleukin-3-dependent cell lines, an effect that was blocked by pharmacological inhibition of PI3K with wortmannin *(30)*. While not specific to AML, substrates involved in cell cycle regulation and DNA repair also appear to be mediated by the PI3K/AKT pathway. One such potential effect on cell cycle involves AKT counteracting DNA damage-induced G1 and G2 checkpoint arrests *(36,37)*, possibly via threonine phosphorylation and inactivation of the cyclin-dependent kinase inhibitors inhibitors p21 and p27 *(38–41)*. AKT can also negate G1/S and G2M arrest by inactivating forkhead transcription factors such as FOXO3a, which protect cells from oxidative stress *(42–44)*. The pro-survival effects of augmented cellular adhesion may be mediated by the AKT-2-related integrin activation *(45)*. With specific regard to AML, overexpression of activated AKT may also occur in primary AML cells, as evidenced by one study in which constitutively activated (phosphorylated) AKT was detected in 17 of 17 leukemic marrow samples, but in none of the 6 normal control marrows *(46)*.

2.2. Rho Proteins

Considerable attention has been given to the potential and controversial role of Rho proteins as potential targets of FTI-mediated antineoplastic effects. The Rho proteins are part of the Ras family of small GTP-binding proteins that coordinate growth factor-induced assembly of intracellular focal adhesions and actin stress fiber formation *(47)*. Posttranslational prenylation occurs in these proteins, leading to both farnesylated and geranylgeranylated forms *(48,49)*, and Rho GTPases appear to be increased in human cancer cells as compared to nonmalignant cells *(50)*. Existing evidence suggests that RhoB might mediate some of the biological consequences of FTI treatment via induction of a preferential increase in the geranylgeranylated (GG) form of Rho B and subsequent cell growth inhibition *(51,52)*. The potential role of RhoB in this setting is also furthered by evidence that growth inhibitory and apoptotic effects elicited by FTIs in *ras*-transformed cells can be abrogated by the introduction of ectopic forms of RhoB *(53,54)*. Other evidence disputes the role of Rho B in FTI-mediated apoptosis. In human pancreatic tumor cells, it was demonstrated that both farnesylated and geranylgeranylated RhoB inhibited anchorage-dependent and -independent growth, induced apoptosis, and suppressed tumor growth.

2.3. Other Farnesylated Proteins

In addition to Ras and Rho, other farnesylated targets may function as important regulators of intracellular function that could be modified by FTIs. Such proteins include the kinetochore-binding centromeric proteins (CENPs) E and F, which are active in the G2 and M phases of the cell cycle and are critical to mitosis *(55,56)*. Although such a proposed mechanism for FTI activity remains largely speculative, FTIs can induce cycle arrest at the G2/M checkpoint in both a p53-dependent and -independent manner *(56–58)*. Furthermore, in human lung cancer cells, it was demonstrated that FTIs inhibit bipolar spindle formation amd subsequent proper chromosomal alignment at the metaphase plate *(59)*.

3. PRECLINICAL STUDIES IN MYELOID LEUKEMIA

FTIs possess variable antileukemia activity when tested in preclinical models, an effect that may relate in part to expression of various Ras isoforms. In one such model using *NF1*-deficient cells, which impart a myeloid leukemic phenotype on the presumptive basis of Ras hyperactivation, the FTI L-744,832 failed to inhibit in vivo leukemic growth, although it did selectively inhibit H-Ras, but not N-Ras or K-Ras, farnesylation *(60)*. These findings suggest that one mechanism by which FTIs fail to inhibit neoplastic growth may be based on the specific Ras isoform driving the disease. Other preclinical studies have demonstrated that in vitro, human AML cells appear to be sensitive to the effects of various FTIs, although evidence to suggest preferential sensitivity compared with normal hematopoietic progenitors is lacking *(61,62)*. It appears doubtful that FTIs are able to inhibit at the leukemic "stem" cell level, as evidenced by experiments in which FTI-treated human AML cells maintained their ability to promote engraftment in NOD-SCID mice at a similar level to untreated leukemic cells *(62)*. Mechanistically, FTI-mediated leukemic cell apoptosis may occur, at least in part, via an inhibitory effect on various Ras-related signaling pathways. For example, in myeloid leukemia cell lines demonstrating constitutive activity of MEK and MAPK, at least one FTI was able to cause growth inhibition *(63)*. More direct evidence for such an effect was demonstrated in experiments wherein the FTI L744832, when combined with a Chk1 inhibitor, provided synergistic pro-apoptotic activity in AML cell lines and primary AML blasts *(64)*. Because this combination elicited a decrease in phosphorylated AKT expression, and because enforced activation of AKT abrogated the pro-apoptotic effect of this combination *(64)*, it is plausible to propose the AKT signaling mechanism as a target for FTIs in AML.

4. CLINICAL TRIALS IN AML

To date, several trials of farnesyltransferase inhibitors in AML have been completed in patients with refractory or relapsed as well as previously untreated disease. As mentioned previously, tipifarnib (Zarnestra®, R115777, Johnson & Johnson PRD) is the most clinically developed of these agents in AML, and the ensuing discussion will focus on its use in AML.

4.1. Relapsed or Refractory AML

Interest in using FTIs to target Ras-mediated signaling spurred the development and implementation of FTIs in acute leukemias, particularly AML. It was not until later that evidence emerged suggesting that Ras may not, in fact, be a primary or exclusive target for FTIs. The initial phase 1 trial of FTI therapy in hematological malignancies using the orally bioavailable FTI tipifarnib was launched in 1999 and enrolled 34 patients primarily with refractory or relapsed acute leukemias *(65)*. In this trial, tipifarnib was orally administered on a twice-daily dosing schedule for 21 days every 4–6 weeks. The findings in this trial have had important implications in the development of future trials with FTIs and in AML specifically. First of all, it was demonstrated that consistent inhibition of farnesyltransferase within the leukemic cells occurred at varying dose levels well below the maximum tolerated dose. Second, overall toxicity was limited, with dose-limiting neurologic toxicity occurring at the 1200 mg bid dosing level. Toxicities rarely occurred at doses below 600 mg bid. Interestingly, bonafide responses occurred in 10 of 34 (29%) evaluable patients, including 2 complete responses. These responses occurred across the entire spectrum of dosing levels and did not seem to correlate with the degree of FTase inhibition in sampled leukemic cells, despite the fact that more consistent inhibition of FTase overall was seen at doses of 300 mg bid and higher. Perhaps the most intriguing finding to emanate from this study was a complete absence of detectable *ras* mutations, despite clinical drug activity, suggesting that the functional target of farnesyltransferase inhibition may not be Ras and that mutated *ras* appears not to be a determining factor in responsiveness to such an agent. Similar findings have been noted in other clinical trials of FTIs *(66,67)*.

In light of the safety and efficacy demonstrated in the aforementioned phase 1 trial, a large, international multicenter phase 2 trial was subsequently undertaken to further and more precisely delineate the antileukemic activity of the FTI tipifarnib *(68)*. Clinical activity, albeit modest, was demonstrated in this group of heavily pretreated patients, with 7% achieving complete response or complete response with incomplete platelet recovery and 14% with reductions in bone marrow blasts by more than 50%. It also appeared that a survival advantage was conveyed to the responding patients, with the median survival of this group being about 1 year, compared with less than 3 months for the entire group. Similar to the original phase 1 trial, safety and tolerability were once again demonstrated, with only rare cases of severe nonhematological adverse events observed.

4.2. Newly Diagnosed AML: Focus on Elderly Patients

The demonstrable safety and efficacy profile of FTIs has made it an intriguing compound to study in selected groups of poor risk AML patients who might otherwise do very poorly with, or perhaps even be ineligible for, standard cytotoxic chemotherapy in the upfront setting. In this context, a large phase 2 trial of tipifarnib in elderly poor risk adults with AML was launched in 2001, and the results wereupdated in December 2004 *(69)*. This clinical trial examined a somewhat unique group of patients in that the median age was 74 yearsand the majority of patients had AML that had evolved from an antecedent hematological disorder, most commonly myelodysplastic syndrome (Fig. 4; *see* Color Plate 14, following p. 174). Patients were treated with tipifarnib at 600 mg twice daily for 21 days, followed by a rest period of up to 6 weeks. The complete response rate for the entire group was 15%, and importantly, complete responders survived for a median of 54 weeks, compared with only 19 weeks for noncomplete responders. Equally important was the fact that the regimen was very safe and well tolerated: the treatment-related death rate was less than 10%, and only one-third of patients required hospitalization at any point during treatment. In addition to the patients experiencing complete response, several others had a partial response or hematological improvement that permitted therapy to continue for a prolonged period of time.

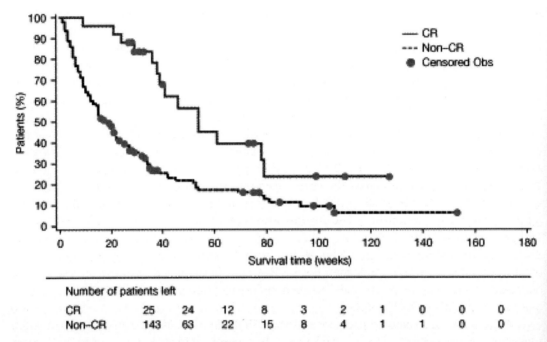

Fig. 4. (Color Plate 14, following p. 174) Overall survival for tipifarnib-treated patients with complete remission (CR) compared with non-CR. (From ref. *69*.)

5. FUTURE DIRECTIONS

5.1. Roles in Other AML Settings

The evidence of promising clinical activity and low toxicity has prompted the development of FTIs along other avenues in AML. One such area is in the postremission setting, in which conventional or higher-dose chemotherapeutic approaches (transplant-excluded) have failed to affect the risk of relapse or improve survival for older patients (70–72). To this end, several studies have been implemented to test the efficacy of FTIs during first complete remission in elderly or otherwise high-risk patients. This postremission strategy has also been undertaken for patients with AML in second or subsequent remission in an ongoing study through the Eastern Cooperative Oncology Group.

5.2. Combination Therapy

For reasons similar to those stated above, there has been great interest in the development of strategies that combine FTIs with traditional cytotoxics and, to a lesser extent, other novel biological agents. Unfortunately, an incomplete understanding of the mechanism that drives the antineoplastic effects of FTIs has limited successful combinatorial strategies in the clinic to date. Nonetheless, this area remains one of active investigation, and several recent publications attest to the fact that synergy with FTIs and cytotoxics or biologics is indeed possible. Taking into consideration the potential of FTIs to induce growth arrest at the G2M checkpoint of the cell cycle has led some investigators to pursue combinations with mitotic poisons such as taxanes and epipodophyllotoxins. One early study combined the FTI L-744,832 with paclitaxel, leading to synergistic inhibition of cell growth in vitro, imdicating that inhibition of protein farnesylation may deregulate a mitotic checkpoint and secondarily resulting in enhanced mitotic sensitivity to paclitaxel *(73)*. Other studies combining FTIs with chemotherapeutic agents such as cisplatin or taxanes have similarly demonstrated highly additive or synergistic effects of the combination *(74,75)*.

In AML there are also emerging data that shed light upon potentially useful combinations. Preliminary data from one group demonstrated synergistic growth inhibition with FTI L-744,832 and topoisomerase II inhibitors, as well as an increased level of apoptosis with the combination *(76)*. Other data indicate synergistic inhibition of leukemic colony growth when the FTI tipifarnib was combined with etoposide (S. Kaufmann, personal communication). From the standpoint of combination strategies between FTIs and biologics, interesting developments are emerging. One study of leukemic cell lines demonstrated synergy between the FTI L-744,832 and several inhibitors of the enzyme geranylgeranyltransferase *(77)*. Because a postulated mechanism of resistance to FTIs may be based upon alternative prenylation, such a combination is particularly intriguing. Taking advantage of the possible cell cycle-inhibitory effects of FTIs, another group of investigators studied the effects of combining an FTI with cyclin-dependent kinase inhibitors and demonstrated synergistic effects upon apoptosis of several cancer cell lines, including AML.

Clinical trials combining FTIs with other agents are just beginning to be implemented. One such study at Johns Hopkins Sidney Kimmel Comprehensive Cancer Center is examining the combination of tipifarnib with etoposide, predicated on the potential synergy demonstrated in vitro, for elderly patients with untreated AML. Another study being performed at the Princess Margaret Hospital in Toronto, Ontario, Canada, combines tipifarnib with standard daunorubicin plus cytarabine. The results of these trials should expand the antileukemic effects of FTIs in a setting that will not create undue toxicity.

6. CHANGING THE TREATMENT PARADIGM

Perhaps the most clinically important aspect of a new, targeted agent lies in its ability to be administered on a "chronic" basis with manageable toxicity. Historically, the successful treatment of AML has depended upon a finite number of cytotoxic chemotherapy cycles given in rapid succession, with the definition of success being complete remission. Given the usual aggressiveness of the underlying disease, in conjunction with an inability to give a prolonged course of toxic treatment, it is not surprising that disease response to treatment that is less than complete would not qualify as meaningful in the majority of cases. While the ultimate efficacy of FTIs in the arena of AML remains to be fully determined, the aforementioned clinical trials raise the question as to whether newer, targeted agents may eventually induce a shift in the traditional goals of therapy in AML, such that disease stabilization with improvement in hematological parameters could allow patients to be treated on an ongoing basis while maintaining a reasonable quality of life. These questions will need to be more definitively addressed in future clinical trials of FTIs and other targeted agents, but the possibility that disease control could be achieved, and survival perhaps lengthened, would surely be a worthwhile goal for a large proportion of elderly patients.

REFERENCES

1. End DW. Farnesyl protein transferase inhibitors and other therapies targeting the Ras signal transduction pathway. Invest New Drugs 1999;17:241–258.
2. Rowinsky EK, Windle JJ, Von Hoff DD. Ras protein farnesyltransferase: a strategic target for anticancer therapeutic development. J Clin Oncol 1999;17:3631–3652.

3. Patnaik A, Rowinsky EK. Early clinical experience with farnesyl protein transferase inhibitors. In: Sebti SM, Hamilton AD, eds. Farnesyltransferase Inhibitors in Cancer Therapy. Totowa: Humana Press; 2001:233–249.

4. Boguski MS, McCormick F. Proteins regulating Ras and its relatives. Nature 1993;366:643–654.

5. Lowy DR, Willumsen BM. Function and regulation of ras. Annu Rev Biochem 1993;62:851–891.

6. Khosravi-Far R, Cox AD, Kato K, Der CJ. Protein prenylation: key to ras function and cancer intervention? Cell Growth Differ 1992;3:461–469.

7. Kiyoi H, Naoe T, Nakano Y, et al. Prognostic implication of FLT3 and N-RAS gene mutations in acute myeloid leukemia. Blood 1999;93:3074–3080.

8. Lee YY, Kim WS, Bang YJ, et al. Analysis of mutations of neurofibromatosis type 1 gene and N-ras gene in acute myelogenous leukemia. Stem Cells 1995;13:556–563.

9. Neubauer A, Dodge RK, George SL, et al. Prognostic importance of mutations in the ras proto-oncogenes in de novo acute myeloid leukemia. Blood 1994;83:1603–1611.

10. Padua RA, Guinn BA, al-Sabah AI, et al. RAS, FMS, and p53 mutations and poor clinical outcome in myelodysplasias: a 10 year follow-up. Leukemia 1998;12:887–892.

11. Paquette RL, Landaw EM, Pierre RV, et al. N-ras mutations are associated with poor prognosis and increased risk of leukemia in myelodysplastic syndrome. Blood 1993;82:590–599.

12. Radich JP, Kopecky KJ, Willman CL, et al. N-ras mutations in adult de novo acute myelogenous leukemia: prevalence and clinical significance. Blood 1990;76:801–807.

13. Reuther GW, Lambert QT, Rebhun JF, et al. RasGRP4 is a novel Ras activator isolated from acute myeloid leukemia. J Biol Chem 2002;277:30,508–30,514.

14. Kardinal C, Konkol B, Lin H, et al. Chronic myelogenous leukemia blast cell proliferation is inhibited by peptides that disrupt Grb2-SoS complexes. Blood 2001;98:1773–1781.

15. Sawyers CL, McLaughlin J, Witte ON. Genetic requirement for Ras in the transformation of fibroblasts and hematopoietic cells by the Bcr-Abl oncogene. J Exp Med 1995;181:307–313.

16. Mizuki M, Fenski R, Halfter H, et al. Flt3 mutations from patients with acute myeloid leukemia induce transformation of 32D cells mediated by the Ras and STAT5 pathways. Blood 2000;96:3907–3914.

17. Dorrell C, Takenaka K, Minden MD, Hawley RG, Dick JE. Hematopoietic cell fate and the initiation of leukemic properties in primitive primary human cells are influenced by Ras activity and farnesyltransferase inhibition. Mol Cell Biol 2004;24:6993–7002.

18. Brtva TR, Drugan JK, Ghosh S, et al. Two distinct Raf domains mediate interaction with Ras. J Biol Chem 1995;270:9809–9812.

19. Marshall M. Interactions between Ras and Raf: key regulatory proteins in cellular transformation. Mol Reprod Dev 1995;42:493–499.

20. Vojtek AB, Hollenberg SM, Cooper JA. Mammalian Ras interacts directly with the serine/threonine kinase Raf. Cell 1993;74:205–214.

21. Dent P, Haser W, Haystead TA, et al. Activation of mitogen-activated protein kinase kinase by v-Raf in NIH 3T3 cells and in vitro. Science 1992;257:1404–1407.

22. Kyriakis JM, App H, Zhang XF, et al. Raf-1 activates MAP kinase-kinase. Nature 1992;358:417–421.

23. Robbins DJ, Zhen E, Owaki H, et al. Regulation and properties of extracellular signal-regulated protein kinases 1 and 2 in vitro. J Biol Chem 1993;268:5097–5106.

24. Davis RJ. Transcriptional regulation by MAP kinases. Mol Reprod Dev 1995;42:459–467.

25. Xing J, Ginty DD, Greenberg ME. Coupling of the RAS-MAPK pathway to gene activation by RSK2, a growth factor-regulated CREB kinase. Science 1996;273:959–963.

26. Bonni A, Brunet A, West AE, et al. Cell survival promoted by the Ras-MAPK signaling pathway by transcription-dependent and -independent mechanisms. Science 1999;286:1358–1362.

27. Jones PF, Jakubowicz T, Pitossi FJ, Maurer F, Hemmings BA. Molecular cloning and identification of a serine/threonine protein kinase of the second-messenger subfamily. Proc Natl Acad Sci USA 1991;88:4171–4175.

28. Qiu RG, Chen J, Kirn D, McCormick F, Symons M. An essential role for Rac in Ras transformation. Nature 1995;374:457–459.

29. Rodriguez-Viciana P, Warne PH, Dhand R, et al. Phosphatidylinositol-3-OH kinase as a direct target of Ras. Nature 1994;370:527–532.

30. Kinoshita T, Shirouzu M, Kamiya A, et al. Raf/MAPK and rapamycin-sensitive pathways mediate the anti-apoptotic function of p21 Ras in IL-3-dependent hematopoietic cells. Oncogene 1997;15:619–627.

31. Alessi DR, Cuenda A, Cohen P, Dudley DT, Saltiel AR. PD 098059 is a specific inhibitor of the activation of mitogen-activated protein kinase kinase in vitro and in vivo. J Biol Chem 1995;270:27,489–27,494.

32. Kim SC, Hahn JS, Min YH, et al. Constitutive activation of extracellular signal-regulated kinase in human acute leukemias: combined role of activation of MEK, hyperexpression of extracellular signal-regulated kinase, and downregulation of a phosphatase, PAC1. Blood 1999;93:3893–3899.

33. Kornblau SM, Milella M, Ball G, et al. ERK2 and Phospho-ERK2 are prognostic for survival in AML and complement the prognostic impact of Bax and BCL-2. Blood 2001;98:716a.

34. Towatari M, Iida H, Iwata H, Hamaguchi M, Saito H. Constitutive activation of mitogen-activated protein kinase pathway in acute leukemia cells. Leukemia 1997;11:479–484.

35. Skorski T, Bellacosa A, Nieborowska-Skorska M, et al. Transformation of hematopoietic cells by BCR/ABL requires activation of a PI-3k/Akt dependent pathway. EMBO J 1997;16:6151–6161.

36. Henry MK, Lynch JT, Eapen AK, Quelle FW. DNA damage-induced cell-cycle arrest of hematopoietic cells is overridden by activation of the PI-3 kinase/Akt signaling pathway. Blood 2001;98:834–841.

37. Kandel ES, Skeen J, Majewski N, et al. Activation of Akt/protein kinase B overcomes a G(2)/m cell cycle checkpoint induced by DNA damage. Mol Cell Biol 2002;22:7831–7841.

38. Liang J, Zubovitz J, Petrocelli T, et al. PKB/Akt phosphorylates p27, impairs nuclear import of p27 and opposes p27-mediated G1 arrest. Nat Med 2002;8:1153–1160.

39. Rossig L, Jadidi AS, Urbich C, et al. Akt-dependent phosphorylation of p21(Cip1) regulates PCNA binding and proliferation of endothelial cells. Mol Cell Biol 2001;21:5644–5657.

40. Shin I, Yakes FM, Rojo F, et al. PKB/Akt mediates cell-cycle progression by phosphorylation of p27(Kip1) at threonine 157 and modulation of its cellular localization. Nat Med 2002;8:1145–1152.

41. Viglietto G, Motti ML, Bruni P, et al. Cytoplasmic relocalization and inhibition of the cyclin-dependent kinase inhibitor p27(Kip1) by PKB/Akt-mediated phosphorylation in breast cancer. Nat Med 2002;8:1136–1144.

42. Brunet A, Bonni A, Zigmond MJ, et al. Akt promotes cell survival by phosphorylating and inhibiting a Forkhead transcription factor. Cell 1999;96:857–868.

43. Kops GJ, Medema RH, Glassford J, et al. Control of cell cycle exit and entry by protein kinase B-regulated forkhead transcription factors. Mol Cell Biol 2002;22:2025–2036.

44. Tran H, Brunet A, Grenier JM, et al. DNA repair pathway stimulated by the forkhead transcription factor FOXO3a through the Gadd45 protein. Science 2002;296:530–534.

45. Jiang K, Coppola D, Crespo NC, et al. The phosphoinositide 3-OH kinase/AKT2 pathway as a critical target for farnesyltransferase inhibitor-induced apoptosis. Mol Cell Biol 2000;20:139–148.

46. Lancet JE, Ryan CP, Abboud CN, et al. Differences in the expression of signal transduction molecules between normal and leukemic bone marrow. Blood 2002;98:111a.

47. Ridley AJ, Hall A. The small Gtp-binding protein Rho regulates the assembly of focal adhesions and actin stress fibers in response to growth-factors. Cell 1992;70:389–399.

48. Armstrong SA, Hannah VC, Goldstein JL, Brown MS. CAAX geranylgeranyl transferase transfers farnesyl as efficiently as geranylgeranyl to RhoB. J Biol Chem 1995;270:7864–7868.

49. Adamson P, Marshall CJ, Hall A, Tilbrook PA. Post-translational modifications of p21rho proteins. J Biol Chem 1992;267:20,033–20,038.

50. Fritz G, Just I, Kaina B. Rho GTPases are over-expressed in human tumors. Int J Cancer 1999;81:682–687.

51. Du W, Lebowitz PF, Prendergast GC. Cell growth inhibition by farnesyltransferase inhibitors is mediated by gain of geranylgeranylated RhoB. Mol Cell Biol 1999;19:1831–1840.

52. Lebowitz PF, Casey PJ, Prendergast GC, Thissen JA. Farnesyltransferase inhibitors alter the prenylation and growth-stimulating function of RhoB. J Biol Chem 1997;272:15,591–15,594.

53. Lebowitz PF, Davide JP, Prendergast GC. Evidence that farnesyltransferase inhibitors suppress Ras transformation by interfering with Rho activity. Mol Cell Biol 1995;15:6613–6622.

54. Lebowitz PF, Sakamuro D, Prendergast GC. Farnesyl transferase inhibitors induce apoptosis of Ras-transformed cells denied substratum attachment. Cancer Res 1997;57:708–713.

55. Ashar HR, James L, Gray K, et al. Farnesyl transferase inhibitors block the farnesylation of CENP-E and CENP-F and alter the association of CENP-E with the microtubules. J Biol Chem 2000;275:30,451–30,457.

56. Ashar HR, James L, Gray K, et al. The farnesyl transferase inhibitor SCH 66336 induces a G(2) --> M or G(1) pause in sensitive human tumor cell lines. Exp Cell Res 2001;262:17–27.

57. Feldkamp MM, Lau N, Guha A. Growth inhibition of astrocytoma cells by farnesyl transferase inhibitors is mediated by a combination of anti-proliferative, pro-apoptotic and anti-angiogenic effects. Oncogene 1999;18:7514–7526.

58. Gu WZ, Tahir SK, Wang YC, et al. Effect of novel CAAX peptidomimetic farnesyltransferase inhibitor on angiogenesis in vitro and in vivo. Eur J Cancer 1999;35:1394–1401.

59. Crespo NC, Ohkanda J, Yen TJ, Hamilton AD, Sebti SM. The farnesyltransferase inhibitor, FTI-2153, blocks bipolar spindle formation and chromosome alignment and causes prometaphase accumulation during mitosis of human lung cancer cells. J Biol Chem 2001;276:16,161–16,167.
60. Mahgoub N, Taylor BR, Gratiot M, et al. In vitro and in vivo effects of a farnesyltransferase inhibitor on *Nf1*-deficient hematopoietic cells. Blood 1999;94:2469–2476.
61. Huang XK, Meyer P, Li B, Raza A, Preisler HD. The effects of the farnesyl transferase inhibitor FTI L-778,123 on normal, myelodysplastic, and myeloid leukemia bone marrow progenitor proliferation in vitro. Leukemia Lymphoma. 2003;44:157–164.
62. Liesveld JL, Lancet JE, Rosell KE, et al. Effects of the farnesyl transferase inhibitor R115777 on normal and leukemic hematopoiesis. Leukemia 2003;17:1806–1812.
63. Morgan MA, Dolp O, Reuter CWM. Cell-cycle-dependent activation of mitogen-activated protein kinase kinase (MEK-1/2) in myeloid leukemia cell lines and induction of growth inhibition and apoptosis by inhibitors of RAS signaling. Blood 2001;97:1823–1834.
64. Dai Y, Rahmani M, Pei XY, et al. Farnesyltransferase inhibitors interact synergistically with the Chk1 inhibitor UCN-01 to induce apoptosis in human leukemia cells through interruption of both Akt and MEK/ERK pathways and activation of SEK1/JNK. Blood 2005;105:1706–1716.
65. Karp JE, Lancet JE, Kaufmann SH, et al. Clinical and biological activity of the farnesyltransferase inhibitor R115777 in adults with refractory and relapsed acute leukemias: a phase I clinical-correlative trial. Blood 2001;97:3361–3369.
66. Kurzrock R, Albitar M, Cortes JE, et al. Phase II study of R115777, a farnesyl transferase inhibitor, in myelodysplastic syndrome. J Clin Oncol 2004;22:1287–1292.
67. Kurzrock R, Verstovsek S, Wright JJ, et al. Phase I study using alternate week administration of the farnesyl transferase inhibitor R115777 (Zarnestra™) in patients with myelodysplastic syndrome. Blood 2004;104:402a.
68. Harousseau J-L, Reiffers J, Lowenberg B, et al. Zarnestra (R115777) in patients with relapsed and refractory acute myelogenous leukemia (AML): results of a multicenter phase 2 study. Blood 2003;102:176a.
69. Lancet JE, Gotlib J, Gojo I, et al. Tipifarnib (ZARNESTRA™) in previously untreated poor-risk AML of the elderly: updated results of a multicenter phase 2 trial. Blood 2004;104:249a.
70. Lowenberg B, Suciu S, Archimbaud E, et al. Use of recombinant GM-CSF during and after remission induction chemotherapy in patients aged 61 years and older with acute myeloid leukemia: final report of AML-11, a phase III randomized study of the Leukemia Cooperative Group of European Organization for the Research and Treatment of Cancer and the Dutch Belgian Hemato-Oncology Cooperative Group. Blood 1997;90: 2952–2961.
71. Lowenberg B, Suciu S, Archimbaud E, et al. Mitoxantrone versus daunorubicin in induction-consolidation chemotherapy—the value of low-dose cytarabine for maintenance of remission, and an assessment of prognostic factors in acute myeloid leukemia in the elderly: final report. European Organization for the Research and Treatment of Cancer and the Dutch-Belgian Hemato-Oncology Cooperative Hovon Group. J Clin Oncol 1998;16:872–881.
72. Stone RM, Berg DT, George SL, et al. Postremission therapy in older patients with de novo acute myeloid leukemia: a randomized trial comparing mitoxantrone and intermediate-dose cytarabine with standard-dose cytarabine. Blood 2001;98:548–553.
73. Moasser MM, Sepp-Lorenzino L, Kohl NE, et al. Farnesyl transferase inhibitors cause enhanced mitotic sensitivity to taxol and epothilones. Proc Natl Acad Sci USA 1998;95:1369–1374.
74. Adjei AA, Davis JN, Bruzek LM, Erlichman C, Kaufmann SH. Synergy of the protein farnesyltransferase inhibitor SCH66336 and cisplatin in human cancer cell lines. Clin Cancer Res 2001;7:1438–1445.
75. Sun JZ, Blaskovich MA, Knowles D, et al. Antitumor efficacy of a novel class of non-thiol-containing peptidomimetic inhibitors of farnesyltransferase and geranylgeranyltransferase I: Combination therapy with the cytotoxic agents cisplatin, taxol, and gemcitabine. Cancer Res 1999;59:4919–4926.
76. Reuter CW, Wegner J, Morgan MA, Ganser A. Co-treating AML cells with FTI potentiates apoptosis induced by topoisomerase II inhibitors. Blood 2002;100:542a.
77. Morgan MA, Wegner J, Aydilek E, Ganser A, Reuter CW. Synergistic cytotoxic effects in myeloid leukemia cells upon cotreatment with farnesyltransferase and geranylgeranyl transferase-I inhibitors. Leukemia 2003;17: 1508–1520.

13 Modulating Gene Expression as a Therapeutic Approach in the Treatment of AML

Tamer Fandy, Hetty Carraway,
and Steven D. Gore

CONTENTS

Summary

Chemotherapy plays an indispensable role in the management of leukemia. However, resistance development and lack of selectivity are major drawbacks. Unfortunate side effects of chemotherapy create a continuous demand for developing other novel strategies for treatment. Epigenetic modulation of gene expression is one of the emerging and promising strategies that has demonstrated successful clinical outcome in acute myeloid leukemis (AML). However, the exact molecular mechanism of action of epigenetic modifiers remains unclear. Ongoing clinical trials are attempting to identify the possible candidate genes that upon re-expression can induce remission and cure in patients. Interestingly, epigenetic modifiers exhibit other pharmacological effects not related to gene expression modulation, including generation of reactive oxygen species and DNA damage induction. It appears that epigenetic therapy is having a promising impact in myelodysplatic syndrome (MDS) and leukemia, but exactly how these epigenetic modifiers achieve clinical responses remains to be elucidated.

Key Words: DNA methylation; demethylating agent; histone deacetylase inhibitor; promoter hypermethylation; histone acetyltransferase; histone methyltransferase; 5-azacytidine; decitabine.

1. INTRODUCTION

1.1. Epigenetics and AML

Epigenetics refers to heritable changes in gene transcription that occur without a change in the sequence of nuclear DNA. The epigenome indicates the overall set of epigenetic modifications, or "epigenetic marks," in a cell. The postgenomic era has shown that both DNA methylation and histone modifications can affect gene expression by remodeling

From: *Contemporary Hematology: Acute Myelogenous Leukemia*
Edited by: J. E. Karp © Humana Press Inc., Totowa, NJ

the chromatin architecture. The important role that epigenetics plays in determining the biological phenotype can be dramatically seen by the ability of epigenetic differences to explain the differences in anthropomorphic features in monozygotic twins *(1)*. Genomic imprinting (a phenomenon in which the expression of certain genes is determined by whether the gene is inherited from the female or male parent) is also effected through epigenetic modifications *(2)*. Silencing of tumor suppressor genes through DNA methylation and/or histone modification has increased the recognition of the role of epigenetics in cancer development *(3)*.

1.2. DNA Methylation

To date, the most extensively characterized epigenetic alteration is DNA methylation. Cytosine methylation of the palindromic CpG dinucleotide sequence has been the most widely known and studied modification, but non-CpG DNA methylation has been also reported in eukaryotes *(4)*. CpG islands are regions of more than 500 base pairs containing a CG content of 55% or more *(5)*. Aberrant *de novo* methylation of CpG islands near the promoter regions of tumor suppressor genes is a hallmark of cancer and is found early during carcinogenesis *(3)*. A transient covalent complex forms between DNA methyltransferases (DNMTs) and the C6 position in cytosine resulting in the activation of C5 position (Fig. 1A). Subsequently, a methyl group from the methyl donor S-adenosyl-L-methionine (SAM) is transferred to the activated C5 position of cytosine followed by the release of DNMT enzyme by β–elimination *(6)*. Hypermethylation of CpG islands near the promoter region of genes usually silences its expression. The biological effects of the loss of gene function caused by promoter hypermethylation and by coding-region mutations are similar. For instance, mutation or epigenetic silencing of *MLH1* causes the form of genomic instability termed microsatellite instability in colon cancer and other tumors. Similarly, both genetic and epigenetic changes in *BRCA1,* a breast cancer susceptibility gene, produce similar DNA microarray patterns of gene expression in breast cancer *(7)*.

1.3. Histone Modifications

Posttranslational modification of histones by acetylation or methylation make up an important set of epigenetic marks, and they are believed to constitute a complex combinatorial "histone code." Histone acetylation/deacetylation is controlled by two sets of enzymes, histone acetyltransferases (HAT) and histone deacetylases (HDAC), respectively. The chromatin architecture is regulated by the activity of these two enzymes, where HAT is associated with the transcriptionally active state (euchromatin), and HDAC is associated with the transcriptionally repressed state (heterochromatin) *(8)*. The recruitment of HDAC by DNA methyltransferase and by specific methyl-binding proteins represses transcription by inducing a transcriptionally repressed state of chromatin *(9)*. Other forms of histone modifications that can induce chromatin remodeling also exist. Methylation of histones, in which a number of lysine residues within histones H3 and H4 are subject to methylation by site-specific enzymes, can affect gene expression. Some methylated lysines are involved in activation, whereas others are involved in repression. Current evidence suggests that methylated lysines within histones direct the recruitment of different methyl-binding proteins, which mediate the biological effects of lysine methylation. The methylation of H3-K9 and H3-K27 has been linked to gene silencing, while K4, K36, and K79 within histone H3 are associated with the positive regulation of gene expression. Recently, studies have provided convincing evidence for the reversal of histone methylation, thereby providing an additional level of epigenetic control. LSD1 (a FAD-dependent amine oxidase with substrate specificity

A

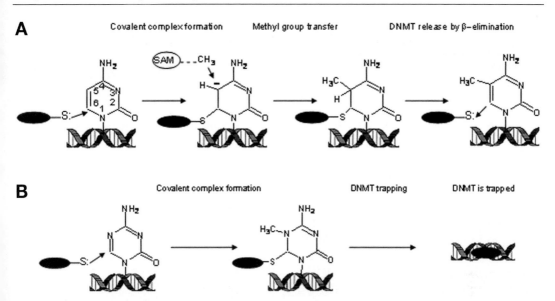

B

Fig. 1. The enzymatic process of cytosine methylation by DNA methyltransferase (DNMT) and the methyl group donor S-adenosyl-L-methionine (SAM). (**A**) DNMT release from cytosine by β-elimination. The black circle with sulfur group represents the DNMT enzyme. (**B**) DNMT is trapped by the nucleoside analog 5-Aza because of the absence of a proton at position 5.

for methylated K4 on histone H3) demethylates H3-K4 and H3-K9 through an amine oxidase reaction and seems to function as both a positive and negative regulator of gene expression *(10)*. It is interesting to note that all *MLL* (mixed leukemia lineage) fusion proteins (a fusion protein associated with high-risk acute leukemia) truncate the histone methyltransferase domain of MLL *(11)*. The implication of this functional change continues to direct us to optimize targeted therapies through epigenetic mechanisms and have optimism about their impact.

Phosphorylation is another covalent posttranslational modification of histones; the main substrate for phosphorylation is histone H3. The ε-amino group of histone lysine residues is also subject to modification by ubiquitin and ubiquitin-like proteins such as SUMO *(12)*. Because of the large size of these modifications, it is not clear whether SUMOylation and ubiquitination directly affects nucleosomal structure or packing or whether this modification serves to promote/inhibit interaction with nonhistone proteins, or both. Histone phosphorylation, ubiquitination, and SUMOylation are not yet known as targets for drug development.

Because inhibitors of HDAC enzymes can induce expression of genes silenced in heterochromatin, they are likely to be beneficial in the treatment of cancer by inducing the expression of tumor suppressor genes and pro-apoptotic genes. While concern has been expressed that nonspecific HDAC inhibitors could lead to the induction of thousands of genes, microarray analysis has shown that only a small percentage of genes were modulated by HDAC inhibitors *(13)*, and surprisingly, both induction and repression of genes were observed. The lack of a global effect after administering HDAC inhibitors could be explained by the dominance of DNA methylation over histone acetylation as an epigenetic modifier *(14)*.

Table 1
Hypermethylated Genes in Hematological Malignancies

Function	Gene	Tumor	Ref.
Cell cycle regulation	p14^{ARF}	Acute lymphoblastic leukemia	83
Cell cycle regulation	p15^{INK4B}	Leukemias/gliomas	15
Cell cycle regulation	p16^{INK4A}	Various tumors	84
Cell cycle regulation/apoptosis	p73	Leukemias/lymphomas	85
Cell cycle regulation	KLF4	Leukemia	86
Cell cycle regulation/apoptosis	GADD45G	Various tumors	87
Apoptosis	DAPK	Various tumors	88
Apoptosis	Apaf-1	Leukemia	89
Apoptosis	ASPP1	Leukemia	90
Apoptosis	WWOX	Leukemias	91
Transcription factor	EGR3	Leukemia	86
Transcription factor	HIC1	Leukemia	92
Signal transduction	SOCS-1	Multiple myeloma	93
Signal transduction	PTPN6 (SHP1)	Multiple myeloma	94
Signal transduction	PTPRG	Lymphoma	95
Putative gene	BCL7a	Lymphoma	95
Nuclear envelope/ DNA replication	Lamin A/C	Leukemias/lymphomas	96
DNA damage	FANCF	Leukemia	97
Metastasis	CDH1	Various	98
Cytokine receptor	IL-12R-β2	Lymphomas	99
Retinoic acid signaling	TIG1	Leukemia	100
Metastasis	TIMP3	Various tumors	88
Calcium metabolism	Calcitonin	Acute lymphoblastic leukemia	101
Estrogen receptor	ER	MDS	102

2. HYPERMETHYLATED GENES

Loss of expression of tumor suppressor genes is usually attributed to genetic causes (mutations or deletions) as well as epigenetic causes such as CpG island hypermethylation. Aberrant methylation of CpG islands in the promoter region of genes is a hallmark of human cancers *(15)*. Two mechanisms have been proposed to describe the silencing effect of CpG islands hypermethylation. First, methylated CpG islands in the promoter region can inhibit the binding of transcription factors to their CpG-containing recognition sites *(16)*. The second mechanism proposes the involvement of methyl CpG-binding proteins like MeCP1 and MeCP2 *(17)*. In the last decade, a myriad of hypermethylated genes were discovered and correlated to tumorigenesis. Table 1 categorizes some of the known hypermethylated genes in hematological malignancies according to their function.

3. CYTOGENETICS, TRANSCRIPTION FACTORS, AND MATURATION ARREST

A variety of genetic defects lead to the development of AML. Accumulation of primitive hematopoietic blast cells in lieu of mature blood cells constitutes the unifying phenotypic feature of this genetically and clinically heterogeneous group of disorders. Maturation arrest has been associated with dysregulated patterns of gene transcription, which may arise through aberrant transcription factors as well as epigenetic silencing of regulatory genes. Cloning of breakpoints at recurring chromosomal translocations led to the best-characterized genetic abnormalities in AML, which led to aberrant transcriptional programs.

The t(8;21) translocation, associated with a subset of AML classified as M2 by the French–American–British classification (FAB) and with a recognizable phenotype by light microscopy and flow cytometry, encodes the chimeric gene AML1-ETO. This subset of AML represents 10–15% of all cases and is associated with a favorable prognosis. The translocation fuses the DNA-binding domain of RUNX1 (core-binding factor [CBF]α) to nearly all of ETO (eight twenty-one, also known as MTG8 myeloid translocation gene on chromosome 8), which functions as a transcriptional co-repressor. The fusion protein is a potent transcriptional repressor, but the direct targets of transcriptional regulation that mediate cellular transformation are unknown *(18–20)*. Expression of the fusion gene inhibits the differentiation of myeloid progenitors by suppressing genes associated with myeloid differentiation. Interestingly, a recent cooperation was suggested between AML1-ETO and Wilms' tumor gene (WT1) to exert its leukemogenic function; WT1 is expressed at high levels in almost all human leukemia *(21)*.

The CBFB-MYH11 fusion gene, encoding the fusion protein CBFβ-SMMHC, is another aberrant transcription factor created by the relatively common inversion of chromosome 16. This fusion protein, which involves the β subunit of CBF (AML1 is the α subunit) also interferes with transcription of genes associated with myeloid differentiation regulated by CBF. Interestingly, the typical leukemia associated with this fusion gene (classified as M4 with abnormal eosinophils, or M4Eo in the FAB classification) shares many clinical features with the other main CBF leukemia AML (AML1-ETO), including preservation of some myeloid differentiation, the presence of dysplastic eosinophils, and high degree of curability with cytarabine intensive chemotherapy regimens *(22)*.

The retinoic acid-signaling pathway is involved in the regulation of hematopoietic myeloid differentiation and is altered in APL, resulting in differentiation blockage of leukemic blasts. The APL-specific RARα fusion proteins PML/RARα and PLZF/RARα bind to and constitutively repress promoters of retinoic acid target genes via aberrant recruitment of multisubunit complexes containing HDAC activities. The impact of epigenetic therapy on these fusion genes is yet to be established, but the functional impact of these fusion genes may be altered with such an approach.

The *MLL* gene located at 11q23 is fused to a variety of partner genes through chromosomal translocations in acute leukemia. Approximately 50 different chromosomal translocations of the human *MLL* gene are currently known and associated with high-risk acute leukemia *(23)*. For a list of the different fusion partners, the *Atlas for Genetics and Cytogenetics in Oncology and Hematology* (www.infobiogen.fr/services/chromcancer/genes) provides a comprehensive guide. The exact role of *MLL* fusion proteins in leukemogenesis is not well defined; however, gain of function is the most plausible mechanism that describes the oncogenic potential of the chimeric *MLL* proteins. The soundness of this mechanism is supported by a series of retroviral transduction experiments showing that only the protein chimeras and not the truncated *MLL* can induce leukemia *(24,25)*. Moreover, knockin animals that express *MLL* fusion protein under the authentic control of the *MLL* promoter and the *bona fide* chromatin environment further supports the gain of function hypothesis *(26,27)*. Because *MLL* positively regulates Hox gene expression, leukemogenic *MLL* fusion proteins are expected to disrupt critical patterns of *HOX* gene expression in hematopoietic progenitor cells in ways that selectively contribute to either myeloid (e.g., *MLL*-AF9) or lymphoid (e.g., *MLL*-AF4) acute leukemias *(28)*. The fact that some of *MLL* translocation partners are not transcriptional factors and express self-association domains prompted the hypothesis that *MLL* dimerization may also be involved in cell transformation *(29,30)*. For instance, β-galactosidase, which oligomerizes into a tetramer in solution and has no known transcriptional activity, induced leukemia when the bacterial lacZ gene was fused to *MLL* and knockin mice embryonic stem cells, albeit with long latency *(31)*. The small oligomerization domain of Gephyrin (GPHN), a neuronal receptor, was shown to be both necessary and sufficient to give the MLL fusion protein transformation capability *(32)*. Taken together, dimerization or oligomerization of *MLL* could also explain the transforming potential of *MLL* fusion proteins.

Chromosome 5 and/or 7 abnormalities are cytogenetic findings indicative of a poor prognosis in patients with AML or MDS. In AML and MDS, monosomy 7 and deletion of chromosome 7q are a few of the most common cytogenetic aberrations. Considerable effort has been made to identify tumor suppressor genes that are deleted in these recurring abnormalities; to date no unifying commonly deleted tumor suppressor genes have been identified.

Trisomy 8 is one of the most frequent numerical chromosomal abnormalities observed in AML and MDS. In contrast, tetrasomy 8 is a rare cytogenetic abnormality reported in only a few cases with myeloid malignancies—mostly AML of monocytic lineage. The biological sequelae of trisomy 8 remain uncertain. The Cancer Genome Anatomy Project (CGAP) provides an excellent tool for learning about different cases of chromosomal abnormalities called the Mitelman Database of Chromosome Aberrations in Cancer (http://cgap.nci.nih.gov/chromosomes/Mitelman). Table 2 summarizes the known chromosomal abnormalities in AML and their associated prognosis.

4. DNMT INHIBITORS

4.1. DNMT Inhibitors in MDS and AML

5-Azacytidine (5-Aza) and 5-aza-2′deoxycytidine (DAC) are well-known DNMT inhibitors. The structural similarity of 5-Aza and DAC with cytosine allows for their incorporation into DNA in lieu of cytosine residues with consequent complex formation with DNMT (Fig. 1A). However, DNMT is not released from 5-Aza or DAC by β–elimination when the nucleoside is incorporated DNA; thus, the DNMT remains trapped as an inactive adduct because of the absence of a proton at the 5 position (Fig. 1B). Consequently, the DNMT pool becomes depleted during the S-phase progression of the cell cycle, and its methylation pattern cannot be transmitted to daughter chromatids. The trapping of DNMT by 5-Aza and DAC was recently visualized and measured by fluorescence recovery after photobleaching *(33)*. Although it is common to consider both 5-Aza and DAC as pharmacological equivalents, they do differ pharmacologically. Specifically, 5-Aza is incorporated into RNA as well as DNA; the biological consequences of this difference are not clear.

MDS is a precursor of a particularly treatment-resistant subset of AML. 5-Aza and DAC are DNA hypomethylating drugs that were tested for their efficacy in the treatment of MDS and AML. DAC was evaluated for efficacy and cytotoxicity in poor prognosis AML and was able to induce differentiation of cells and clinical response in 40% of the patients with minimal cytotoxicity *(34)*. Low doses of DAC were also shown to be more efficacious than high doses in different hematological malignancies *(35)*. DAC was also shown to induce hematologic and cytogenetic remissions in MDS patients *(36–38)*. Furthermore, 5-Aza treatment of MDS patients resulted in significantly higher response rates, improved quality of life,

Table 2
Karyotype as a Prognostic Factor in AML

Chromosomal abnormality	Affected genes	Prognosis
–7	Multiple	Poor
–5	Multiple	Poor
Miscellaneous	Multiple	Intermediate–Poor
11q23	MLL	Intermediate–Poor
Trisomy/Tetrasomy 8	Multiple	Intermediate–Poor
t(8;21)(q22;q22)	AML1/ETO	Good
inv(16)(p13;q22)	CBFb/MYH11	Good

and reduced risk of leukemic transformation compared with supportive care *(39)*. Both 5-Aza (FDA approved in 2004) and DAC (FDA approved in 2006) are used for the treatment of MDS and are available commercially.

Hypermethylation and subsequent transcriptional silencing of tumor suppressor genes are found in various tumor entities. Genes involved in cell cycle regulation, tumor suppression, cell growth, and differentiation are possible targets for DNMT inhibitors because of their pivotal role in the initiation and progression of hematological disorders. One of the most commonly methylated genes in AML and MDS is $p15^{INK4b}$, an inhibitor of the cyclin-dependent kinases 4 and 6. The in vivo methylation and protein expression changes of $p15^{INK4b}$ in elderly MDS patients during treatment with low-dose decitabine were studied *(40)*. Nine of 12 patients with initially hypermethylated $p15^{INK4b}$ showed a decrease in methylation after one or more cycles of decitabine therapy. The observed clinical remission may correlate with demethylation; however, responses including complete remissions were also seen in patients with unmethylated $p15^{INK4b}$. This implies that $p15^{INK4b}$ hypermethylation is not mandatory for therapeutic success. Indeed, a similar study showed no correlation between $p15^{INK4b}$ methylation level and clinical response *(35)*. On the other hand, in 12 patients treated with 5-Aza followed by the HDAC inhibitor phenylbutyrate, reversal of promoter methylation of $p15^{INK4b}$ and/or *CDH-1* following 10 or 14 days of 5-Aza was demonstrated in 6 of 6 patients who achieved a clinical response but 0 of 6 nonresponders *(41)*.

Creative novel strategies for using DNMT inhibitors should be adapted in the future. The use of DNA methyltransferase inhibitors either as maintenance therapy after induction with chemotherapy or as preparation for patients with MDS/high-risk AML for stem cell transplantation is ongoing. The optimal duration of DNA methyltransferase inhibitor therapy for MDS has not been determined. However, some investigators advocate prolonged maintenance therapy *(42,43)*.

4.2. Methylation-Independent Effects of DNMT Inhibitors

The molecular mechanisms underpinning the clinical activity of DNMT inhibitors remain unclear. Administration of low doses of DNMT inhibitors is clearly associated with reversal of methylation of promoters of genes that may be biologically important; data on the re-expression of these genes is less clear *(40,41,44)*. Other potential mechanisms must be considered, including the ability of DNMT inhibitors to induce DNA damage. The DNA damage response involves the activation of the genome guardian p53, which transactivates a myriad of genes resulting in cell cycle arrest and/or apoptosis. The complex network of activated/suppressed genes in the context of the DNA damage pathway could lower the tumor

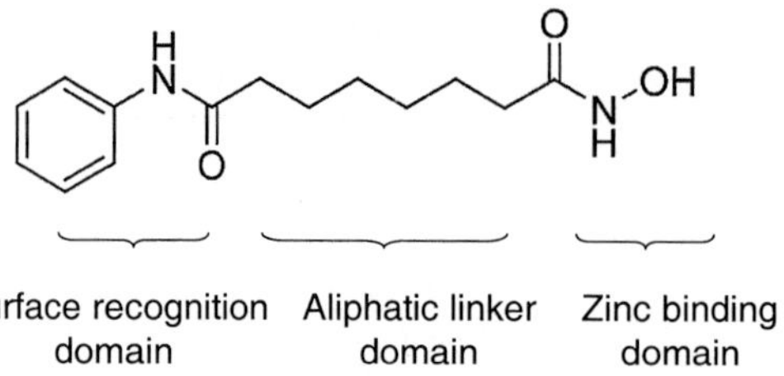

Fig. 2. The chemical structure of Vorinostat (SAHA) showing the three different pharmacophoric domains.

burden by inducing apoptosis in leukemia progenitors. Several reports highlighted the importance of the methylation-independent effects of DNMT inhibitors *(45–48)*. The dissection of the signaling pathway of DNMT inhibitor-induced apoptosis remains to be elucidated in the forthcoming years; the involvement of the mitochondria and caspase 3 rather than the death receptors was reported recently *(48)*. Better understanding of the molecular mechanisms required for clinical response is critical for the development of more active and selective congeners of DNMT inhibitors as well as for the rational design of strategies combining DNMT inhibitors with other selective and nonselective antineoplastic agents.

5. HDAC INHIBITORS IN AML

5.1. Introduction

HDACs are divided into three classes: class I HDACs, including HDAC1, HDAC2, HDAC3, and HDAC8, are localized in the nucleus and can recruit transcriptional cofactors and repressors. Class II members, including HDAC4, HDAC5, HDAC6, HDAC7, and HDAC9, can shuttle between the cytoplasm and the nucleus. Class III HDACs, also known as Sirtuins, form a structurally distinct class of NAD-dependent enzymes that are similar to the yeast SIR2 proteins.

HDAC inhibitors showed promising significant in vitro and in vivo activity against a variety of hematological and solid tumor model systems *(49,50)*. HDAC inhibitors inhibit HDACs with varying degrees of class specificity, resulting in histone hyperacetylation and easier access of transcription factors with consequent increase in gene expression which could explain their anticancer effect.

The direct interaction of HDAC inhibitors with the active zinc site of HDAC enzymes (Class I and II only) appears to be a prerequisite for their inhibitory activity *(51)*. The chemical structure of HDAC inhibitors can be divided into three pharmacophoric domains: the zinc metal-binding domain, represented by the hydroxamic acid moiety in a compound like suberoylanilide hydroxamic acid (Vorinostat; Fig. 2), the linker domain, represented by 5–6 aliphatic carbon chain, and the surface recognition domain, represented by a hydrophobic cap moiety that interacts with the edge of the catalytic pocket of HDACs enzymes.

5.2. Chemical Classification of HDAC Inhibitors

HDAC inhibitors can be categorized under five distinct groups based on chemical structure. Table 3 illustrates the five different groups and shows examples of different compounds within each group. The IC_{50}s of these compounds differ markedly from the high millimolar range to the low nanomolar concentrations.

Table 3
Chemical Classification of HDAC Inhibitors

Chemical group	Examples	Chemical structure
Hydroxamic acids	Suberoylanilide hydroxamic acid (SAHA), trichostatin A (TSA), NVP-LAQ824, pyroxamide, scriptaid, oxamflatin, CHAPs	TSA
Benzamides	MS-275, CI-994	MS-275
Cyclic peptides	FK-228, trapoxin A/B, chlamydocin, apicidin	Trapoxin B
Short-chain fatty acids	Phenylbutyrate, sodium butyrate, valproic acid, phenyl acetate	Phenylbutyrate
Miscellaneous	Depudecin, psammaplins	Depudecin

5.3. Mechanism of Action of HDAC Inhibitors

Extensive research involving HDAC inhibitors in the last decade has shown that these agents have pleotropic effects in addition to modulation of gene expression through chromatin remodeling; thus, focusing on the latter mechanism as a unique target is likely to be inadequate to explain the actions of HDAC inhibitors. HDAC inhibitors are selective agents that can induce cell cycle arrest, differentiation, and apoptosis. It is not clearly understood how HDAC inhibitors have a selective action for neoplastic vs normal cells. However, defective cell cycle checkpoints in cancer cells may help explain this (52). HDAC inhibitors can induce acetylation of other protein targets, including transcription factors and heat shock proteins, which may contribute to cell death. Generation of reactive oxygen species (ROS) has been associated with HDAC inhibitor-induced apoptosis (53). ROS generation was explained by the ability of HDAC inhibitors to modulate the expression of thioredoxin and glutathione *(54)*. The co-administration of ROS scavengers reduced the cytotoxicity of HDAC inhibitors and emphasized the role of ROS in HDAC inhibitor-induced apoptosis. Interestingly, it was observed that the thioredoxin levels were selectively increased in normal cells and not neoplastic cells, resulting in a selective oxidative damage in neoplastic cells only and providing another plausible explanation for the selectivity of HDAC inhibitors.

The effect of HDAC inhibitors on the extrinsic (death receptors) and the intrinsic (mitochondrial) death signaling pathways was extensively studied. The reported changes differed according to the tumor and cell type. For instance, exposure of leukemia or multiple myeloma cells to HDAC inhibitors upregulated the expression of tumor necrosis factor (TNF)-α-related apoptosis inducing ligand (TRAIL) receptors (DR4/5) and TRAIL itself *(55,56)*. On the other hand, other leukemia cell lines did not show any alteration in the death receptors expression *(57)*.

The dissipation of the mitochondrial membrane potential is a common event of HDAC inhibitors; however, the downstream effectors differ widely based on the tumor and cell type. For example, in leukemia cells, HDAC-inhibitor-induced apoptosis was caspase dependent *(58)*, whereas in myeloma cells it was caspase-independent *(55)*. The release of different apoptogenic factors from the mitochondria like Omi/HtrA2 and AIF was also reported in leukemia cells *(59)*.

Other possible mechanisms that may contribute to HDAC-inhibitor-induced apoptosis, including NF-κB activation, generation of ceramide, and modulating heat shock protein expression, are described in detail elsewhere *(60)*.

5.4. Use of HDAC Inhibitors to Target Leukemia Fusion Genes

In leukemia cells, the oncogenic fusion proteins AML1-ETO and PML-RARα form complexes with HDACs to repress the transcription of genes *(61)*. The administration of *all-trans*-retinoic acid (ATRA) with HDAC inhibitors resulted in marked increase in its activity *(62)*. In the absence of ligand, wild-type RARα binds to retinoic acid response elements (RARE) as a heterodimer with RXR, recruiting a multiprotein transcriptional repression complex. This complex includes HDAC1. The removal of acetyl groups from lysine moieties in the tails of histones leads to changes in chromatin conformation, which are prohibitive for transcription of genes downstream from the RARE *(63)*. Upon binding of ligand, the transcriptional repression complex is released and co-activating proteins are recruited, including those with HAT activity, enabling transcription. Like wild-type RARα, PML-RARα binds to RARE, recruiting the transcriptional repression complex *(61)*. While the subsequent transcriptional repression can be reversed by pharmacological concentrations of ATRA, significantly higher concentrations of ATRA are required compared to the wild-type receptor *(64)*. Synergistic transcriptional activation can be achieved with the addition of HDAC inhibitors *(64)*; such synergy is also seen in differentiation assays.

The APL variant associated with the chromosomal translocation t(11;17) and fusion gene PLZF-RARα is clinically resistant to ATRA induction *(65)*. The PLZF gene has a POZ domain, which is maintained in the fusion gene; this domain appears to recruit components of the transcriptional repression complex in a retinoid-independent fashion *(64)*. This second receptor–co-repressor interaction may explain the retinoid resistance of this APL variant. Addition of HDAC inhibitors restores retinoid sensitivity of this APL variant, although not necessarily to the degree of typical PML-RARα. HDAC inhibitors also restore retinoid sensitivity to ATRA-resistant APL cell lines *(66)*. HDAC inhibitors could thus be critical adjuncts to ATRA-based differentiation therapy of APL. HDAC inhibitors could potentially increase the already high response rate of primary APL, increase the sensitivity of ATRA-resistant APL variants such as PLZF-RARα, and restore retinoid sensitivity to ATRA-resistant relapsed PML-RARα APL.

The t(8;21) is one of the most frequent chromosomal translocations associated with acute leukemia. This translocation creates a fusion protein consisting of the AML-1 transcription factor and the ETO co-repressor (AML1-ETO), which represses transcription through AML1 (RUNX1) DNA-binding sites and immortalizes hematopoietic progenitor cells. ETO is capable of making multiple contacts with the mSin3 and nuclear hormone co-repressors and binds to histone deacetylases-1, -2, and -3 *(67)*. p14^{ARF} (MDM2 antagonist) was shown to be a direct target for repression by AML1-ETO with consequent downregulation of p53 *(67)*. HDAC inhibitors could relieve the repression of p14^{ARF}, leading to p53 upregulation and restoration of growth arrest and apoptosis in response to cytotoxic agents. Collectively, it is possible that HDAC inhibitors may have a future role in treating the malignant pheonotype identified by fusion proteins, resulting from chromosomal translocations, because HDACs appear to be recruited and essential for the transcriptional co-repressor complexes.

5.5. Synergistic Interactions of HDAC Inhibitors in AML

HDAC inhibitors may best be exploited through biologically rational combination strategies. Synergy between TSA and ATRA or vitamin D$_3$ in differentiation induction was demonstrated in AML *(50)*. Sodium butyrate synergized phorbol myristate acetate (PMA) induced apoptosis and impaired differentiation induction in AML cells *(68)*. Vorinostat (SAHA) and flavopiridol interacted synergistically to induce apoptosis in human leukemia cells *(69)*. Also, SAHA enhanced the cytotoxic effect of imatinib mesylate (Gleevec) in Bcr-Abl-positive human acute leukemia *(70,71)*. The combination of TSA or the depsipeptide FR901228 with DAC induced higher cytotoxicity than either agent alone *(72)*. SAHA or sodium butyrate synergized apoptosis induction by the proteasome inhibitor Bortezomib (Velcade) in human leukemia *(73)*. Co-administration of the heat shock protein (Hsp) 90 antagonists 17-allylamino-17-demethoxygeldanamycin (17-AAG) with SAHA or sodium butyrate synergized apoptosis induction and predicted a novel antileukemic therapy *(74)*. Furthermore, the simultaneous activation of the mitochondrial (intrinsic) death pathway by SAHA or sodium butyrate and the death receptor (extrinsic) pathway by TRAIL interacted synergistically in inducing mitochondrial damage and apoptosis (57). Inactivation of ERK 1/2 by the alkyl-lysophospholipid perifosine synergized SAHA or TSA induced mitochondrial damage and apoptosis *(75)*.

5.6. Clinical Evaluation of HDAC Inhibitors in MDS and AML

The development of HDAC inhibitors as antileukemic agents is progressing rapidly. Several clinical trials have been conducted to investigate their potential as antitumor agents. The butyrates were the first class of histone deacetylase inhibitors used in the clinic *(76)*. A phase I clinical trial with sodium phenylbutyrate in MDS and AML patients showed some hematological improvement without partial or complete remission *(77)*. Prolonged infusion with phenylbutyrate was also well tolerated by the patients *(78)*. However, sodium phenylbutyrate was not an ideal candidate because of its nonspecific biological effects and requirements for near millimolar administration. Other agents, including SAHA and MS-275, were shown to be orally bioavailable with minimal toxicity. Oral SAHA showed linear pharmacokinetics and good bioavailability and demonstrated a broad range of antitumor activity against solid and hematological malignancies *(79)*. The long half-life of MS-275 (39–80 hours) makes it an attractive oral candidate because of the expected low frequency of administration. A recent trial with MS-275 described its linear pharmacokinetics and demonstrated its tolerability *(80)*.

The combination of DNA hypomethylating agents and HDAC inhibitors could, at least theoretically, re-express important silenced tumor suppressor genes; therefore, it is tempting to clinically evaluate this combination. A phase I trial sequencing 5-Aza with sodium phenyl-butyrate in MDS and AML patients was completed *(41)*; a similar trial utilizing MS-275 is underway. Robust clinical responses were observed in the earlier study; however, the enhanced effect of the combination therapy over monotherapy needs to be confirmed. Confirmation of the additional benefit of DNMT/HDAC inhibitor combinations compared to DNMT inhibitors alone will require confirmation in a randomized trial.

Valproic acid (VPA) is another HDAC inhibitor that has been used as monotherapy or in combination with ATRA in MDS and AML *(81)*. VPA was clinically useful in low-risk MDS, but for patients with high-risk MDS, VPA was combined with chemotherapy or demethylating drugs. ATRA induced a prolonged second response in relapsed patients whom initially responded to VPA *(81,82)*.

6. CONCLUSION

The inadequate cure rate in response to cytotoxic agents in patients with AML has indicated a need for the development of novel therapeutic moieties. HDACs and DNMT inhibitors show promising results in MDS and AML treatment, but their exact mechanism of action demands further elucidation. Chromosomal abnormalities leading to fusion gene products often associate with HDACs for repressive activity and gene silencing and suggest there may be utility in exploring and manipulating the role of epigenetics in leukemogenesis. Single-agent therapy with a demethylating agent has been promising, and its optimal dosing schedule is likely to be defined shortly. Ideal combination therapies with various HDAC inhibitors and demethylating agents are also exciting and are actively being pursued and tested. Epigenetic changes resulting in reactivation of silenced genes may be possible via other modifications of histones not yet realized, such as manipulation of chromatin structure via phosphorylation, ubiqutination, and SUMOylation. The alternative hypothesis of triggering DNA damage pathways in addition to reactivation of epigenetically silenced genes needs to be further addressed for better understanding of the mechanism involved in curing effects of epigenetic therapy.

REFERENCES

1. Fraga MF, Ballestar E, Paz MF, et al. Epigenetic differences arise during the lifetime of monozygotic twins. Proc Natl Acad Sci USA 2005;102(30):10,604–10,609.
2. Swales AK, Spears N. Genomic imprinting and reproduction. Reproduction 2005;130(4):389–399.
3. Jones PA, Baylin SB. The fundamental role of epigenetic events in cancer. Nat Rev Genet 2002;3(6): 415–428.
4. Clark SJ, Harrison J, Frommer M. CpNpG methylation in mammalian cells. Nat Genet 1995;10(1):20–27.
5. Takai D, Jones PA. Comprehensive analysis of CpG islands in human chromosomes 21 and 22. Proc Natl Acad Sci USA 2002;99(6):3740–3745.
6. Chen L, MacMillan AM, Chang W, Ezaz-Nikpay K, Lane WS, Verdine GL. Direct identification of the active-site nucleophile in a DNA (cytosine-5)-methyltransferase. Biochemistry 1991;30(46):11,018–11,025.
7. Herman JG, Baylin SB. Gene silencing in cancer in association with promoter hypermethylation. N Engl J Med 2003;349(21):2042–2054.

8. Marks P, Rifkind RA, Richon VM, Breslow R, Miller T and Kelly WK. Histone deacetylases and cancer: causes and therapies. Nat Rev Cancer 2001;1(3):194–202.

9. Robertson KD, Ait-Si-Ali S, Yokochi T, Wade PA, Jones PL, Wolffe AP. DNMT1 forms a complex with Rb, E2F1 and HDAC1 and represses transcription from E2F-responsive promoters. Nat Genet 2000;25(3): 338–342.

10. Shi Y, Lan F, Matson C, et al. Histone demethylation mediated by the nuclear amine oxidase homolog LSD1. Cell 2004;119(7):941–953.

11. Slany RK. When epigenetics kills: MLL fusion proteins in leukemia. Hematol Oncol 2005;23(1):1–9.

12. Santos-Rosa H, Caldas C. Chromatin modifier enzymes, the histone code and cancer. Eur J Cancer 2005; 41(16):2381–2402.

13. Van Lint C, Emiliani S, Verdin E. The expression of a small fraction of cellular genes is changed in response to histone hyperacetylation. Gene Expr 1996;5(4–5):245–253.

14. Cameron EE, Bachman KE, Myohanen S, Herman JG, Baylin SB. Synergy of demethylation and histone deacetylase inhibition in the re-expression of genes silenced in cancer. Nat Genet 1999;21(1):103–107.

15. Herman JG, Jen J, Merlo A, Baylin SB. Hypermethylation-associated inactivation indicates a tumor suppressor role for p15INK4B. Cancer Res 1996;56(4):722–727.

16. Iguchi-Ariga SM, Schaffner W. CpG methylation of the cAMP-responsive enhancer/promoter sequence TGACGTCA abolishes specific factor binding as well as transcriptional activation. Genes Dev 1989;3(5): 612–619.

17. Bird AP, Wolffe AP. Methylation-induced repression—belts, braces, and chromatin. Cell 1999;99(5):451–454.

18. Nimer SD, Moore MA. Effects of the leukemia-associated AML1-ETO protein on hematopoietic stem and progenitor cells. Oncogene 2004;23(24):4249–4254.

19. Tonks A, Tonks AJ, Pearn L, et al. Expression of AML1-ETO in human myelomonocytic cells selectively inhibits granulocytic differentiation and promotes their self-renewal. Leukemia 2004;18(7):1238–1245.

20. Peterson LF, Zhang DE. The 8;21 translocation in leukemogenesis. Oncogene 2004;23(24):4255–4262.

21. Nishida S, Hosen N, Shirakata T, et al. AML1-ETO rapidly induces acute myeloblastic leukemia in cooperation with Wilms' tumor gene, WT1. Blood 2006;107(8):3303–3312.

22. Castilla LH, Garrett L, Adya N, et al. The fusion gene Cbfb-MYH11 blocks myeloid differentiation and predisposes mice to acute myelomonocytic leukaemia. Nat Genet 1999;23(2):144–146.

23. Meyer C, Schneider B, Reichel M, et al. Diagnostic tool for the identification of MLL rearrangements including unknown partner genes. Proc Natl Acad Sci USA 2005;102(2):449–454.

24. DiMartino JF, Ayton PM, Chen EH, Naftzger CC, Young BD, Cleary ML. The AF10 leucine zipper is required for leukemic transformation of myeloid progenitors by MLL-AF10. Blood 2002;99(10): 3780–3785.

25. DiMartino JF, Miller T, Ayton PM, et al. A carboxy-terminal domain of ELL is required and sufficient for immortalization of myeloid progenitors by MLL-ELL. Blood 2000;96(12):3887–3893.

26. Forster A, Pannell R, Drynan LF, et al. Engineering de novo reciprocal chromosomal translocations associated with Mll to replicate primary events of human cancer. Cancer Cell 2003;3(5):449–458.

27. Corral J, Lavenir I, Impey H, et al. An Mll-AF9 fusion gene made by homologous recombination causes acute leukemia in chimeric mice: a method to create fusion oncogenes. Cell 1996;85(6):853–861.

28. Look AT. Oncogenic transcription factors in the human acute leukemias. Science 1997;278(5340): 1059–1064.

29. Martin ME, Milne TA, Bloyer S, et al. Dimerization of MLL fusion proteins immortalizes hematopoietic cells. Cancer Cell 2003;4(3):197–207.

30. Sano K. Structure of AF3p21, a new member of mixed lineage leukemia (MLL) fusion partner proteins-implication for MLL-induced leukemogenesis. Leuk Lymphoma 2001;42(4):595–602.

31. Dobson CL, Warren AJ, Pannell R, Forster A, Rabbitts TH. Tumorigenesis in mice with a fusion of the leukaemia oncogene Mll and the bacterial lacZ gene. EMBO J 2000;19(5):843–851.

32. Eguchi M, Eguchi-Ishimae M, Greaves M. The small oligomerization domain of gephyrin converts MLL to an oncogene. Blood 2004;103(10):3876–3882.

33. Schermelleh L, Spada F, Easwaran HP, et al. Trapped in action: direct visualization of DNA methyltransferase activity in living cells. Nat Methods 2005;2(10):751–756.

34. Petti MC, Mandelli F, Zagonel V, et al. Pilot study of 5-aza-2'-deoxycytidine (Decitabine) in the treatment of poor prognosis acute myelogenous leukemia patients: preliminary results. Leukemia 1993;7 (suppl 1): 36–41.

35. Issa JP, Garcia-Manero G, Giles FJ, et al. Phase 1 study of low-dose prolonged exposure schedules of the hypomethylating agent 5-aza-2′-deoxycytidine (decitabine) in hematopoietic malignancies. Blood 2004; 103(5):1635–1640.

36. van den Bosch J, Lubbert M, Verhoef G, Wijermans PW. The effects of 5-aza-2′-deoxycytidine (Decitabine) on the platelet count in patients with intermediate and high-risk myelodysplastic syndromes. Leuk Res 2004;28(8):785–790.

37. Claus R, Almstedt M, Lubbert M. Epigenetic treatment of hematopoietic malignancies: in vivo targets of demethylating agents. Semin Oncol 2005;32(5):511–520.

38. Hackanson B, Robbel C, Wijermans P, Lubbert M. In vivo effects of decitabine in myelodysplasia and acute myeloid leukemia: review of cytogenetic and molecular studies. Ann Hematol 2005;84 (suppl 13):32–38.

39. Silverman LR, Demakos EP, Peterson BL, et al. Randomized controlled trial of azacitidine in patients with the myelodysplastic syndrome: a study of the cancer and leukemia group B. J Clin Oncol 2002;20(10): 2429–2440.

40. Daskalakis M, Nguyen TT, Nguyen C, et al. Demethylation of a hypermethylated P15/INK4B gene in patients with myelodysplastic syndrome by 5-Aza-2′-deoxycytidine (decitabine) treatment. Blood 2002; 100(8):2957–2964.

41. Gore SD, Baylin S, Sugar E, et al. Combined DNA methyltransferase and histone deacetylase inhibition in the treatment of myeloid neoplasms. Cancer Res 2006;66(12):6361–6369.

42. Silverman LR, Mufti GJ. Methylation inhibitor therapy in the treatment of myelodysplastic syndrome. Nat Clin Pract Oncol 2005;2 (suppl 10):S12–23.

43. Ruter B, Wijermans PW, Lubbert M. Superiority of prolonged low-dose azanucleoside administration?: results of 5-aza-2′-deoxycytidine retreatment in high-risk myelodysplasia patients. Cancer 2006;106(8): 1744–1750.

44. Oki Y, Kantarijan H, Davis J, et al. Hypomethylation induction in MDS after treatment with decitabine at three different doses. ASCO Annual Meeting 2005;Abstract No: 6546.

45. Bouchard J. Mechanism of action of 5-AZA-dC: induced DNA hypomethylation does not lead to aberrant gene expression in human leukemic CEM cells. Leuk Res 1989;13(8):715–722.

46. Zhu WG, Hileman T, Ke Y, et al. 5-Aza-2′-deoxycytidine activates the p53/p21Waf1/Cip1 pathway to inhibit cell proliferation. J Biol Chem 2004;279(15):15,161–15,166.

47. Schmelz K, Wagner M, Dorken B, Tamm I. 5-Aza-2′-deoxycytidine induces p21WAF expression by demethylation of p73 leading to p53-independent apoptosis in myeloid leukemia. Int J Cancer 2005;114(5): 683–695.

48. Tamm I, Wagner M, Schmelz K. Decitabine activates specific caspases downstream of p73 in myeloid leukemia. Ann Hematol 2005;84 (suppl 13):47–53.

49. Sambucetti LC, Fischer DD, Zabludoff S, et al. Histone deacetylase inhibition selectively alters the activity and expression of cell cycle proteins leading to specific chromatin acetylation and antiproliferative effects. J Biol Chem 1999;274(49):34,940–34,947.

50. Kosugi H, Towatari M, Hatano S, et al. Histone deacetylase inhibitors are the potent inducer/enhancer of differentiation in acute myeloid leukemia: a new approach to anti-leukemia therapy. Leukemia 1999;13(9): 1316–1324.

51. Finnin MS, Donigian JR, Cohen A, et al. Structures of a histone deacetylase homologue bound to the TSA and SAHA inhibitors. Nature 1999;401(6749):188–193.

52. Johnstone RW, Licht JD. Histone deacetylase inhibitors in cancer therapy: is transcription the primary target? Cancer Cell 2003;4(1):13–18.

53. Ruefli AA, Ausserlechner MJ, Bernhard D, et al. The histone deacetylase inhibitor and chemotherapeutic agent suberoylanilide hydroxamic acid (SAHA) induces a cell-death pathway characterized by cleavage of Bid and production of reactive oxygen species. Proc Natl Acad Sci USA 2001;98(19):10,833–10,838.

54. Butler LM, Zhou X, Xu WS, et al. The histone deacetylase inhibitor SAHA arrests cancer cell growth, up-regulates thioredoxin-binding protein-2, and down-regulates thioredoxin. Proc Natl Acad Sci USA 2002;99(18):11,700–11,705.

55. Fandy TE, Shankar S, Ross DD, Sausville E, Srivastava RK. Interactive effects of HDAC inhibitors and TRAIL on apoptosis are associated with changes in mitochondrial functions and expressions of cell cycle regulatory genes in multiple myeloma. Neoplasia 2005;7(7):646–657.

56. Insinga A, Monestiroli S, Ronzoni S, et al. Inhibitors of histone deacetylases induce tumor-selective apoptosis through activation of the death receptor pathway. Nat Med 2005;11(1):71–76.

57. Rosato RR, Almenara JA, Dai Y, Grant S. Simultaneous activation of the intrinsic and extrinsic pathways by histone deacetylase (HDAC) inhibitors and tumor necrosis factor-related apoptosis-inducing ligand (TRAIL) synergistically induces mitochondrial damage and apoptosis in human leukemia cells. Mol Cancer Ther 2003;2(12):1273–1284.

58. Amin HM, Saeed S, Alkan S. Histone deacetylase inhibitors induce caspase-dependent apoptosis and downregulation of daxx in acute promyelocytic leukaemia with t(15;17). Br J Haematol 2001;115(2): 287–297.

59. Guo F, Sigua C, Tao J, et al. Cotreatment with histone deacetylase inhibitor LAQ824 enhances Apo-2L/tumor necrosis factor-related apoptosis inducing ligand-induced death inducing signaling complex activity and apoptosis of human acute leukemia cells. Cancer Res 2004;64(7):2580–2589.

60. Rosato RR, Grant S. Histone deacetylase inhibitors: insights into mechanisms of lethality. Expert Opin Ther Targets 2005;9(4):809–824.

61. Lin RJ, Nagy L, Inoue S, Shao W, Miller WH, Jr, Evans RM. Role of the histone deacetylase complex in acute promyelocytic leukaemia. Nature 1998;391(6669):811–814.

62. Jing Y, Xia L, Waxman S. Targeted removal of PML-RARalpha protein is required prior to inhibition of histone deacetylase for overcoming all-trans retinoic acid differentiation resistance in acute promyelocytic leukemia. Blood 2002;100(3):1008–1013.

63. Redner RL, Wang J, Liu JM. Chromatin remodeling and leukemia: new therapeutic paradigms. Blood 1999; 94(2):417–428.

64. Guidez F, Ivins S, Zhu J, Soderstrom M, Waxman S, Zelent A. Reduced retinoic acid-sensitivities of nuclear receptor corepressor binding to PML- and PLZF-RARalpha underlie molecular pathogenesis and treatment of acute promyelocytic leukemia. Blood 1998;91(8):2634–2642.

65. Licht JD, Chomienne C, Goy A, et al. Clinical and molecular characterization of a rare syndrome of acute promyelocytic leukemia associated with translocation (11;17). Blood 1995;85(4):1083–1094.

66. He LZ, Guidez F, Triboli C, et al. Distinct interactions of PML-RARalpha and PLZF-RARalpha with co-repressors determine differential responses to RA in APL. Nat Genet 1998;18(2):126–135.

67. Linggi B, Muller-Tidow C, van de Locht L, et al. The t(8;21) fusion protein, AML1 ETO, specifically represses the transcription of the p14(ARF) tumor suppressor in acute myeloid leukemia. Nat Med 2002; 8(7):743–750.

68. Rahmani M, Dai Y, Grant S. The histone deacetylase inhibitor sodium butyrate interacts synergistically with phorbol myristate acetate (PMA) to induce mitochondrial damage and apoptosis in human myeloid leukemia cells through a tumor necrosis factor-alpha-mediated process. Exp Cell Res 2002;277(1): 31–47.

69. Almenara J, Rosato R, Grant S. Synergistic induction of mitochondrial damage and apoptosis in human leukemia cells by flavopiridol and the histone deacetylase inhibitor suberoylanilide hydroxamic acid (SAHA). Leukemia 2002;16(7):1331–1343.

70. Nimmanapalli R, Fuino L, Stobaugh C, Richon V, Bhalla K. Cotreatment with the histone deacetylase inhibitor suberoylanilide hydroxamic acid (SAHA) enhances imatinib-induced apoptosis of Bcr-Abl-positive human acute leukemia cells. Blood 2003;101(8):3236–3239.

71. Yu C, Rahmani M, Almenara J, et al. Histone deacetylase inhibitors promote STI571-mediated apoptosis in STI571-sensitive and -resistant Bcr/Abl+ human myeloid leukemia cells. Cancer Res 2003;63(9):2118–2126.

72. Shaker S, Bernstein M, Momparler LF, Momparler RL. Preclinical evaluation of antineoplastic activity of inhibitors of DNA methylation (5-aza-2′-deoxycytidine) and histone deacetylation (trichostatin A, depsi-peptide) in combination against myeloid leukemic cells. Leuk Res 2003;27(5):437–444.

73. Yu C, Rahmani M, Conrad D, Subler M, Dent P, Grant S. The proteasome inhibitor bortezomib interacts synergistically with histone deacetylase inhibitors to induce apoptosis in Bcr/Abl+ cells sensitive and resist-ant to STI571. Blood 2003;102(10):3765–3774.

74. Rahmani M, Yu C, Dai Y, et al. Coadministration of the heat shock protein 90 antagonist 17-allylamino-17-demethoxygeldanamycin with suberoylanilide hydroxamic acid or sodium butyrate synergistically induces apoptosis in human leukemia cells. Cancer Res 2003;63(23):8420–8427.

75. Rahmani M, Reese E, Dai Y, et al. Coadministration of histone deacetylase inhibitors and perifosine synergistically induces apoptosis in human leukemia cells through Akt and ERK1/2 inactivation and the generation of ceramide and reactive oxygen species. Cancer Res 2005;65(6):2422–2432.

76. Gore SD, Carducci MA. Modifying histones to tame cancer: clinical development of sodium phenylbutyrate and other histone deacetylase inhibitors. Expert Opin Investig Drugs 2000;9(12):2923–2934.

77. Gore SD, Weng LJ, Zhai S, et al. Impact of the putative differentiating agent sodium phenylbutyrate on myelodysplastic syndromes and acute myeloid leukemia. Clin Cancer Res 2001;7(8):2330–2339.
78. Gore SD, Weng LJ, Figg WD, et al. Impact of prolonged infusions of the putative differentiating agent sodium phenylbutyrate on myelodysplastic syndromes and acute myeloid leukemia. Clin Cancer Res 2002; 8(4):963–970.
79. Kelly WK, O'Connor OA, Krug LM, et al. Phase I study of an oral histone deacetylase inhibitor, suberoyl-anilide hydroxamic acid, in patients with advanced cancer. J Clin Oncol 2005;23(17):3923–3931.
80. Ryan QC, Headlee D, Acharya M, et al. Phase I and pharmacokinetic study of MS-275, a histone deacety-lase inhibitor, in patients with advanced and refractory solid tumors or lymphoma. J Clin Oncol 2005; 23(17):3912–3922.
81. Kuendgen A, Strupp C, Aivado M, et al. Treatment of myelodysplastic syndromes with valproic acid alone or in combination with all-trans retinoic acid. Blood 2004;104(5):1266–1269.
82. Kuendgen A, Knipp S, Fox F, et al. Results of a phase 2 study of valproic acid alone or in combination with all-trans retinoic acid in 75 patients with myelodysplastic syndrome and relapsed or refractory acute myeloid leukemia. Ann Hematol 2005;84 (suppl 13):61–66.
83. Roman-Gomez J, Jimenez-Velasco A, Castillejo JA, et al. Promoter hypermethylation of cancer-related genes: a strong independent prognostic factor in acute lymphoblastic leukemia. Blood 2004;104(8):2492–2498.
84. Otterson GA, Khleif SN, Chen W, Coxon AB, Kaye FJ. CDKN2 gene silencing in lung cancer by DNA hypermethylation and kinetics of p16INK4 protein induction by 5-aza 2'deoxycytidine. Oncogene 1995; 11(6):1211–1216.
85. Kawano S, Miller CW, Gombart AF, et al. Loss of p73 gene expression in leukemias/lymphomas due to hypermethylation. Blood 1999;94(3):1113–1120.
86. Yasunaga J, Taniguchi Y, Nosaka K, et al. Identification of aberrantly methylated genes in association with adult T-cell leukemia. Cancer Res 2004;64(17):6002–6009.
87. Ying J, Srivastava G, Hsieh WS, et al. The stress-responsive gene GADD45G is a functional tumor suppres-sor, with its response to environmental stresses frequently disrupted epigenetically in multiple tumors. Clin Cancer Res 2005;11(18):6442–6449.
88. Esteller M, Corn PG, Baylin SB, Herman JG. A gene hypermethylation profile of human cancer. Cancer Res 2001;61(8):3225–3229.
89. Furukawa Y, Sutheesophon K, Wada T, et al. Methylation silencing of the Apaf-1 gene in acute leukemia. Mol Cancer Res 2005;3(6):325–334.
90. Agirre X, Roman-Gomez J, Jimenez-Velasco A, et al. ASPP1, a common activator of TP53, is inactivated by aberrant methylation of its promoter in acute lymphoblastic leukemia. Oncogene 2006;25(13):1862–1870.
91. Ishii H, Vecchione A, Furukawa Y, et al. Expression of FRA16D/WWOX and FRA3B/FHIT genes in hematopoietic malignancies. Mol Cancer Res 2003;1(13):940–947.
92. Issa JP, Zehnbauer BA, Kaufmann SH, Biel MA, Baylin SB. HIC1 hypermethylation is a late event in hematopoietic neoplasms. Cancer Res 1997;57(9):1678–1681.
93. Galm O, Yoshikawa H, Esteller M, Osieka R, Herman JG. SOCS-1, a negative regulator of cytokine signaling, is frequently silenced by methylation in multiple myeloma. Blood 2003;101(7):2784–2788.
94. Chim CS, Fung TK, Cheung WC, Liang R, Kwong YL. SOCS1 and SHP1 hypermethylation in multiple myeloma: implications for epigenetic activation of the Jak/STAT pathway. Blood 2004;103(12): 4630–4635.
95. van Doorn R, Zoutman WH, Dijkman R, et al. Epigenetic profiling of cutaneous T-cell lymphoma: promoter hypermethylation of multiple tumor suppressor genes including BCL7a, PTPRG, and p73. J Clin Oncol 2005;23(17):3886–3896.
96. Agrelo R, Setien F, Espada J, et al. Inactivation of the lamin A/C gene by CpG island promoter hyper-methylation in hematologic malignancies, and its association with poor survival in nodal diffuse large B-cell lymphoma. J Clin Oncol 2005;23(17):3940–3947.
97. Tischkowitz M, Ameziane N, Waisfisz Q, et al. Bi-allelic silencing of the Fanconi anaemia gene FANCF in acute myeloid leukaemia. Br J Haematol 2003;123(3):469–471.
98. Yoshiura K, Kanai Y, Ochiai A, Shimoyama Y, Sugimura T, Hirohashi S. Silencing of the E-cadherin invasion-suppressor gene by CpG methylation in human carcinomas. Proc Natl Acad Sci USA 1995;92(16): 7416–7419.
99. Airoldi I, Di Carlo E, Banelli B, et al. The IL-12Rbeta2 gene functions as a tumor suppressor in human B cell malignancies. J Clin Invest 2004;113(11):1651–1659.

100. Youssef EM, Chen XQ, Higuchi E, et al. Hypermethylation and silencing of the putative tumor suppressor Tazarotene-induced gene 1 in human cancers. Cancer Res 2004;64(7):2411–2417.

101. Roman J, Castillejo JA, Jimenez A, et al. Hypermethylation of the calcitonin gene in acute lymphoblastic leukaemia is associated with unfavourable clinical outcome. Br J Haematol 2001;113(2):329–338.

102. Aggerholm A, Holm MS, Guldberg P, Olesen LH, Hokland P. Promoter hypermethylation of p15INK4B, HIC1, CDH1, and ER is frequent in myelodysplastic syndrome and predicts poor prognosis in early-stage patients. Eur J Haematol 2006;76(1):23–32.

14   Differentiation Therapy in AML

Tara L. Lin and William Matsui

CONTENTS

Summary

Defective or aberrant differentiation is a hallmark of acute leukemias. This chapter addresses the current strategies being explored in the clinical arena to overcome the "differentiation blockade" by manipulating critical biological and molecular attributes of the leukemic cell. These strategies include the manipulation of cell cycle kinetics, alteration in the balance between pro-survival and pro-death pathways, and chromatin remodeling with resultant modulation of the expression of genes whose products may drive the differentiation process.

Key Words: Leukemia; myelodysplastic syndrome; differentiation; growth factors; cell cycle; retinoic acid; vitamin D; histone deacetylase; DNA methylation; bryostatin-1.

1. INTRODUCTION

The complex genetic changes responsible for the formation of human cancers may result in specific cellular features that are common to many tumors regardless of their stage, grade, or originating tissue *(1)*. For example, cancer cells may exhibit unregulated growth, resistance to apoptosis, or genetic instability compared to their normal counterparts. In addition, many tumor cells also display varying degrees of differentiation and often express antigens or genes typical of earlier stages of development. Despite blocks in maturation, it appears that some neoplastic cells are able to complete the differentiation process; a striking example of this are teratomas persisting after systemic treatment of germ cell tumors that consist of fully mature cellular elements. Terminal differentiation results in the loss of long-term proliferative capacity and the induction of apoptosis, and the potential to force the completion of disrupted maturation programs underlies the concept of differentiation therapy. Acute myeloid leukemia (AML) has served as the prototypical disease for studying the induction of tumor cell differentiation and has provided many of the best studied laboratory models to identify both pharmacological and biological differentiating agents. In addition, a distinct subtype of AML, acute promyelocytic leukemia (APL), remains the only example of clinically effective differentiation

From: *Contemporary Hematology: Acute Myelogenous Leukemia*
Edited by: J. E. Karp © Humana Press Inc., Totowa, NJ

therapy. It is likely that these model systems will continue to provide further insight into the cellular and molecular processes that govern tumor cell differentiation and improve the clinical efficacy of differentiation therapy in both AML and other cancers.

2. APL: THE IDEAL MODEL OF DIFFERENTIATION THERAPY

APL is characterized by the clonal expansion of leukemic blasts blocked at the promyelocytic stage of myeloid differentiation *(2)*. In the majority of cases, APL cells carry a distinctive chromosomal translocation involving the promyelocytic leukemia gene (*PML*) on chromosome 15 and the retinoic acid receptor α gene (*RARα*) on chromosome 17 that produces the novel fusion protein PML-RARα *(3–6)*. Less common cytogenetic variants of APL have also been described that involve the amino-terminal portions of the promyelocytic leukemia zinc finger (*PLZF*), nucleophosmin, nuclear mitotic apparatus, or the signal transducer and activator of transcription 5b gene products encoded on chromosome 11, 5, 11, or 17, respectively *(7–9)*. However, the fusion partner in each of these cases invariably consists of the carboxy-terminal portion of RARα that harbors the ligand- and DNA-binding domains. The uniform involvement of RARα highlights its importance in the pathogenesis of APL, and the resulting chimeric receptors exert a dominant negative effect on normal RARα signaling regardless of the specific fusion partner *(8,9)*. As a result, RARα–mediated transcriptional activation of genes required for normal myeloid development is inhibited, resulting in the characteristic promyelocytic maturation arrest. Exposure of APL cells to pharmacologically achievable levels of the natural RARα ligand all-*trans*-retinoic acid (ATRA) relieves transcriptional repression and induces terminal granulocytic maturation *(6,10)*.

The finding that APL cells undergo terminal differentiation in response to ATRA *in vitro* prompted clinical trials examining its activity *in vivo*. These initial trials demonstrated that ATRA produced high rates of complete remission (CR) when used as a single agent in patients with both newly diagnosed and relapsed APL *(10–13)*. Furthermore, the clinical characteristics of these responses were unique compared to those achieved with standard antileukemic cytotoxic chemotherapy because low rates of alopecia, infectious complications, and bone marrow aplasia were observed. Instead, bone marrow examination revealed that leukemic cells underwent progressive morphological maturation similar to the *in vitro* responses to ATRA *(11)*. Numerous clinical studies have subsequently established the clinical efficacy of differentiation therapy in APL, and patients receiving ATRA during induction, consolidation, or maintenance experience dramatically improved long-term survival rates *(14)*. Furthermore, the combined use of ATRA and standard cytotoxic chemotherapy has resulted in disease-free survival (DFS) rates in excess of 70% and has transformed APL into the most curable form of AML *(15)*. Despite its efficacy in APL, ATRA has not demonstrated significant activity in other cancers, including other subtypes of AML. However, the success of differentiation therapy in APL provides the proof of principal that this strategy may be broadly effective in many tumor types and has stimulated intense examination of the cellular mechanisms involved in this process as well as the identification of novel differentiating agents.

3. PHARMACOLOGICAL DIFFERENTIATING AGENTS

The functional DNA and ligand-binding domains contained within PML-RARα are thought to mediate the unique sensitivity of APL cells to ATRA. However, a variety of unrelated pharmacological agents that do not signal directly through RARα, such as vitamin D, phorbol esters, bryostatin-1, arsenic trioxide, and even some typical cytotoxic anticancer agents have also been found to induce the differentiation of APL cells *in vitro (16–21)*. Other leukemia-based systems, such as murine erythroleukemia (MEL) cells, and human cell lines derived from primary patient samples, such as HL-60, U937, and K562, have also allowed the identification of a wide variety of agents that possess differentiating activity. Furthermore, many of these agents are active against tumor types *in vitro*, suggesting that they may be widely applicable. The following sections will examine broad classes of pharmacological differentiating agents that include those currently under investigation in AML.

3.1. Retinoids

Retinoids are involved in the regulation of growth and differentiation of many tissues, including the hematopoietic system *(22)*. As a class, retinoids exert their effects through two major classes of intracellular receptors, the retinoic acid receptors (RAR) and retinoid X receptors (RXR). These receptors bind as RAR-RAR homodimers or RAR-RXR hetero-dimers to specific DNA sequences, retinoic acid response elements (RAREs), located within the promoters of specific target genes. Following ligand binding, RARE-containing promoters become transcriptionally activated. Similar to its activity in APL, ATRA has been found to induce the differentiation of a number of non-APL AML cell lines *in vitro* associated with cell cycle arrest and activation of a number of intracellular signaling pathways normally utilized by growth factor receptors *(23–27)*.

These laboratory studies and the success of ATRA in APL prompted the clinical examination of ATRA in patients with non-APL AML. There are few reports on the use of ATRA alone in AML, although a single case report has described the achievement of a sustained CR with ATRA alone *(28)*. ATRA has been studied as a single agent in myelodysplastic syndrome (MDS), primarily in small single-armed trials. A dose-escalation trial of ATRA in patients with MDS described only 1 of 29 evaluable patients experiencing improved neutrophil and platelet counts *(29)*. In another dose-escalation trial, 3 of 15 patients had decreased transfusion requirements and another had an increase in neutrophil and platelet counts *(30)*. A multi-institutional trial of single agent ATRA in MDS demonstrated improvements in hemoglobin in 3 of 23 patients and increased neutrophil counts and decreased bone marrow blasts in two others *(31)*.

The majority of clinical studies in AML have investigated ATRA in combination with traditional antileukemic cytotoxic chemotherapy, at both standard and low doses, as well as with other differentiation agents. A pilot study compared 19 newly diagnosed patients with AML who received ATRA during induction chemotherapy to 29 historical control patients and found no difference in CR, DFS, or overall survival (OS) rates *(32)*. Bolanos-Meade and colleagues similarly examined the addition of ATRA to timed-sequential chemotherapy (TST) in a larger study of 63 patients with newly diagnosed AML *(33)*. Compared to the outcome of historical controls treated with TST induction and consolidation, no improvement in DFS or OS was observed. A randomized phase II study examined 95 high-risk AML patients receiving induction chemotherapy consisting of idarubicin and cytosine arabinoside (ara-c) with or without ATRA *(34)*. Again, there was no statistical difference between the groups in terms of CR, DFS, or OS rates. A phase II study compared the addition of ATRA and/or granulocyte colony-stimulating factor (G-CSF) to induction chemotherapy consisting of fludarabine, ara-c, and idarubicin to chemotherapy alone in 215 patients with poor prognosis AML or high-grade MDS *(35)*. Although the addition of G-CSF improved the CR rate, neither ATRA nor G-CSF improved DFS or OS rates. Although these early trials showed no improvement in DFS or OS, further studies have been undertaken. In the only published phase III trial of ATRA plus chemotherapy, 242 patients 61 years or older with *de novo* or secondary AML or high-grade MDS were randomized to receive induction and consolidation chemotherapy with or without ATRA *(36)*. There was a significant improvement in the initial CR rate in patients receiving ATRA (52% vs 39%, $p = 0.05$), and following first consolidation, those achieving CR were randomized again to either intensive consolidation or oral maintenance therapy. A significant difference in OS was observed with a median survival of 11.3 months in the ATRA arm compared to 7.0 months in the chemotherapy alone arm $(p = 0.01)$, suggesting that the addition of ATRA to multiple phases of treatment may benefit patients with high risk AML. The combination of low-dose ara-c and ATRA was studied as a novel induction regimen in 33 patients with high-risk AML *(37)*. A CR rate of 48% was observed and correlated with blast percentage in the bone marrow at the time of treatment. Because low-dose ara-C may induce AML differentiation *in vitro*, the efficacy of this combination suggests that the use of multiple differentiating agents may improve clinical efficacy. The conflicting results of these studies in both AML and MDS may be a result of the differences in the administration of ATRA, the particular patient populations studied, and the specific regimens of chemotherapy used. However, further studies are warranted to better clarify the role of ATRA in non-AML APL.

Other steroisomers of ATRA, namely 13-*cis*-retinoic acid and 9-*cis*-retinoic acid, demonstrate different binding affinities for RAR and RXR receptors *(38)*. Like ATRA, these agents have been found to have activity against AML *in vitro (39)*. Small single-armed clinical trials of 13-*cis*-retinoic acid in patients with MDS have shown an improvement in peripheral blood counts, reduced peripheral or bone marrow blast counts, and even improved survival in some patients *(40–44)*. In particular, one report reviewed four patients with AML and four patients with MDS treated with 13-*cis*-retinoic acid *(45)*. No responses were observed in the MDS patients, but three of four patients with AML had normalization of their peripheral blood counts. However, a randomized study of 13-*cis*-retinoic acid in 68 MDS patients showed no benefit over placebo in terms of hematological response or progression-free survival *(46)*, and in AML, a phase II study of 18 elderly patients failed to observe any responses *(47)*. Two trials have studied 9-*cis*-retinoic acid in APL. In the first, 7 patients with relapsed APL following ATRA therapy were treated with 9-*cis*-retinoic acid, and a single patient experienced a CR *(48)*. In the second, 18 patients with APL, including 13 with relapsed disease (11 with prior ATRA therapy) and 5 who were newly diagnosed, were evaluated *(49)*. Four of 5 newly diagnosed patients and 4 of 13 relapsed patients attained a CR. Therefore, 9-*cis*-retinoic acid clearly has activity in APL, but like 13-*cis*-retinoic acid, the *in vivo* activity of this retinoid in other subtypes of AML is yet to be determined.

3.2. Vitamin D

The active metabolite of vitamin D, 1,25-dihydroxyvitamin D, plays a critical role in calcium homeostasis, but it is also thought to play a role in the regulation of normal hematopoiesis *(50)*. Like RARs, the vitamin D receptor is a member of the intracellular steroid hormone receptor superfamily and forms heterodimers with RXRs to activate the transcription of target genes *(51,52)*. Vitamin D has been found to induce the monocytic differentiation of a number of AML cell lines as well as the APL cell line NB4 in combination with other agents *(18,53–55)*. Small, nonrandomized clinical trials of vitamin D in AML have shown both CR and partial response (PR) when given in combination with low-dose ara-c (CR 17%, PR 45%) or low-dose ara-c and hydroxyurea (CR 45%, PR 34%) *(56,57)*. The dose-limiting toxicity of 1,25-dihydroxy vitamin D is hypercalcemia. Therefore, several vitamin D derivatives with fewer effects on calcium metabolism have been developed and studied as anticancer agents. Two of these derivatives, CB1093 and EB1089, have been shown to be active against AML *in vitro* (*55,58–60*). EB1089 has been clinically examined in patients with solid tumors and found to be well tolerated (*61,62*), and given the results of trials with vitamin D, these agents show promise in AML.

3.3. Protein Kinase C Agonists

3.3.1. PHORBOL MYRISTATE ACETATE (PMA)

Phorbol myristate acetate (PMA; 12-tetradecanoylphorbol-13-acetate) is the prototypical phorbol ester initially found to promote the formation tumors within the skin of mice (*63,64*). However, PMA was also among the first compounds found to induce the differentiation of both AML cell lines and primary samples (*65–67*). PMA binds directly to protein kinase C (PKC) and induces its translocation to the nucleus where it activates a number of transcription factors involved in myeloid differentiation. The carcinogenic properties of PMA limited enthusiasm regarding its clinical use as a differentiating agent. However, recent studies in patients with refractory AML have been reported. Han and colleagues reported a trial of PMA in 12 patients with AML, chronic myeloid leukemia (CML), in blast crisis or high-grade MDS (*68*). All evaluable patients had a reduction in circulating blasts and marked improvement in performance status, but the duration of responses was limited and ranged from 26 days to 8 months.

3.3.2. BRYOSTATIN-1

The tumorgenicity of PMA promoted the search for other activators of PKC and led to the discovery of bryostatin-1. Bryostatin-1 is macrocyclic lactone originally isolated from the marine bryozoan *Bugula neritina*. Like PMA, bryostatin-1 induces the activation of PKC, but it appears to lack carcinogenic potential, possibly because of its ability to activate different isoforms of PKC compared to PMA or its ability to downregulate PKC with prolonged exposure (*69–73*). Bryostatin-1 has a wide variety of biological effects, including the ability to induce the differentiation of AML cells and limit their clonogenic potential *in vitro* (*74–76*). Interestingly, it appears to have differential effects on normal and leukemic cells in that it promotes the growth of normal hematopoietic progenitors by inducing the release of stimulating cytokines by supporting bone marrow cells (*77,78*). The cellular mechanisms responsible for the induction of leukemic differentiation are unknown, but bryostatin-1 is potent inducer of cell cycle arrest at G_1 or both G_1 and G_2/M, which is mediated by the inhibition of cyclin-dependent kinase 2 (CDK2) and the upregulation of the cyclin-dependent kinase (CDK) inhibitors p21$^{cip1/waf1}$ and p27^{kip1} (*79,80*). Promising results were seen in a phase I study of bryostatin-1 combined with high-dose ara-c in 23 patients with relapsed or refractory acute leukemia (*81*). Four patients achieved a CR, one patient achieved CR but was excluded from the final analysis because she did not complete the full course of therapy, and an additional patient had a 5-month leukemia-free interval although continuing to be persistent dependent on transfusions. Therefore, PMA and bryostatin-1 may be effective in the treatment of AML, especially when combined with other agents.

3.4. Histone Deacetylase Inhibitors

3.4.1. SODIUM BUTYRATE, PHENYLBUTYRATE, AND VALPROIC ACID

Local chromosomal structure plays an important role in the regulation of gene expression and may be influenced by the acetylation of histones that is modulated by two classes of enzymes: histone acetyltransferases (HATs) and histone deacetylases (HDACs) *(82–84)*. HDACs are found in association with transcriptional co-repressors and act by producing hypoacetylated histones that bind tightly to DNA, thereby restricting access by the transcriptional machinery. Furthermore, HDACs can induce hypoacetylation of a number of transcription factors, which inhibits their activity *(85,86)*. In contrast, HATs are associated with transcriptional co-activators and induce histone hyperacetylation characteristic of highly active promoters. Although mutation of HDAC genes has not been detected in human cancers, HDACs are involved in the pathogenesis of APL *(87)*. HDACs are normally found at target promoters within complexes containing RARα and transcriptional co-repressors *(88,89)*. In the presence of ATRA, transcriptional co-activators replace co-repressors and allow the assembly of active transcription complexes. Wild-type RARα mediates this process at physiological ATRA levels. However, at these ATRA concentrations, co-repressors and HDACs remain associated with PML-RARα, resulting in continued transcriptional repression at promoters required for myeloid differentiation and the characteristic promyelocytic maturation arrest *(90,91)*. Superphysiological, but pharmacologically achievable, levels of ATRA can overcome repression by PML-RARα and allow the completion of myeloid differentiation. A broader role for HDACs in AML is illustrated by examining the t(8;21) translocation found in a portion of cases with the M2 subtype of AML *(92)*. This translocation creates a novel fusion protein derived from the AML1 and ETO gene products that associates with HDACs and represses the transcription of genes required for myeloid differentiation *(92)*.

A variety of compounds with the ability to inhibit HDAC activity have been developed and examined in AML. The short-chain fatty acid sodium butyrate was one of the first compounds found to inhibit HDAC activity *(93,94)*. Later, the aromatic fatty acid butyrate derivative phenylbutyrate (PB), a pro-drug for phenylacetate, was developed, and recently, the short chain fatty acid valproic acid (VPA), extensively utilized as an anticonvulsant agent, has also been found to inhibit HDAC activity *(95–97)*. Each of these agents has been shown to induce the differentiation of AML cells as well as augment the differentiating effects of ATRA in APL *(95,96,98–103)*. In addition to the inhibition of HDACs, these agents have a wide range of biological activities that include the inhibition of cell cycling, activation of cAMP- and PKC-mediated signaling pathways, and augmentation of apoptosis induced by cytotoxic chemotherapeutic agents *(104–107)*. Therefore, it is unclear whether their differentiating effects arise solely through HDAC inhibition.

Two studies of PB in patients with AML and MDS have been reported. In the first, 27 patients with either MDS or AML received PB as a 7-day continuous infusion *(108)*. Although no patients achieved a CR or PR, hematological improvements in granulocytes and platelets were observed in 4 patients. In the second, two dosing schedules of PB were studied (7-day continuous infusion with 7-day drug holiday and 21-day continuous infusion with 7-day drug holiday) *(109)*. There were no responses on the 7-day continuous infusion arm, and 2 patients with MDS had improvements in their platelet count for 10 months and 3 months on the 21-day continuous infusion arm. Kuendgen and colleagues conducted a trial of VPA with or without ATRA in MDS and AML patients *(110)*. Of the 23 patients enrolled, 18 received VPA alone with planned ATRA for lack of response or relapse, and 5 received VPA plus ATRA as initial therapy. Hematological improvement was seen in 7 patients, and one partial response was observed. Three patients had ongoing responses of 4, 4, and 9 months at the time of publication. Four patients were given VPA and ATRA after relapse on VPA alone, and 2 experienced responses that persisted for 11 and 16 months.

3.4.2. SUBEROYLANILIDE HYDROXAMIC ACID AND MS-275

Suberoylanilide hydroxamic acid (SAHA) is a second-generation hybrid polar compound that is an effective inducer of differentiation in AML cells *(111,112)*. Like the prototypical hybrid polar compound hexamethylamine bisacetamide (HMBA), it induces cell cycle inhibition, but it also has significant HDAC-inhibitory activity *(113)*. Studies of SAHA against human AML cell lines *in vitro* have demonstrated that it has a limited differentiating capacity, but also a potent ability to induce apopotosis *(114)*. MS-275 is a synthetic benzamide with leukemic differentiating activity *in vitro (115)*. In comparison to sodium butyrate and PB, both SAHA and MS-275 have potent HDAC inhibition that is easily achievable *in vivo*, and these agents have recently begun to enter clinical trials in AML. Phase I data with both SAHA and MS-275 are emerging, and each of these compounds appears to be relatively well tolerated *(116,117)*. These agents are in the early stages of clinical trials, and the results for HDAC inhibition in AML are eagerly awaited.

3.5. Hypomethylation Agents

In addition to histone acetylation, the methylation of DNA CpG motifs contained within promoter elements may influence local chromosomal structure and transcriptional activity *(118,119)*. Methylation of the DNA template results in transcriptional inactivity by a variety of mechanisms that include directly interfering with the binding of transcriptional regulators, interactions with HDACs, and recruitment of repressive methyl-CpG binding proteins *(120)*. In many tumors the methylation of specific promoters is strikingly abnormal compared to that in normal tissue. As a result, genes that regulate processes such as DNA repair and cell cycle control are silenced. Strategies to reverse aberrant hypermethylation include the cytidine analogs 5-azacytidine and 5-aza-2′-deoxycytidine. Both of these agents have the ability to induce the maturation of leukemic cell lines, either alone or in combination with other differentiating agents *(121–126)*.

Both 5-azacytidine and 5-aza-2′-deoxycytidine have been extensively examined for activity in AML, but these trials utilized intermediate to high doses of either agent that are primarily cytotoxic rather than acting as demethylating agents *(127)*. 5-Azacytidine was recently examined at lower doses and approved by the U.S. Food and Drug Administration for the treatment of MDS following a phase III study of 191 patients with high-risk MDS *(128)*. Patients were randomized to either treatment with 5-azacytidine or best supportive care. In the treatment arm, the overall response rate was 60%, with 7% CR, 16% PR, and 37% with improvement in blood counts, compared to the supportive care arm, in which only 5% had improvement in blood counts and none with CR or PR ($p < 0.001$). Encouraging data have also emerged from a phase II study of 5-aza-2′-deoxycytidine in 66 high-risk MDS patients in which 49% of patients had some response (13 CR, 3 PR, and 16 patients with hematological improvement) *(129)*. Therefore, these agents clearly are active in MDS at doses that primarily induce DNA demethylation and are currently under active study in AML *(130)*.

3.6. Polar Planar Molecules

3.6.1. DIMETHYLSULFOXIDE

Dimethylsulfoxide (DMSO) is a hybrid polar compound originally found to induce the differentiation of Friend MEL cells *(131)*. This study described erythroid maturation of isolated splenic hematopoietic cells transformed by the Friend leukemia virus in response to DMSO and is notable because it provides the first evidence that neoplastic cells may be chemically induced to undergo terminal differentiation. Furthermore, DMSO is active against HL-60 APL cells (132,133). The cellular mechanisms leading to differentiation induction by DMSO are poorly understood, but it has been found to induce cell cycle arrest primarily through the induction of CDK inhibitors such as p21[cip/waf1] (134). Despite its ability to induce differentiation, DMSO has not been specifically studied as an antitumor agent, although peak plasma levels well above those required to induce differentiation *in vitro* have been detected in patients undergoing reinfusion of cryopreserved stem cell grafts during autologous transplantation (135). Therefore, clinical studies utilizing this agent as a differentiation inducer in AML may be feasible.

3.6.2. HEXAMETHYLAMINE BISACETAMIDE

Similar to DMSO, HMBA was initially identified by its ability to induce the differentiation of MEL cells, and it has activity against human HL60 and U937 cells (136,137). The mechanisms by which HMBA promotes cellular maturation are unknown, but it is also a potent inhibitor of cell cycling (138). Furthermore, MEL cells treated with HMBA appear to activate PKC, suggesting that this signal transduction pathway plays a role in its activity (139). Andreeff and colleagues observed responses in 9 of 41 patients with AML or MDS in a phase II trial. Of these, 3 patients experienced a CR with a median duration of 6.8 months (range 1.3–16 months), and 6 patients demonstrated a PR with a median duration of 3.7 months (range 1–7 months). Furthermore, in some responders investigators were able to demonstrate that circulating neutrophils contained the cytogenetic abnormality seen in the malignant hematopoietic precursors as evidence of differentiation by HMBA (140).

3.7. Low-Dose Cytotoxic Chemotherapy

The primary action of cytotoxic chemotherapeutic agents is the induction of apoptosis, but it is well recognized that these agents primarily induce differentiation rather than cell death when utilized at low doses. Several studies have demonstrated that several compounds, including ara-C, aphidicolin, deoxyadenosine analogs, anthracyclines, and vincristine, can induce the differentiation of AML cells in vitro (20,141–143). The mechanisms by which these agents induce differentiation are unknown, but they induce cell cycle arrest, and clinical strategies examining the use of low-dose cytoxic agents have been investigated.

Several cytotoxic agents have been used at low doses in an attempt to induce differentiation of leukemic cells; the majority have studied low-dose ara-c (LDAC) in AML and MDS. An extensive review by Cheson and Simon included 59 clinical trials of 846 patients treated with doses of ara-c from 5 to 25 mg/m² daily (144). Patients with *de novo* AML had a 32% CR rate compared to 16% for secondary AML and 17% for MDS. Rates were similar whether LDAC was administered intermittently or by continuous infusion. The median duration of response was 9, 10, and 10 months for each group, respectively. Tilly and colleagues published results of a randomized trial of LDAC vs intensive induction chemotherapy in 87 elderly patients with *de novo* AML (145). Although more CR were observed in the intensive chemotherapy group (52% vs 32% with LDAC, p <0.001), there were also significantly more early deaths than in the LDAC arm (31% with intensive chemotherapy compared to 10% with LDAC, p <0.001). Overall survival was not significantly different between the two groups (12.8 months with intensive chemotherapy, 8.8 months with LDAC, p >0.12). One phase III study of LDAC vs best supportive care in 141 patients with MDS showed no difference in survival despite an overall response rate of 32% (11% CR and 21% PR) (146). Despite the large number of studies of LDAC, questions remain regarding the patient populations that are likely to benefit and the optimal dose and schedule of LDAC.

4. GROWTH FACTORS: BIOLOGICAL DIFFERENTIATING AGENTS

Normal hematopoiesis consists of distinct cellular compartments organized in a hierarchical manner. Self-renewing stem cells are long lived and give rise to all hematopoietic lineages. These cells in turn give rise to progenitors that have undergone lineage commitment and have limited proliferative potential. Finally, progenitors produce mature cells such as neutrophils and erythrocytes that serve as effectors and are terminally differentiated. Multiple growth factors and cytokines play an important role in maintaining hematopoietic homeostasis that ensures the adequate production of normal effectors, and myeloid growth factors, such as granulocyte-macrophage colony-stimulating factor (GM-CSF) and G-CSF, appear to exert biological effects at multiple stages of maturation *(147)*. Furthermore, these growth factors may influence the fate of AML cells, as case reports have described complete remissions utilizing only myeloid growth factors as a single agent *(148)*.

In addition to pharmacological differentiating agents, myeloid growth factors may play a significant role in the differentiation of APL. Several case reports have described complete remissions in APL utilizing G-CSF as a single agent *(149,150)*, and the overexpression of G-CSF receptors in a murine cell line model of APL allows differentiation to occur in response to G-CSF in the absence of ATRA *(151)*. G-CSF and GM-CSF have also been shown to enhance the activity of ATRA *(152–155)* as well as restore ATRA sensitivity in resistant t(15;17) APL cases expressing PML-RARα *(156–158)*. PML-RARα retains the carboxy-terminal portions of RARα that harbor the DNA and ligand-binding domains responsible for the modulation of transcriptional activity by ATRA. Although these domains are identically shared in the PLZF-RARα fusion protein that is encoded by the less common t(11;17) APL variant, ATRA is clinically ineffective in this setting *(7,159,160)*. However, the addition of G-CSF also appears to restore ATRA responsiveness to these resistant cells both *in vitro* and *in vivo* *(156–158)*. We examined the role of myeloid growth factors in the differentiation of APL by ATRA *(21)*. G-CSF alone had little effect on the differentiation of APL cells, but like others, we found that the differentiation of both the NB4 APL cell line and primary clinical samples derived from the blood or bone marrow of patients with APL by ATRA was enhanced by the addition of G-CSF. Furthermore, when the activity of growth factors thought to be elaborated by the leukemic cells themselves or contained within the serum used to propagate cells *in vitro* was neutralized using monoclonal antibodies against G-CSF, GM-CSF, and interleukin-3, ATRA had little effect on phenotypic differentiation. Since multiple studies have demonstrated that leukemic blasts from APL patients express significantly higher levels of myeloid growth factor receptors than other types of AML *(161,162)*, the unique sensitivity of APL cells to differentiation therapy, not only with ATRA but also with other unrelated pharmacological differentiating agents, may in part result from an increased cellular sensitivity to growth factors.

We have also examined the role of growth factors in the differentiation of non-APL AML and found similar results. We studied the differentiation of two AML cell lines, HL-60 and U937, and AML clinical samples induced by three distinct pharmacological agents, bryostatin-1, hydroxyurea, and phenylburyate *(163)*. Each of these agents induced terminal AML differentiation manifested by the upregulation of myeloid maturation markers as well as the inhibition of subsequent clonogenic growth. As in our studies of APL, GM-CSF had little effect when used alone, but the activity of each pharmacological agent was significantly augmented by the addition of the growth factor. Our findings are similar to those of other reports in which combinations of differentiating agents and serum-derived growth factors induced the differentiation of AML cells *(164–166)*. Moreover, myeloid growth factors were required for the differentiating effects of all of the tested agents in that neutralizing monoclonal antibodies against myeloid growth factors inhibited differentiation. Therefore, growth factors appear to be necessary for the activity of pharmacological differentiating agents *in vitro*, and the maximal induction of terminal differentiation requires the activities of both of these classes of agents.

The exact interaction between myeloid growth factors and pharmacological differentiating agents in AML is unclear, but most differentiating agents share the ability to induce cell cycle arrest. We found that this property was critical in mediating their effects because all the pharmacological differentiating agents tested were active only at concentrations that were cytostatic *(21,163)*. There is ample evidence suggesting that cellular differentiation is closely linked to regulation of the cell cycle *(167,168)*. Signals that stimulate cell cycle progression, such as the overexpression of c-myc, c-myb, or E2F-1, inhibit differentiation *(169–171)*; conversely, the inhibition of cell cycle progression promotes differentiation *(169,172–174)*. Further evidence that the cell cycle plays a role in differentiation is apparent by examining the genetic changes that lead to tumorigenesis in a variety of malignancies. Newly diagnosed aggressive hematological malignancies like AML, that phenotypically resemble undifferentiated hematological progenitors, commonly harbor mutations or epigenetic modification of genes that result in the deregulation of G_1- to S-cell cycle transitions, such as the CDK inhibitors $p15^{Ink4b}$ and $p16^{Ink4a}$ *(175–177)*. On the other hand, mutations in genes regulating the G_1/S transition are infrequent in newly diagnosed patients with indolent hematological disorders, such as multiple myeloma and CML, that retain the ability to differentiate *(175,176,178)*. Interestingly, deregulation of these genes is common during disease transformation or progression and is associated with a corresponding block in differentiation (e.g., blast crisis CML and plasma cell leukemia) *(179–181)*. These findings suggest that the inhibition of cell cycling may, in fact, be a prerequisite step in the induction of differentiation. Furthermore, the induction of cell cycle arrest may be the major mechanism responsible for the activity of pharmacological differentiating agents.

Myeloid growth factors are pleotropic and can enhance proliferation and inhibit programmed cell death in addition to inducing differentiation. It has not been possible to uncouple these individual effects, and in the setting of the genetic changes responsible for leukemic transformation, the proliferative action of growth factors likely prevails and may lead to the acceleration of clinical disease. However, our results suggest that the inhibition of cell cycling by pharmacological differentiating agents may block the proliferative effects of growth factors and preferentially augment their differentiating activity, which would ultimately result in elimination of the malignant clone. Our results also suggest that both pharmacological differentiating agents at doses that inhibit cell cycling, such as ATRA and bryostatin-1, and myeloid growth factors are necessary, but not sufficient, for the differentiation of AML.

Thus, it appears that a specific interaction between pharmacological differentiating agents, myeloid growth factors, and the cell cycle is critical to the determination of leukemic cell fate *(21)*. Evidence suggests that the decision to proliferate and undergo DNA replication and cell division or, alternatively, to differentiate and enter a quiescent state (G_0) is made within G_1 *(182–184)*. In APL, the expression of PML-RARα appears to favor cell proliferation, possibly by inducing the overexpression of cyclin A1 that likely enhances the entry into the S phase, thereby irreversibly committing the cell to undergo division *(184–186)*. ATRA may interfere with this process by inducing expression of the CDK inhibitors p21$^{wafl/cip1}$ and p27^{kip1}, resulting in cell cycle arrest at G$_1$ *(25,27)*. The expression of p21$^{wafl/cip1}$ and p27^{kip1} appears to be required for differentiation, but these cell cycle inhibitors are not sufficient, and it is likely that other signals are required *(187,188)*. Growth factors also appear to exert their action within G$_1$ to promote proliferation or induce lineage-specific differentiation *(182,184, 189,190)*. Therefore, it is possible that pharmacological differentiating agents may modulate the cellular response to growth factors during this cell cycle phase. Both bryostatin-1 and phenylbutyrate, which block cell cycling at G$_1$, and hydroxyurea, which inhibits S phase, augmented the differentiating effects of growth factors *(21,163)*. Furthermore, the expression of p210$^{bcr-abl}$ in CML cells inhibits cell cycle progression at G$_2$/M, and these cells differentiate in response to growth factors alone *(191,192)*, suggesting that the specific phase of cell cycle inhibition may not be of critical importance.

Our data suggest two potential explanations for the discordance between the *in vitro* activity and clinical ineffectiveness of differentiation therapy. The first is that adequate cell cycle inhibition may not be achieved clinically. However, several reports have demonstrated that combinations of pharmacological differentiating agents may augment both cell cycle arrest and differentiation *in vitro*, suggesting that the clinical use of multiple agents may be able to produce the desired cytostatic effect *(18,193–195)*. Furthermore, low-dose chemotherapy has also been shown to augment both cell cycle arrest and differentiation of APL cells in response to ATRA, and these findings could explain recent clinical data indicating that maintenance therapy combining ATRA with low doses of methotrexate or 6-mercaptopurine may produce the best long-term results in APL patients *(20,196,197)*. A second possible reason for the clinical inactivity of pharmacological differentiation agents is that growth factors active in a particular tumor cell type may not be present at adequate levels *in vivo* to induce differentiation. Accordingly, ATRA-insensitive cases of APL may undergo clinical remissions when exogenous G-CSF is administered *(156–158)*. Therefore, therapeutic strategies combining growth factors that are active in a specific malignancy with pharmacological differentiating agents that effectively inhibit cell cycling *in vivo* may improve the clinical activity of differentiation therapy.

5. CLINICAL IMPLICATIONS OF DIFFERENTIATION THERAPY

Several studies have demonstrated that the cellular organization of AML mirrors normal hematopoiesis, with self-renewing leukemic stem cells giving rise to blasts with little long-term replicative potential *(198,199)*. CRs in response to induction therapy indicate that leukemic blasts are sensitive to the effects of standard cytotoxic agents, but relapse suggests that AML stem cells are spared. Given the hierarchical organization of AML, the induction of terminal differentiation may promote the loss of self-renewal and lead to long-term remissions. However, because cancer stem cells in AML form only a small proportion of the total tumor burden, therapies that affect only stem cells and halt the production of new tumor cells may be delayed and clinically detected only after mature cells that form the bulk of the tumor undergo spontaneous apoptosis *(200)*. Therefore, it is likely that effective clinical strategies with the potential to produce long-term remissions may initially require treatment with agents, such as cytotoxic chemotherapy, to reduce the burden of leukemic blasts followed by novel strategies, such as differentiation therapy with combinations of pharmacological agents and myeloid growth factors to eliminate AML stem cells.

REFERENCES

1. Hanahan D, Weinberg RA. The hallmarks of cancer. Cell 2000;100(1):57–70.
2. Warrell RP, Jr., de The H, Wang ZY, Degos L. Acute promyelocytic leukemia. N Engl J Med 1993;329(3): 177–189.
3. Rowley J, Golomb H, Dougherty C. 15/17 translocation, a consistent chromosomal change in acute promyelocytic leukaemia. Lancet 1977;309(8010):549–550.
4. Larson RA, Kondo K, Vardiman JW, Butler AE, Golomb HM, Rowley JD. Evidence for a 15;17 translocation in every patient with acute promyelocytic leukemia. Am J Med 1984;76(5):827–841.
5. de The H, Lavau C, Marchio A, Chomienne C, Degos L, Dejean A. The PML-RAR alpha fusion mRNA generated by the t(15;17) translocation in acute promyelocytic leukemia encodes a functionally altered RAR. Cell 1991;66(4):675–684.
6. Kakizuka A, Miller WH, Jr., Umesono K, et al. Chromosomal translocation t(15;17) in human acute promyelocytic leukemia fuses RAR alpha with a novel putative transcription factor, PML. Cell 1991;66(4): 663–674.
7. Redner RL. Variations on a theme: the alternate translocations in APL. Leukemia 2002;16(10):1927–1932.
8. Lin RJ, Egan DA, Evans RM. Molecular genetics of acute promyelocytic leukemia. Trends in Genetics 1999;15(5):179–184.
9. Melnick A, Licht JD. Deconstructing a disease: RAR alpha, its fusion partners, and their roles in the patho-genesis of acute promyelocytic leukemia. Blood 1999;93(10):3167–3215.
10. Huang ME, Ye YC, Chen SR, et al. Use of all-trans retinoic acid in the treatment of acute promyelocytic leukemia. Blood 1988;72(2):567–572.
11. Warrell RP, Jr., Frankel SR, Miller WH, Jr., et al. Differentiation therapy of acute promyelocytic leukemia with tretinoin (all-trans-retinoic acid). N Engl J Med 1991;324(20):1385–1393.
12. Castaigne S, Chomienne C, Daniel MT, et al. All-trans retinoic acid as a differentiation therapy for acute promyelocytic leukemia. I. Clinical results. Blood 1990;76(9):1704–1709.
13. Degos L, Wang ZY. All trans retinoic acid in acute promyelocytic leukemia. Oncogene 2001;20(49): 7140–7145.
14. Tallman MS, Andersen JW, Schiffer CA, et al. All-trans retinoic acid in acute promyelocytic leukemia: long-term outcome and prognostic factor analysis from the North American Intergroup protocol. Blood 2002;100(13):4298–4302.
15. Tallman MS, Andersen JW, Schiffer CA, et al. All-trans-retinoic acid in acute promyelocytic leukemia. N Engl J Med 1997;337(15):1021–1028.
16. Muto A, Kizaki M, Yamato K, et al. 1,25-Dihydroxyvitamin D3 induces differentiation of a retinoic acid-resistant acute promyelocytic leukemia cell line (UF-1) associated with expression of p21(WAF1/CIP1) and p27(KIP1). Blood 1999;93(7):2225–2233.
17. Bhatia M, Kirkland JB, Meckling-Gill KA. M-CSF and 1,25 dihydroxy vitamin D3 synergize with 12-O-tetradecanoylphorbol-13-acetate to induce macrophage differentiation in acute promyelocytic leukemia NB4 cells. Leukemia 1994;8(10):1744–1749.
18. Song XD, Norman AW. Bryostatin-1 and 1alpha,25-dihydroxyvitamin D3 synergistically stimulate the differentiation of NB4 acute promyelocytic leukemia cells. Leukemia 1999;13(2):275–281.
19. Miller WH, Jr., Schipper HM, Lee JS, Singer J, Waxman S. Mechanisms of action of arsenic trioxide. Cancer Res 2002;62(14):3893–3903.
20. Niitsu N, Higashihara M, Honma Y. The catalytic DNA topoisomerase II inhibitor ICRF-193 and all-trans retinoic acid cooperatively induce granulytic differentiation of acute promyelocytic leukemia cells: candi-date drugs for chemo-differentiation therapy against acute promyelocytic leukemia. Exp Hematol 2002; 30(11):1273–1282.
21. Matsui W, Smith BD, Vala M, et al. Requirement for myeloid growth factors in the differentiation of acute promyelocytic leukaemia. Br J Haematol 2005;128(6):853–862.
22. Collins SJ. The role of retinoids and retinoic acid receptors in normal hematopoiesis. Leukemia 2002; 16(10):1896–1905.
23. Colombat P, Santini V, Delwel R, Krefft J, Bredmond JL, Lowenberg B. Primary human acute myeloblastic leukaemia: an analysis of in vitro granulytic maturation following stimulation with retinoic acid and G- CSF. Br J Haematol 1991;79(3):382–389.
24. Santini V, Colombat P, Delwel R, van Gurp R, Touw I, Lowenberg B. Induction of granulytic maturation in acute myeloid leukemia by G-CSF and retinoic acid. Leuk Res 1991;15(5):341–350.

25. Liu M, Iavarone A, Freedman LP. Transcriptional activation of the human p21(WAF1/CIP1) gene by retinoic acid receptor. Correlation with retinoid induction of U937 cell differentiation. J Biol Chem 1996; 271(49):31,723–31,728.

26. Ketley NJ, Allen PD, Kelsey SM, Newland AC. Modulation of idarubicin-induced apoptosis in human acute myeloid leukemia blasts by all-trans retinoic acid, 1,25(OH)$_2$ vitamin D3, and granulocyte-macrophage colony-stimulating factor. Blood 1997;90(11):4578–4587.

27. Dimberg A, Bahram F, Karlberg I, Larsson LG, Nilsson K, Oberg F. Retinoic acid-induced cell cycle arrest of human myeloid cell lines is associated with sequential down-regulation of c-Myc and cyclin E and post-transcriptional up-regulation of p27(Kip1). Blood 2002;99(6):2199–2206.

28. Griggs JJ, Henley SE, Rowe JM. Treatment of refractory undifferentiated acute myelogenous leukemia with all-trans-retinoic acid. Am J Hematol 1994;45(2):177–180.

29. Kurzrock R, Estey E, Talpaz M. All-trans retinoic acid: tolerance and biologic effects in myelodysplastic syndrome. J Clin Oncol 1993;11(8):1489–1495.

30. Aul C, Runde V, Gattermann N. All-trans retinoic acid in patients with myelodysplastic syndromes: results of a pilot study. Blood 1993;82(10):2967–2974.

31. Ohno R, Naoe T, Hirano M, et al. Treatment of myelodysplastic syndromes with all-trans retinoic acid. Leukemia Study Group of the Ministry of Health and Welfare. Blood 1993;81(5):1152–1154.

32. Bassan R, Chiodini B, Lerede T, et al. Prolonged administration of all-trans retinoic acid in combination with intensive chemotherapy and G-CSF for adult acute myelogenous leukemia: single-centre pilot study in different risk groups. Hematol J 2002;3(4):193–200.

33. Bolanos-Meade J, Karp JE, Guo C, et al. Timed sequential therapy of acute myelogenous leukemia in adults: a phase II study of retinoids in combination with the sequential administration of cytosine arabinoside, idarubicin and etoposide. Leuk Res 2003;27(4):313–321.

34. Belhabri A, Thomas X, Wattel E, et al. All trans retinoic acid in combination with intermediate-dose cytarabine and idarubicin in patients with relapsed or refractory non promyelocytic acute myeloid leukemia: a phase II randomized trial. Hematol J 2002;3(1):49–55.

35. Estey EH, Thall PF, Pierce S, et al. Randomized phase II study of fludarabine + cytosine arabinoside + idarubicin +/– all-trans retinoic acid +/– granulocyte colony-stimulating factor in poor prognosis newly diagnosed acute myeloid leukemia and myelodysplastic syndrome. Blood 1999;93(8):2478–2484.

36. Schlenk RF, Frohling S, Hartmann F, et al. Phase III study of all-trans retinoic acid in previously untreated patients 61 years or older with acute myeloid leukemia. Leukemia 2004;18(11):1798–1803.

37. Venditti A, Stasi R, Del Poeta G, et al. All-trans retinoic acid and low-dose cytosine arabinoside for the treatment of 'poor prognosis' acute myeloid leukemia. Leukemia 1995;9(7):1121–1125.

38. Bastien J, Rochette-Egly C. Nuclear retinoid receptors and the transcription of retinoid-target genes. Gene 2004;328:1–16.

39. Shiohara M, Dawson MI, Hobbs PD, et al. Effects of novel RAR- and RXR-selective retinoids on myeloid leukemic proliferation and differentiation in vitro. Blood 1999;93(6):2057–2066.

40. Gold EJ, Mertelsmann RH, Itri LM, et al. Phase I clinical trial of 13-*cis*-retinoic acid in myelodysplastic syndromes. Cancer Treat Rep 1983;67(11):981–986.

41. Greenberg BR, Durie BG, Barnett TC, Meyskens FL, Jr. Phase I-II study of 13-*cis*-retinoic acid in myelodysplastic syndrome. Cancer Treat Rep 1985;69(12):1369–1374.

42. Picozzi VJ, Jr., Swanson GF, Morgan R, Hecht F, Greenberg PL. 13-*cis* Retinoic acid treatment for myelodysplastic syndromes. J Clin Oncol 1986;4(4):589–595.

43. Kerndrup G, Bendix-Hansen K, Pedersen B, Ellegaard J, Hokland P. 13-*cis* Retinoic acid treatment of myelodysplastic syndromes. Leuk Res 1987;11(1):7–16.

44. Clark RE, Jacobs A, Lush CJ, Smith SA. Effect of 13-*cis*-retinoic acid on survival of patients with myelodysplastic syndrome. Lancet 1987;1(8536):763–765.

45. Hoffman SJ, Robinson WA. Use of differentiation-inducing agents in the myelodysplastic syndrome and acute non-lymphocytic leukemia. Am J Hematol 1988;28(2):124–127.

46. Koeffler HP, Heitjan D, Mertelsmann R, et al. Randomized study of 13-*cis* retinoic acid v placebo in the myelodysplastic disorders. Blood 1988;71(3):703–708.

47. Kramer ZB, Boros L, Wiernik PH, et al. 13-*cis*-Retinoic acid in the treatment of elderly patients with acute myeloid leukemia. A phase II pilot study of the Eastern Cooperative Oncology Group. Cancer 1991;67(6):1484–1486.

48. Miller WJ, Jakubowski A, Tong WP, et al. 9-*cis* Retinoic acid induces complete remission but does not reverse clinically acquired retinoid resistance in acute promyelocytic leukemia. Blood 1995;85(11):3021–3027.

49. Soignet SL, Benedetti F, Fleischauer A, et al. Clinical study of 9-*cis* retinoic acid (LGD1057) in acute promyelocytic leukemia. Leukemia 1998;12(10):1518–1521.

50. Grande A, Montanari M, Tagliafico E, et al. Physiological levels of 1 alpha, 25 dihydroxyvitamin D3 induce the monocytic commitment of CD34+ hematopoietic progenitors. J Leukoc Biol 2002;71(4):641–651.

51. Baker AR, McDonnell DP, Hughes M, et al. Cloning and expression of full-length cDNA encoding human vitamin D receptor. Proc Natl Acad Sci USA 1988;85(10):3294–3298.

52. Aranda A, Pascual A. Nuclear hormone receptors and gene expression. Physiol Rev 2001;81(3):1269–1304.

53. Song X, Sheppard HM, Norman AW, Liu X. Mitogen-activated protein kinase is involved in the degradation of p53 protein in the bryostatin-1-induced differentiation of the acute promyelocytic leukemia NB4 cell line. J Biol Chem 1999;274(3):1677–1682.

54. Hughes PJ, Steinmeyer A, Chandraratna RA, Brown G. 1Alpha,25-dihydroxyvitamin D3 stimulates steroid sulphatase activity in HL60 and NB4 acute myeloid leukaemia cell lines by different receptor-mediated mechanisms. J Cell Biochem 2005;94(6):1175–1189.

55. James SY, Williams MA, Kelsey SM, Newland AC, Colston KW. The role of vitamin D derivatives and retinoids in the differentiation of human leukaemia cells. Biochem Pharmacol 1997;54(5):625–634.

56. Petrini M, Caracciolo F, Corini M, Valentini P, Sabbatini AR, Grassi B. Low-dose ARA-C and 1(OH) D3 administration in acute non lymphoid leukemia: pilot study. Haematologica 1991;76(3):200–203.

57. Slapak CA, Desforges JF, Fogaren T, Miller KB. Treatment of acute myeloid leukemia in the elderly with low-dose cytarabine, hydroxyurea, and calcitriol. Am J Hematol 1992;41(3):178–183.

58. Jung CW, Kim ES, Seol JG, et al. Antiproliferative effect of a vitamin D3 analog, EB1089, on HL-60 cells by the induction of TGF-[beta] receptor. Leuk Res 1999;23(12):1105–1112.

59. James SY, Williams MA, Kelsey SM, Newland AC, Colston KW. Interaction of vitamin D derivatives and granulocyte-macrophage colony-stimulating factor in leukaemic cell differentiation. Leukemia 1997;11(7):1017–1025.

60. Pakkala I, Savli H, Knuutila S, Binderup L, Pakkala S. CB1093, a novel vitamin D analog; effects on differentiation and clonal growth on HL-60 and de novo leukemia cells. Leuk Res 1997;21(4):321–326.

61. Evans TR, Colston KW, Lofts FJ, et al. A phase II trial of the vitamin D analogue Seocalcitol (EB1089) in patients with inoperable pancreatic cancer. Br J Cancer 2002;86(5):680–685.

62. Gulliford T, English J, Colston KW, Menday P, Moller S, Coombes RC. A phase I study of the vitamin D analogue EB 1089 in patients with advanced breast and colorectal cancer. Br J Cancer 1998;78(1):6–13.

63. Bhisey RA, Sirsat SM. Selective promoting activity of phorbol myristate acetate in experimental skin carcinogenesis. Br J Cancer 1976;34(6):661–665.

64. Baird WM, Boutwell RK. Tumor-promoting activity of phorbol and four diesters of phorbol in mouse skin. Cancer Res 1971;31(8):1074–1079.

65. Sachs L. Control of normal cell differentiation and the phenotypic reversion of malignancy in myeloid leukaemia. Nature 1978;274(5671):535–539.

66. Koeffler HP, Bar-Eli M, Territo M. Phorbol diester-induced macrophage differentiation of leukemic blasts from patients with human myelogenous leukemia. J Clin Invest 1980;66(5):1101–1108.

67. Huberman E, Callaham MF. Induction of terminal differentiation in human promyelocytic leukemia cells by tumor-promoting agents. PNAS 1979;76(3):1293–1297.

68. Han ZT, Zhu XX, Yang RY, et al. Effect of intravenous infusions of 12-O-tetradecanoylphorbol-13-acetate (TPA) in patients with myelocytic leukemia: preliminary studies on therapeutic efficacy and toxicity. Proc Natl Acad Sci USA 1998;95(9):5357–5361.

69. Hennings H, Blumberg PM, Pettit GR, Herald CL, Shores R, Yuspa SH. Bryostatin 1, an activator of protein kinase C, inhibits tumor promotion by phorbol esters in SENCAR mouse skin. Carcinogenesis 1987;8(9):1343–1346.

70. Kraft AS, Baker VV, May WS. Bryostatin induces changes in protein kinase C location and activity without altering c-myc gene expression in human promyelocytic leukemia cells (HL-60). Oncogene 1987;1(2):111–118.

71. Jones RJ, Sharkis SJ, Miller CB, Rowinsky EK, Burke PJ, May WS. Bryostatin 1, a unique biologic response modifier: anti-leukemic activity in vitro. Blood 1990;75(6):1319–1323.

72. Gebbia V, Citarrella P, Miserendino V, et al. The effects of the macrocyclic lactone bryostatin-1 on leukemic cells in vitro. Tumori 1992;78(3):167–171.

73. Jalava A, Lintunen M, Heikkila J. Protein kinase C-alpha but not protein kinase C-epsilon is differentially down-regulated by bryostatin 1 and tetradecanoyl phorbol 13-acetate in SH-SY5Y human neuroblastoma cells. Biochem Biophys Res Commun 1993;191(2):472–478.

74. Kraft AS, William F, Pettit GR, Lilly MB. Varied differentiation responses of human leukemias to bryostatin 1. Cancer Res 1989;49(5):1287–1293.

75. Grant S, Pettit GR, Howe C, McCrady C. Effect of the protein kinase C activating agent bryostatin 1 on the clonogenic response of leukemic blast progenitors to recombinant granulocyte-macrophage colony-stimulating factor. Leukemia 1991;5(5):392–398.

76. Asiedu C, Biggs J, Lilly M, Kraft AS. Inhibition of leukemic cell growth by the protein kinase C activator bryostatin 1 correlates with the dephosphorylation of cyclin-dependent kinase 2. Cancer Res 1995;55(17): 3716–3720.

77. May WS, Sharkis SJ, Esa AH, et al. Antineoplastic bryostatins are multipotential stimulators of human hematopoietic progenitor cells. Proc Natl Acad Sci USA 1987;84(23):8483–8487.

78. Sharkis SJ, Jones RJ, Bellis ML, et al. The action of bryostatin on normal human hematopoietic progenitors is mediated by accessory cell release of growth factors. Blood 1990;76(4):716–720.

79. Schwaller J, Peters UR, Pabst T, et al. Up-regulation of p21WAF1 expression in myeloid cells is activated by the protein kinase C pathway. Br J Cancer 1997;76(12):1554–1557.

80. Vrana JA, Saunders AM, Chellappan SP, Grant S. Divergent effects of bryostatin 1 and phorbol myristate acetate on cell cycle arrest and maturation in human myelomonocytic leukemia cells (U937). Differentiation 1998;63(1):33–42.

81. Cragg LH, Andreeff M, Feldman E, et al. Phase I trial and correlative laboratory studies of bryostatin 1 (NSC 339555) and high-dose 1-B-D-arabinofuranosylcytosine in patients with refractory acute leukemia. Clin Cancer Res 2002;8(7):2123–2133.

82. Kouzarides T. Histone acetylases and deacetylases in cell proliferation. Curr Opin Gen Dev 1999;9(1): 40–48.

83. Struhl K. Histone acetylation and transcriptional regulatory mechanisms. Genes Dev 1998;12(5):599–606.

84. Tsukiyama T, Wu C. Chromatin remodeling and transcription. Curr Opin Gen Dev 1997;7(2):182–191.

85. Boyes J, Byfield P, Nakatani Y, Ogryzko V. Regulation of activity of the transcription factor GATA-1 by acetylation. Nature 1998;396(6711):594–598.

86. Imhof A, Yang XJ, Ogryzko VV, Nakatani Y, Wolffe AP, Ge H. Acetylation of general transcription factors by histone acetyltransferases. Curr Biol 1997;7(9):689–692.

87. Lin RJ, Nagy L, Inoue S, Shao W, Miller WH, Jr., Evans RM. Role of the histone deacetylase complex in acute promyelocytic leukaemia. Nature 1998;391(6669):811–814.

88. Alland L, Muhle R, Hou H, Jr., et al. Role for N-CoR and histone deacetylase in Sin3-mediated transcriptional repression. Nature 1997;387(6628):49–55.

89. Heinzel T, Lavinsky RM, Mullen TM, et al. A complex containing N-CoR, mSin3 and histone deacetylase mediates transcriptional repression. Nature 1997;387(6628):43–48.

90. Grignani F, De Matteis S, Nervi C, et al. Fusion proteins of the retinoic acid receptor-alpha recruit histone deacetylase in promyelocytic leukaemia. Nature 1998;391(6669):815–818.

91. Grignani F, Ferrucci PF, Testa U, et al. The acute promyelocytic leukemia-specific PML-RAR alpha fusion protein inhibits differentiation and promotes survival of myeloid precursor cells. Cell 1993;74(3):423–431.

92. Wang J, Hoshino T, Redner RL, Kajigaya S, Liu JM. ETO, fusion partner in t(8;21) acute myeloid leukemia, represses transcription by interaction with the human N-CoR/mSin3/HDAC1 complex. PNAS 1998;95(18): 10,860–10,865.

93. Kruh J. Effects of sodium butyrate, a new pharmacological agent, on cells in culture. Mol Cell Biochem 1982;42(2):65–82.

94. Cousens LS, Gallwitz D, Alberts BM. Different accessibilities in chromatin to histone acetylase. J Biol Chem 1979;254(5):1716–1723.

95. Lea MA, Tulsyan N. Discordant effects of butyrate analogues on erythroleukemia cell proliferation, differentiation and histone deacetylase. Anticancer Res 1995;15(3):879–883.

96. Gottlicher M, Minucci S, Zhu P, et al. Valproic acid defines a novel class of HDAC inhibitors inducing differentiation of transformed cells. EMBO J 2001;20(24):6969–6978.

97. Phiel CJ, Zhang F, Huang EY, Guenther MG, Lazar MA, Klein PS. Histone deacetylase is a direct target of valproic acid, a potent anticonvulsant, mood stabilizer, and teratogen. J Biol Chem 2001;276(39):36,734–36,741.

98. DiGiuseppe JA, Weng LJ, Yu KH, et al. Phenylbutyrate-induced G1 arrest and apoptosis in myeloid leukemia cells: structure-function analysis. Leukemia 1999;13(8):1243–1253.

99. Gore SD, Samid D, Weng LJ. Impact of the putative differentiating agents sodium phenylbutyrate and sodium phenylacetate on proliferation, differentiation, and apoptosis of primary neoplastic myeloid cells. Clin Cancer Res 1997;3(10):1755–1762.

100. Rius C, Zorrilla A, Mata F, Aller P. Comparative effects of butyrate and N6, 2′-O-dibutyryladenosine-3′:5′-cyclic monophosphate on growth, differentiation and gene expression in U937 human monoblastoid cells. Biochem Int 1991;23(3):555–562.

101. Rubio MA, Lopez-Rodriguez C, Nueda A, et al. Granulocyte-macrophage colony-stimulating factor, phorbol ester, and sodium butyrate induce the CD11c integrin gene promoter activity during myeloid cell differentiation. Blood 1995;86(10):3715–3724.

102. Santini V, Scappini B, Gozzini A, et al. Butyrate-stable monosaccharide derivatives induce maturation and apoptosis in human acute myeloid leukaemia cells. Br J Haematol 1998;101(3):529–538.

103. Witt O, Sand K, Pekrun A. Butyrate-induced erythroid differentiation of human K562 leukemia cells involves inhibition of ERK and activation of p38 MAP kinase pathways. Blood 2000;95(7):2391–2396.

104. Tai G, Eun-Young J, Yuji H, et al. Different effects of cyclic AMP and butyrate on eosinophilic differentiation, apoptosis and bcl-2 expression of a human eosinophilic leukemia cell line, EoL-1. Hematol Oncol 1996;14(4):181–192.

105. Rickard KL, Gibson PR, Young GP, Phillips WA. Activation of protein kinase C augments butyrate-induced differentiation and turnover in human colonic epithelial cells in vitro. Carcinogenesis 1999;20(6):977–984.

106. Archer SY, Meng S, Shei A, Hodin RA. p21(WAF1) is required for butyrate-mediated growth inhibition of human colon cancer cells. Proc Natl Acad Sci USA 1998;95(12):6791–6796.

107. Bhatia U, Traganos F, Darzynkiewicz Z. Induction of cell differentiation potentiates apoptosis triggered by prior exposure to DNA-damaging drugs. Cell Growth Differ 1995;6(8):937–944.

108. Gore SD, Weng LJ, Zhai S, et al. Impact of the putative differentiating agent sodium phenylbutyrate on myelodysplastic syndromes and acute myeloid leukemia. Clin Cancer Res 2001;7(8):2330–2339.

109. Gore SD, Weng LJ, Figg WD, et al. Impact of prolonged infusions of the putative differentiating agent sodium phenylbutyrate on myelodysplastic syndromes and acute myeloid leukemia. Clin Cancer Res 2002;8(4):963–970.

110. Kuendgen A, Strupp C, Aivado M, et al. Treatment of myelodysplastic syndromes with valproic acid alone or in combination with all-trans retinoic acid. Blood 2004;104(5):1266–1269.

111. Richon VM, Webb Y, Merger R, et al. Second generation hybrid polar compounds are potent inducers of transformed cell differentiation. Proc Natl Acad Sci USA 1996;93(12):5705–5708.

112. Sakajiri S, Kumagai T, Kawamata N, Saitoh T, Said JW, Koeffler HP. Histone deacetylase inhibitors profoundly decrease proliferation of human lymphoid cancer cell lines. Exp Hematol 2005;33(1):53–61.

113. Richon VM, Emiliani S, Verdin E, et al. A class of hybrid polar inducers of transformed cell differentiation inhibits histone deacetylases. Proc Natl Acad Sci USA 1998;95(6):3003–3007.

114. Vrana JA, Decker RH, Johnson CR, et al. Induction of apoptosis in U937 human leukemia cells by suberoylanilide hydroxamic acid (SAHA) proceeds through pathways that are regulated by Bcl-2/Bcl-x(L), c-Jun, and p21(CIP1), but independent of p53. Oncogene 1999;18(50):7016–7025.

115. Saito A, Yamashita T, Mariko Y, et al. A synthetic inhibitor of histone deacetylase, MS-27-275, with marked in vivo antitumor activity against human tumors. PNAS 1999;96(8):4592–4597.

116. Kelly W, Richon VM, O'Connor O, et al. Phase I clinical trial of histone deacetylase inhibitor: suberoylanilide hydroxamic acid administered intravenously. Clin Cancer Res 2003;9(10):3578–3588.

117. Gojo I, Gore S, Jiemjit A, et al. Phase I study of histone deacetylase inhibitor (HDI) MS-275 in adults with refractory or realpsed hematologic malignancies. Blood 2004;102(11):388a.

118. Jones PA, Baylin SB. The fundamental role of epigenetic events in cancer. Nat Rev Genet 2002;3(6):415–428.

119. Herman JG, Baylin SB. Gene silencing in cancer in association with promoter hypermethylation. N Engl J Med 2003;349(21):2042–2054.

120. Baylin SB. Mechanisms underlying epigenetically mediated gene silencing in cancer. Semin Cancer Biol 2002;12(5):331–337.

121. Cheng JC, Matsen CB, Gonzales FA, et al. Inhibition of DNA methylation and reactivation of silenced genes by zebularine. J Natl Cancer Inst 2003;95(5):399–409.

122. Christman JK, Mendelsohn N, Herzog D, Schneiderman N. Effect of 5-azacytidine on differentiation and DNA methylation in human promyelocytic leukemia cells (HL-60). Cancer Res 1983;43(2):763–769.

123. Gambari R, Del Senno L, Barbieri R, et al. Human leukemia K-562 cells: induction of erythroid differentiation by 5-azacytidine. Cell Differ 1984;14(2):87–97.

124. Creusot F, Acs G, Christman JK. Inhibition of DNA methyltransferase and induction of Friend erythroleukemia cell differentiation by 5-azacytidine and 5-aza-2′-deoxycytidine. J Biol Chem 1982;257(4):2041–2048.

125. Momparler RL, Dore BT, Momparler LF. Effect of 5-aza-2′-deoxycytidine and retinoic acid on differentiation and c-myc expression in HL-60 myeloid leukemic cells. Cancer Lett 1990;54(1–2):21–28.

126. Dore BT, Chomienne C, Momparler RL. Effect of 5-aza-2′-deoxycytidine and vitamin D3 analogs on growth and differentiation of human myeloid leukemic cells. Cancer Chemother Pharmacol 1998;41(4): 275–280.

127. Santini V, Kantarjian HM, Issa JP. Changes in DNA methylation in neoplasia: pathophysiology and therapeutic implications. Ann Intern Med 2001;134(7):573–586.

128. Silverman LR, Demakos EP, Peterson BL, et al. Randomized controlled trial of azacitidine in patients with the myelodysplastic syndrome: a study of the cancer and leukemia group B. J Clin Oncol 2002;20(10): 2429–2440.

129. Wijermans P, Lubbert M, Verhoef G, et al. Low-dose 5-aza-2′-deoxycytidine, a DNA hypomethylating agent, for the treatment of high-risk myelodysplastic syndrome: a multicenter phase II study in elderly patients. J Clin Oncol 2000;18(5):956–962.

130. Issa JP, Garcia-Manero G, Giles FJ, et al. Phase 1 study of low-dose prolonged exposure schedules of the hypomethylating agent 5-aza-2′-deoxycytidine (decitabine) in hematopoietic malignancies. Blood 2004;103(5):1635–1640.

131. Friend C, Scher W, Holland JG, Sato T. Hemoglobin synthesis in murine virus-induced leukemic cells in vitro: stimulation of erythroid differentiation by dimethyl sulfoxide. Proc Natl Acad Sci USA 1971; 68(2):378–382.

132. Santos-Beneit AM, Mollinedo F. Expression of genes involved in initiation, regulation, and execution of apoptosis in human neutrophils and during neutrophil differentiation of HL-60 cells. J Leukoc Biol 2000; 67(5):712–724.

133. Arcangeli A, Carla M, Bene MRD, Becchetti A, Wanke E, Olivotto M. Polar/apolar compounds induce leukemia cell differentiation by modulating cell-surface potential. PNAS 1993;90(12):5858–5862.

134. Jiang H, Lin J, Su ZZ, Collart FR, Huberman E, Fisher PB. Induction of differentiation in human promyelocytic HL-60 leukemia cells activates p21, WAF1/CIP1, expression in the absence of p53. Oncogene 1994; 9(11):3397–3406.

135. Egorin MJ, Rosen DM, Sridhara R, Sensenbrenner L, Cottler-Fox M. Plasma concentrations and pharmacokinetics of dimethylsulfoxide and its metabolites in patients undergoing peripheral-blood stem-cell transplants. J Clin Oncol 1998;16(2):610–615.

136. Gambari R, Rifkind RA, Marks PA. Stability of alpha and beta globin messenger RNA during induced differentiation of mouse erythroleukemia cells. Blood 1979;54(4):933–939.

137. Haces A, Breitman TR, Driscoll JS. Chemical differentiating agents. Differentiation of HL-60 cells by hexamethylenebisacetamide analogues. J Med Chem 1987;30(2):405–409.

138. Kiyokawa H, Richon VM, Venta-Perez G, Rifkind RA, Marks PA. Hexamethylenebisacetamide-induced erythroleukemia cell differentiation involves modulation of events required for cell cycle progression through G1. Proc Natl Acad Sci USA 1993;90(14):6746–6750.

139. Leng L, Yu F, Dong L, Busquets X, et al. Differential modulation of protein kinase C isoforms in erythroleukemia during induced differentiation. Cancer Res 1993;53(22):5554–5558.

140. Andreeff M, Stone R, Michaeli J, et al. Hexamethylene bisacetamide in myelodysplastic syndrome and acute myelogenous leukemia: a phase II clinical trial with a differentiation- inducing agent. Blood 1992; 80(10):2604–2609.

141. Griffin J, Munroe D, Major P, Kufe D. Induction of differentiation of human myeloid leukemia cells by inhibitors of DNA synthesis. Exp Hematol 1982;10(9):774–781.

142. Jeannesson P, Lahlil R, Chenais B, et al. Anthracyclines as tumor cell differentiating agents: Effects on the regulation of erythroid gene expression. Leukemia Lymphoma 1997;26(5–6):575–587.

143. Leung MF, Sartorelli AC. The effects of microtubule disrupting drugs on the differentiation of HL-60 leukemia cells. Leuk Res 1992;16(9):929–935.

144. Cheson BD, Simon R. Low-dose ara-C in acute nonlymphocytic leukemia and myelodysplastic syndromes: a review of 20 years' experience. Semin Oncol 1987;14(2 suppl 1):126–133.

145. Tilly H, Castaigne S, Bordessoule D, et al. Low-dose cytarabine versus intensive chemotherapy in the treatment of acute nonlymphocytic leukemia in the elderly. J Clin Oncol 1990;8(2):272–279.

146. Miller KB, Kim K, Morrison FS, et al. The evaluation of low-dose cytarabine in the treatment of myelodysplastic syndromes: a phase-III intergroup study. Ann Hematol 1992;65(4):162–168.

147. Ikebuchi K, Ihle JN, Hirai Y, Wong GG, Clark SC, Ogawa M. Synergistic factors for stem cell proliferation: further studies of the target stem cells and the mechanism of stimulation by interleukin-1, interleukin-6, and granulocyte colony-stimulating factor. Blood 1988;72(6):2007–2014.

148. Camera A, Volpicelli M, Villa MR, Risitano AM, Rossi M, Rotoli B. Complete remission induced by high dose erythropoietin and granulocyte colony stimulating factor in acute erythroleukemia (AML-M6 with maturation). Haematologica 2002;87(11):1225–1227.

149. Yamasaki Y, Izumi Y, Sawada H, Fujita K. Probable in vivo induction of differentiation by recombinant human granulocyte colony stimulating factor (rhG-CSF) in acute promyelocytic leukaemia (APL). Br J Haematol 1991;78(4):579–580.

150. Vaickus L, Villalona-Calero MA, Caligiuri T. Acute progranulocytic leukemia (APL): possible in vivo differentiation by granulocyte colony-stimulating factor (G-CSF). Leukemia 1993;7(10):1680–1681.

151. Maun NA, Gaines P, Khanna-Gupta A, et al. G-CSF signaling can differentiate promyelocytes expressing a defective retinoic acid receptor: evidence for divergent pathways regulating neutrophil differentiation. Blood 2004;103(5):1693–1701.

152. Nakamaki T, Sakashita A, Sano M, et al. Granulocyte-colony stimulating factor and retinoic acid cooperatively induce granulocyte differentiation of acute promyelocytic leukemia cells in vitro. Jpn J Cancer Res 1989;80(11):1077–1082.

153. Imaizumi M, Sato A, Koizumi Y, et al. Potentiated maturation with a high proliferating activity of acute promyelocytic leukemia induced in vitro by granulocyte or granulocyte/macrophage colony-stimulating factors in combination with all-trans retinoic acid. Leukemia 1994;8(8):1301–1308.

154. Gianni M, Terao M, Zanotta S, Barbui T, Rambaldi A, Garattini E. Retinoic acid and granulocyte colony-stimulating factor synergistically induce leukocyte alkaline phosphatase in acute promyelocytic leukemia cells. Blood 1994;83(7):1909–1921.

155. Miyauchi J, Inatomi Y, Ohyashiki K, Asada M, Mizutani S, Toyama K. The in vitro effects of all-trans-retinoic acid and hematopoietic growth factors on the clonal growth and self-renewal of blast stem cells in acute promyelocytic leukemia. Leuk Res 1997;21(4):285–294.

156. Tsurumi H, Tojo A, Takahashi T, Moriwaki H, Asano S, Muto Y. The combined effects of all-trans retinoic acid and granulocyte colony-stimulating factor as a differentiation induction therapy for acute promyelocytic leukemia. Intern Med 1993;32(8):648–650.

157. Jansen JH, de Ridder MC, Geertsma WM, et al. Complete remission of t(11;17) positive acute promyelocytic leukemia induced by all-trans retinoic acid and granulocyte colony-stimulating factor. Blood 1999; 94(1):39–45.

158. Higuchi T, Kizaki M, Omine M. Induction of differentiation of retinoic acid-resistant acute promyelocytic leukemia cells by the combination of all-trans retinoic acid and granulocyte colony-stimulating factor. Leuk Res 2004;28(5):525–532.

159. Chen Z, Brand NJ, Chen A, et al. Fusion between a novel Kruppel-like zinc finger gene and the retinoic acid receptor-alpha locus due to a variant t(11;17) translocation associated with acute promyelocytic leukaemia. EMBO J 1993;12(3):1161–1167.

160. Licht JD, Chomienne C, Goy A, et al. Clinical and molecular characterization of a rare syndrome of acute promyelocytic leukemia associated with translocation (11;17). Blood 1995;85(4):1083–1094.

161. Katayama N, Kita K, Kawakami K, et al. Granulocyte colony-stimulating factor and its receptor in acute promyelocytic leukemia. Am J Hematol 1998;58(1):31–35.

162. de Gentile A, Toubert ME, Dubois C, et al. Induction of high-affinity GM-CSF receptors during all-trans retinoic acid treatment of acute promyelocytic leukemia. Leukemia 1994;8(10):1758–1762.

163. Matsui WH, Gladstone DE, Vala MS, et al. The role of growth factors in the activity of pharmacological differentiation agents. Cell Growth Differ 2002;13(6):275–283.

164. Bloch A. Dynamics of interaction between DNA-specific antitumor agents and serum-contained cytokines in the initiation of ML-1 human myeloblastic leukemia cell differentiation. Leukemia 1993;7(8):1219–1224.

165. Honma Y, Honma C, Bloch A. Mechanism of interaction between antineoplastic agents and natural differentiation factors in the induction of human leukemic cell maturation. Cancer Res 1986;46(12 pt 1): 6311–6315.

166. Roddie PH, Horton Y, Turner ML. Primary acute myeloid leukaemia blasts resistant to cytokine-induced differentiation to dendritic-like leukaemia cells can be forced to differentiate by the addition of bryostatin-1. Leukemia 2002;16(1):84–93.

167. Coffman FD, Studzinski GP. Differentiation-related mechanisms which suppress DNA replication. Exp Cell Res 1999;248:58–73.

168. Studzinski GP, Harrison LE. Differentiation-related changes in the cell cycle traverse. Int Rev Cytol 1999;189:1–59.

169. Prochownik EV, Kukowska J, Rodgers C. c-myc Antisense transcripts accelerate differentiation and inhibit G1 progression in murine erythroleukemia cells. Mol Cell Biol 1988;8(9):3683–3695.

170. Bloch A, Liu XM, Wang LG. Regulation of c-myb expression in ML-1 human myeloblastic leukemia cells by c-ets-1 protein. Adv Enzyme Regul 1995;35:35–41.

171. Amanullah A, Hoffman B, Liebermann DA. Deregulated E2F-1 blocks terminal differentiation and loss of leukemogenicity of M1 myeloblastic leukemia cells without abrogating induction of p15(INK4B) and p16(INK4A). Blood 2000;96(2):475–482.

172. Asada M, Yamada T, Fukumuro K, Mizutani S. p21Cip1/WAF1 is important for differentiation and survival of U937 cells. Leukemia 1998;12(12):1944–1950.

173. Furukawa Y. Cell cycle regulation of hematopoietic stem cells. Hum Cell 1998;11(2):81–92.

174. Cenciarelli C, De Santa F, Puri PL, et al. Critical role played by cyclin D3 in the MyoD-mediated arrest of cell cycle during myoblast differentiation. Mol Cell Biol 1999;19(7):5203–5217.

175. Hangaishi A, Ogawa S, Imamura N, et al. Inactivation of multiple tumor-suppressor genes involved in negative regulation of the cell cycle, MTS1/p16INK4A/CDKN2, MTS2/p15INK4B, p53, and Rb genes in primary lymphoid malignancies. Blood 1996;87(12):4949–4958.

176. Ragione FD, Iolascon A. Inactivation of cyclin-dependent kinase inhibitor genes and development of human acute leukemias. Leuk Lymphoma 1997;25(1–2):23–35.

177. Herman JG, Civin CI, Issa JP, Collector MI, Sharkis SJ, Baylin SB. Distinct patterns of inactivation of p15INK4B and p16INK4A characterize the major types of hematological malignancies. Cancer Res 1997; 57(5):837–841.

178. Imamura J, Miyoshi I, Koeffler HP. p53 in hematologic malignancies. Blood 1994;84(8):2412–2421.

179. Ahuja H, Bar-Eli M, Advani SH, Benchimol S, Cline MJ. Alterations in the p53 gene and the clonal evolution of the blast crisis of chronic myelocytic leukemia. Proc Natl Acad Sci USA 1989;86(17):6783–6787.

180. Quesnel B, Guillerm G, Vereecque R, et al. Methylation of the p15(INK4b) gene in myelodysplastic syndromes is frequent and acquired during disease progression. Blood 1998;91(8):2985–2990.

181. Corradini P, Inghirami G, Astolfi M, et al. Inactivation of tumor suppressor genes, p53 and Rb1, in plasma cell dyscrasias. Leukemia 1994;8(5):758–767.

182. Blagosklonny MV, Pardee AB. The restriction point of the cell cycle. Cell Cycle 2002;1(2):103–110.

183. Gutierrez C, Ramirez-Parra E, Castellano MM, del Pozo JC. G(1) to S transition: more than a cell cycle engine switch. Curr Opin Plant Biol 2002;5(6):480–486.

184. Sherr CJ. The Pezcoller lecture: cancer cell cycles revisited. Cancer Res 2000;60(14):3689–3695.

185. Blanchard JM. Cyclin A2 transcriptional regulation: modulation of cell cycle control at the G1/S transition by peripheral cues. Biochem Pharmacol 2000;60(8):1179–1184.

186. Muller C, Yang R, Park DJ, Serve H, Berdel WE, Koeffler HP. The aberrant fusion proteins PML-RAR alpha and PLZF-RAR alpha contribute to the overexpression of cyclin A1 in acute promyelocytic leukemia. Blood 2000;96(12):3894–3899.

187. Harvat BL, Wang A, Seth P, Jetten AM. Up-regulation of p27Kip1, p21WAF1/Cip1 and p16Ink4a is associated with, but not sufficient for, induction of squamous differentiation. J Cell Sci 1998;111 (pt 9):1185–1196.

188. Sgambato A, Cittadini A, Faraglia B, Weinstein IB. Multiple functions of p27(Kip1) and its alterations in tumor cells: a review. J Cell Physiol 2000;183(1):18–27.

189. Lotem J, Sachs L. Cytokine control of developmental programs in normal hematopoiesis and leukemia. Oncogene 2002;21(21):3284–3294.

190. Oberg F, Wu S, Bahram F, Nilsson K, Larsson LG. Cytokine-induced restoration of differentiation and cell cycle arrest in v-Myc transformed U-937 monoblasts correlates with reduced Myc activity. Leukemia 2001; 15(2):217–227.

191. Bedi A, Barber JP, Bedi GC, et al. BCR-ABL-mediated inhibition of apoptosis with delay of G2/M transition after DNA damage: a mechanism of resistance to multiple anticancer agents. Blood 1995;86(3):1148–1158.

192. Bedi A, Zehnbauer BA, Griffin CA, et al. Eradication of chronic myeloid leukemia (CML) progenitors by growth factor (GF)-induced terminal differentiation. Blood 1993;82:330a.

193. Darwiche N, El Sabban M, Bazzi R, et al. Retinoic acid dramatically enhances the arsenic trioxide-induced cell cycle arrest and apoptosis in retinoic acid receptor alpha-positive human T-cell lymphotropic virus type-I-transformed cells. Hematol J 2001;2(2):127–135.

194. Zheng X, Chang RL, Cui XX, et al. Synergistic effects of clinically achievable concentrations of 12-O-tetradecanoylphorbol-13-acetate in combination with all-trans retinoic acid, 1alpha,25-dihydroxyvitamin D3, and sodium butyrate on differentiation in HL-60 cells. Oncol Res 2000;12(9–10):419–427.

195. James SY, Williams MA, Newland AC, Colston KW. Leukemia cell differentiation: cellular and molecular interactions of retinoids and vitamin D. Gen Pharmacol 1999;32(1):143–154.
196. Fenaux P, Chastang C, Chevret S, et al. A randomized comparison of all transretinoic acid (ATRA) followed by chemotherapy and ATRA plus chemotherapy and the role of maintenance therapy in newly diagnosed acute promyelocytic leukemia. The European APL Group. Blood 1999;94(4):1192–1200.
197. de Botton S, Coiteux V, Chevret S, et al. Outcome of childhood acute promyelocytic leukemia with all-trans-retinoic acid and chemotherapy. J Clin Oncol 2004;22(8):1404–1412.
198. Bonnet D, Dick JE. Human acute myeloid leukemia is organized as a hierarchy that originates from a primitive hematopoietic cell. Nat Med 1997;3(7):730–737.
199. Lapidot T, Sirard C, Vormoor J, et al. A cell initiating human acute myeloid leukaemia after transplantation into SCID mice. Nature 1994;367(6464):645–648.
200. Jones RJ, Matsui WH, Smith BD. Cancer stem cells: Are we missing the target? J Natl Cancer Inst 2004;96(8):583–585.

15 Stem Cell Transplantation for AML

Javier Bolaños-Meade and Richard J. Jones

CONTENTS

Summary

Bone marrow transplantation is the treatment of choice for some patients with acute myeloid leukemia (AML) and myelodysplastic syndrome (MDS). Patients with high-risk disease such as those with MDS, in second (or subsequent) complete remission, or those with poor risk cytogenetics will benefit the most with this approach. With current transplant techniques, outcomes have improved over recent years. Even when relapse and graft-vs-host disease still are important problems faced by these patients, novel approaches have been developed to decrease the risk of complications. In this chapter, the current state of the art on transplantation for AML will be discussed.

Key Words: Acute myeloid leukemia; myelodysplastic syndrome; promyelocytic leukemia; bone marrow transplantation; graft-vs-host disease.

1. INTRODUCTION

In humans, the infusion of bone marrow as a therapeutic tool goes back to the mid-twentieth century, when it was successfully used to rescue patients after a nuclear catastrophe *(1)*. E. D. Thomas and G. W. Santos in the United States were among the early investigators attempting to use blood and marrow transplantation (BMT) for the therapy of malignant disorders *(2,3)*, including acute myeloid leukemia (AML) *(3–7)*. Over the past three decades, allogeneic and autologous BMT have become the standard treatment for selected patients with AML. The present chapter will discuss the role of autologous and allogeneic BMT strategies for patients with AML and myelodysplastic syndrome (MDS).

From: *Contemporary Hematology: Acute Myelogenous Leukemia*
Edited by: J. E. Karp © Humana Press Inc., Totowa, NJ

2. WHO NEEDS A BONE MARROW TRANSPLANT?

The treatment of newly diagnosed AML is divided into two broad phases: induction and postremission (consolidation or augmentation) therapy. Induction therapy is aimed at eliminating the overt leukemia and its severe toxicities resulting from infiltration of the marrow and other tissues. Although induction therapy is now very effective, with complete remission rates greater than 70%, the long-term disease-free survival of patients after just one cycle of induction therapy is only about 10% (8,9). However, one or more additional cycles of postremission therapy, aimed at the minimal residual leukemia remaining after induction therapy, will substantially reduce the relapse rate (8–13). Both conventional chemotherapy approaches and BMT are effective postremission therapies. Comparative studies have not conclusively defined the relative roles these different postremission therapies should play in patients with AML. This is at least partly because AML is a heterogeneous disease and there appear to be subsets of patients who are likely to benefit more from one type of therapy than another. However, emerging data suggest that it should be possible to integrate BMT into a comprehensive treatment plan that optimizes AML patients' chances for cure.

Age, FLT3 status, white blood cell count at diagnosis (perhaps related to FLT3 mutation), performance status, a preceding MDS, and particularly cytogenetics influence treatment results (11–20). Newly diagnosed patients with favorable risk karyotype (including t(15;17), t(8;21), or inv(16)) have reasonable outcomes with conventional chemotherapy regimens alone. In contrast, patients with adverse cytogenetics (complex karyotype or with abnormalities on chromosomes 5 or 7) have an unacceptably high risk of relapse with just chemotherapy (12,21,22). Therefore, patients with adverse cytogenetics should be considered potential candidates for BMT. Patients with an antecedent MDS or treatment-related AML (both sometimes called secondary AML) are also rarely cured by postremission therapy with chemotherapy alone and should also be considered for allografting (11,12). The use of BMT in AML patients in first complete remission with intermediate risk cytogenetics remains a matter of debate and will depend greatly on the individual patient.

Upon relapse, it is clear that almost everyone should be considered a potential transplant candidate. Breems et al. designed a prognostic index for patients in first relapse (23). In their study they found that even patients in the favorable group had less than 50% overall survival at 5 years. Therefore, it is clear that aggressive therapies are needed in these patients.

Once all these factors have been contemplated for a given patient, the next question is if the patient is a candidate for the procedure. It is clear that not everyone who needs a transplant is a candidate for the procedure because of a myriad of factors, such as age, comorbidities, lack of donors, and performance status. However, the recent development of reduced-intensity conditioning regimens has broadened the application of allogeneic BMT to older and less fit patients.

3. TYPE AND TIMING OF TRANSPLANT

Autologous and matched related allogeneic grafts after myeloablative conditioning have been the most widely used transplants for AML. More recently, matched unrelated and haploidentical related transplants and reduced intensity conditioning are also being employed. A discussion on the type and timing of the transplant will follow.

3.1. Transplantation in First Complete Remission

The use of BMT as consolidation for patients with AML has been explored extensively. Six randomized studies have been reported comparing autologous BMT *vs* chemotherapy *(24–29)*. Five of these studies also included an allogeneic BMT comparison arm *(24–28)*.

Burnett et al. reported a study comparing autologous BMT as late intensification against observation in patients in first complete remission *(29)*. After three courses of intensive chemotherapy, patients underwent a bone marrow harvest. They were then randomized to receive, after one more course of chemotherapy, no further treatment or an autologous BMT after preparation with cyclophosphamide and total-body irradiation. Three-hundred and eighty-one patients were randomized (38% of those eligible), and of the 190 patients allocated to autologous BMT, 126 received it. On intention-to-treat analysis the number of relapses was substantially lower in the autotransplant group than in the group assigned no further treatment (37% vs 58%, $p = 0.0007$), resulting in superior disease-free survival at 7 years (53 vs 40%; $p = 0.04$).

In 1989 Reiffers et al. reported 85 patients under the age of 50 who were entered into a prospective study comparing the effectiveness of allogeneic or autologous BMT and intensive chemotherapy for patients in first complete remission *(24)*. Fifty-eight patients who were in remission were assigned to the three different therapies. Fifty-two patients were assessable: 20 patients with an HLA-identical sibling donor underwent allogeneic BMT within 3 months after achievement of complete remission; the other 32 patients were randomized to receive autologous BMT or intensive chemotherapy. The actuarial risk of relapse at 3 years was 18% for the allogeneic patients, 50% for the autologous patients, and 83% in the chemotherapy group. The difference was highly significant ($p < 0.0002$). The disease-free survival was, respectively, 66, 41, and 16% ($p < 0.004$). However, the certainty of the findings is compromised by the small size of the trial.

Reiffers et al. published another study with 204 adult patients with *de novo* AML and prospectively compared allogeneic BMT, autologous BMT, and chemotherapy *(25)*. Of the 135 patients who were still in first complete remission at study entry, 36 had an HLA-identical sibling donor and were allocated to allogeneic BMT (group I); of the 99 patients not eligible for allograft, 77 were randomized to either autotransplant (39 patients) or chemotherapy (38 patients). There was no statistical difference between autologous BMT and chemotherapy for either disease-free or overall survival, and these two groups were combined for analysis (group II). The actuarial risk of relapse at 3 years was significantly lower for group I patients (24%) than for the group II patients (56%; $p < 0.009$). The 3-year disease-free survival was higher for group I patients (66.5%) than for the group II patients (42.4%) ($p < 0.05$ by multivariate analysis); the disease-free survival and risk of relapse were influenced by the initial white count, the number of chemotherapy courses to obtain a remission, and the type of postinduction treatment.

Harousseau et al. studied patients between the ages of 15 and 50 *(28)*. After achieving remission, patients up to the age of 40 and having an HLA-identical sibling were assigned to undergo an allogeneic BMT. All the other patients received one course of high-dose cytarabine and an anthracycline; they were then randomized to either a second course of chemotherapy with amsacrine and etoposide or a combination of busulfan and cyclophosphamide followed by an unpurged autologous BMT. Of 367 in remission, only 219 actually received the planned intensive postremission treatment (73 allografts, 75 autotransplants, and 71 intensive chemotherapy). With a median follow-up of 62 months, the 4-year disease-free survival of the group was 39.5%. The type of postremission therapy had no significant impact on the outcome. There was no difference in the 4-year disease-free and overall survival between 88 patients for whom an allogeneic transplant was scheduled (44% and 53%, respectively) and 134 patients of the same age category without an HLA-identical sibling (38% and 53%, respectively). Similarly, there was no difference in the outcome between autologous BMT and chemotherapy.

Cassileth et al. compared high-dose cytarabine with autologous or allogeneic BMT as consolidation during first remission in patients aged 16–55 (26). After complete remission was achieved, one cycle of consolidation with idarubicin and cytarabine was given to all patients. Those with HLA-identical siblings were assigned to allogeneic BMT, whereas the remaining patients were randomized to receive a single course of high-dose cytarabine or transplantation of autologous marrow purged with 4-hydroperoxycyclophosphamide. The conditioning regimen for both allogeneic and autologous BMT was oral busulfan and intravenous cyclophosphamide. In an intention-to-treat analysis, no significant differences in disease-free survival were found among patients. Survival after complete remission was somewhat better after chemotherapy than after autologous marrow transplantation ($p = 0.05$). There was a marginal advantage in terms of overall survival with chemotherapy as compared with allogeneic BMT ($p = 0.04$). However, a reanalysis showed that the postremission therapies appeared to have different efficacies by cytogenetic risk groups (30). Patients with favorable cytogenetics did significantly better following autologous BMT and allogeneic BMT than with chemotherapy alone. Perhaps the most notable difference between postremission therapies was in patients with unfavorable cytogenetics, who did significantly better with allogeneic BMT (30). In fact, allogeneic BMT produced similar outcomes in all risk groups of first-remission AML.

Zittoun et al. also compared chemotherapy with autologous and allogeneic BMT (27). Patients with an HLA-identical sibling were assigned to undergo allogeneic BMT; the others were randomized to undergo unpurged autologous BMT or a second course of intensive chemotherapy with high-dose cytarabine and daunorubicin. A total of 144 patients were assigned to allogeneic BMT, and 95 were randomized to autologous BMT and 104 to intensive chemotherapy. The relapse rate was highest in the intensive chemotherapy group and lowest in the allogeneic BMT patients, whereas the mortality rate was, as expected, highest after allogeneic BMT and lowest after intensive chemotherapy. The projected rate of disease-free survival at 4 years was 55% for allogeneic transplantation, 48% for autologous transplantation, and 30% for intensive chemotherapy. However, the overall survival after complete remission was similar in the three groups, as many who relapsed after chemotherapy were salvaged with autologous BMT.

Studies prospectively comparing allogeneic BMT with intensive chemotherapy or autologous BMT as consolidation for first-remission AML have been criticized because the allocation to allogeneic BMT is always a "genetic" randomization (i.e., patients with matched sibling donors will receive allogeneic transplant). Nevertheless, such an allocation is justified because only a minority of patients will have a matched sibling donor and the presence of a matched donor should not produce a selection bias. However, these studies generally only studied younger patients, so caution must be exerted when these results are extrapolated to older populations. Also, only 54–87% of the patients randomized to autologous BMT actually received this therapy. Five studies reported overall survival results; none showed a difference between autologous BMT and chemotherapy, although there was a trend favoring autologous BMT in three (25,27,29) and chemotherapy in two (26,28). In terms of disease-free survival, all six studies reported a trend favoring autologous BMT over chemotherapy, but only the study by Zittoun et al. reported a statistically better outcome (27). A recent meta-analysis of these data confirmed the favorable disease-free survival associated with autologous BMT, but also showed no difference in overall survival between the two strategies (31). Therefore, either intensive chemotherapy or autologous BMT would appear to be a reasonable choice for consolidation of patients in first complete remission.

Clearly, allogeneic BMT as consolidation of patients in first complete remission produces a better leukemia-free survival, although the high therapy-related mortality can obscure a benefit in terms of overall survival (24,25,27). Thus, many centers will not consider allogeneic BMT in patients with favorable-risk AML (e.g., those with t(8;21), inv(16), or t(15;17) chromosomal abnormalities). In contrast, AML patients with unfavorable features (those with adverse cytogenetics, secondary AML, and possibly those with FLT3 mutations) are rarely cured by postremission therapy with chemotherapy alone (21,22). However, allogeneic BMT produces similar outcomes in all risk groups of first remission AML (30). Thus, AML patients with unfavorable characteristics should strongly be considered potential candidates for allogeneic BMT in first remission.

3.2. Transplantation at Relapse

Gale et al. compared the 3-year disease-free survival in 485 AML patients receiving chemotherapy or allogeneic BMT in second complete remission (32). The chemotherapy cohort included 244 patients treated on trials of the British Medical Research Council, Eastern Cooperative Oncology Group, and MD Anderson Hospital. The allogeneic BMT cohort included 257 persons transplanted worldwide and reported to the International Bone Marrow Transplant Registry. Subjects were selected for comparable age and year of treatment. Preliminary analyses identified two factors correlated with disease-free survival: age and duration of first remission. Although the treatment-related mortality was higher for allogeneic BMT (56% vs 7% for chemotherapy), it produced a better (26% vs 17%) 3-year disease-free survival. Allogeneic BMT during early relapse (before a patient's clinical status deteriorates) appears to produce results similar to BMT in second remission, possibly with less toxicity (33). Donor lymphocyte infusions are usually considered the treatment of choice for patients who relapse after allogeneic BMT for AML (34,35). Toxicity is high because successful treatment is essentially only seen in the setting of graft-vs-host disease (GVHD). However, 20–30% of patients will achieve long-term remissions.

3.3. Transplantation for Resistant Disease

Allogeneic BMT is the only potentially curative option for patients with AML that is refractory to induction therapy. The City of Hope group reported their experience in 68 patients who consecutively underwent allogeneic transplantation between July 1978 and August 2000 with primary refractory disease (36). With a median follow-up of 3 years, the 3-year probabilities of disease-free survival, overall survival, and relapse rate were 31, 30, and 51%, respectively. However, most other studies of allogeneic BMT for primary resistant AML demonstrate a disease-free survival of only 10–20% at 5 years (37). The results of allogeneic BMT in patients with refractory relapse (unable to induce a remission with salvage therapy at relapse) are even worse.

4. ALLOGENEIC BMT FOR MDS

Similar to AML arising from an antecedent MDS, intensive chemotherapy and autologous BMT play limited roles in the treatment of MDS. Complete responses are seen in up to 50% of patients with intensive chemotherapy, but cures are rarely, if ever, seen, and it is not even clear that survival is extended *(38,39)*. Reports of successful treatment of MDS by intensive chemotherapy can probably be explained by the inclusion of "oligoblastic" or "smoldering" AML as MDS *(40)*; although these patients met FAB criteria for MDS by having low blast counts, many had normal or favorable (i.e., t(8:21)) cytogenetics as well as limited phenotypic dysplasia. It is now clear that such patients have low blast count *de novo* AML, rather than MDS, with a behavior and prognosis similar to usual AML *(40–42)*.

The success of allogeneic BMT in MDS is largely dependent on the stage of the disease at the time of transplantation. Sierra et al. published detailed data on 452 recipients of HLA-identical sibling transplants for MDS reported to the International Bone Marrow Transplant Registry from 1989 to 1997 *(43)*. Sixty percent had refractory anemia with excess blasts (136 patients) or with excess blasts in transformation (136 patients—these patients are now classified as AML by World Health Organization criteria). Conditioning regimens included total body irradiation in 44% of the cases, and the marrow grafts were T-cell depleted in 13%. The cumulative incidence of grades II–IV acute and chronic GVHD was 36%. Three-year transplantation-related mortality, relapse, disease-free survival, and overall survival rates were 37, 23, 40, and 42%, respectively. Multivariate analyses showed that young age and platelet counts higher than $100 \times 10^9/L$ at transplantation were associated with lower transplant-related mortality and higher disease-free and overall survival rates. Relapse incidence was higher in patients with high percentages of blasts in the, with high International Prognostic Scoring System scores at diagnosis, and with T-cell-depleted transplants. Importantly, this was a very young group of MDS patients, with a median age of 38.

De Witte et al. reported an analysis of 1378 autologous, related, and unrelated allogeneic transplants for MDS reported to the European Group for Blood and Marrow Transplantation *(44)*. The estimated disease-free survival and estimated relapse risk at 3 years were both 36% for 885 patients transplanted from matched siblings. In the multivariate analysis, age and stage of disease had independent prognostic significance for disease-free survival, survival, and treatment-related mortality. The estimated disease-free survival at 3 years was 25% for the 198 patients with matched unrelated donors, 28% for the 91 patients with mismatched family donors, and 33% for the 126 patients autografted in first complete remission. The nonrelapse mortality was 58% for patients with unrelated donors, 66% for patients with nonidentical family donors, and 25% for autografted patients. The relapse rate was 18% was for patients with mismatched family donors, 41% for patients with unrelated donors, and 55% for patients treated with autologous BMT.

The Seattle group reported their experience in the 251 MDS patients (median age 38) transplanted from 1981 to 1996 *(45)*. The overall disease-free survival rate was 40%, with an 18% relapse rate. The 5-year disease-free survival was 60, 36, and 28% for low- and intermediate-1 risk, intermediate-2 risk, and high-risk patients, respectively. Factors that increased transplant-related mortality in a multivariate analysis were older age, increasing disease duration, mismatched donors, male gender, and therapy-related MDS. Increasing disease duration, morphology, and cytogenetics predicted relapse. Increasing age, disease morphology, and cytogenetics were significant in determining disease-free survival.

Determining the optimal timing for BMT in these patients is a challenge. Cutler et al. examined the timing of BMT in newly diagnosed MDS patients *(46)*. For low and intermediate-1 International Prognostic Scoring System groups, delayed transplantation maximized overall survival. However, transplantation prior to leukemic evolution was associated with a greater number of life years than transplantation at the time of leukemic progression. In a cohort of patients under the age of 40 years, an even more marked survival advantage for delayed transplantation was noted. For intermediate-2 and high International Prognostic Scoring System groups, transplantation at diagnosis maximized overall survival.

5. REDUCED INTENSITY CONDITIONING

Allogeneic BMT is associated with high treatment-related mortality, especially in older patients. The use of reduced-intensity conditioning can decrease the early transplant-related toxicity, which should be of particular benefit to older and debilitated patients *(47)*. Ruiz-Argüelles et al. published a prospective study of allogeneic BMT with reduced intensity conditioning in 24 patients with AML *(48)*. All patients engrafted with a median time to achieve an absolute neutrophil count over $0.5 \times 10^9/L$ of 12 days and a median time to a platelet count greater than $20 \times 10^9/L$ of 13 days. With a median follow-up of 450 days (range 33–2670), the median posttransplant overall survival has not been reached, and both overall and progression-free survival are 66%. In 14 patients, GVHD complicated the posttransplant recovery. Grade I–II GVHD occurred in 12 patients, and fatal grade IV developed in 2 patients. Forty-seven percent of patients had limited chronic GVHD. The transplant-related mortality was 8%, and in 22 cases the procedure was completed fully on an outpatient basis. The median age of patients in this report was 35.

Giralt et al. reported 15 patients (13 with acute myeloid leukemia and 2 with MDS) treated with reduced intensity conditioning *(49)*. All patients had an HLA-identical or one-antigen-mismatched related donor, and the median age was 59 years. Twelve patients were either refractory to therapy or beyond first relapse. The conditioning regimens included purine analogs in the majority of patients. Treatment was well tolerated. Eight patients achieved complete remissions that lasted a median of 60 days. Grade II or higher acute GVHD occurred in 3 patients. Chimerism analysis of bone marrow cells in patients achieving remission showed >90% donor cells between 14 and 30 days after BMT, and 3 of 4 patients remaining in remission beyond 60 and 90 days maintained >80% donor cells.

Although the follow-up is short in these studies, the results appear promising, especially in patients transplanted in complete remission.

6. SOURCE OF THE GRAFT

Perhaps few issues are as controversial as what constitutes the optimal graft source, peripheral blood vs bone marrow, for allogeneic transplantation *(50–52)*. Peripheral blood offers a faster rate of engraftment and possibly more potent graft-vs-leukemia activity. Conversely, GVHD may also be higher with peripheral blood. Of the eight published randomized trials comparing peripheral blood and bone marrow allografts (involving multiple malignancies) *(53–61)*, only one reported a statistically significant increase in grades II–IV acute GVHD with the use of peripheral blood (52 vs 39%) *(59)*. However, most studies have found an increase in chronic GVHD with peripheral blood. The meta-analysis published by Cutler et al. found that both acute and chronic GVHD were more common after peripheral blood than after bone marrow *(51)*. Nevertheless, most studies have shown little difference in day 100 transplant-related mortality, disease-free survival, and relapse rates *(59)*. The advantages (faster engraftment and enhanced graft-vs-leukemia) and disadvantages (more chronic GVHD) of peripheral blood may ultimately lead to its being used in certain subsets of patients. A recent International Bone Marrow Transplant Registry analysis shows higher mortality in children after peripheral blood *(52)*. Patients transplanted in first remission may do better with bone marrow *(62)*, whereas patients with more advanced AML at the time of BMT may benefit from peripheral blood *(63,64)*.

Because the majority of patients will not have HLA-identical siblings, alternative donors are becoming increasingly studied, especially in patients beyond first remission where autologous BMT and nontransplant approaches have had limited activity. The Seattle group has reported an approx 30% disease-free survival after unrelated BMT in second-remission AML *(65)*. In cases without either a matched sibling or an unrelated donor, haploidentical grafts are an option because almost everybody will have a donor *(66–68)*. As in unrelated BMT, GVHD is a limiting factor. In animal models of haploidentical BMT, a high dose of cyclophosphamide post-BMT selectively eliminates host-vs-graft and graft-vs-host reactive T cells, thereby preventing graft rejection and reducing GVHD *(69,70)*. To test the activity of post-BMT cyclophosphamide (one or two doses), 56 patients (median age 48 years) with advanced hematological malignancies (18 with AML and 8 with MDS) received cyclophosphamide 50 mg/kg iv either once (on day 3, 20 patients) or twice (on days 3 and 4, 36 patients) after nonmyeloablative conditioning and haploidentical BMT at Johns Hopkins *(66)*. All were conditioned as outpatients with fludarabine, cyclophosphamide, and total body irradiation, transplanted with non-T-cell-depleted marrow, and treated with growth factors, tacrolimus, and mycophenolate mofetil beginning the day after the last dose of cyclophosphamide. Compared to patients receiving a single dose of post-BMT cyclophosphamide, those receiving two doses had significantly less grade II–IV (43% vs 78%; $p = 0.01$) and grade III–IV acute GVHD (20% vs 53%; $p = 0.006$) by day 200 after BMT. Death from GVHD occurred in 5 of 13 assessable patients receiving one dose vs 2 of 28 assessable patients receiving two doses of post-BMT cyclophosphamide. At a median follow-up of 172 days (range 32–1440 days), 21 patients remained alive without disease progression. The toxicity profile of this novel approach, including GVHD, compares favorably to matched sibling BMT.

Umbilical cord blood has also been a source of stem cells, especially because of cell yield, in children and young adults. Because children tolerate mismatches better than adults, interpretation of risk in this group is difficult. It seems that the rate of acute GVHD is lower with this approach, but no randomized studies exist to clarify this issue *(71–73)*.

7. GVHD

A detailed discussion on acute and chronic GVHD is beyond the scope of this chapter, and these entities have been recently reviewed *(74–77)*. However, it is important to review some basic aspects related to these complications. Many factors can play a role in the risk developing GVHD. HLA matching is the greatest determinant of risk for the development of GVHD. The incidence of acute GVHD increases with the level of HLA mismatch *(78–80)*. Utilizing DNA testing, it is known that mismatch in HLA-A, -B, -C, or -DRB1 increases the risk of GVHD and has a negative effect on survival *(81–85)*, and HLA-DRB1 has been associated with an increase in severe acute GVHD *(86)*. However, the mismatch causes not just increased acute GVHD, but also higher rates of other transplant-related toxicities. Donor and host factors other than HLA type, such as minor histocompatibility antigens, cytokine polymorphisms, or KIR typing, also play important roles. Age of the recipient is also very important: the older the patient is, the higher the risk of developing the disease *(87,88)*. Donor parity and sex mismatch and cytomegalovirus positivity have also been associated with an increased risk of acute GVHD and decreased survival in some but not all studies *(89–93)*. The use of higher doses of total body irradiation have been associated with the development of acute GVHD *(94)*.

Prophylaxis of GVHD is more effective than therapy of active GVHD. In high-risk malignancies, avoidance of GVHD prophylaxis to favor a graft-vs-leukemia effect has been tested. However, the results have been poor, suggesting that even patients with high-risk disease need to receive some form of prophylaxis to lessen the side effects of GVHD *(95,96)*. Removing T-cells from the graft may be the most effective means to reduce the incidence of GVHD *(97,98)*. However, most studies have consistently shown higher rates of relapse, graft failure, and infections after T-cell depletion *(99–101)*. Whether the decrease in GVHD associated with T-cell depletion counterbalances the increase in relapse rate and graft failure is unclear, but excellent results have been reported with T-cell depletion, especially first remission *(102,103)*.

The backbone for the therapy of GVHD is the use of steroids *(104–106)*. Steroids have multiple mechanisms that theoretically can explain their effectiveness, including their ability to kill lymphocytes and inhibit the release of inflammatory cytokines. Because of the availability of an intravenous formulation, methylprednisolone is commonly used as first-line agent, usually at a dose of 2 mg/kg/day *(107)*. Once therapy has been started, a rapid taper is often enough to control disease while minimizing side effects *(108)*. Once steroids are given, it is expected that 20–70% of patients will respond and 20–40% will have durable responses. Other immunosuppressive therapies, including tumor necrosis factor blockade, mycophenolate mofetil, and photopheresis, have either not been found to be better than steroids alone or have not been compared directly to steroid therapy in large, randomized trials *(109–112)*.

If a patient fails to respond to steroids, the prognosis is often poor, not only from the GVHD itself, but also from opportunistic infections *(104,113)*. For steroid-refractory acute GVHD, ATG, sirolimus, visilizumab, infliximab alemtuzumab, daclizumab, denileukin diftitox, mycophenolate mofetil, and pentostatin have all been used, but no therapy can be considered a standard of care *(106,113–121)*.

8. CONCLUSIONS

Without question, BMT is an effective treatment for patients with AML and MDS. Strategies to decrease toxicities, especially better antibiotics and supportive care, have improved the results over time. It is expected that the use of "alternative" donor sources (e.g., haploidentical family members and umbilical cord cells) will expand the use of this curative approach to patients who otherwise would not be candidates for the procedure.

REFERENCES

1. Mathé G, Jammet H, Pendic B, et al. Transfusions et greffes de moelle osseuse homologue chez des humains irradiés a haute dose accidentellement. Rev Franç Études Clin Biol 1959;4(3):226–238.
2. Thomas ED, Lochte HL, Jr., Lu WC, Ferrebee JW. Intravenous infusion of bone marrow in patients receiving radiation and chemotherapy. N Engl J Med 1957;257(11):491–496.
3. Santos GW, Sensenbrenner LL, Burke PJ, et al. Marrow transplanation in man following cyclophosphamide. Transplant Proc 1971;3(1):400–404.

4. Graw RG, Jr., Santos GW. Bone marrow transplantation in patients with leukemia. Incidence and severity of graft-vs-host disease in successful HL-A-matched transplants. Transplantation 1971;11(2): 197–199.

5. Thomas ED, Buckner CD, Rudolph RH, et al. Allogeneic marrow grafting for hematologic malignancy using HL-A matched donor-recipient sibling pairs. Blood 1971;38(3):267–287.

6. Thomas ED, Buckner CD, Clift RA, et al. Marrow transplantation for acute nonlymphoblastic leukemia in first remission. N Engl J Med 1979;301(11):597–599.

7. Santos GW, Burke PJ, Sensenbrenner LL, Owens AH. Bone marrow transplantation in an adult with acute leukemia. Cancer Chemother Rep Part 1 1969;53(1):93.

8. Cassileth PA, Harrington DP, Hines JD, et al. Maintenance chemotherapy prolongs remission duration in adult acute nonlymphocytic leukemia. J Clin Oncol 1988;6(4):583–587.

9. Vaughan WP, Karp JE, Burke PJ. Two-cycle timed-sequential chemotherapy for adult acute nonlymphocytic leukemia. Blood 1984;64(5):975–980.

10. Mayer RJ, Davis RB, Schiffer CA, et al. Intensive postremission chemotherapy in adults with acute myeloid leukemia. Cancer and Leukemia Group B. N Engl J Med 1994;331(14):896–903.

11. Bolaños-Meade J, Karp JE, Guo CF, et al. Timed sequential therapy of acute myelogenous leukemia in adults: a phase II study of retinoids in combination with the sequential administration of cytosine arabinoside, idarubicin and etoposide. Leukemia Research 2003;27(4):313–321.

12. Bolaños-Meade J, Guo C, Gojo I, Karp JE. A phase II study of timed sequential therapy of acute myelogenous leukemia (AML) for patients over the age of 60: two cycle timed sequential therapy with topotecan, ara-C and mitoxantrone in adults with poor-risk AML. Leuk Res 2004;28(6):571–577.

13. Castaigne S, Chevret S, Archimbaud E, et al. Randomized comparison of double induction and timed-sequential induction to a "3 + 7" induction in adults with AML: long-term analysis of the Acute Leukemia French Association (ALFA) 9000 study. Blood 2004;104(8):2467–2474.

14. Byrd JC, Mrozek K, Dodge RK, et al. Pretreatment cytogenetic abnormalities are predictive of induction success, cumulative incidence of relapse, and overall survival in adult patients with de novo acute myeloid leukemia: results from Cancer and Leukemia Group B (CALGB 8461). Blood 2002;100(13): 4325–4336.

15. Farag SS, Ruppert AS, Mrozek K, et al. Outcome of induction and postremission therapy in younger adults with acute myeloid leukemia with normal karyotype: a cancer and leukemia group B study. J Clin Oncol 2005;23(3):482–493.

16. Farag SS, Archer KJ, Mrozek K, et al. Isolated trisomy of chromosomes 8, 11, 13 and 21 is an adverse prognostic factor in adults with de novo acute myeloid leukemia: results from Cancer and Leukemia Group B 8461. Int J Oncol 2002;21(5):1041–1051.

17. Marcucci G, Mrozek K, Ruppert AS, et al. Abnormal cytogenetics at date of morphologic complete remission predicts short overall and disease-free survival, and higher relapse rate in adult acute myeloid leukemia: results from cancer and leukemia group B study 8461. J Clin Oncol 2004;22(12):2410–2418.

18. Swirsky DM, de Bastos M, Parish SE, Rees JK, Hayhoe FG. Features affecting outcome during remission induction of acute myeloid leukaemia in 619 adult patients. Br J Haematol 1986;64(3):435–453.

19. Craddock C, Tauro S, Moss P, Grimwade D. Biology and management of relapsed acute myeloid leukaemia. Br J Haematol 2005;129(1):18–34.

20. Keung YK, Cobos E, Bolaños-Meade J, Issarachai S, Brideau A, Morgan D. Evans syndrome after autologous bone marrow transplant for recurrent Hodgkin's disease. Bone Marrow Transplant 1997;20(12): 1099–1101.

21. Grimwade D, Walker H, Oliver F, et al. The importance of diagnostic cytogenetics on outcome in AML: analysis of 1,612 patients entered into the MRC AML 10 trial. The Medical Research Council Adult and Children's Leukaemia Working Parties. Blood 1998;92(7):2322–2333.

22. Wheatley K, Burnett AK, Goldstone AH, et al. A simple, robust, validated and highly predictive index for the determination of risk-directed therapy in acute myeloid leukaemia derived from the MRC AML 10 trial. United Kingdom Medical Research Council's Adult and Childhood Leukaemia Working Parties. Br J Haematol 1999;107(1):69–79.

23. Breems DA, van Putten WL, Huijgens PC, et al. Prognostic index for adult patients with acute myeloid leukemia in first relapse. J Clin Oncol 2005;23(9):1969–1978.

24. Reiffers J, Gaspard MH, Maraninchi D, et al. Comparison of allogeneic or autologous bone marrow transplantation and chemotherapy in patients with acute myeloid leukaemia in first remission: a prospective controlled trial. Br J Haematol 1989;72(1):57–63.

25. Reiffers J, Stoppa AM, Attal M, et al. Allogeneic vs autologous stem cell transplantation vs chemotherapy in patients with acute myeloid leukemia in first remission: the BGMT 87 study. Leukemia 1996;10(12): 1874–1882.

26. Cassileth PA, Harrington DP, Appelbaum FR, et al. Chemotherapy compared with autologous or allogeneic bone marrow transplantation in the management of acute myeloid leukemia in first remission. N Engl J Med 1998;339(23):1649–1656.

27. Zittoun RA, Mandelli F, Willemze R, et al. Autologous or allogeneic bone marrow transplantation compared with intensive chemotherapy in acute myelogenous leukemia. European Organization for Research and Treatment of Cancer (EORTC) and the Gruppo Italiano Malattie Ematologiche Maligne dell'Adulto (GIMEMA) Leukemia Cooperative Groups. N Engl J Med 1995;332(4):217–223.

28. Harousseau JL, Cahn JY, Pignon B, et al. Comparison of autologous bone marrow transplantation and intensive chemotherapy as postremission therapy in adult acute myeloid leukemia. The Groupe Ouest Est Leucemies Aigues Myeloblastiques (GOELAM). Blood 1997;90(8):2978–2986.

29. Burnett AK, Goldstone AH, Stevens RM, et al. Randomised comparison of addition of autologous bone-marrow transplantation to intensive chemotherapy for acute myeloid leukaemia in first remission: results of MRC AML 10 trial. UK Medical Research Council Adult and Children's Leukaemia Working Parties. Lancet 1998;351(9104):700–708.

30. Slovak ML, Kopecky KJ, Cassileth PA, et al. Karyotypic analysis predicts outcome of preremission and postremission therapy in adult acute myeloid leukemia: a Southwest Oncology Group/Eastern Cooperative Oncology Group Study. Blood 2000;96(13):4075–4083.

31. Nathan PC, Sung L, Crump M, Beyene J. Consolidation therapy with autologous bone marrow transplantation in adults with acute myeloid leukemia: a meta-analysis. J Natl Cancer Inst 2004;96(1):38–45.

32. Gale RP, Horowitz MM, Rees JK, et al. Chemotherapy vs transplants for acute myelogenous leukemia in second remission. Leukemia 1996;10(1):13–19.

33. Appelbaum FR, Clift RA, Buckner CD, et al. Allogeneic marrow transplantation for acute nonlymphoblastic leukemia after first relapse. Blood 1983;61(5):949–953.

34. Collins RH, Jr., Shpilberg O, Drobyski WR, et al. Donor leukocyte infusions in 140 patients with relapsed malignancy after allogeneic bone marrow transplantation. J Clin Oncol 1997;15(2):433–444.

35. Porter DL, Collins RH, Jr., Hardy C, et al. Treatment of relapsed leukemia after unrelated donor marrow transplantation with unrelated donor leukocyte infusions. Blood 2000;95(4):1214–1221.

36. Fung HC, Stein A, Slovak M, et al. A long-term follow-up report on allogeneic stem cell transplantation for patients with primary refractory acute myelogenous leukemia: impact of cytogenetic characteristics on transplantation outcome. Biol Blood Marrow Transplant 2003;9(12):766–771.

37. Song KW, Lipton J. Is it appropriate to offer allogeneic hematopoietic stem cell transplantation to patients with primary refractory acute myeloid leukemia? Bone Marrow Transplant, in press.

38. Beran M. Intensive chemotherapy for patients with high-risk myelodysplastic syndrome. Int J Hematol 2000;72(2):139–150.

39. Kurzrock R. Myelodysplastic syndrome overview. Semin Hematol 2002;39(3):18–25.

40. Bernstein SH, Brunette VL, Davey FR, et al. Acute myeloid leukemia-type chemotherapy for newly diagnosed patients without antecedent cytopenias having myelodysplastic syndrome as defined by French-American-British criteria: a cancer and leukemia group B study. J Clin Oncol 1996;14(9):2486–2494.

41. Xue YQ, Yu F, Zhou ZG, Guo Y, Xie X, Lin BJ. Translocation-(8,21) in oligoblastic leukemia—is this a true myelodysplastic syndrome? Leukemia Res 1994;18(10):761–765.

42. Chan GCF, Wang WC, Raimondi SC, et al. Myelodysplastic syndrome in children: differentiation from acute myeloid leukemia with a low blast count. Leukemia 1997;11(2):206–211.

43. Sierra J, Perez WS, Rozman C, et al. Bone marrow transplantation from HLA-identical siblings as treatment for myelodysplasia. Blood 2002;100(6):1997–2004.

44. de Witte T, Hermans J, Vossen J, et al. Haematopoietic stem cell transplantation for patients with myelodysplastic syndromes and secondary acute myeloid leukaemias: a report on behalf of the Chronic Leukaemia Working Party of the European Group for Blood and Marrow Transplantation (EBMT). Br J Haematol 2000;110(3):620–630.

45. Appelbaum FR, Anderson J. Allogeneic bone marrow transplantation for myelodysplastic syndrome: Outcomes analysis according to IPSS score. Leukemia 1998;12:S25–S29.

46. Cutler CS, Lee SJ, Greenberg P, et al. A decision analysis of allogeneic bone marrow transplantation for the myelodysplastic syndromes: delayed transplantation for low-risk myelodysplasia is associated with improved outcome. Blood 2004;104(2):579–585.

47. Jacobsohn DA, Duerst R, Tse W, Kletzel M. Reduced intensity haemopoietic stem-cell transplantation for treatment of non-malignant diseases in children. Lancet 2004;364(9429):156–162.
48. Ruiz-Argüelles GJ, Gómez-Almaguer D, Gómez-Rangel J, et al. Allogeneic hematopoietic stem cell transplantation with non-myeloablative conditioning in patients with acute myelogenous leukemia eligible for conventional allografting: a prospective study. Leuk Lymphoma 2004;45(6):1191–1195.
49. Giralt S, Estey E, Albitar M, et al. Engraftment of allogeneic hematopoietic progenitor cells with purine analog-containing chemotherapy: harnessing graft-vs-leukemia without myeloablative therapy. Blood 1997;89(12):4531–4536.
50. Arai S, Klingemann HG. Hematopoietic stem cell transplantation: bone marrow vs mobilized peripheral blood. Arch Med Res 2003;34(6):545–553.
51. Cutler C, Giri S, Jeyapalan S, Paniagua D, Viswanathan A, Antin JH. Acute and chronic graft-vs-host disease after allogeneic peripheral-blood stem-cell and bone marrow transplantation: a meta-analysis. J Clin Oncol 2001;19(16):3685–3691.
52. Eapen M, Horowitz MM, Klein JP, et al. Higher mortality after allogeneic peripheral-blood transplantation compared with bone marrow in children and adolescents: the histocompatibility and alternate stem cell source working committee of the international bone marrow transplant registry. J Clin Oncol 2004;22(24):4872–4880.
53. Vigorito AC, Azevedo WM, Marques JF, et al. A randomised, prospective comparison of allogeneic bone marrow and peripheral blood progenitor cell transplantation in the treatment of haematological malignancies. Bone Marrow Transplant 1998;22(12):1145–1151.
54. Mahmoud H, Fahmy O, Kamel A, Kamel M, El Haddad A, El Kadi D. Peripheral blood vs bone marrow as a source for allogeneic hematopoietic stem cell transplantation. Bone Marrow Transplant 1999;24(4):355–358.
55. Blaise D, Kuentz M, Fortanier C, et al. Randomized trial of bone marrow vs lenograstim-primed blood cell allogeneic transplantation in patients with early-stage leukemia: a report from the Societe Francaise de Greffe de Moelle. J Clin Oncol 2000;18(3):537–546.
56. Heldal D, Tjonnfjord G, Brinch L, et al. A randomised study of allogeneic transplantation with stem cells from blood or bone marrow. Bone Marrow Transplant 2000;25(11):1129–1136.
57. Powles R, Mehta J, Kulkarni S, et al. Allogeneic blood and bone-marrow stem-cell transplantation in haematological malignant diseases: a randomised trial. Lancet 2000;355(9211):1231–1237.
58. Bensinger WI, Martin PJ, Storer B, et al. Transplantation of bone marrow as compared with peripheral-blood cells from HLA-identical relatives in patients with hematologic cancers. N Engl J Med 2001;344(3):175–181.
59. Schmitz N, Beksac M, Hasenclever D, et al. Transplantation of mobilized peripheral blood cells to HLA-identical siblings with standard-risk leukemia. Blood 2002;100(3):761–767.
60. Couban S, Simpson DR, Barnett MJ, et al. A randomized multicenter comparison of bone marrow and peripheral blood in recipients of matched sibling allogeneic transplants for myeloid malignancies. Blood 2002;100(5):1525–1531.
61. Schmitz N, Beksac M, Bacigalupo A, et al. Filgrastim-mobilized peripheral blood progenitor cells vs bone marrow transplantation for treating leukemia: 3-year results from the EBMT randomized trial. Haematologica 2005;90(5):643–648.
62. Gorin NC, Labopin M, Rocha V, et al. Marrow vs peripheral blood for geno-identical allogeneic stem cell transplantation in acute myelocytic leukemia: influence of dose and stem cell source shows better outcome with rich marrow. Blood 2003;102(8):3043–3051.
63. Champlin RE, Schmitz N, Horowitz MM, et al. Blood stem cells compared with bone marrow as a source of hematopoietic cells for allogeneic transplantation. IBMTR Histocompatibility and Stem Cell Sources Working Committee and the European Group for Blood and Marrow Transplantation (EBMT). Blood 2000;95(12):3702–3709.
64. Horan JT, Liesveld JL, Fernandez ID, et al. Survival after HLA-identical allogeneic peripheral blood stem cell and bone marrow transplantation for hematologic malignancies: meta-analysis of randomized controlled trials. Bone Marrow Transplant 2003;32(3):293–298.
65. Sierra J, Storer B, Hansen JA, et al. Unrelated donor marrow transplantation for acute myeloid leukemia: an update of the Seattle experience. Bone Marrow Transplant 2000;26(4):397–404.
66. Fuchs EJ, Luznik L, Chen AR, et al. Post-transplantation cyclophosphamide (Cy) reduces graft rejection and graft-vs-host disease (GVHD) after non-myeloablative, partially HLA-mismatched (haploidentical) bone marrow transplantation (BMT). Blood 2004;104(11).

67. Aversa F, Tabilio A, Velardi A, et al. Treatment of high-risk acute leukemia with T-cell-depleted stem cells from related donors with one fully mismatched HLA haplotype. N Engl J Med 1998;339(17):1186–1193.

68. Ortin M, Raj R, Kinning E, Williams M, Darbyshire PJ. Partially matched related donor peripheral blood progenitor cell transplantation in paediatric patients adding fludarabine and anti-lymphocyte gamma-globulin. Bone Marrow Transplant 2002;30(6):359–366.

69. Luznik L, Jalla S, Engstrom LW, Iannone R, Fuchs EJ. Durable engraftment of major histocompatibility complex-incompatible cells after nonmyeloablative conditioning with fludarabine, low-dose total body irradiation, and posttransplantation cyclophosphamide. Blood 2001;98(12):3456–3464.

70. Luznik L, Engstrom LW, Iannone R, Fuchs EJ. Posttransplantation cyclophosphamide facilitates engraftment of major histocompatibility complex-identical allogeneic marrow in mice conditioned with low-dose total body irradiation. Biol Blood Marrow Transplant 2002;8(3):131–138.

71. Kurtzberg J, Laughlin M, Graham ML, et al. Placental blood as a source of hematopoietic stem cells for transplantation into unrelated recipients. N Engl J Med 1996;335(3):157–166.

72. Laughlin MJ, Barker J, Bambach B, et al. Hematopoietic engraftment and survival in adult recipients of umbilical-cord blood from unrelated donors. N Engl J Med 2001;344(24):1815–1822.

73. Thomson BG, Robertson KA, Gowan D, et al. Analysis of engraftment, graft-vs-host disease, and immune recovery following unrelated donor cord blood transplantation. Blood 2000;96(8):2703–2711.

74. Higman MA, Vogelsang GB. Chronic graft vs host disease. Br J Haematol 2004;125(4):435–454.

75. Vogelsang GB. How I treat chronic graft-vs-host disease. Blood 2001;97(5):1196–1201.

76. Bolaños-Meade J, Vogelsang GB. Novel strategies for steroid-refractory acute graft-vs-host disease. Curr Opin Hematol 2005;12(1):40–44.

77. Bolaños-Meade J, Vogelsang GB. Acute graft-vs-host disease. Clin Adv Hematol Oncol 2004;2(10): 672–682.

78. Beatty PG, Clift RA, Mickelson EM, et al. Marrow transplantation from related donors other than HLA-identical siblings. N Engl J Med 1985;313(13):765–771.

79. Kernan NA, Bartsch G, Ash RC, et al. Analysis of 462 transplantations from unrelated donors facilitated by the National Marrow Donor Program. N Engl J Med 1993;328(9):593–602.

80. Szydlo R, Goldman JM, Klein JP, et al. Results of allogeneic bone marrow transplants for leukemia using donors other than HLA-identical siblings. J Clin Oncol 1997;15(5):1767–1777.

81. Flomenberg N, Baxter-Lowe LA, Confer D, et al. Impact of HLA-class I and class II high resolution matching on outcomes of unrelated donor BMT. Blood 2001;98(11):813A.

82. Petersdorf EW, Gooley TA, Anasetti C, et al. Optimizing outcome after unrelated marrow transplantation by comprehensive matching of HLA class I and II alleles in the donor and recipient. Blood 1998;92(10): 3515–3520.

83. Petersdorf EW, Gooley T, Malkki M, et al. The biological significance of HLA-DP gene variation in haematopoietic cell transplantation. Br J Haematol 2001;112(4):988–994.

84. Petersdorf EW, Hansen JA, Martin PJ, et al. Major-histocompatibility-complex class I alleles and antigens in hematopoietic-cell transplantation. N Engl J Med 2001;345(25):1794–1800.

85. Sasazuki T, Juji T, Morishima Y, et al. Effect of matching of class I HLA alleles on clinical outcome after transplantation of hematopoietic stem cells from an unrelated donor. Japan Marrow Donor Program. N Engl J Med 1998;339(17):1177–1185.

86. Petersdorf EW, Kollman C, Hurley CK, et al. Effect of HLA class II gene disparity on clinical outcome in unrelated donor hematopoietic cell transplantation for chronic myeloid leukemia: the US National Marrow Donor Program Experience. Blood 2001;98(10):2922–2929.

87. Sullivan KM, Storb R, Buckner CD, et al. Graft-vs-host disease as adoptive immunotherapy in patients with advanced hematologic neoplasms. N Engl J Med 1989;320(13):828–834.

88. Klingemann HG, Storb R, Fefer A, et al. Bone marrow transplantation in patients aged 45 years and older. Blood 1986;67(3):770–776.

89. Flowers ME, Pepe MS, Longton G, et al. Previous donor pregnancy as a risk factor for acute graft-vs-host disease in patients with aplastic anaemia treated by allogeneic marrow transplantation. Br J Haematol 1990; 74(4):492–496.

90. Weisdorf D, Hakke R, Blazar B, et al. Risk factors for acute graft-vs-host disease in histocompatible donor bone marrow transplantation. Transplantation 1991;51(6):1197–1203.

91. Bross DS, Tutschka PJ, Farmer ER, et al. Predictive factors for acute graft-vs-host disease in patients transplanted with HLA-identical bone marrow. Blood 1984;63(6):1265–1270.

92. Nash RA, Pepe MS, Storb R, et al. Acute graft-vs-host disease: analysis of risk factors after allogeneic marrow transplantation and prophylaxis with cyclosporine and methotrexate. Blood 1992;80(7):1838–1845.

93. Larsson K, Aschan J, Remberger M, Ringden O, Winiarski J, Ljungman P. Reduced risk for extensive chronic graft-vs-host disease in patients receiving transplants with human leukocyte antigen-identical sibling donors given polymerase chain reaction-based preemptive therapy against cytomegalovirus. Transplantation 2004;77(4):526–531.

94. Clift RA, Buckner CD, Appelbaum FR, et al. Allogeneic marrow transplantation in patients with acute myeloid leukemia in first remission: a randomized trial of two irradiation regimens. Blood 1990;76(9): 1867–1871.

95. Fassas AB, Morris C, Badros A, Van Rhee F, Tricot G. Separating graft-vs-tumor from graft-vs-host reactions. Leuk Lymphoma 2002;43(4):725–733.

96. Fassas AB, Rapoport AP, Cottler-Fox M, Chen T, Tricot G. Encouraging preliminary results in 12 patients with high-risk haematological malignancies by omitting graft-vs-host disease prophylaxis after allogeneic transplantation. Br J Haematol 2000;111(2):662–667.

97. Przepiorka D, Huh YO, Khouri I, et al. Graft failure and graft-vs-host disease after subtotal T-cell-depleted marrow transplantation: correlations with marrow hematopoietic and lymphoid subsets. Prog Clin Biol Res 1994;389:557–563.

98. Ho VT, Soiffer RJ. The history and future of T-cell depletion as graft-vs-host disease prophylaxis for allogeneic hematopoietic stem cell transplantation. Blood 2001;98(12):3192–3204.

99. Marmont AM, Horowitz MM, Gale RP, et al. T-cell depletion of HLA-identical transplants in leukemia. Blood 1991;78(8):2120–2130.

100. Goldman JM, Gale RP, Horowitz MM, et al. Bone marrow transplantation for chronic myelogenous leukemia in chronic phase. Increased risk for relapse associated with T-cell depletion. Ann Intern Med 1988;108(6):806–814.

101. Martin PJ, Hansen JA, Buckner CD, et al. Effects of in vitro depletion of T cells in HLA-identical allogeneic marrow grafts. Blood 1985;66(3):664–672.

102. Soiffer RJ, Fairclough D, Robertson M, et al. CD6-depleted allogeneic bone marrow transplantation for acute leukemia in first complete remission. Blood 1997;89(8):3039–3047.

103. Papadopoulos EB, Carabasi MH, Castro-Malaspina H, et al. T-cell-depleted allogeneic bone marrow transplantation as postremission therapy for acute myelogenous leukemia: freedom from relapse in the absence of graft-vs-host disease. Blood 1998;91(3):1083–1090.

104. Martin PJ, Schoch G, Fisher L, et al. A retrospective analysis of therapy for acute graft-vs-host disease: secondary treatment. Blood 1991;77(8):1821–1828.

105. Martin PJ, Schoch G, Fisher L, et al. A retrospective analysis of therapy for acute graft-vs-host disease: initial treatment. Blood 1990;76(8):1464–1472.

106. Weisdorf D, Haake R, Blazar B, et al. Treatment of moderate/severe acute graft-vs-host disease after allogeneic bone marrow transplantation: an analysis of clinical risk features and outcome. Blood 1990;75(4): 1024–1030.

107. Van Lint MT, Uderzo C, Locasciulli A, et al. Early treatment of acute graft-vs-host disease with high- or low-dose 6-methylprednisolone: a multicenter randomized trial from the Italian Group for Bone Marrow Transplantation. Blood 1998;92(7):2288–2293.

108. Hings IM, Filipovich AH, Miller WJ, et al. Prednisone therapy for acute graft-vs-host disease: short- vs long-term treatment. A prospective randomized trial. Transplantation 1993;56(3):577–580.

109. Uberti JP, Ayash L, Levine JE, et al. Phase I/II trial on the use of etanercept (Enbrel (R)) and solumedrol as primary treatment for acute graft-vs-host disease (aGVHD). Blood 2003;102(11):243A.

110. Greinix HT, Volc-Platzer B, Rabitsch W, et al. Successful use of extracorporeal photochemotherapy in the treatment of severe acute and chronic graft-vs-host disease. Blood 1998;92(9):3098–3104.

111. Ilhan O, Celebi H, Arat M, et al. Treatment of acute and chronic graft vs host disease with mycophenolate mofetil. Blood 1999;94:368B.

112. Le Blanc K, Rasmusson I, Sundberg B, et al. Treatment of severe acute graft-vs-host disease with third party haploidentical mesenchymal stem cells. Lancet 2004;363(9419):1439–1441.

113. Arai S, Margolis J, Zahurak M, Anders V, Vogelsang GB. Poor outcome in steroid-refractory graft-vs-host disease with antithymocyte globulin treatment. Biol Blood Marrow Transplant 2002;8(3):155–160.

114. Jacobsohn DA, Hallick J, Anders V, McMillan S, Morris L, Vogelsang GB. Infliximab for steroid-refractory acute GVHD: a case series. Am J Hematol 2003;74(2):119–124.

115. Benito AI, Furlong T, Martin PJ, et al. Sirolimus (rapamycin) for the treatment of steroid-refractory acute graft-vs-host disease. Transplantation 2001;72(12):1924–1929.

116. Ho VT, Zahrieh D, Hochberg E, et al. Safety and efficacy of denileukin diftitox in patients with steroid-refractory acute graft-vs-host disease after allogeneic hematopoietic stem cell transplantation. Blood 2004; 104(4):1224–1226.

117. Przepiorka D, Kernan NA, Ippoliti C, et al. Daclizumab, a humanized anti-interleukin-2 receptor alpha chain antibody, for treatment of acute graft-vs-host disease. Blood 2000;95(1):83–89.

118. Carella AM, Beltrami G, Scalzulli PR, Carella AM, Jr., Corsetti MT. Alemtuzumab can successfully treat steroid-refractory acute graft-vs-host disease (aGVHD). Bone Marrow Transplant 2004;33(1):131–132.

119. Carpenter PA, Appelbaum FR, Corey L, et al. A humanized non-FcR-binding anti-CD3 antibody, visilizumab, for treatment of steroid-refractory acute graft-vs-host disease. Blood 2002;99(8):2712–2719.

120. Kim JG, Sohn SK, Kim DH, et al. Different efficacy of mycophenolate mofetil as salvage treatment for acute and chronic GVHD after allogeneic stem cell transplant. Eur J Haematol 2004;73(1):56–61.

121. Bolaños-Meade J, Jacobsohn DA, Margolis J, et al. Pentostatin in steroid-refractory acute graft-vs-host disease. J Clin Oncol 2005;23(12):2661–2668.

16 Tumor Vaccines in Leukemia

Ivan Borrello

CONTENTS

Summary

The goal of cancer vaccination is to elicit an active systemic immune response against antigen(s) expressed by tumor cells, with that response resulting in a therapeutically useful antitumor effect. This goal is being realized through the identification of tumor-associated antigens, the discovery of critical immunological effector cells, and a growing understanding of the complex cellular and molecular mechanisms that determine immune-based host–tumor interactions. Vaccine clinical trials in leukemias are examining diverse antigenic targets, new vaccine formulations, and a spectrum of clinical settings in which immunomodulation may be optimally conducted. The ability to integrate vaccines with other immunomodulatory strategies in earlier stages of disease, particularly in the minimal residual disease state or in combination with adoptive T-cell therapies, may optimize clinical application and overall clinical effect.

1. INTRODUCTION

Despite the recent development of a myriad of novel therapies in the treatment of leukemias, a significant number of patients afflicted with these diseases still succumb to it. As such, a measurable and sustainable antitumor effect requires treatment regimens designed to integrate non-cross-reactive therapies in the appropriate sequence and setting. Immunotherapy represents such an alternative. The clinical benefit of allogeneic transplantation in inducing and maintaining remissions in patients with myeloid leukemias coupled to the impact of donor lymphocyte infusions (DLI) *(1)* provide direct evidence of the therapeutic efficacy of T-cell immunity. In chronic myeloid leukemia (CML), DLI induces both hematological as well as cytogenetic responses in approx 75% of patients in chronic phase, whereas the response rate goes down to 33% in patients that transformed to accelerated phase or blast crisis *(2,3)*. A commonly held belief is that graft-vs-leukemia (GVL) is unattainable in the absence of graft-vs-host disease (GVHD), thus supporting the notion of a nonspecific, allogeneic T-cell response directed in large against non-tumor-specific host antigens. However, in CML the

From: *Contemporary Hematology: Acute Myelogenous Leukemia*
Edited by: J. E. Karp © Humana Press Inc., Totowa, NJ

disease response occurs in 70–90% of DLI recipients with evidence of an antitumor response even in patients not experiencing GVHD *(4)*. These data demonstrate separation of GVL from GVHD and suggest the presence of tumor-specific antigens as well as their recognition by allogeneic T-cells.

Increasing evidence suggests the presence of an intrinsic immune-mediated antitumor response. Recent data comparing tumor development in genetically immunodeficient mice vs wild-type mice clearly demonstrate the ability of the normal immune system to decrease the incidence of chemically induced as well as spontaneous tumors and to vastly alter the immunogenicity of those tumors that escape immune recognition *(5)*. Furthermore, clinical evidence to support the hypothesis of immune surveillance was described in solid malignancies where the extent of tumor infiltration by lymphocytes directly correlated with improved survival *(6,7)*. Additionally, data demonstrating a direct correlation between lymphocyte recovery following autologous stem cell transplantation and improved tumor-free survival further support the hypothesis of an endogenous, immune-mediated, tumor-specific response *(8,9)*.

Despite the evidence strongly suggesting in vivo antitumor immunity, the mere presence of detectable cancers is proof of the inability to mount clinically meaningful tumor-specific immune responses. Recent advances in our understanding of a failed antitumor immune response have shed light on various pathways of tumor escape. Such mechanisms include (1) failure to express tumor-associated antigens (TAAs) capable of being recognized by the immune system *(10)*, (2) downregulation of the expression of major histocompatibility complex (MHC) molecules on the tumor cell surface necessary for antigen presentation *(11)*, (3) insufficient expression of costimulatory molecules by the tumor capable of binding their cognate receptors on tumor-specific T-cells *(12)*, (4) overexpression of inhibitory molecules on tumor-specific T-cells *(13,14)*, (5) lack of co-localization of tumor-specific T-cells and the tumor *(15)*, and (6) a complexity of tumor–host interactions within the tumor microenvironment caused by immunosuppressive cells and cytokines.

Effective immunotherapy must, therefore, be able to both overcome or eliminate the suppressive elements within the host environment and also generate or enhance the tumor-specific response. Strategies aimed at overcoming these suppressive elements are reviewed elsewhere *(16)* and are not the subject of this discussion. In contrast, the generation or augmentation of a tumor-specific immune response can be achieved through a variety of approaches, including (1) the adoptive transfer of tumor-specific T-cells, (2) the administration of immunomodulatory cytokines, and (3) vaccination strategies aimed at generating cytotoxic effector T-cells and increasing their precursor frequency within the host.

2. LEUKEMIA VACCINES: OBJECTIVES AND STRATEGIES

A major objective of cancer vaccination is to elicit an active systemic immune response against antigen(s) expressed by tumor cells that result in a therapeutically useful antitumor effect. Studies utilizing this approach were initially reported by William Coley in the late 19th century. In these early studies, patients with advanced cancer were treated with bacterial extracts, Coley's toxin, in an attempt to activate a nonspecific systemic immune response that would hopefully impart an immune-mediated antitumor effect *(17)*. This concept was subsequently expanded by using killed tumor cells or tumor cell lysates mixed with adjuvants such as bacille Calmette-Guérin (BCG) and *Corynebacterium parvum* to augment tumor-specific immune responses *(18)*. However, the lack of clinical efficacy generated skepticism about the validity of this approach in cancer treatment. Recently, advances in the identification of tumor-associated antigens *(19,20)* coupled with the growing understanding of the cellular and molecular mechanisms regulating host–tumor interactions *(21–23)* and the discovery of immunologically relevant molecules have provided the appropriate framework for a more rationale vaccine development.

An ideal tumor vaccine should generate an active tumor-specific, systemic immune response in the cancer-bearing host capable of eradicating preexisting malignant cells and providing long-lived immunological memory that protects the vaccinated host against relapse. However, one major obstacle for the development of such a vaccine thus far has been the identification of appropriate antigen(s) to target.

2.1. Identification of Appropriate Antigen(s) to Target

Several broad categories of tumor antigens recognized by T-cells have been identified through the establishment of T-cell lines or clones from cancer-bearing patients *(24,25)*. Antigens identified in this fashion fall into the following general categories:

1. Unique tumor antigens expressed exclusively in the tumor from which they were identified.
2. Shared tumor-specific antigens expressed in many tumors but not in normal adult tissue.
3. Tissue-specific differentiation antigens expressed by the normal tissue from which the tumor arose.
4. Oncogene and tumor supressor gene products as tumor antigens.
5. Viral-associated antigens.

As with most malignancies, the relative immunogenicity of the antigens expressed by leukemic cells has yet to be defined. In addition, as described below, each category of these tumor antigens presents interesting features and challenges in the design of effective vaccine strategies.

2.1.1. Unique Tumor Antigens

Unique tumor antigens are not considered suitable targets in the formulation of generic vaccines because of their patient-restricted expression. However, if they were able to mediate major immune responses, these vaccine strategies would be highly effective *(26)*. A common finding in leukemia is the presence of chromosomal translocations that result in the generation of fusion genes encoding chimeric proteins. The joining region of these chimeric proteins represent true tumor-specific antigens and are, therefore, appealing targets for immunotherapy *(27)*. Furthermore, for certain gene products, tumor escape through antigen loss in response to selective immunological pressure may not occur if the fusion protein is required for transformation. The chimeric protein bcr/abl resulting from a t(9;22) chromosomal translocation in patients with CML represents by far the best example in this category of unique tumor antigens. Indeed, bcr/abl is tumor-specific, essential for the malignant transformation, and displays a limited variability with only two breakpoints *(28)*. As a potential target for immunotherapy, the cytoplasmic location of this chimeric protein and the lack of evidence that protease cleavage can generate candidate antigenic peptides for effective presentation to T-cells had initially diminished enthusiasm towards bcr/abl as a suitable target for vaccination *(29)*. Recently however, Clark et al. provided direct proof that human CML cells can process and present HLA-associated immunogenic peptides derived from the bcr/abl fusion protein. Furthermore, these peptides were recognized by antigen-specific cytotoxic T-cells resulting in the destruction of autologous leukemic cells *(30)*. These findings, together with the results of a recently completed clinical trial in patients with CML showing that vaccination with bcr-abl breakpoint fusion peptides led to peptide-specific T-cell-mediated immune responses has revived the interest in vaccine strategies targeting unique tumor antigens *(28)*. Additional putative unique tumor antigens in leukemia include the DEK-CAN fusion peptide derived from t(6;9) in patients with AML *(31)* as well as the products of the AML/ETO or the PML-RARα gene rearrangement *(32,33)*.

2.1.2. SHARED TUMOR ANTIGENS

These antigens are commonly present on various samples of the same histological subtype of malignancy and on different tumor types, but not in normal tissues except for testis and placenta. Because they are not patient-restricted, shared tumor antigens represent prime candidates for the development of broadly applicable vaccine formulations *(34)*. Although the cancer testis antigens (i.e., MAGE, BAGE) were initially identified in the early 1990s in patients with solid malignancies (especially patients with melanoma) *(35,36)*, the presence of these shared tumor antigens in AML samples in hematological tumors have been recently documented. PRAME (preferentially expressed antigen of melanoma), another cancer testis antigen, is selectively expressed in 47% of AML patients but not in healthy volunteers *(37)*.

2.1.3. OVEREXPRESSED TUMOR ANTIGENS

Although not truly tumor specific, proteinase 3 and Wilms' tumor gene-encoded transcription factor-1 (WT1) are markedly overexpressed in various myeloid leukemias. PR3, a primary neutrophilic granule protein, is abundant in leukemic progenitors from patients with acute myeloid leukemia (AML) and CML, but is minimally expressed by normal marrow progenitors. Interestingly, it also plays a critical role in maintaining a leukemic phenotype since its inhibition resulted in growth arrest and terminal differentiation of the HL-60 promyelocytic cell line *(38)*. This protein has the interesting immunological attribute of being the target autoantigen in Wegener's granulomatosis. Using algorithms based on HLA class I peptide-binding motifs, Molldrem et al. have identified proteinase 3 peptides that bind common HLA alleles. These peptides have been used to stimulate T-cell populations leading to the generation of PR-3-specific cytotoxic T-cells able to recognize and kill unmodified AML cells while sparing normal bone marrow cells *(39)*. Furthermore, by using PR-1/HLA-A*0201 tetrameric complexes, CD8+ T-cells specific for a peptide derived from PR-3 have been identified in CML patients that achieved remission following allogeneic bone marrow transplant or interferon treatment *(40)*. Given these results, these candidate peptides are currently explored for their ability to amplify leukemia-specific T-cell populations for adoptive therapy and are being used directly in a Phase I vaccine trial.

A second candidate antigen is WT1, also markedly overexpressed by most human leukemias, including AML, CML, and acute lymphocytic leukemia (ALL). WT1 is a zinc finger transcription factor involved in leukemogenesis. This critical role in malignant transformation makes the generation of tumor escape by antigen loss less likely with this target *(41)*. An HLA A201-restricted epitope of WT1 has recently been identified. Furthermore, T-cells specific for this epitope have been generated and shown to lyse leukemia cell lines and inhibit colony formation by transformed CD34+ progenitor cells from CML patients, while not affecting normal CD34+ progenitors *(42,43)*.The recent demonstration that antibodies against WT1 are present in the serum of patients with AML *(43)* makes this antigen an enticing target for vaccine strategies aimed at generating both cellular and humoral antileukemic immune responses.

As a result of the identification of tumor antigens expressed by hematological tumors, an increasing number of vaccine strategies have been developed and are currently being evaluated in preclinical models and/or clinical trials.

3. GENERATION OF IMMUNE RESPONSES AGAINST TUMOR ANTIGENS TO WHICH THE IMMUNE SYSTEM HAS BEEN EXPOSED

In contrast to vaccination against infectious agents in which immunization seeks to prime an immune response to antigens the immune system has not yet encountered (prophylactic vaccination), cancer vaccination is aimed at eliciting immune responses against tumor antigens to which the immune system has already been exposed (therapeutic vaccination). In the clinical arena, it should be pointed out that by the time a patient is diagnosed with cancer, the immune system has been already exposed to tumor antigens and is still allowing tumor growth *(26)*. Although the basis for this failure of the immune system to control tumors arising *de novo* is not completely understood, it is plausible that the patient's immune system may well have been rendered "tolerant or unresponsive to the tumor." This explanation was first evoked after a set of surprising experimental findings in human tumors demonstrating that most of the human tumor antigens identified are not neo-antigens uniquely expressed by cancer cells, but rather tissue-specific differentiation antigens also expressed in normal tissues. Therefore, it is possible that the immune system may see tumors more as a "self" than as a "foreign," resulting in tolerance to tumor antigens in a fashion similar to the induction of peripheral tolerance to self-antigens *(44)*. Recently, studies in experimental models in which T-cells specific for tumor-associated antigens could be marked and monitored in vivo are providing increasing evidence that the natural response of the immune system to tumor antigens seems to be tolerance induction rather than immune activation. Indeed, utilizing T-cell receptor (TCR) transgenic mice specific for a model tumor antigen, we have obtained direct evidence supporting the existence of tumor antigen-specific tolerance that develops during B-cell lymphoma progression. In these studies, early in the course of growth of the murine lymphoma, A20, tumor-specific CD4[+] T-cells lost their naïve phenotype (indicative of having encountered tumor antigen in vivo) and even became partially activated. Despite this initial activation, the T-cells rapidly become unresponsive to subsequent antigenic stimulation suggestive of impaired function *(45)*. Furthermore, by using parent-into-F1 bone marrow chimeras, we have unambiguously demonstrated that tumor antigen processing and presentation by bone marrow-derived antigen-presenting cells (APCs), and not direct presentation by lymphoma cells, is the dominant mechanism underlying the development of tumor antigen-specific T-cell tolerance *(46)*. Importantly, the induction of this unresponsive state was associated with an impaired response to therapeutic vaccination, pointing, therefore, to tumor-induced immune tolerance as a critical barrier to be faced in the design of effective cancer vaccines.

Needless to say, similar findings of tumor antigen-specific tolerance have been recently described in patients with metastatic cancer. Lee et al., using peptide/HLA-A*0201 tetramers, have shown that circulating T-cells specific for the tumor-associated antigens MART-1 or tyrosinase are rendered unresponsive in the cancer-bearing host and thus unable to control melanoma growth *(47)*. Taken together, these sobering findings of tumor-induced antigen-specific immune tolerance raise the bar for establishing effective therapeutic vaccination, since tolerance must be broken in order for cancer vaccines to trigger meaningful immune responses against established tumors.

The requirement for bone-marrow-derived APCs in both the induction of tolerance to tumor antigens *(46)* as well as priming effective anti-tumor T-cell responses not only places APCs at the crossroads of these highly divergent outcomes but also points to modulation of these cells as a critical strategy to overcome tumor-induced tolerance *(21,48)*. Indeed, current strategies using genetically modified tumor cells as vaccines are largely based on engaging

APCs in several ways, including attracting APCs to the vaccine site (i.e., granulocyte-macrophage colony-stimulating factor [GM-CSF] tumor cell-based vaccines) *(49)*, enhancing APC function (i.e., GM-CSF/CD40 ligand tumor cell-based vaccine) *(50)*, and converting the tumor itself into an APC through fusion of dendritic cells with the autologous tumor *(51)*.

4. VACCINE FORMULATIONS

4.1. Antigen-Specific Strategies

4.1.1. ACUTE MYELOID LEUKEMIA

Although tumor-rejection antigens have yet to be formally identified in AML, several candidates are being explored. Proteinase 3, a primary neutrophilic granule protein, is markedly overexpressed in myeloid leukemias. Proteinase 3-specific cytotoxic T-cells have been generated capable of recognizing and killing myeloid leukemic cells in an antigen-specific fashion *(39)*. Furthermore, the presence of polymorphisms in the proteinase 3 gene was analyzed in 23 HLA-A2 patients and their HLA-identical donors. In four donor-recipient pairs in which at least one allele was absent, no relapse was detected. In contrast, 7 of 15 of the remaining patients in which no allelic differences were detected relapsed *(52)*. These data suggest a role of proteinase 3-specific T-cell responses in the GVL effect of allogeneic transplants and underscores the role of this protein as an immunogen in AML vaccine trials.

Another potential tumor antigen is the WT1 markedly overexpressed in AML, CML, and several solid tumors. As with proteinase 3, T-cells have also been generated to recognize HLA-restricted WT1 peptides capable of selectively killing WT1 leukemia cells *(53)*. PML-RARα HLA-DR-restricted peptides can generate CD4[+] lymphocytes with specific cytotoxicity against autologous peptide pulsed acute promyelocytic leukemic cells. These data demonstrate the ability of neoplastic cells to process and present intracellular proteins on its surface *(33)*. However, the absence of peptide-specific immune responses upon vaccination with a 25mer PML-RARα peptide likely reflects the inability of an HLA-class II-negative cell to present the peptides on the leukemia blast cell surface *(54)*. The role these proteins will have in developing vaccine strategies remains to be determined.

4.1.2. CHRONIC MYELOID LEUKEMIA

CML has demonstrated significant immune susceptibility through its ability to respond to donor lymphocyte infusions with sustained remissions in patients that relapsed following an allogeneic T-cell-depleted bone marrow transplant *(1,55)*. While this response is largely mediated by minor histocompatibility antigen differences between the donor and recipient, the presence of a measurable clinical benefit in CML as compared to other myeloid leukemias suggests a tumor-specific response. A vaccination strategy with greater tumor specificity and significantly lower toxicity than that associated with allogeneic transplantation and donor lymphocyte infusions has, therefore, considerable appeal.

One possible tumor antigen candidate is the bcr-abl fusion protein (p210). This chimeric protein is uniquely expressed in CML, and the junctional amino acid sequence is not expressed on any normal protein. Bocchia et al. recently reported their findings utilizing five b3a2 breakpoint-derived HLA class I and class II-restricted peptides in patients with persistent disease on either imatinib or interferon-α for at least 12 months *(56)*. Complete cytogenetic response (CCR) was observed in 5 of 10 patients on imatinib treatment, with 3 of these 5 achieving molecular remission. In the group receiving interferon-α, two of six patients achieved CCR in response to vaccination. Interestingly, these responses appeared to correlate with evidence of the induction of peptide-specific immunity.

4.2. Tumor-Cell Based Vaccine Strategies

One limitation of an antigen-specific vaccine approach is the possibility of limiting the therapeutic effect to priming immune responses to a single antigen and the subsequent risk of relapsing with tumors no longer expressing the antigens against which they were vaccinated, a phenomenon known as "antigen escape variants." Furthermore, with few exceptions, it is still not clear whether the tumor-specific antigens identified to date represent immunodominant proteins to which effective immune responses can be generated. With this in mind, a vaccine formulation using the tumor cell itself as an antigen source offers the advantage of expressing a broad spectrum of tumor antigens present on the tumor cell's surface (polyvalent vaccination) that can potentially serve as targets for the immune system *(57)*. The efficacy of this approach relies on the ability to induce stronger immunity against tumor-selective antigens than against normal tissue antigens present on the tumor cell's surface. Critical to vaccine development is the ability to modify the tumor cell with genes encoding immunologically relevant molecules and producing a sustained, local release of its product leading to local inflammation at the vaccine site without systemic toxicity. The initial studies using genetically altered tumors to enhance their immunogenicity were performed by Lindenmann and Klein in the late 1960s *(58)*. In these studies, vaccination with lysates of influenza-infected tumor cells resulted in the generation of systemic immune responses. In contrast, nonvirally infected tumor lysates alone or admixed with the same virus elicited no measurable immune response. More recently, because of the significant advances in gene-transfer techniques, a variety of tumor cells have been genetically modified to either secrete cytokines locally or express new or increased levels of cell-membrane molecules such as adhesion or costimulatory molecules. With this approach, the immunogenicity of malignant cells is increased either by enhancing the presentation of tumor antigens and/or by providing enhanced co-stimulatory signals to the T-cell arm of the immune system *(57)*. In preclinical models, these tumor-cell-based vaccine strategies prime systemic immune responses capable of rejecting a subsequent tumor challenge or eradicate established micrometastatic tumors. A systemic comparison of 10 different cytokines or cell surface molecule-based tumor vaccines showed that immunization with tumors transduced with a retroviral vector expressing granulocyte-macrophage colony-stimulating factor (GM-CSF) produced the greatest degree of systemic immunity, which was enhanced relative to irradiated nontransduced tumors *(59)*. Priming with GM-CSF-transduced tumor cells led to a potent, long-lived antitumor immunity that required the participation of both CD4[+] and CD8[+] T-cells. Further dissection of the mechanisms mediating this strong antitumor effect showed that GM-CSF produced at the vaccine site promotes the recruitment and activation of host's APCs, which efficiently take up, process, and present tumor antigens to antigen-specific T-cells, leading to strong antitumor responses *(21)*. Multiple reports have since confirmed the bioactivity of GM-CSF-transduced tumor cells in a number of different tumor model systems, including hematological malignancies *(49)*.

4.2.1. GM-CSF TUMOR-CELL-BASED VACCINE STRATEGIES

To date, GM-CSF-secreting vaccines that have been tested clinically have fallen into two categories: autologous tumors virally transduced to secrete GM-CSF (renal cell carcinoma, melanoma, prostate carcinoma, and lung cancer) and GM-CSF-producing allogeneic tumor cell lines (pancreatic carcinoma and prostate carcinoma). In the former scenario, vaccine development was hampered by the ability to harvest adequate amounts of tumor, expense, labor intensity, and GM-CSF variability of each patient's vaccine formulation. With the latter, the strategy relies on the ability to prime immune responses to shared tumor antigens of similar histologies and is ideal in situations in which tumor tissue is limited. This strategy relies on the requirement of antigen processing and presentation by host APCs, and thus MHC compatibility between host and vaccinating tumor is not required *(60)*. However, one limitation to this approach is the possible generation of allogeneic responses to the tumor vaccine itself, which could ultimately reduce cell viability and, more importantly, antitumor efficacy with subsequent vaccinations.

The relative ease with which tumor can be obtained from leukemia patients greatly facilitates the use of autologous tumor vaccines in this disease. In an effort to simplify vaccine production, we have recently shown that although GM-CSF secretion is a critical parameter in the generation of systemic antitumor responses, autocrine secretion is not required and paracrine production is equally effective *(61)*. We have therefore developed an allogeneic bystander cell line that secretes large and stable amounts of GM-CSF (K562/GM-CSF). This cell line was chosen because it can be easily grown in suspension and has no detectable levels of either HLA class I or class II expression, thereby minimizing the likelihood of anti-bystander allogeneic responses with multiple vaccinations. This universal bystander vaccine approach thus obviates the requirement of gene modification for each individual tumor source and guarantees uniform cytokine production.

4.2.2. Clinical Implementation of GM-CSF-Based Leukemia Vaccines

As described above, a variety of different vaccine approaches are currently being examined. This is especially relevant when considering the absence of significant clinical benefit of tumor vaccines in most of the trials published to date. In addition to increasing the number of antigens delivered in the vaccine formulation, we need to optimize numerous other conditions in an effort to improve the therapeutic benefit of tumor vaccines. Parameters being examined include, but are not limited to, (1) immune adjuvants, including cytokines (GM-CSF, interleukin [IL]-4, IL-12), co-stimulatory molecules (B7-1, B7-2) *(62,63)* or Toll-like receptor (TLR) agonists *(64)* to augment immunogenicity of the vaccine, (2) inhibitors of immuno-suppressive pathways such as CTLA-4 blockade *(65,66)*, (3) abolition of regulatory T-cells (Tregs) *(67)*, (4) utilization of tumor vaccines in a setting of minimal residual disease, and (5) integration of tumor vaccines in the autologous transplant setting with the addition of adoptive immunotherapy *(68,69)*.

Bone marrow transplantation has demonstrated a significant clinical benefit in the treatment of many hematological malignancies. Nevertheless, the long-term benefit of this modality remains limited in that many patients ultimately succumb to their disease or suffer the consequences of the morbidity and mortality of GVHD associated with allogeneic transplantation. Integration of cancer vaccines in the autologous transplant setting offers several theoretical as well as real advantages. The posttransplant setting is a period of minimal residual disease in which the likelihood of vaccine strategies to impart a clinically effective response is greatest. Furthermore, the adaptive transfer of tumor-specific immunity from the pretransplant period through the infusion of "primed" lymphocytes, the skewing of the developing immune repertoire with vaccinations during the period of immune reconstitution, and the abolition of tolerogenic mechanisms as a result of the myeloablative regimen are all theoretical advantages that must counterbalance by the global immunosuppression accompanying the early post-transplant period.

In an attempt to model the integration of GM-CSF-based tumor cell vaccines in the autologous bone marraow transplantation setting, we recently established a syngeneic murine model *(68)*. This model demonstrates the effectiveness of antitumor vaccines as measured by the ability to cure a preestablished tumor burden when such vaccines were administered early posttransplant long before full immune reconstitution. Surprisingly, the ability to elicit effective antitumor responses was significantly greater in the transplanted mice than in their nontransplanted counterparts with an equivalent tumor burden. In the model of minimal residual disease, T-cells were found to undergo a significant clonal expansion and activation early posttransplant that declined with the development of macroscopic disease. Interestingly, vaccination with irradiated GM-CSF producing autologous tumor during the period of immune reconstitution maintained T-cell responsiveness and enhanced survival. These data demonstrate the presence of an "autologous graft vs host" effect in the posttransplant period, which is normally transient but can be prolonged following vaccination.

A recent trial in AML utilized autologous tumor admixed with the K562/GM-CSF producing bystander cell administered to patients in a complete remission following induction and consolidation chemotherapy and went on to receive an autologous stem cell transplant. A pretransplant vaccination was administered followed 2 weeks later by leukapheresis. This pretransplant vaccine serves the purpose of priming tumor-specific lymphocytes that are collected and reinfused together with the stem cells following the myeloablative preparative regimen. The patients then received eight posttransplant vaccinations starting 6 weeks after bone marrow transplant. Clearly, determinations of the relative contribution of the vaccine vs the autologous transplant to the clinical outcome are difficult in a clinical study in which the two therapies are overlapping. However, changes in tumor burden between the pretransplant vaccination and leukapheresis likely reflect the immunotherapeutic intervention because no cytotoxic therapy is administered at that time. WT1 transcript levels were followed in these patients as a measure of minimal residual disease. Of the 20 evaluable patients, 11 had a measurable decrease in WT1 transcripts following the pretransplant vaccine that was associated with a longer time to relapse. However, a more reliable measure of immune responsiveness is the development of a delayed-type hypersensitivity (DTH) reaction to the tumor antigens. Patients with positive leukemia-specific DTH reactions (6/20) had 100% relapse-free survival with a median follow-up of 23 months as compared to 60% in patients in whom no DTH reactions were observed. These preliminary data provide evidence of our ability to prime leukemia-specific immune responses with possible clinical benefit.

5. CONCLUSIONS

The role of the immune system in the treatment of leukemia has been well documented in a variety of settings. Specifically, the increased antitumor effect of allogeneic transplants over autologous and the ability to reinduce remissions with donor lymphocyte infusions in a substantial number of patients all point to the critical role of the immune system in these diseases. However, what these interventions have accomplished in clinical efficacy, they lack in tumor specificity. Nevertheless, these data contribute to a growing body of literature supporting the role of immunotherapy in this disease. It is incumbent upon us to refine these treatment paradigms to obtain greater tumor specificity and reduced toxicity. Early clinical studies utilizing cancer vaccines have demonstrated the ability to achieve such a goal but have thus far shown limited success in imparting clinically significant benefits. Reasons for this are multifactorial and include the inability to overcome the inherent tumor-specific tolerogenic mechanisms of cancer-bearing hosts, ineffective vaccine formulations, and excessive tumor burdens. New studies are being conducted or planned testing different vaccine formulations and/or targets as well as settings in which immunomodulation could result in enhanced therapeutic efficacy. Fortunately, the ability to integrate these therapies with immunomodulatory agents in earlier stages of disease, in patients with minimal residual disease, or in combination with adoptive T-cell therapy will significantly improve the therapeutic efficacy of vaccine approaches. The recent successes of antibody therapies in the treatment of leukemias have convinced many skeptics of the important antitumor role the immune system plays. We can only hope that our increased understanding of the mechanisms that enhance antitumor immune responsiveness will translate into the delivery of immunotherapy with greater tumor specificity and reduced toxicity.

REFERENCES

1. Kolb HJ, Holler E. Adoptive immunotherapy with donor lymphocyte transfusions. Curr Opin Oncol 1997;9:139–145.
2. Michallet AS, Nicolini F, Furst S, et al. Outcome and long-term follow-up of alloreactive donor lymphocyte infusions given for relapse after myeloablative allogeneic hematopoietic stem cell transplantations (HSCT). Bone Marrow Transplant 2005.
3. Collins RH, Jr., Shpilberg O, Drobyski WR, et al. Donor leukocyte infusions in 140 patients with relapsed malignancy after allogeneic bone marrow transplantation. J Clin Oncol 1997;15:433–444.
4. Giralt SA, Kolb HJ. Donor lymphocyte infusions. Curr Opin Oncol 1996;8:96–102.
5. Shankaran V, Ikeda H, Bruce AT, et al. IFNgamma and lymphocytes prevent primary tumour development and shape tumour immunogenicity. Nature 2001;410:1107–1111.
6. Nakano O, Sato M, Naito Y, et al. Proliferative activity of intratumoral CD8(+) T-lymphocytes as a prognostic factor in human renal cell carcinoma: clinicopathologic demonstration of antitumor immunity. Cancer Res 2001;61:5132–5136.
7. Zhang L, Conejo-Garcia JR, Katsaros D, et al. Intratumoral T cells, recurrence, and survival in epithelial ovarian cancer. N Engl J Med 2003;348:203–213.
8. Porrata LF, Gertz MA, Inwards DJ, et al. Early lymphocyte recovery predicts superior survival after autologous hematopoietic stem cell transplantation in multiple myeloma or non- Hodgkin lymphoma. Blood 2001;98:579–585.
9. Porrata LF, Litzow MR, Tefferi A, et al. Early lymphocyte recovery is a predictive factor for prolonged survival after autologous hematopoietic stem cell transplantation for acute myelogenous leukemia. Leukemia 2002;16:1311–1318.
10. Dunn GP, Old LJ, Schreiber RD. The immunobiology of cancer immunosurveillance and immunoediting. Immunity 2004;21:137–148.
11. Garrido F, Ruiz-Cabello F, Cabrera T, et al. Implications for immunosurveillance of altered HLA class I phenotypes in human tumours. Immunol Today 1997;18:89–95.
12. Sotomayor EM, Borrello I, Tubb E, et al. Conversion of tumor-specific CD4+ T-cell tolerance to T-cell priming through in vivo ligation of CD40. Nat Med 1999;5:780–787.
13. Sotomayor EM, Borrello I, Tubb E, Allison JP, Levitsky HI. In vivo blockade of CTLA-4 enhances the priming of responsive T cells but fails to prevent the induction of tumor antigen-specific tolerance. Proc Natl Acad Sci USA 1999;96:11,476–11,481.
14. Egen JG, Kuhns MS, Allison JP. CTLA-4: new insights into its biological function and use in tumor immunotherapy. Nat Immunol 2002;3:611–618.
15. Dudley ME, Rosenberg SA. Adoptive-cell-transfer therapy for the treatment of patients with cancer. Nat Rev Cancer 2003;3:666–675.
16. Zou W. Immunosuppressive networks in the tumour environment and their therapeutic relevance. Nat Rev Cancer 2005;5:263–274.
17. Nauts HC. Bacteria and cancer–antagonisms and benefits. Cancer Surv 1989;8:713–723.

18. Berd D, Maguire HC, Jr., McCue P, Mastrangelo MJ. Treatment of metastatic melanoma with an autologous tumor-cell vaccine: clinical and immunologic results in 64 patients. J Clin Oncol 1990;8:1858–1867.

19. Boon T, van der Bruggen P. Human tumor antigens recognized by T lymphocytes. J Exp Med 1996; 183:725–729.

20. Rosenberg SA. A new era for cancer immunotherapy based on the genes that encode cancer antigens. Immunity 1999;10:281–287.

21. Huang AY, Golumbek P, Ahmadzadeh M, Jaffee E, Pardoll D, Levitsky H. Role of bone marrow-derived cells in presenting MHC class I-restricted tumor antigens. Science 1994;264:961–965.

22. Leach DR, Krummel MF, Allison JP. Enhancement of antitumor immunity by CTLA-4 blockade [see comments]. Science 1996;271:1734–1736.

23. Sogn JA. Tumor immunology: the glass is half full. Immunity 1998;9:757–763.

24. van der Bruggen P, Traversari C, Chomez P, et al. A gene encoding an antigen recognized by cytolytic T lymphocytes on a human melanoma. Science 1991;254:1643–1647.

25. Topalian SL, Rivoltini L, Mancini M, et al. Human CD4+ T cells specifically recognize a shared melanoma-associated antigen encoded by the tyrosinase gene. Proc Natl Acad Sci USA 1994;91:9461–9465.

26. Pardoll DM. Cancer vaccines. Nat Med 1998;4:525–531.

27. Disis ML, Cheever MA. Oncogenic proteins as tumor antigens. Curr Opin Immunol 1996;8:637–642.

28. Pinilla-Ibarz J, Cathcart K, Korontsvit T, et al. Vaccination of patients with chronic myelogenous leukemia with bcr-abl oncogene breakpoint fusion peptides generates specific immune responses. Blood 2000;95: 1781–1787.

29. Pinilla-Ibarz J, Cathcart K, Scheinberg DA. CML vaccines as a paradigm of the specific immunotherapy of cancer. Blood Rev. 2000;14:111–120.

30. Clark RE, Dodi IA, Hill SC, et al. Direct evidence that leukemic cells present HLA-associated immunogenic peptides derived from the BCR-ABL b3a2 fusion protein. Blood 2001;98:2887–2893.

31. von Lindern M, Fornerod M, van Baal S, et al. The translocation (6;9), associated with a specific subtype of acute myeloid leukemia, results in the fusion of two genes, dek and can, and the expression of a chimeric, leukemia-specific dek-can mRNA. Mol Cell Biol 1992;12:1687–1697.

32. Downing JR, Head DR, Curcio-Brint AM, et al. An AML1/ETO fusion transcript is consistently detected by RNA-based polymerase chain reaction in acute myelogenous leukemia containing the (8;21)(q22;q22) translocation. Blood 1993;81:2860–2865.

33. Gambacorti-Passerini C, Grignani F, Arienti F, Pandolfi PP, Pelicci PG, Parmiani G. Human CD4 lymphocytes specifically recognize a peptide representing the fusion region of the hybrid protein pml/RAR alpha present in acute promyelocytic leukemia cells. Blood 1993;81:1369–1375.

34. Robbins PF, Kawakami Y. Human tumor antigens recognized by T cells. Curr Opin Immunol 1996;8: 628–636.

35. Traversari C, van der Bruggen P, Luescher IF, et al. A nonapeptide encoded by human gene MAGE-1 is recognized on HLA-A1 by cytolytic T lymphocytes directed against tumor antigen MZ2-E. J Exp Med 1992;176:1453–1457.

36. Boel P, Wildmann C, Sensi ML, et al. BAGE: a new gene encoding an antigen recognized on human melanomas by cytolytic T lymphocytes. Immunity 1995;2:167–175.

37. Greiner J, Ringhoffer M, Simikopinko O, et al. Simultaneous expression of different immunogenic antigens in acute myeloid leukemia. Exp Hematol 2000;28:1413–1422.

38. Bories D, Raynal MC, Solomon DH, Darzynkiewicz Z, Cayre YE. Down-regulation of a serine protease, myeloblastin, causes growth arrest and differentiation of promyelocytic leukemia cells. Cell 1989;59:959–968.

39. Molldrem JJ, Clave E, Jiang YZ, et al. Cytotoxic T lymphocytes specific for a nonpolymorphic proteinase 3 peptide preferentially inhibit chronic myeloid leukemia colony-forming units. Blood 1997;90:2529–2534.

40. Molldrem JJ, Lee PP, Wang C, et al. Evidence that specific T lymphocytes may participate in the elimination of chronic myelogenous leukemia. Nat Med 2000;6:1018–1023.

41. Bergmann L, Maurer U, Weidmann E. Wilms tumor gene expression in acute myeloid leukemias. Leuk Lymphoma 1997;25:435–443.

42. Ohminami H, Yasukawa M, Fujita S. HLA class I-restricted lysis of leukemia cells by a CD8(+) cytotoxic T-lymphocyte clone specific for WT1 peptide. Blood 2000;95:286–293.

43. Gao L, Bellantuono I, Elsasser A, et al. Selective elimination of leukemic CD34(+) progenitor cells by cytotoxic T lymphocytes specific for WT1. Blood 2000;95:2198–2203.

44. Pardoll D. T cells and tumours. Nature 2001;411:1010–1012.

45. Staveley-O' Carroll K, Sotomayor E, Montgomery J, et al. Induction of antigen-specific T cell anergy: An early event in the course of tumor progression. Proc Natl Acad Sci USA 1998;95:1178–1183.
46. Sotomayor EM, Borrello I, Rattis FM, et al. Cross-presentation of tumor antigens by bone marrow-derived antigen-presenting cells is the dominant mechanism in the induction of T-cell tolerance during B-cell lymphoma progression. Blood 2001;98:1070–1077.
47. Lee PP, Yee C, Savage PA, et al. Characterization of circulating T cells specific for tumor-associated antigens in melanoma patients. Nat Med 1999;5:677–685.
48. Hsu FJ, Benike C, Fagnoni F, et al. Vaccination of patients with B-cell lymphoma using autologous antigen-pulsed dendritic cells. Nat Med 1996;2:52–58.
49. Levitsky HI, Montgomery J, Ahmadzadeh M, et al. Immunization with granulocyte-macrophage colony-stimulating factor- transduced, but not B7-1-transduced, lymphoma cells primes idiotype- specific T cells and generates potent systemic antitumor immunity. J Immunol 1996;156:3858–3865.
50. Chiodoni C, Paglia P, Stoppacciaro A, Rodolfo M, Parenza M, Colombo MP. Dendritic cells infiltrating tumors cotransduced with granulocyte/macrophage colony-stimulating factor (GM-CSF) and CD40 ligand genes take up and present endogenous tumor-associated antigens, and prime naive mice for a cytotoxic T lymphocyte response. J Exp Med 1999;190:125–133.
51. Gong J, Chen D, Kashiwaba M, Kufe D. Induction of antitumor activity by immunization with fusions of dendritic and carcinoma cells. Nat Med 1997;3:558–561.
52. Clave E, Molldrem J, Hensel N, Raptis A, Barrett AJ. Donor-recipient polymorphism of the proteinase 3 gene: a potential target for T-cell alloresponses to myeloid leukemia. J Immunother 1999;22:1–6.
53. Ohminami H, Yasukawa M, Fujita S. HLA class I-restricted lysis of leukemia cells by a CD8(+) cytotoxic T- lymphocyte clone specific for WT1 peptide. Blood 2000;95:286–293.
54. Dermime S, Bertazzoli C, Marchesi E, et al. Lack of T-cell-mediated recognition of the fusion region of the pml/RAR-alpha hybrid protein by lymphocytes of acute promyelocytic leukemia patients. Clin Cancer Res 1996;2:593–600.
55. Li Y, Bendandi M, Deng Y, et al. Tumor-specific recognition of human myeloma cells by idiotype-induced CD8(+) T cells. Blood 2000;96:2828–2833.
56. Bocchia M, Gentili S, Abruzzese E, et al. Effect of a p210 multipeptide vaccine associated with imatinib or interferon in patients with chronic myeloid leukaemia and persistent residual disease: a multicentre observational trial. Lancet 2005;365:657–662.
57. Pardoll DM. New strategies for enhancing the immunogenicity of tumors. Curr Opin Immunol 1993;5:719–725.
58. Lindenmann J, Klein PA. Viral oncolysis: increased immunogenicity of host cell antigen associated with influenza virus. J Exp Med 1967;126:93–108.
59. Dranoff G, Jaffee E, Lazenby A, et al. Vaccination with irradiated tumor cells engineered to secrete murine granulocyte-macrophage colony-stimulating factor stimulates potent, specific, and long-lasting anti-tumor immunity. Proc Natl Acad Sci USA 1993;90:3539–3543.
60. Toes RE, Blom RJ, van der Voort E, Offringa R, Melief CJ, Kast WM. Protective antitumor immunity induced by immunization with completely allogeneic tumor cells. Cancer Res 1996;56:3782–3787.
61. Borrello I, Sotomayor EM, Cooke S, Levitsky HI. A universal granulocyte-macrophage colony-stimulating factor-producing bystander cell line for use in the formulation of autologous tumor cell-based vaccines. Hum Gene Ther 1999;10:1983–1991.
62. Chan L, Hardwick N, Darling D, et al. IL-2/B7.1 (CD80) fusagene transduction of AML blasts by a self-inactivating lentiviral vector stimulates T cell responses in vitro: a strategy to generate whole cell vaccines for AML. Mol Ther 2005;11:120–131.
63. Koya RC, Kasahara N, Pullarkat V, Levine AM, Stripecke R. Transduction of acute myeloid leukemia cells with third generation self-inactivating lentiviral vectors expressing CD80 and GM-CSF: effects on proliferation, differentiation, and stimulation of allogeneic and autologous anti-leukemia immune responses. Leukemia 2002;16:1645–1654.
64. Baldridge JR, McGowan P, Evans JT, et al. Taking a Toll on human disease: Toll-like receptor 4 agonists as vaccine adjuvants and monotherapeutic agents. Expert Opin Biol Ther 2004;4:1129–1138.
65. Hurwitz AA, Yu TF, Leach DR, Allison JP. CTLA-4 blockade synergizes with tumor-derived granulocyte-macrophage colony-stimulating factor for treatment of an experimental mammary carcinoma. Proc Natl Acad Sci USA 1998;95:10,067–10,071.
66. Dranoff G. CTLA-4 blockade: unveiling immune regulation. J Clin Oncol 2005;23:662–664.

67. Cohen IR, Quintana FJ, Mimran A. Tregs in T cell vaccination: exploring the regulation of regulation. J Clin Invest 2004;114:1227–1232.
68. Borrello I, Sotomayor EM, Rattis FM, Cooke SK, Gu L, Levitsky HI. Sustaining the graft-versus-tumor effect through posttransplant immunization with granulocyte-macrophage colony-stimulating factor (GM-CSF)-producing tumor vaccines. Blood 2000;95:3011–3019.
69. Kwak LW, Neelapu SS, Bishop MR. Adoptive immunotherapy with antigen-specific T cells in myeloma: a model of tumor-specific donor lymphocyte infusion. Semin Oncol 2004;31:37–46.

V SPECIAL CHALLENGES

17 Treatment, Outcomes, and Challenges of Newly Diagnosed AML in Children and Adolescents

Robert J. Arceci

CONTENTS

Summary

Acute myeloid leukemia (AML) in children encompasses a distinctive set of diseases with special considerations related to age, drug metabolism, and both short- and long-term sequelae. This chapter will emphasize inherited syndromes that predispose to leukemogenesis, development of secondary AML, and the roles of dose intensification and stem cell transplantation in the ongoing improvement in cure rates. The importance of risk stratification in the design of clinical trials, based on cytogenetic and molecular characteristics, is critical to optimizing the balance between curability, quality of life, and minimization of long-term sequelae for children with AML.

Key Words: Inherited predisposition; familial syndromes; chromosomal instability; age-dependent drug metabolism; risk group stratification.

1. INTRODUCTION

At the heart of a chapter on pediatric acute myeloid leukemia (AML) in the context of a general text on myeloid leukemias are the issues of what distinguishes pediatric AML and its treatment from that of adult patients. This is particularly important in light of the debate regarding the optimal treatment of adolescents and young adults with a variety of different cancers. This debate has been fueled in part by studies that have concluded that young adults with cancer have improved outcomes when treated on protocols designed for pediatric patients compared to those designed for adults. A second contributor to this debate includes the impact of genomic approaches to understanding cancer. A natural outgrowth of such studies

From: *Contemporary Hematology: Acute Myelogenous Leukemia*
Edited by: J. E. Karp © Humana Press Inc., Totowa, NJ

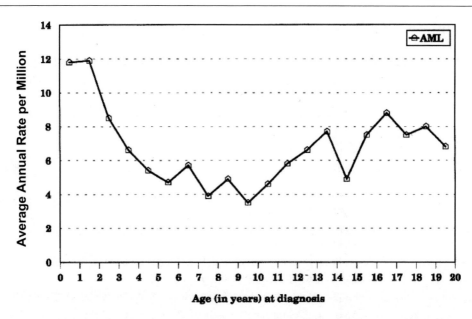

Fig. 1. SEER data on pediatric AML rate per million by age. (From ref. *1*.)

is the ability to ask whether specific types of cancer characterized by distinctive cytogenetic or molecular abnormalities are the same disease when found in a 5-, 25-, or 55-year-old individual. The answer to this question has a profound impact on the potential for therapeutic drug development in children. Third, there is the issue of what the age-specific characteristics are in terms of pharmacological metabolism of therapeutic agents and toxicity considerations. This issue is critical in the design of clinical trials in terms of chemotherapeutic dosing, but also in terms of which short- and long-term adverse sequelae would be expected and acceptable as risks. In addition, this issue has relevance to how one defines a "pediatric" patient, both in terms of physiology as well as psychosocial needs. Although the answers to these questions are not yet completely apparent, this chapter will address some of the essential aspects of pediatric AML along with its treatment, outcomes, and challenges in order to help establish areas that are distinct and shared with AML in young or older adults.

2. EPIDEMIOLOGY

Approximately 6500 children younger than 20 years develop acute leukemia annually in the United States. AML represents about 15% of these cases, resulting in just fewer than 1000 cases per year *(1)*. The other 85% of acute leukemia in children and adolescents is represented by lymphoblastic leukemia (ALL) along with a few percent of patients with chronic myelo- genous leukemia as well as myelodysplastic and myeloproliferative disorders. There is small peak incidence of AML in infants followed by a decline that stays stable until adulthood (Fig. 1). In adults, the opposite ratio exists, with AML accounting for approx 80% of acute leukemia and lymphoblastic the remaining 20%. AML in adults increases with age, and particularly beyond age 55 there is a dramatic increase in AML, in large part caused by secondary AML and myelodysplastic syndromes. There does not appear to be a predilection for male or female in pediatric AML.

There are racial and ethnic background differences in the incidence of AML in children. For example, black children have a slightly higher incidence than white children, whereas Hispanic children have the highest incidence *(2–4)*. This difference is in part a result of the higher incidence of acute promyelocytic leukemia (APL) in Hispanic patients during childhood and young childhood. A higher incidence of AML in Asian children has also been reported *(2)*. The incidence of secondary AML resulting from exposures to chemotherapy and radiation therapy given for other malignancies is a growing concern in survivors of childhood cancer *(5–7)*.

3. INHERITED PREDISPOSITION

Certain inherited syndromes predispose some children to the development of AML. The determination of the genetic pathways affected in these children has led to important insights into the molecular origins of many cancers, including AML. In addition, these children often present significant challenges in terms of treatment.

3.1. Abnormal Chromosome Number

Trisomy 21, or Down syndrome (DS), is the most common inherited condition that predisposes to the development of leukemia, with an approx 14-fold risk compared to the general population *(8)*. Within the first 3 years of life, AML, and particularly acute megakaryoblastic leukemia (AMKL), predominates in children with DS *(9)*.

Infants with DS also have an increased predisposition for a condition known as transient myeloproliferative disorder (TMD), sometimes referred to as preleukemia. Approximately 10% of newborns with DS develop TMD. Although clinically indistinguishable from congenital leukemia, TMD usually spontaneously resolves over several weeks to months. Of clinical importance, phenotypically normal children who are mosaic for trisomy 21 also have an increased risk of developing TMD and subsequent leukemia *(9,10)*. Approximately 20–30% of children with DS and TMD will go onto develop AMKL *(8,9,11,12)*.

The close association between DS, TMD, and AMKL strongly suggests that trisomy 21, along with possibly other shared genetic abnormalities, cooperate to cause AML. Although the *aml1* gene is located on chromosome 21 and has been strongly associated with the development of AML, its expression, mutation, and gene dosage effect in children with DS and AML have not been definitively shown to be causative in the AMKL of DS. Mouse transgenic models harboring increased copies of chromosome regions synteic to those of trisomy 21 in humans may help unravel this important predisposition question *(13)*. A nearly uniform finding has been the identification of GATA-1 gene mutations in both the TMD and AMKL of DS *(14)*. These mutations are most commonly the result of a premature stop codon leading to the truncation of the GATA-1 protein before the amino-terminal activation domain, thus abrogating transcriptional activity *(14)*. In addition, such GATA-1 mutations have been identified both at the time of birth and even prenatally in DS *(15,16)*. These results demonstrate the high probability that mutations in GATA-1 represent an early event in the development of TMD and AMKL in children with DS *(17)*.

Important questions include why the majority of children with DS and TMD have a spontaneous regression of their disease and why a minority go on to develop AMKL. RNA transcript expression analysis of TMD and AMKL samples from patients with DS are beginning to shed light on possible pathways contributing to progression to overt leukemia *(16,18,19)*. A GATA1 mutation in an adult with AML has been reported, although systematic studies have not yet been reported in large numbers of adult samples with AML *(20)*. In addition to DS, there has also been an association with developing AML in Klinefelter syndrome (XXY) and Turner syndrome (XO), but the number of cases is low and molecular mechanisms have not been reported *(21,22)*.

3.2. Inherited Marrow Failure and Chromosome Instability Syndromes

An increased risk for developing AML is characteristic of several inherited syndromes characterized by bone marrow failure and congenital abnormalities. Many of these disorders are characterized by defects in DNA repair, apoptosis, or cell cycle regulation.

Fanconi anemia (FA), an autosomal-recessive inherited disorder, is frequently characterized by congenital abnormalities of the skeleton, short stature, microcephaly, cardiac abnormalities, genitourinary tract abnormalities, café-au-lait spots, and mental retardation along with progressive, hematopoietic failure. It has been estimated that patients with FA have a 15,000-fold greater risk than the general population for developing AML and an actuarial risk of myelodysplastic syndrome (MDS) or AML of about 50% by 40 years of age *(23–25)*. Multiple gene defects give rise to FA, all of which appear to be related to either the same multiprotein complex or related proximal or distal pathways involved in detecting and repairing DNA damage *(26)*. These FA gene mutations result in hypersensitivity to genotoxic agents and chromosomal instability *(26–28)*. The identification of somatic mutations of several FA genes in AML further strengthens an etiological role of these pathways in AML.

Dyskeratosis congenita (DC), most frequently inherited in a X-linked fashion, is in many cases a result of mutations of the DKC1 gene, which codes for a protein called dyskerin, a catalytic subunit of nucleolar RNA particles and a component of the telomerase complex *(29–31)*. DC represents an interesting spectrum of disorders that link marrow failure with alterations of skin pigmentation, nail dystrophy, and mucosal leucoplakia to MDS and AML. Bloom syndrome (BS) represents a disorder characterized by chromosomal instability resulting from mutations in the *blm* helicase gene as well an increased risk of developing leukemia *(32,33)*. Ataxia-telangiectasia (AT), a syndrome characterized by immunodeficiency and increased sensitivity to genotoxic agents, is also associated with increased frequency of leukemia. The *ATM* gene plays a fundamental role in the recognition of DNA damage and recruitment of DNA repair mechanisms *(34,35)*.

3.3. Ayndromes With Alterations in Cell Signaling and Survival Pathways

Some inherited syndromes are associated with cell signaling and survival pathways. For example, the familial platelet disorder with a propensity to develop AML (FPD/AML) and congenital amegakaryocytic thrombocytopenia (CAMT) are both inherited syndromes with a predisposition for developing MDS/AML *(36,37)*. FDP/AML is caused by mutations in the transcription factor CFFA2 *(36)*. CAMT is caused by mutations in the thrombopoietin receptor (c-mpl) *(38)*.

Patients with severe congenital neutropenia (Kostmann syndrome) are characterized by inherited granulocytopenias and an increased risk of developing MDS/AML *(39–41)*. The frequency of AML developing in these patients increases with age. Kostmann syndrome and cyclic neutropenia have been linked to inherited mutations in the elastase gene *(42,43)*. Mutations of the elastase gene in these two syndromes affect different parts of the protein; of interest, only Kostmann syndrome has been associated with an increased incidence of MDS/AML *(43)*. Somatic activating mutations of the granulocyte colony-stimulating factor (G-CSF) receptor have been observed before the development of AML in some patients with Kostmann syndrome *(44)*. These G-CSF receptor mutations usually manifest themselves by a rising white blood cell count in patients on a stable dose of G-CSF and with previously stable white blood cell counts. The introduction of G-CSF cytokine therapy in patients with Kostmann syndrome has prolonged and improved the clinical outcomes, although controversy remains as to whether the AML developing in these patients is in part the result of chronic cytokine stimulation, is simply a natural consequence of patients living longer, or is a combination effect *(41,45,46)*.

Shwachman-Diamond syndrome (SDS), an inherited, autosomal recessive disorder, is also characterized by granulocytopenia as well as pancreatic insufficiency, skeletal abnormalities and an increased risk of developing MDS/AML *(47)*. Mutations in the SBDS gene are found in most patients with Shwachman-Diamond syndrome and are associated with ribosome biosynthesis and function as well as chromosome changes leading to marrow failure and MDS/AML *(48–50)*. Diamond-Blackfan anemia (DBA) is an inherited syndrome characterized by congenital anemia, skeletal and urogenital abnormalities, sometimes progressive bone marrow failure, and an increased risk of developing MDS and AML *(51)*. Mutations in the RPS19 gene, which codes for a small ribosomal subunit protein, have been reported to occur in approx 25% of cases *(52–54)*. Another potential locus leading to DBA, representing another 25–30% of cases, has been localized on chromosome 8 *(55)*. Although it is unclear how alterations in ribosome biosynthesis can lead to AML and other forms of cancer, experimental evidence is accumulating that such pathways are indeed cancer predisposing when altered *(56,57)*. For instance, zebrafish models of insertional mutagenesis have strongly linked ribosomal protein genes to the development of various tumors *(58)*. Furthermore, extraribosomal functions of these ribosomal genes, including important interactions with the p53 pathway, have been described *(56,57)*.

Neurofibromatosis type 1 (NF1) and Noonan syndrome are related disorders caused by different molecular lesions, both of which lead to increased activation of RAS gene pathways and have a predisposition for developing myeloid leukemias, including juvenile myelomonocytic leukemia (JMML), MDS, and AML *(59–61)*. NF1 can be caused by mutations in the gene coding for neurofibromin, a guanosine triphosphatase. Neurofibromin converts activated guanosine triphosphate–RAS to inactive guanosine diphosphate–RAS; however, mutated forms lead to the accumulation of activated guanosine triphosphate–RAS, which in turn leads to persistent stimulation and proliferation of myeloid progenitors and an increased risk of developing leukemia *(59,61)*.

Mutations in the gene coding for PTPN11 phosphatase account for approximately one-third of the cases of Noonan syndrome *(62)*. While germline mutations of PTPN11 have been shown to cause Noonan syndrome and JMML, somatic gain-of-function mutations of PTPN11 may account for approximately one-third of acquired JMML and a low percentage of patients with MDS or AML *(63,64)*.

These inherited syndromes have thus linked inherited developmental disorders affecting chromosome instability, cell signaling pathways, as well as regulation of cell cycle and survival mechanisms to the etiology of myeloid leukemias. In many cases these pathways have also been shown to be relevant to the development of leukemia when somatically mutated. The identification of these pathways has also provided potential new therapeutic targets in AML.

3.4. Twins and Familial AML

An increased frequency of both AML and ALL in siblings of patients with leukemia has been recognized for nearly a century. The nearly 100% concordance of leukemia in identical twins is a result of transplacental transfer *(65–67)*. Further confirmation of these observations and the common origin of leukemia in identical twins comes from the demonstration of the same molecular defects characterizing the leukemia in both twins *(65,68)*. Close clinical follow-up of the normal twin is therefore essential; some clinicians suggest follow-up with physical examination and peripheral blood cell counts every 2–4 weeks for several months and then every 1–2 months until approx 2 years of age. Bone marrow examinations should be done only when clinically indicated. The risk of developing acute leukemia for non-identical twins has been estimated to be a two- to fourfold increase until approx 6 years of age. After that time, the risk becomes similar to that of the general population *(69)*. Cases of familial leukemia suggest yet other hereditary contributions in the etiology of AML. Familial cases have been reported to be associated with constitutional translocations involving t(7;20)(p13;p12) and t(3;6)(p14;p11) as well as familial monosomy 7 *(70–72)*.

4. ACQUIRED PREDISPOSITION AND ENVIRONMENTAL CAUSES

4.1. Acquired Predispositions

Up to 20% of patients with severe aplastic leukemia treated with immunosuppressive agents may develop MDS or AML *(73,74)*. Acquired forms of amegakaryocytic thrombocytopenia (AAMT) have been described to have an increased risk of MDS/AML *(75,76)*. Paroxysmal nocturnal hemoglobinuria, an acquired pancytopenic condition, may also lead to MDS/AML, as can acquired monosomy 7 *(77)*.

4.2. Environmental Risks

Although children do not have the same risk of lengthy exposure to environmental genotoxic agents as adults, it is expected that similar exposures, such as to ionizing radiation or genotoxic chemicals, including benzene and pesticides, would increase the risk of MDS and AML as in older individuals *(78–80)*. Interestingly, no increase in leukemia was observed in children exposed prenatally to the ionizing radiation from the atomic bombs at Nagasaki and Hiroshima during World War II *(81,82)*. Prenatal exposure to diagnostic X-rays and any link to increased risk of cancer to the offspring remains controversial. Definitive evidence that prenatal or postnatal exposure to ultrasound or the effects of electrical power lines increases the risk of AML is lacking *(83,84)*.

Prenatal exposure to some genotoxic chemicals has, however, been reported to increase postnatal incidence AML. For example, maternal alcohol consumption has been associated with an increased risk of AML in offspring, although there have also been dissenting reports on this association *(85)*. An association between parental smoking of tobacco or marijuana has been made with an increased incidence of AML in offspring, while other reports have not found such links *(86–88)*. Excess maternal ingestion of foods and vegetables with high contents of topoisomerase II inhibitors has been reported to be associated with the development of AML in exposed offspring, particularly the subtype characterized by MLL gene rearrangements *(89–91)*.

An increasingly worrisome concern of pediatric oncologists is the development of secondary AML in patients treated for other malignancies or even nonmalignant conditions with genotoxic chemotherapeutic agents. Furthermore, these exposures take on increased impact for children, adolescents, and young adults, who will have longer periods of risk than older adults. Exposure to alkylating agents, commonly used to treat brain tumors, lymphomas, and other solid tumors, results in an increased incidence of secondary AML, with a peak incidence at 4–5 years, but with an at-risk period extending 12 years *(92–94)*. The increasing use of multiple, tandem autologous hematopoietic stem cell transplants with or without radiation exposures may produce increased risk of developing MDS and AML *(95,96)*. The increased risk of secondary AML after exposure to epipodophyllotoxins, such as etoposide (VP-16), is well established *(97,98)*. And although the initial reports concerned children with ALL and relatively long exposures with high cumulative doses of VP-16, it is well recognized that significantly lower exposures can lead to secondary AML *(99)*. The development of secondary AML in children treated initially for their primary cancers may be one of the most compelling reasons to develop alternative and less genotoxic therapeutic paradigms.

5. CELLULAR AND MOLECULAR ORIGINS

Although much less extensively studied in children than in adults, the cellular origins of AML are believed to be similar in the most common subtypes of AML. Thus, AML in children and adults develops as a result of genetic changes, which are inherited or acquired, in primitive hematopoietic precursor cells that result in the expansion of leukemic cells displaying an incomplete block in differentiation *(100,101)*. The heterogeneity of myeloid leukemias is likely to arise from the different types of genetic changes that have occurred as well as the stage of maturation during which the leukemic self-initiating precursor cell (also termed the leukemia stem cell) undergoes transformation *(100–102)*.

For example, a t(8;21) abnormality may lead to M1 AML with minimal differentiation, whereas an inv(16) abnormality may result in an M4eo subtype, despite occurrence in an early progenitor cell of the same maturational stage. Initiating events may primarily affect the ability of the leukemic stem cell to differentiate but retain the ability to self-replicate *(103,104)*. In contrast, other genetic mutations, such as those affecting pathways regulating apoptosis, cell survival, and proliferation, may change the phenotype of the leukemia as well as provide the proliferative advantage of the leukemia *(105)*. These secondary changes commonly affect the function of growth and survival factor receptors, such as FLT-3 or c-KIT, and cooperate with the products of chromosomal translocations to generate leukemic self-renewing stem cells *(106,107)*.

While the cellular origin of AML in children and adults is of great importance in terms of identifying potential surrogate markers of minimal residual disease, the molecular differences between the self-renewing leukemic stem cell and its normal counterparts has immense therapeutic importance in terms of the development of treatments that selectively target that leukemic stem cell *(108–111)*. The identification of the changes characterizing leukemic stem cells is also likely to expand our understanding of the molecular heterogeneity of AML, which presents significant challenges for definitively testing new, targeted therapies in clinical trials.

6. TREATING CHILDREN AND ADOLESCENTS WITH AML: APPROACHES AND OUTCOMES

The overall goal of treatment for children and adolescents with AML is to eradicate their leukemia without causing significant short- or long-term adverse sequelae that would prevent them from leading normal lives. We have not yet achieved this goal for the majority of children with AML. However, significant improvements have been made.

Before 1970, nearly all children and adolescents with AML died. The initial attempts to treat AML with relatively low-dose antimetabolite therapy that was being used successfully to treat children with ALL failed. Based on animal models of leukemia and the predicted effectiveness of dose intensity in AML, subsequent treatment approaches were developed that used more intensive dosing of multiple, non-cross-resistant chemotherapeutic agents. The results of these approaches from the 1970s and 1980s led to overall cure rates of 25–35% in children and adolescents with AML (112–114).

Based on the partial success of these approaches, clinical trials in the pediatric cooperative groups in the 1990s continued to dose intensify chemotherapy timing or length of exposure as well as utilize hematopoietic stem cell transplantation (HSCT). In addition, with the rise of dose intensification, the role of preemptive and aggressive supportive care measures has taken on an increasingly important role. In addition, during this period, the heterogeneity of AML became more evident such that some initial attempts to risk stratify patients began. Results from these dose-intensified trials have brought the overall cure rate of AML in children and adolescents to approx 50% (115).

6.1. Remission Induction

The combination of cytarabine arabinoside (AraC) and an anthracycline in the 1960s and 1970s led to remission rates of approx 60–70%. The "7 and 3" combination, consisting of 7 days of intravenous infusion of 100 mg/m^2 of AraC along with 3 days of bolus daunomycin at 45 mg/m^2/day, became a standard backbone and approach for most cooperative, clinical trial groups. Subsequently, the addition of other agents such as etoposide or 6-thioguanine, along with improved supportive care measures, led to remission induction rates of 70–85% (116,117). Several remission-induction questions have been addressed in more recent studies, including: Which anthracycline is best? Can the dose of AraC be intensified? Can additional agents be added to the backbone of "7 and 3" to improve remission outcomes? Would the introduction of supportive care measures, such as cytokines, improve remission rates?, and Could intensification of remission therapy be achieved without significantly increasing treatment-related mortality?

The introduction of different anthracyclines or related agents, such as idarubicin and mitoxantrone, has not produced consistent improvements. A Berlin–Frankfurt–Münster (BFM) pilot study showed evidence that idarubicin was superior to daunomycin in induction (118), yet the CCG-2941 trial showed that idarubicin was too toxic to be used in sequential courses of intensively timed IdaDCTER therapy (119). An MRC/ICRF meta-analysis of several randomized trials comparing idarubicin or mitoxantrone vs daunomycin reported that there was a statistically significant improvement in remission rate with idarubicin and a trend for mitoxantrone being better than daunomycin (120–122). However, the overall DFS was not different among the different groups. Of note, a detailed analysis by age was not done, although there was a suggestion that idarubicin was more advantageous in younger patients (120). On the other hand, other trials have not achieved higher remission rates by introducing idarubicin (118,123). A possible reason for differences in the conclusions from such studies as well as a challenge for future trials of this type is the issue of dose equivalency and how to adjust for this among different anthracyclines. Thus, there is no consensus or definitive evidence as to which anthracycline is best.

Increasing the dose of the AraC during induction has not been shown to consistently improve remission rates. Randomized studies in adults with AML have not demonstrated significant differences with AraC at 100–200 mg/m^2 or at doses 20–30 times those amounts (i.e., 1000–3000 mg/m^2 every 12 hours for 8–12 doses) in terms of improved remission rates (124–128).

Although the addition of other agents to the "7 and 3" backbone appears to have resulted in improved remission rates from 70 to 85%, no randomized trial has demonstrated superiority of a particular agent or combination of agents over any other combination. For example, the Medical Research Council (MRC) AML 10 trial tested 6-thioguanine vs etoposide in combination with daunomycin and cytarabine; the results showed no statistically significant difference in remission rate between the two induction regimens although the toxicity profiles differed *(129)*.

Several studies have examined the potential role of cytokines, such as G-CSF or granulocyte-macrophage colony-stimulating factor (GM-CSF), to reduce the period of neutropenia and serious infections. Although the results have shown that the use of such cytokines following induction and possibly consolidation therapy reduces periods of neutropenia, the effect on the incidence of infections and hospitalization has been variable *(130–134)*. Most studies have not shown a consistent effect on the remission rate, the duration of response, and the incidence of relapse. The addition of G-CSF in a nonrandomized fashion to intensively timed DCTER on the CCG-2891 study appeared to reduce the frequency of fatal infectious complications and thus improve the remission rate to 82% *(135)*. However, the use of cytokines during remission induction or even at other times during treatment in children with AML is not currently recommended unless prolonged neutropenia and/or life-threatening infections develop. Finally, although there does not appear to be an impact on relapse rates with the use of cytokine support, this issue should continue to be closely analyzed, especially in subgroups of patients *(136)*.

Based in part on observations that AML is responsive to dose intensification as well as on data that kinetically mediated approaches might increase leukemic cell killing, several different strategies were tested in pediatric trials. One approach, used primarily by European cooperative groups, increased the total initial exposure to AraC and an anthracycline. For example, the Cancer and Leukemia Group B showed that a "7 and 3" induction gave improved results compared to a shorter "5 and 2" regimen *(137)*. The MRC AML 9 trial showed that a "10 and 3" plus 6-thioguanine regimen produced improved results compared to a "5 and 1" plus 6-thioguanine combination *(138)*. As noted above, the MRC AML 10 trial compared 10 days of AraC along with anthracycline in combination with either etoposide or 6-thioguanine *(122,129)*. There was no significant difference in remission rate for either etoposide or 6-thioguanine, both giving a remission rate of approx 85% following one or two courses of therapy and 92% following four cycles of treatment. The LAME 89/91 study utilized AraC at 1000 mg/m^2 for 5 days and replaced the standard 3 days of daunomycin with 5 days of mitoxantrone and demonstrated a remission rate of 87% *(139)*. The BFM trials 83 and 87 as well as several Nordic trials increased the exposure to AraC during the first 14 days of treatment and demonstrated a similar remission rate to other studies *(140–143)*.

An alternative approach, tested in the CCG-2891 trial, attempted to test the hypothesis that intensively timed chemotherapy would recruit and kill leukemic cells based on cell cycle kinetic studies. The CCG-2891 trial randomized a "standard" vs "intensive" timing induction using the five-drug DCTER (dexamethasone, cytarabine, thioguanine, etoposide, rubidomyicin) regimen *(144,145)*. Intensively timed induction therapy gave the second course of DCTER on days 10–13 regardless of bone marrow status, while standard timing delivered the second course of chemotherapy following bone marrow recovery, usually at about 30 days. The complete remission rate for the intensive and standard timing arm was 78% and 74%, respectively, which was not statistically significant *(144,145)*. However, despite the similar remission rate, the intensively timed arm had a lower relapse rate and a significantly improved event-free survival (EFS) and overall survival (OS) compared to the standard timing arm regardless of postinduction therapy *(144,145)*. This study therefore demonstrated that increased timing intensity during remission induction therapy was associated with a greater toxicity but an overall more favorable outcome, suggesting that a higher-quality remission has an impact on outcome regardless of the type of postremission treatment.

With the limits of intensification essentially reached at this time, the major challenge for improving remission rates is to introduce novel agents that are more effective against the relevant leukemic cells while not introducing additional and especially, overlapping toxicities. Such agents being tested in pediatric trials include anti-CD33–calicheamicin antibody conjugates (gemtuzomab ozagomicin) *(146)* and inhibitors of activated tyrosine kinases, such as FLT3, or their downstream signaling pathways *(147)*. The promise of molecularly characterizing leukemias at the time of diagnosis in order to direct initial treatment is also a much-anticipated possibility. Such an approach would avoid exposing all patients to the considerable toxicity of currently used remission induction treatments.

6.2. Postremission Treatment

Although there are no definitive data as to how many postremission courses of therapy are required to effectively cure AML, without any postremission therapy, nearly all patients will have a relapse of their disease. The type and length of postremission therapy have been the subject of multiple, pivotal clinical trials.

6.3. Intensification or Maintenance

Several early studies from Saint Jude Children's Research Hospital (SJCRH AML-76), the Children's Cancer Group (CCG-241), and the German cooperative groups demonstrated that postremission therapy resulted in a 20–25% 2-year relapse-free survival, but that patients who did not receive postremission therapy nearly all died from leukemia *(148–150)*. The DFCI 80-035 and the SJCRH AML-80 studies both gave non-cross-resistant combination chemotherapy sequentially for about 1 year but did not achieve significantly better results than previous trials giving less therapy *(151–154)*. The BFM-78 trial used 2 years of mainte-nance therapy after induction and consolidation courses of therapy and showed an EFS of 35% (150).

The MRC AML8 trial from the 1970s used a common induction regimen for children and adults consisting of daunorubicin, cytarabine, and 6-thioguanine (DAT 1+5). The remission rate was 67%. One portion of this trial randomized patients to two or six cycles of consolidation therapy with DAT. A second portion of the protocol randomized patients who were still in remission at the end of 1 year to cytarabine and 6-thioguanine maintenance therapy or late intensification with cyclophosphamide, vincristine, cytarabine, and prednisolone. There was no significant difference in outcome between the short or long courses of consolidation therapy and only a marginally significant improvement for patients given late intensification compared with continued maintenance therapy. Relapse-free survival for all patients enrolled on the study was only 18% *(155,156)*.

The POG-8101 trial randomized patients between two postremission maintenance arms, which differed in that one group received daunomycin/AraC and 6TG/Ara-C/5AZ in addition to AraC/6TG and COAP. The maintenance period lasted 2 years and showed results similar to previous trials of that period *(124)*. Another important study of that era was the LAME 89/91 study, which randomized children to 18 months of maintenance therapy with low-dose mercaptopurine and cytarabine vs more intensive postremission therapy; the maintenance

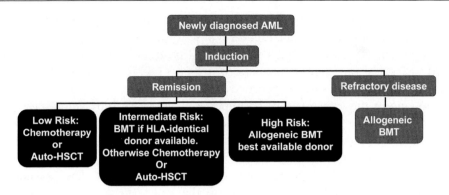

Fig. 2. Flow algorithm for risk-based assignment of treatment for pediatric patients with newly diagnosed acute myeloid leukemia (AML). Of note, in MRC and BFM clinical trials (*see* text), patients with intermediate risk AML are considered for allogeneic hematopoietic stem cell transplantation (HSCT) in CR2. In the United States and in COG trials, patients in the intermediate risk group are offered an allogeneic HSCT in CR1. (Please *see* text for details.)

regimen had a significantly lower OS *(157)*. Several studies in adults also strongly suggested that increasing the intensity of postremission therapy, especially with high-dose AraC, resulted in a lower relapse rate than that observed with less intense maintenance therapy, especially in patients with favorable cytogenetics such as t(8;21) or inv(16) *(158,159)*.

The CCG-213 trial, which ran from 1985 through 1989, assigned patients to a 4-month postremission intensification treatment and then randomized patients to 2 years of maintenance therapy or no further treatment *(160)*. This study and the CCG-213P trial showed that intensification of postremission therapy resulted in a better outcome. Other contemporary studies, such as the SJCRH AML-83, BFM-83, BFM-87, and POG-8498, also pointed to increased dose intensity, particularly with AraC, as being responsible for a lower relapse rate and longer DFS than obtained with more conventional, lower dose AraC *(140,150,154,161)*. As noted above, in the CCG-2891 trial, patients who received induction therapy with intensively timed DCTER had a statistically significant survival advantage compared to that observed for standard timing DCTER regardless of the type of postremission therapy received *(145,162)*. Thus, several studies have demonstrated that increased intensity of early treatment appears to abrogate the benefit of maintenance, lower dose chemotherapy. The BFM study group still uses maintenance chemotherapy based on the results of thr BFM-87 trial, in which a maintenance phase was beneficial to a low-risk group of patients not receiving HSCT although the outcome for patients who received maintenance therapy was worse following relapse *(142)*. Another exception is APL, in which maintenance therapy has been shown to improve outcomes; this has been true in pediatric as well as adult patients *(163)*.

6.4. How Many Cycles of Postremission Therapy Are Necessary?

The above trials, using fewer, more intensive courses compared to a greater number of less intensive courses of treatment, have demonstrated that shorter intense therapy precludes the necessity to have prolonged maintenance phases. However, very little information is available on the optimal number of courses of therapy.

Tallman et al., examined the impact of the number of postremission cycles of chemotherapy before HLA-matched sibling donor bne marrow transplant on the survival of adult patients with AML *(164)*. This study concluded that there was no survival advantage for patients who received postremission chemotherapy compared with patients who proceeded directly to bone marrow transplant as soon as remission was achieved. Unfortunately, one needs to be cautious in interpreting the conclusions of this report because it was based on a retrospective nonrandomized design and did not require a standardized postremission treatment regimen. The MRC AML 12 study randomized patients to a total of four vs five courses of therapy. Preliminary results from this study suggest no difference between four and five courses *(121)*. Longer follow-up of these results will be important. The CCG-2961 study gave patients a total of three courses of intensive chemotherapy with comparable results to other trials, suggesting that fewer courses may be adequate *(165)*. This question is particularly significant in light of the morbidity and mortality associated with each course of intensive chemotherapy. With only approx 50% of all patients being cured and surviving, any consideration of decrease in therapy may need to be studied in only the very best risk groups, such as younger children with DS or possibly those with rapid early responses without evidence for minimal residual disease and inv(16).

6.5. Do All Patients With AML Require an Allogeneic HSCT in First Remission? The Importance of Risk Group Stratification

While both autologous and allogeneic HSCT represent alternative approaches to intensification, allogeneic transplantation also provides the potential advantage of immune-mediated antileukemia responses. However, HSCT is associated with increased acute and long-term morbidity and mortality. Several randomized studies in pediatrics have shown no advantage of autologous bone marrow transplantation compared to chemotherapy alone *(139,144,166)*. Thus, in terms of OS, either treatment approach appears equivalent. On the other hand, a majority of clinical trials have demonstrated a consistent advantage for allogeneic HSCT in terms of DFS, but not always in OS *(139,144,167–169)*. The lack of an advantage in OS in some reports is in part a result of the significant short- and long-term morbidity and mortality associated with this type of transplant *(168,169)*.

Given the potential for improved disease control and the potential complications of transplantation, significant questions are when and in which patients should allogeneic HSCT be offered *(167,168,170)*. To provide answers to these questions, a prospective analysis of prognostic factors and subgroups comparing outcomes for patients being treated with chemotherapy alone (or with autologous HSCT) vs those being treated with allogeneic HSCT would be key. Such information would provide the basis for a stratification analysis with transplant vs chemotherapy outcomes compared across different subsets of patients. Another important issue is to evaluate the impact of patient selection in which not all patients receive the initially intended treatment. Third, the evaluation of outcomes for patients receiving chemotherapy vs transplant can also provide insight into which subgroups would receive a selective advantage from one or the other type of postremission therapy. For example, if a subset of patients were to benefit from HSCT compared to chemotherapy alone, then the factor(s) identifying, for instance, that group of patients as high risk upon receiving chemotherapy alone would lose its significance when transplantation was used. Therefore, it is important to understand the characteristics and outcomes of different subgroups of patients with newly diagnosed AML who are treated with chemotherapy alone or with allogeneic HSCT.

The European Bone Marrow Transplantation group reviewed the outcomes of patients with newly diagnosed AML who received a HSCT in CR1 from 1980 to 1995. The analysis included 846 patients who received an autologous HSCT and 826 patients who received a matched sibling donor HSCT *(171)*. The impact of cytogenetics was closely examined, with "good" cytogenetics being those that included t(15;17), t(8;21), or inv(16) chromosome abnormalities and "poor" cytogenetics being those that included abnormalities of chromosomes 5 and/or 7, 11q or had hypodiploidy. All other patients were considered to have "standard" risk cytogenetics. The EFS was the same (46%) for patients with "good" or "standard" cytogenetics who received autologous HSCT. For those patients receiving matched sibling donor allografts, there was a small EFS and relapse advantage in the "good" risk compared to the "standard" risk cytogenetic group (62% vs 58%, respectively, and 12% vs 24 incidence of relapse, respectively). Patients with poor risk cytogenetics did relatively poorly regardless of transplant type with a 26% and 27% EFS after autologous vs allogeneic transplant, respectively. In addition, patients with poor risk cytogenetics had a higher relapse rate compared to patients with standard risk cytogenetics with either autologous (73% vs 49%, respectively) or allografts (62% vs 24%, respectively). A multivariate analysis of the characteristics of this large patient population showed that longer interval from diagnosis to CR1 of more than 39 days was significantly associated with worse EFS for both autologous and allogeneic HSCT. These results suggest that time to remission, i.e., initial response to therapy, is important across all cytogenetic risk groups. In addition, these analyses suggest that allogeneic HSCT does not benefit all cytogenetic risk groups equally. This conclusion further emphasized that some poor prognosis, biological characteristics of different AML subgroups may be less likely to be overcome with allogeneic HSCT than other types.

The importance of cytogenetics in predicting outcome for patients with AML has been demonstrated in multiple studies independent of what the postremission therapy includes. "Favorable" cytogenetics, including the t(8;21), t(15;17) and inv(16) chromosome abnormalities, can be contrasted with "poor" cytogenetics, which primarily include abnormalities of chromosomes 5 and/or 7. "Standard" risk cytogenetics include the group of patients whose AML contains chromosome abnormalities not present in favorable or poor risk groups. Favorable cytogenetics portend a significantly improved outcome in both adult and pediatric patients *(172–178)*. For example, in the MRC AML 10 trial, patients with favorable cytogenetics (whether pediatric or adult) had a significantly improved response to induction therapy, relapse rate, and survival than patients with standard or poor risk cytogenetics *(176)*. Of note, however, is that in the pediatric age group, the difference was less marked and the relapse-free survival was similar between the favorable and standard risk groups *(122)*. The outcomes have not shown a significant advantage in OS of HSCT in first remission compared to chemotherapy alone in either the favorable or standard cytogenetic risk groups in the MRC 10 and the subsequent trials thus far reported *(121,122,169)*.

The POG 8821 study demonstrated that patients with AML having a t(8;21) or inv(16) abnormality had a significantly improved remission rate compared to patients with a normal karyotype *(179)*. Interestingly, patients with an inv(16) abnormality had a better OS (75%) than patients with a normal karyotype (54%), but patients with a t(8;21) abnormality had a higher relapse rate compared to those with inv(16). Nevertheless, the overall outcome was similar in those patients with inv(16) because of the higher salvage rate for patients with t(8;21) compared to patients with a normal karyotype. Similar findings were observed in the subsequent POG 9421 trial *(128)*. The CCG 2891 trial also demonstrated an advantage of favorable cytogenetics in terms of outcome. Although there was a suggestion that allogeneic HSCT improved survival in the favorable cytogenetics group compared to chemotherapy, the number of patients in the subgroups was insufficient to make definitive conclusions *(180)*.

Unfavorable cytogenetics as defined above have been associated with a poor prognosis in multiple clinical trials for children or adults. However, children with these adverse karyotypes appear to have better accounts than adults with these abnormalities; these results suggest that either the adult host (age, comorbidities) or the intrinsic characteristics of the adult AML (acquisition of additional resistance pathways) differ from that of children as the treatment on the MRC trials is essentially the same for all age groups *(122,176,181)*.

The potential role of molecular markers identifiable at the time of diagnosis or soon thereafter in helping to risk-stratify patients to chemotherapy or autologous HSCT vs allogeneic HSCT is becoming increasingly important. For example, the internal tandem duplication (ITD) mutations in the FLT3 receptor have been strongly associated with a very poor prognosis in patients with AML *(182–189)*. The correlation with poor outcome is particularly strong in cases in which there is a high allelic ratio of FLT3-ITD to normal alleles *(185,188)*. Thus, the allelic ratio appears to be a continuous variable, but with a survival reported to be essentially 0% with an allelic ratio of >0.78 compared to 60% for an allelic ratio of <0.78. In pediatrics, a FLT3-ITD–to–normal allelic ratio of >0.69 was reported to have an extremely poor prognosis compared to those with a lower ratio, which in turn was not different from that in patients without a FLT3-ITD mutation *(185,188)*. Point mutations involving the 835/836 codons in the tyrosine kinase domain of FLT3 do not carry a poor prognosis *(185,187,190)*. Additional work has demonstrated by microarray RNA analysis that patients with a low RUNX3-to-ATRX transcript expression ratio had a 70% survival, while a high ratio predicted an extremely poor prognosis *(191)*. Results such as these emphasize the complexity of using a single marker to serve as a prognostic factor in which to stratify treatment. Furthermore, while some data suggest that allogeneic HSCT can overcome the resistance of patients with FLT3-ITDs, these data are not extensive, prospective, or without controversy *(192)*. This remains an important issue to be addressed.

However, a group of patients with mutations of either tyrosine kinase receptors (e.g., FLT3-ITD, c-KIT, c-fms) or RAS was shown to have an approx 70% DFS with allogeneic HSCT compared to only 23% DFS when postremission therapy included only chemotherapy or autologous HSCT *(189)*. In contrast, mutation-negative patients had a 55% DFS with allogeneic HSCT and 40% DFS with chemotherapy alone or autologous HSCT, suggesting that there was a selective effect of allogeneic HSCT in the group with such mutations. These data also suggest that allogeneic HSCT may provide a better outcome for patients with these mutations compared to patients with complex cytogenetics.

Mutations in the nucleophosmin (NPM) gene have been associated with an improved prognosis in adult AML, which has a normal karyotype and absence of FLT3-ITD mutations *(193–198)*. Such information would potentially provide information that would lead to a recommendation that the better risk standard cytogenetic group should not receive an allogeneic HSCT in CR1. At this time, however, insufficient pediatric data are available to confirm the NPM results observed in adults or to make informed recommendations for changes in treatment *(198,199)*. Similarly, activating mutations of c-KIT have now been correlated with a worse outcome for patients with core-binding factor AML than those without c-KIT mutations *(200–202)*. Whether or not allogeneic HSCT is able to make a significant difference in outcome for these patients is unclear.

The type of and response to induction therapy has been shown to affect the outcome following HSCT. As noted above, the group of patients receiving intensively timed DCTER in the CCG-2891 study showed an improved EFS after allogeneic BMT compared to those randomized to receive the same induction but with standard timing *(145,162)*. This has suggested that the "depth" of remission is an important prognostic factor regardless of the postremission therapy a patient receives. Minimal residual disease (MRD) has been associated with a significant risk of relapse in AML and APL *(203–205)*. The analysis of Nagler et al. *(206–209)* showed that the presence of MRD as assessed by multiparameter flow cytometry before HSCT was associated with a higher relapse rate among 21 patients undergoing transplant (46% vs 25%, respectively). Although this study had a small number of patients, other studies have also strongly suggested MRD positivity prior to transplant, even in the relapse setting, to be a poor prognostic factor *(210–212)*. In a French study the number of chemotherapy courses received prior to HSCT was associated with a worse EFS, suggesting that the heavily pretreated patients had either more resistant disease or the greater number of courses of chemotherapy selected for more transplant resistant disease *(213)*. Some data support the idea that HSCT can overcome MRD *(214)*.

Most pediatric cooperative groups now recommend reserving allogeneic HSCT for patients with favorable risk cytogenetics and good early responses to induction therapy after relapse and achievement of a second remission. Furthermore, these groups also mostly recommend HLA matched or one antigen mismatched family donor allogeneic HSCT for patients with high-risk cytogenetics or those patients not achieving remission after two courses of induction therapy, and those with refractory disease after one course of induction therapy. Some groups, notably the MRC and BFM groups, reserve allogeneic HSCT for patients with standard cytogenetic risk with good responses to remission induction treatment, while the COG trials recommend allogeneic HSCT in CR1 for all patients with standard or high-risk cytogenetic AML. The COG trials are also piloting an approach that will allow essentially any form of donor (e.g., HLA matched or partially matched family donors, cord blood, matched unrelated, mismatched unrelated, or haploidentical) for patients with monosomy 7 or with primary refractory disease. It remains unclear what the role of allogeneic HSCT is in this setting of highly refractory disease. Also, HSCT is not recommended in CR1 for patients with APL or patients less than 4 years of age with DS and megakaryoblastic leukemia because of the distinctive biology of the leukemia and/or host that are associated with excellent outcomes.

6.6. Quality of Life

The issue of acute and long-term adverse sequelae of children treated for AML with chemotherapy and/or HSCT remains an important concern and challenge. Leung et al. reported 77 patients treated for AML with a 10-year-from-diagnosis follow-up *(215)*. They showed that patients who received a HSCT experienced the most significant adverse sequelae, particularly involving stature, endocrine problems, infertility, learning difficulties, cataracts, cardiomyopathy, and restrictive lung disease. Of note is that patients who received total body irradiation (TBI) had an overall lower cumulative dose of anthracyclines (204 mg/m^2) compared to those who did not receive TBI (335 mg/m^2), but the frequency of cardiomyopathy was similar. The increased academic difficulties observed in the HSCT group were similar to those observed in patients who received chemotherapy plus cranial radiation.

A study by Michel et al. examined the late effects at a median of nearly 6 years following allogeneic HSCT for 45 children with AML in CR1 *(216)*. Of this group, 26 received busulfan plus cyclophosphamide, while 19 received TBI-containing regimens (9 with fractionated and 10 with single-dose TBI). There was a significant correlation of decreased height, increased incidence of cataracts, and higher frequency of hypothyroidism in the group receiving TBI. Leahey et al. compared the late effects in pediatric patients with AML who received chemotherapy alone or HSCT *(217)*. In this study, patients who received a HSCT had a higher frequency of gonadal failure, but height, renal, and cardiac function were similar between the two groups.

Patients in the POG 8821 study were analyzed for their time without symptoms or toxicity (TWiST) *(218)*. In contrast to other studies, the best TWiST outcomes were observed in

Table 1
Prognostic Factors and Risk Stratification in Pediatric AML

		Prognostic factors		
Risk group	Clinical	Cytogenetic/Molecular	Response to therapy	Molecular
Favourable risk	WBC < 20,000 μL Down Syndrome (<4 years ago)	t(15;17), inv(16), t(8;21), t(9;11)	Rapid response MRD negative	NPM mutations CEBPα mutations Gene expression profiling
Intermediate risk		Normal	<15% blasts after course 1	NPM mutations Gene expression profiling
High risk	WBC > 200,000 μL Secondary AML	5q-, monosomy 5 to 7 Abnormal 3 t(6;9) High	Poor response MRD positive	FLT3-ITD/Normal AR c-KIT mutations c-fms mutations RAS mutations High WT1 expression High VEGF expression High BAALC expression Gene expression profiling Race

patients who underwent an HLA-matched sibling donor HSCT in CR1 compared to patients who received chemotherapy alone or autologous HSCT. Of note, the overall and relapse-free survival were better in the group who received an allogeneic HSCT compared to those who received chemotherapy alone or an autologous HSCT. While such data suggest that if allogeneic transplantation goes well in terms of short- and long-term adverse sequelae, it offers significant advantages in terms of both disease control as well as quality of life. However, a cross-sectional analysis of MRC AML 10 survivors demonstrated that allogeneic or autologous HSCT was associated with decreased sexual functioning and infertility compared to chemotherapy-only regimens *(219)*. While such studies have inherent bias in terms of patient selection, they raise both critical questions in terms of future investigations as well as possibly useful interventions, such as gamete banking prior to HSCT, psychological support, and hormonal status monitoring.

6.7. Areas for Future Research

There are practical and immediately relevant questions that should be answered for children with AML. For example, it is imperative to develop evidence-based recommendations for when and in whom to use allogeneic HSCT from HLA matched or mismatched family or unrelated donors. Another critical question is how to determine in which patients nonmyeloablative allogeneic HSCT can be used, as this approach has the potential of significantly decreasing short- and long-term adverse sequelae. The nonablative approach to HSCT may also provide a platform on which posttransplantation therapies, such as small molecule inhibitors as well as immunostimulatory approaches, can be effectively tested. Whether immunostimulatory approaches can be developed in the setting of autologous HSCT or postchemotherapy is an important adjunctive question to test. In pediatric patients with AML, there is also a significant need to replace cardiotoxic agents with equally effective but non-cardiotoxic drugs. Alternatively, immediate consideration of testing cardioprotectants in this group of patients should be done, as has been the case in pediatric patients with ALL *(220)*.

Clearly, a major hope is that more molecularly targeted therapies will be developed that will increase antileukemic activity without adding significant toxicity. Some of these agents, such as antibody-directed therapies and tyrosine kinase inhibitors, are currently in Phase III or randomized Phase II clinical trials. Whether these approaches will have a future in terms of becoming part of standard treatment regimens will need to await the results of these and confirmatory clinical trials. In addition, while premature in most types of AML, an extended goal of targeted therapy should be to ultimately eliminate the need to use currently available cytotoxic chemotherapy with its inherent short- and long-term associated adverse sequelae. In the cases of APL or M7 AML in the young child with DS, such approaches are already being tested *(9,221,222)*. The subtypes of AML with distinctive molecular signatures, such as those with chromosomal translocations, mutations of signaling pathways, or distinct protein expression patterns, should also be able to be effectively targeted using leukemia-selective or -specific agents. Furthermore, as has been pointed out in many publications, the identification, therapeutic targeting, and tracking of leukemic self-repopulating progenitors or stem cells must be integrated into new agent development and clinical testing. In addition to small molecule development, more effective antibody-mediated or immunostimulatory approaches to leukemic cell killing need to be developed and tested.

How best to definitively test these current and future approaches will be a significant challenge. There is a tremendous need for more predictive in vitro and animal models for the many subtypes of AML. Whether RNA and protein expression analyses or genomic/epigenomic patterns will be able to truly predict whether modulating specific pathways results in clinical efficacy remains unclear. Nevertheless, these are areas in need of significant future investment. At this point in time, and in the conceivable future, the definitive proof that a drug improves outcomes in patients involves demonstrating this in the context of a well-designed and statistically powered clinical trial.

The increasing emphasis on subgroup analysis, prognostic factor stratification, and patient (host) characteristics is pushing the concept that "personalized treatment" will be a requirement for future therapeutic approaches. Thus, the historical approach of using one or two hammers to hit a heterogeneous group of nails is now challenged by the biologically based need to test new selective/specific treatments in increasingly smaller subgroups of patients with AML. Several solutions have been proposed to deal with this important issue. They include the use of standard or modified randomized Phase II trials that employ "pick-the-winner," Bayesian or adjustment of false-positive/negative error approaches to allow decisions of relative efficacy to be made *(223–229)*. The comparison to historical controls is another approach being used in groups with very small numbers of patients; clearly this approach has significant bias, but can be useful especially when one is dealing with extremes in outcomes such as when mortality is extremely high. In such a situation, small numbers of patients with a high success rate make it clear that something has worked. If any of these approaches can increase our ability to bring agents with a greater likelihood of showing efficacy in randomized Phase III trials, this will be a significant advance.

The accrual to Phase III trials will also continue to be a challenge, with diminishing numbers of patients characterized by specific subgroups. However, while often forgotten, it needs to be remembered that about 85% of children with cancer reside in developing countries. Thus, while significant cultural and policy obstacles may need to be overcome, it is essential that mechanisms for effective international trials be established. A potentially large benefit from molecularly targeted therapies is likely to be for patients in developing parts of the world because of the predicted decreased toxicities.

Another approach that has been used in some centers, most notably in the MRC trials, is to include pediatric and adult patients in the same clinical trial. However, such trials need to include more biological investigations into the molecular, genetic, and pharmacological differences between patients of different ages and their leukemias. A de-emphasis on chronological age accompanied by more emphasis on biological similarities and differences may provide a particularly useful approach to testing new agents. This type of approach also has the potential of increasing more timely access to novel agents for children and adolescents.

We are a long way from the day when leukemia and patient genetic profiling will be efficiently determined at the time of diagnosis and subsequently lead to a decision of precisely what combinations, doses, and schedules of nontoxic agents will be used to cure a patient. Until that time, we should be rapidly breaking down any obstacles that stand in the way of developing and testing less toxic approaches to AML. Short of prevention, this is the only hope for improving patient outcomes.

ACKNOWLEDGEMENTS

I am indebted to Drs. Allen Chen, Soheil Meshinchi, Frank Smith, William Woods, Beverly Lange, Irv Bernstein, Eric Sievers, Gary Dahl, Yaddanapudi Ravindranath, and Howard Weinstein for their input and dialogue on AML.

REFERENCES

1. Smith MA, Gloeckler-Ries LA, Gurney JG, Ross JA. Leukemia. In: Ries LAG, et al., eds. Cancer Incidence and Survival Among Children and Adolescents: United States SEER Program 1975-1995. National Cancer Institute, SEER Program. Bethesda, MD: NIH, 1999:17–34.

2. Parkin DM, Stiller CA, Draper GJ, et al. International Incidence of Childhood Cancer. Lyon: IARC Scientific Publication No. 87, 1988.

3. Ross JA, Davies SM, Potter JD. Epidemiology of childhood leukemia, with a focus on infants. Epidemiol Rev 1994;16:243–272.

4. Robison LL, Ross JA. Epidemiology of leukaemias and lymphomas in childhood. In: Chessels J, Hann I, eds. Bailliere's Clinical Paediatrics. London: W.B. Saunders Co., 1995:639–657.

5. Le Deley MC, Leblanc T, Shamsaldin A, et al. Risk of secondary leukemia after a solid tumor in childhood according to the dose of epipodophyllotoxins and anthracyclines: a case-control study by the Societe Francaise d'Oncologie Pediatrique. J Clin Oncol 2003;21(6):1074–1081.

6. Micallef IN, Lillington DM, Apostolidis J, et al. Therapy-related myelodysplasia and secondary acute myelogenous leukemia after high-dose therapy with autologous hematopoietic progenitor-cell support for lymphoid malignancies. J Clin Oncol 2000;18(5):947–955.

7. Smith MA, McCaffrey RP, Karp JE. The secondary leukemias: challenges and research directions. J Natl Cancer Inst 1996;88(7):407–418.

8. Ross JA, Spector LG, Robison LL, Olshan AF. Epidemiology of leukemia in children with Down syndrome. Pediatr Blood Cancer 2005;44(1):8–12.

9. Gamis AS. Acute myeloid leukemia and Down syndrome evolution of modern therapy—state of the art review. Pediatr Blood Cancer 2005;44(1):13–20.

10. Massey GV, Zipursky A, Chang MN, et al. A prospective study of the natural history of transient leukemia (TL) in neonates with Down syndrome (DS): Children's Oncology Group (COG) study POG-9481. Blood 2006;107(12):4606–4613.

11. Doyle JJ, Thorner P, Poon A, Tanswell K, Kamel-Reid S, Zipursky A. Transient leukemia followed by megakaryoblastic leukemia in a child with mosaic Down syndrome. Leuk Lymphoma 1995;17(3–4): 345–350.

12. Cushing T, Clericuzio CL, Wilson CS, et al. Risk for leukemia in infants without Down syndrome who have transient myeloproliferative disorder. J Pediatr 2006;148(5):687–689.

13. Reeves RH. Down syndrome mouse models are looking up. Trends Mol Med 2006;12(6):237–240.

14. Crispino JD. GATA1 mutations in Down syndrome: implications for biology and diagnosis of children with transient myeloproliferative disorder and acute megakaryoblastic leukemia. Pediatr Blood Cancer 2005; 44(1):40–44.

15. Shimada A, Xu G, Toki T, Kimura H, Hayashi Y, Ito E. Fetal origin of the GATA1 mutation in identical twins with transient myeloproliferative disorder and acute megakaryoblastic leukemia accompanying Down syndrome. Blood 2004;103(1):366.

16. Taub JW, Mundschau G, Ge Y, et al. Prenatal origin of GATA1 mutations may be an initiating step in the development of megakaryocytic leukemia in Down syndrome. Blood 2004;104(5):1588–1589.

17. Hitzler JK, Zipursky A. Origins of leukaemia in children with Down syndrome. Nat Rev Cancer 2005;5(1): 11–20.

18. Ge Y, Dombkowski AA, LaFiura KM, et al. Differential gene expression, GATA1 target genes, and the chemotherapy sensitivity of Down syndrome megakaryocytic leukemia. Blood 2006;107(4):1570–1581.

19. Lightfoot J, Hitzler JK, Zipursky A, Albert M, Macgregor PF. Distinct gene signatures of transient and acute megakaryoblastic leukemia in Down syndrome. Leukemia 2004;18(10):1617–123.

20. Harigae H, Xu G, Sugawara T, Ishikawa I, Toki T, Ito E. The GATA1 mutation in an adult patient with acute megakaryoblastic leukemia not accompanying Down syndrome. Blood 2004;103(8):3242–3243.

21. Chaganti RS, Bailey RB, Jhanwar SC, Arlin ZA, Clarkson BD. Chronic myelogenous leukemia in the monosomic cell line of a fertile Turner syndrome mosaic (45,X/46,XX). Cancer Genet Cytogenet 1982; 5(3):215–221.

22. Oguma N, Takemoto M, Oda K, et al. Chronic myelogenous leukemia and Klinefelter's syndrome. Eur J Haematol 1989;42(2):207–208.

23. Auerbach AD. Fanconi anemia and leukemia: tracking the genes. Leukemia 1992;6(suppl 1):1–4.

24. Rosenberg PS, Huang Y, Alter BP. Individualized risks of first adverse events in patients with Fanconi anemia. Blood 2004;104(2):350–355.

25. Alter BP. Cancer in Fanconi anemia, 1927–2001. Cancer 2003;97(2):425–440.

26. D'Andrea AD. The Fanconi road to cancer. Genes Dev 2003;17(16):1933–1936.

27. Gurtan AM, D'Andrea AD. Dedicated to the core: Understanding the Fanconi anemia complex. DNA Repair 2006;5(9–10):1119–1125.

28. Taniguchi T, D'Andrea AD. Molecular pathogenesis of Fanconi anemia: recent progress. Blood 2006; 107(11):4223–4233.

29. Marrone A, Dokal I.Dyskeratosis congenita: molecular insights into telomerase function, ageing and cancer. Expert Rev Mol Med 2004;6(26):1–23.

30. Vulliamy TJ, Knight SW, Mason PJ, Dokal I. Very short telomeres in the peripheral blood of patients with X-linked and autosomal dyskeratosis congenita. Blood Cells Mol Dis 2001;27(2):353–357.

31. Polychronopoulou S, Koutroumba P. Telomere length variation and telomerase activity expression in patients with congenital and acquired aplastic anemia. Acta Haematol 2004;111(3):125–131.

32. Fundia A, Gorla N, Larripa I. Non-random distribution of spontaneous chromosome aberrations in two Bloom syndrome patients. Hereditas, 1995;122(3):239–243.

33. Poppe B, Van Limbergen H, Van Roy N, et al. Chromosomal aberrations in Bloom syndrome patients with myeloid malignancies. Cancer Genet Cytogenet 2001;128(1):39–42.

34. Viniou N, Terpos E, Rombos J, et al. Acute myeloid leukemia in a patient with ataxia-telangiectasia: a case report and review of the literature. Leukemia 2001;15(10):1668–1670.

35. Khanna KK. Cancer risk and the ATM gene: a continuing debate. J Natl Cancer Inst 2000;92(10):795–802.

36. Buijs A, Poddighe P, van Wijk R, et al. A novel CBFA2 single-nucleotide mutation in familial platelet disorder with propensity to develop myeloid malignancies. Blood 2001;98(9):2856–2858.

37. Song WJ, Sullivan MG, Legare RD, et al. Haploinsufficiency of CBFA2 causes familial thrombocytopenia with propensity to develop acute myelogenous leukaemia (see comments). Nat Genet 1999;23(2):166–175.

38. Tonelli R, Scardovi AL, Pession A, et al. Compound heterozygosity for two different amino-acid substitution mutations in the thrombopoietin receptor (c-mpl gene) in congenital amegakaryocytic thrombocytopenia (CAMT). Hum Genet 2000;107(3):225–233.

39. Zeidler C, Schwinzer B, Welte K. Congenital neutropenias. Rev Clin Exp Hematol 2003;7(1):72–83.

40. Horwitz M, Li FQ, Albani D, et al. Leukemia in severe congenital neutropenia: defective proteolysis suggests new pathways to malignancy and opportunities for therapy. Cancer Invest 2003;21(4):579–587.

41. Carlsson G, Aprikyan AA, Goransdotter Ericson K, et al. Neutrophil elastase and granulocyte colony-stimulating factor receptor mutation analyses and leukemia evolution in severe congenital neutropenia patients belonging to the original Kostmann family in northern Sweden. Haematologica 2006;91(5):589–595.

42. Dale DC, Person RE, Bolyard AA, et al. Mutations in the gene encoding neutrophil elastase in congenital and cyclic neutropenia. Blood 2000;96(7):2317–2322.

43. Dale DC, Bolyard AA, Aprikyan A. Cyclic neutropenia. Semin Hematol 2002;39(2):89–94.

44. Hunter MG, Avalos BR. Granulocyte colony-stimulating factor receptor mutations in severe congenital neutropenia transforming to acute myelogenous leukemia confer resistance to apoptosis and enhance cell survival. Blood 2000;95(6):2132–2137.

45. Zeidler C, Boxer L, Dale DC, Freedman MH, Kinsey S, Welte K. Management of Kostmann syndrome in the G-CSF era. Br J Haematol 2000;109(3):490–495.

46. Zeidler C, Welte K. Kostmann syndrome and severe congenital neutropenia. Semin Hematol 2002; 39(2):82–88.

47. Dror Y. Shwachman-Diamond syndrome. Pediatr Blood Cancer 2005;45(7):892–901.

48. Kawakami T, Mitsui T, Kanai M, et al. Genetic analysis of Shwachman-Diamond syndrome: phenotypic heterogeneity in patients carrying identical SBDS mutations. Tohoku J Exp Med 2005;206(3):253–259.

49. Majeed F, Jadko S, Freedman MH, Dror Y. Mutation analysis of SBDS in pediatric acute myeloblastic leukemia. Pediatr Blood Cancer 2005;45(7):920–924.

50. Nicolis E, Bonizzat A, Assael BM, Cipoli M. Identification of novel mutation in patients with Shwachman-Diamond Syndrome. Hum Mutat 2005;25(4):410.

51. Nicolis A, Klein GW, Lipton JM. The Diamond Blackfan Anemia Registry: tool for investigating the epidemiology and biology of Diamond-Blackfan anemia. J Pediatr Hematol Oncol 2001;23(6):377–382.

52. Willig TN, Draptchinskaia N, Dianzani I, et al. Mutations in ribosomal protein S19 gene and diamond blackfan anemia: wide variations in phenotypic expression. Blood 1999;94(12):4294–4306.

53. Draptchinskaia N, Gustavsson P, Andersson B, et al. The gene encoding ribosomal protein S19 is mutated in Diamond-Blackfan anaemia. Nat Genet 1999;21(2):169–175.

54. Cmejla R, Blafkova J, Stopka T, et al. Ribosomal protein S19 gene mutations in patients with diamond-blackfan anemia and identification of ribosomal protein S19 pseudogenes. Blood Cells Mol Dis 2000;26(2):124–132.
55. Gazda H, Lipton JM, Willig TN, et al. Evidence for linkage of familial Diamond-Blackfan anemia to chromosome 8p23.3-p22 and for non-19q non-8p disease. Blood 2001;97(7):2145–2150.
56. Liu JM, Ellis SR. Ribosomes and marrow failure: coincidental association or molecular paradigm? Blood 2006;107(12):4583–4588.
57. Ellis SR, Massey AT. Diamond Blackfan anemia: a paradigm for a ribosome-based disease. Med Hypotheses 2006;66(3):643–648.
58. Amsterdam A, Sadler KC, Lai K, et al. Many ribosomal protein genes are cancer genes in zebrafish. PLoS Biol 2004;2(5):E139.
59. Dasgupta B, Gutmann DH. Neurofibromatosis 1: closing the GAP between mice and men. Curr Opin Genet Dev 2003;13(1):20–27.
60. Shannon KM, Watterson J, Johnson P, et al. Monosomy 7 myeloproliferative disease in children with neurofibromatosis, type 1: epidemiology and molecular analysis. Blood 1992;79(5):1311–1318.
61. Nakai H, Misawa S, Horiike S, et al. Analysis of mutations and expression of GAP-related domain of the neurofibromatosis type 1 (NF1) gene in the progression of chronic myelogenous leukemia. Leukemia 1994;8(6):1027–1033.
62. Baralle D, Mattocks C, Kalidas K, et al. Different mutations in the NF1 gene are associated with Neurofibromatosis-Noonan syndrome (NFNS). Am J Med Genet 2003;119A(1):1–8.
63. Loh ML, Vattikuti S, Schubbert S, et al. Mutations in PTPN11 implicate the SHP-2 phosphatase in leukemogenesis. Blood 2004;103(6):2325–2331.
64. Tartaglia M, Niemeyer CM, Fragale A, et al. Somatic mutations in PTPN11 in juvenile myelomonocytic leukemia, myelodysplastic syndromes and acute myeloid leukemia. Nat Genet 2003;28:28.
65. Greaves MF, Maia AT, Wiemels JL, Ford AM. Leukemia in twins: lessons in natural history. Blood 2003;102(7):2321–2333.
66. Greaves MF, Wiemels J. Origins of chromosome translocations in childhood leukaemia. Nat Rev Cancer 2003;3(9):639–649.
67. Greaves M. Prenatal origins of childhood leukemia. Rev Clin Exp Hematol 2003;7(3):233–245.
68. Maia AT, Ford AM, Jalali GR, et al. Molecular tracking of leukemogenesis in a triplet pregnancy. Blood 2001;98(2):478–482.
69. Horwitz M. The genetics of familial leukemia. Leukemia 1997;11(8):1347–1359.
70. Riccardi VM, Humbert JR, Peakman D. Acute leukemia associated with trisomy 8 mosaicism and a familial translocation 46,XY,t(7;20)(p13;p12). Am J Med Genet 1978;2(1):15–21.
71. Markkanen A, Ruutu T, Rasi V, Franssila K, S Knuutila, de la Chapelle A. Constitutional translocation t(3;6)(p14;p11) in a family with hematologic malignancies. Cancer Genet Cytogenet 1987;25(1):87–95.
72. Minelli A, Maserati E, Giudici G, et al. Familial partial monosomy 7 and myelodysplasia: different parental origin of the monosomy 7 suggests action of a mutator gene. Cancer Genet Cytogenet 2001;124(2): 147–151.
73. Socie G, Henry-Amar M, Bacigalupo A, et al. Malignant tumors occurring after treatment of aplastic anemia. N Engl J Med 1993;329:1152–1157.
74. Maciejewski JP, Selleri C. Evolution of clonal cytogenetic abnormalities in aplastic anemia. Leuk Lymphoma 2004;45(3):433–440.
75. Geissler D, Thaler J, Konwalinka G, Peschel C. Progressive preleukemia presenting amegakaryocytic thrombocytopenic purpura: association of the 5q- syndrome with a decreased megakaryocytic colony formation and a defective production of Meg-CSF. Leuk Res 1987;11(8):731–737.
76. Xue Y, Zhang R, Guo Y, Gu J, Lin B. Acquired amegakaryocytic thrombocytopenic purpura with a Philadelphia chromosome. Cancer Genet Cytogenet 1993;69(1):51–56.
77. Harris JW, Koscick R, Lazarus HM, Eshleman JR, Medof ME. Leukemia arising out of paroxysmal nocturnal hemoglobinuria. Leuk Lymphoma 1999;32(5–6):401–426.
78. McBride ML. Childhood cancer and environmental contaminants. Can J Public Health 1998;89 (suppl 1): S53–62, S58–68.
79. Yin SN, Hayes RB, Linet MS, et al. A cohort study of cancer among benzene-exposed workers in China: overall results. Am J Ind Med 1996;29(3):227–235.
80. Yin SN, Hayes RB, Linet MS, et al. An expanded cohort study of cancer among benzene-exposed workers in China. Benzene Study Group. Environ Health Perspect, 1996;104 (suppl 6):1339–1341.

81. Shimizu Y, Schull WI, Kato H. Cancer risk among atomic bomb survivors: the RERF Life Span Study. JAMA 1990;264:601.

82. Jablon S, Kato H. Childhood cancer in relation to prenatal exposure to atomic-bomb radiation. Lancet 1970;2:1000.

83. Linet MS, Hatch EE, Kleinerman, RA, et al. Residential exposure to magnetic fields and acute lymphoblastic leukemia in children. N Engl J Med 1997;337(1):1–7.

84. Theriault G, Goldberg M, Miller AB, et al. Cancer risks associated with occupational exposure to magnetic fields among electric utility workers in Ontario and Quebec, Canada. Am J Epidemiol 1994;139:550.

85. Shu XO, Ross JA, Pendergrass TW, Reaman GH, Lampkin B, Robison LL. Parental alcohol consumption, cigarette smoking, and risk of infant leukemia: a Childrens Cancer Group study. J Natl Cancer Inst 1996;88(1):24–31.

86. Stjernfeldt M, Berglund K, Lindsten J, Ludvigsson J. Maternal smoking and irradiation during pregnancy as risk factors for child leukemia. Cancer Detect PRev 1992;16(2):129–135.

87. John EM, Savitz DA, Sandler DP. Prenatal exposure to parents' smoking and childhood cancer. Am J Epidemiol 1991;133(2):123–132.

88. Robison LL, Buckley JD, Daigle AE, et al. Maternal drug use and risk of childhood nonlymphoblastic leukemia among offspring. An epidemiologic investigation implicating marijuana (a report from the Childrens Cancer Study Group). Cancer 1989;63(10):1904–1911.

89. Alexander FE, Patheal SL, Biondi A, et al. Transplacental chemical exposure and risk of infant leukemia with MLL gene fusion. Cancer Res 2001;61(6):2542–2546.

90. Ross JA. Dietary flavonoids and the MLL gene: A pathway to infant leukemia? Proc Natl Acad Sci USA 2000;97(9):4411–4413.

91. Strick R, Strissel PL, Borgers S, Smith SL, Rowley JD. Dietary bioflavonoids induce cleavage in the MLL gene and may contribute to infant leukemia. Proc Natl Acad Sci USA 2000;97(9):4790–4795.

92. van Leeuwen FE. Risk of acute myelogenous leukaemia and myelodysplasia following cancer treatment. Baillieres Clin Haematol 1996;9(1):57–85.

93. Stine KC, Saylors RL, Sawyer JR, Becton DL. Secondary acute myelogenous leukemia following safe exposure to etoposide. J Clin Oncol 1997;15(4):1583–1586.

94. Duffner PK, Krischer JP, Horowitz ME, et al. Second malignancies in young children with primary brain tumors following treatment with prolonged postoperative chemotherapy and delayed irradiation: a Pediatric Oncology Group study. Ann Neurol 1998;44(3):313–316.

95. Kletzel M, Katzenstein HM, Haut PR, et al. Treatment of high-risk neuroblastoma with triple-tandem high-dose therapy and stem-cell rescue: results of the Chicago Pilot II Study. J Clin Oncol 2002;20(9): 2284–2292.

96. George RE, Li S, Medeiros-Nancarrow, C, et al. High-risk neuroblastoma treated with tandem autologous peripheral-blood stem cell-supported transplantation: long-term survival update. J Clin Oncol 2006;24(18):2891–2896.

97. Sandoval C, Pui CH, Bowman LC, et al. Secondary acute myeloid leukemia in children previously treated with alkylating agents, intercalating topoisomerase II inhibitors, and irradiation. J Clin Oncol 1993;11(6):1039–1045.

98. Relling MV, Yanishevski Y, Nemec J, et al. Etoposide and antimetabolite pharmacology in patients who develop secondary acute myeloid leukemia. Leukemia 1998;12(3):346–352.

99. Megonigal MD, Cheung NK, Rappaport EF, et al. Detection of leukemia-associated MLL-GAS7 transloca-tion early during chemotherapy with DNA topoisomerase II inhibitors. Proc Natl Acad Sci USA 2000;97(6):2814–2819.

100. Lapidot T, Sirard C, Vormoor J, et al. A cell initiating human acute myeloid leukaemia after transplantation into SCID mice. Nature 1994;367(6464):645–648.

101. Bonnet D, Dick JE. Human acute myeloid leukemia is organized as a hierarchy that originates from a primitive hematopoietic cell. Nat Med 1997;3(7):730–737.

102. Sutherland HJ, Blair A, Zapf RW. Characterization of a hierarchy in human acute myeloid leukemia progenitor cells. Blood 1996;87(11):4754–4761.

103. Hope KJ, Jin L, Dick JE. Acute myeloid leukemia originates from a hierarchy of leukemic stem cell classes that differ in self-renewal capacity. Nat Immunol 2004;5(7):738–743.

104. Dick JE. Acute myeloid leukemia stem cells. Ann NY Acad Sci 2005;1044:1–5.

105. Warner JK, Wang JC, Takenaka K, et al. Direct evidence for cooperating genetic events in the leukemic transformation of normal human hematopoietic cells. Leukemia 2005;19(10):1794–1805.

106. Chan IT, Kutok JL, Williams IR, et al. Oncogenic K-ras cooperates with PML-RAR alpha to induce an acute promyelocytic leukemia-like disease. Blood 2006;108(9):1708–1715.

107. Gilliland DG, Jordan CT, Felix CA. The molecular basis of leukemia. Hematology (Am Soc Hematol Educ Program), 2004:80–97.

108. Jordan CT. The potential of targeting malignant stem cells as a treatment for leukemia. Future Oncol 2005;1(2):205–207.

109. Jordan CT. A new approach to treatment of acute myelogenous leukemia using targeted therapy in combination with standard chemotherapy. Leuk Res 2004;28(11):1121–1122.

110. Guzman ML, Swiderski CF, Howard DS, et al. Preferential induction of apoptosis for primary human leukemic stem cells. Proc Natl Acad Sci USA 2002;99(25):16,220–16,225.

111. Huntly BJ, Gilliland DG. Leukaemia stem cells and the evolution of cancer-stem-cell research. Nat Rev Cancer 2005;5(4):311–321.

112. Kersey JH. Fifty years of studies of the biology and therapy of childhood leukemia. Blood 1997;90(11): 4243–4251.

113. Arceci RJ. Progress and controversies in the treatment of pediatric acute myelogenous leukemia. Curr Opin Hematol 2002;9(4):353–360.

114. Clark JJ, Smith FO, Arceci RJ. Update in childhood acute myeloid leukemia: recent developments in the molecular basis of disease and novel therapies. Curr Opin Hematol 2003;10(1):31–39.

115. Arceci RJ, Golub T. Acute myelogenous leukemia In: P. Pizzo and D. Poplack, Editors. Principles and Practice of Pediatric Oncology. Lippincott Williams and Wilkins: Philadelphia, 2006:591–644.

116. Yates J, Glidewell O, Wiernik P, et al. Cytosine arabinoside with daunorubicin or adriamycin for therapy of acute myelocytic leukemia: a CALGB study. Blood 1982;60(2):454–462.

117. Buckley JD, Lampkin BC, Nesbit ME, et al. Remission induction in children with acute non-lymphocytic leukemia using cytosine arabinoside and doxorubicin or daunorubicin: a report from the Childrens Cancer Study Group. Med Pediatr Oncol 1989;17(5):382–390.

118. Creutzig U, Korholz D, Niemeyer CM, et al. Toxicity and effectiveness of high-dose idarubicin during AML induction therapy: results of a pilot study in children. Klin Padiatr 2000;212(4):163–168.

119. Lange BJ, Dinndorf P, Smith FO, et al. Pilot study of idarubicin-based intensive-timing induction therapy for children with previously untreated acute myeloid leukemia: Children's Cancer Group Study 2941. J Clin Oncol 2004;22(1):150–156.

120. Wheatley K. Meta-analysis of randomized trials of idarubicin (IDAR) or metozantrone (Mito) vs daunorubicin (DNR) as induction therapy for acute myeloid leukaemia (AML). Blood 1995;86:43A.

121. Gibson BE, Wheatley K, Hann IM, et al. Treatment strategy and long-term results in paediatric patients treated in consecutive UK AML trials. Leukemia 2005;19(12):2130–2138.

122. Hann IM, Webb DK, Gibson BE, Harrison CJ. MRC trials in childhood acute myeloid leukaemia. Ann Hematol 2004;83 (suppl 1):S108–112.

123. Volger WR, Weiner RS, Moore JO, Omura GA, Bartolucci AA, Stagg M. Long-term follow-up of a randomized post-induction therapy trial in acute myelogenous leukemia (a Southeastern Cancer Study Group trial). Leukemia 1995;9(9):1456–1460.

124. Steuber CP, Civin C, Krischer J, et al. A comparison of induction and maintenance therapy for acute nonlymphocytic leukemia in childhood: results of a Pediatric Oncology Group study. J Clin Oncol 1991;9(2):247–258.

125. Dillman RO, Davis RB, Green MR, et al. A comparative study of two different doses of cytarabine for acute myeloid leukemia: a phase III trial of Cancer and Leukemia Group B. Blood 1991;78(10): 2520–2526.

126. Bishop JF, Matthews JP, Young GA, et al. A randomized study of high-dose cytarabine in induction in acute myeloid leukemia. Blood 1996;87(5):1710–1717.

127. Weick JK, Kopecky KJ, Appelbaum FR, et al. A randomized investigation of high-dose vs standard-dose cytosine arabinoside with daunorubicin in patients with previously untreated acute myeloid leukemia: a Southwest Oncology Group study. Blood 1996;88(8):2841–2851.

128. Becton D, Dahl GV, Ravindranath Y, et al. Randomized use of cyclosporin A (CsA) to modulate P-glycoprotein in children with AML in remission: Pediatric Oncology Group Study 9421. Blood 2006;107(4):1315–1324.

129. Hann IM, Stevens RF, Goldstone AH, et al. Randomized comparison of DAT vs ADE as induction chemotherapy in children and younger adults with acute myeloid leukemia. Results of the Medical Research Council's 10th AML trial (MRC AML10). Adult and Childhood Leukaemia Working Parties of the Medical Research Council. Blood 1997;89(7):2311–2318.

130. Heil G, Hoelzer D, Sanz MA, et al. A randomized, double-blind, placebo-controlled, phase III study of filgrastim in remission induction and consolidation therapy for adults with de novo acute myeloid leukemia. The International Acute Myeloid Leukemia Study Group. Blood 1997;90(12):4710–4718.
131. Takeshita A, Ohno R, Hirashima K, et al. A randomized double-blind controlled study of recombinant human granulocyte colony-stimulating factor in patients with neutropenia induced by consolidation chemotherapy for acute myeloid leukemia. (rG-CSF clinical study group). Rinsho Ketsueki, 1995;36(6):606–614.
132. Ganser A, Heil G. Use of hematopoietic growth factors in the treatment of acute myelogenous leukemia. Curr Opin Hematol 1997;4(3):191–195.
133. Witz F, Sadoun A, Perrin MC, et al. A placebo-controlled study of recombinant human granulocyte-macrophage colony-stimulating factor administered during and after induction treatment for de novo acute myelogenous leukemia in elderly patients. Groupe Ouest Est Leucemies Aigues Myeloblastiques (GOELAM). Blood 1998;91(8):2722–2730.
134. Ozkaynak MF, Krailo M, Chen Z, Feusner J. Randomized comparison of antibiotics with and without granulocyte colony-stimulating factor in children with chemotherapy-induced febrile neutropenia: a report from the Children's Oncology Group. Pediatr Blood Cancer 2005;45(3):274–280.
135. Alonzo TA, Kobrinsky NL, Aledo A, Lange BJ, Buxton AB, Woods WG. Impact of granulocyte colony-stimulating factor use during induction for acute myelogenous leukemia in children: a report from the Children's Cancer Group. J Pediatr Hematol Oncol 2002;24(8):627–635.
136. Moon HW, Shin S, Kim HY, et al. Therapeutic use of granulocyte-colony stimulating factor could conceal residual malignant cells in patients with AML1/ETO(+) acute myelogenous leukemia. Leukemia 2006; 20(8):1408–1413.
137. Schiffer CA, Dodge R, Larson RA. Long-term follow-up of Cancer and Leukemia Group B studies in acute myeloid leukemia. Cancer 1997;80(11 suppl):2210–2214.
138. Rees JK. Chemotherapy of acute myeloid leukaemia (AML) in UK: past, present and future. Bone Marrow Transplant 1989;4 (suppl 1):110–113.
139. Michel G, Leverger G, Leblanc T, et al. Allogeneic bone marrow transplantation vs aggressive post-remission chemotherapy for children with acute myeloid leukemia in first complete remission. A prospective study from the French Society of Pediatric Hematology and Immunology (SHIP). Bone Marrow Transplant 1996;17(2):191–196.
140. Creutzig U, Ritter J, Schellong G. Identification of two risk groups in childhood acute myelogenous leukemia after therapy intensification in study AML-BFM-83 as compared with study AML-BFM-78. AML-BFM Study Group. Blood 1990;75(10):1932–1940.
141. Sartori PC, Taylor MH, Stevens MC, Darbyshire PJ, Mann JR. Treatment of childhood acute myeloid leukaemia using the BFM-83 protocol. Med Pediatr Oncol 1993;21(1):8–13.
142. Creutzig U, Ritter J, Zimmermann M, Schellong G. Does cranial irradiation reduce the risk for bone marrow relapse in acute myelogenous leukemia? Unexpected results of the Childhood Acute Myelogenous Leukemia Study BFM-87. J Clin Oncol 1993;11(2):279–286.
143. Lie SO, Abrahamsson J, Clausen N, et al. Treatment stratification based on initial in vivo response in acute myeloid leukaemia in children without Down's syndrome: results of NOPHO-AML trials. Br J Haematol 2003;122(2):217–225.
144. Woods WG, Neudorf S, Gold S, et al. A comparison of allogeneic bone marrow transplantation, autologous bone marrow transplantation, and aggressive chemotherapy in children with acute myeloid leukemia in remission: a report from the Children's cancer group. Blood 2001;97(1):56–62.
145. Woods WG, Kobrinsky N, Buckley JD, et al. Timed-sequential induction therapy improves postremission outcome in acute myeloid leukemia: a report from the Children's Cancer Group. Blood 1996;87(12):4979–4989.
146. Arceci RJ, Sande J, Lange B, et al. Safety and efficacy of gemtuzumab ozogamicin in pediatric patients with advanced CD33+ acute myeloid leukemia. Blood 2005;106(4):1183–1188.
147. Gilliland DG. Targeted therapies in myeloid leukemias. Ann Hematol 2004;83 (suppl 1):S75–76.
148. Dahl GV, Kalwinsky DK, Mirro J, Look AT. A comparison of cytokinetically based vs intensive chemotherapy for childhood acute myelogenous leukemia. Hämatol Bluttransfus 1987;30:83–87.
149. Baehner RL, Kennedy A, Sather H, Chard RL, Hammond D. Characteristics of children with acute nonlymphocytic leukemia in long-term continuous remission: a report for Childrens Cancer Study Group. Med Pediatr Oncol 1981;9(4):393–403.
150. Ritter J, Creutzig U, Schellong G. Treatment results of three consecutive German childhood AML trials: BFM- 78, -83, and -87. AML-BFM-Group. Leukemia 1992;6 (suppl 2):59–62.
151. Weinstein HJ, Mayer RJ, Rosenthal DS, Coral FS, Camitta BM, Gelber RD. Chemotherapy for acute myelogenous leukemia in children and adults: VAPA update. Blood 1983; 62(2):315–319.

152. Weinstein HJ, Mayer RJ, Rosenthal DS, et al. Treatment of acute myelogenous leukemia in children and adults. N Engl J Med 1980;303(9):473–478.

153. Grier HE, Gelber RD, Link MP, Camitta BP, Clavell LA, Weinstein HJ. Intensive sequential chemotherapy for children with acute myelogenous leukemia: VAPA, 80-035, and HI-C-Daze. Leukemia 1992;6 (suppl 2): 48–51.

154. Dahl GV, Kalwinsky DK, Mirro J, et al. Allogeneic bone marrow transplantation in a program of intensive sequential chemotherapy for children and young adults with acute nonlymphocytic leukemia in first remission. J Clin Oncol 1990;8(2):295–303.

155. Rees JK, Gray RG, Swirsky D, Hayhoe FG. Principal results of the Medical Research Council's 8th acute myeloid leukaemia trial. Lancet 1986;2(8518):1236–1241.

156. Rees JK, Gray RG, Wheatley K. Dose intensification in acute myeloid leukaemia: greater effectiveness at lower cost. Principal report of the Medical Research Council's AML9 study. MRC Leukaemia in Adults Working Party. Br J Haematol 1996;94(1):89–98.

157. Perel Y, Auvrignon A, Leblanc T, et al. Impact of addition of maintenance therapy to intensive induction and consolidation chemotherapy for childhood acute myeloblastic leukemia: results of a prospective randomized trial, LAME 89/91. Leucamie Aique Myeloide Enfant. J Clin Oncol 2002;20(12):2774–2782.

158. Preisler HD, Raza A, Rustum Y, Browman G. The treatment of patients with acute nonlymphocytic leukemia in remission. Semin Oncol 1985;12 (2 suppl 3):91–97.

159. Buchner T, Urbanitz D, Hiddemann W, et al. Intensified induction and consolidation with or without maintenance chemotherapy for acute myeloid leukemia (AML): two multicenter studies of the German AML Cooperative Group. J Clin Oncol 1985;3(12):1583–1589.

160. Wells RJ, Woods WG, Lampkin BC, et al. Impact of high-dose cytarabine and asparaginase intensification on childhood acute myeloid leukemia: a report from the Childrens Cancer Group. J Clin Oncol 1993;11(3): 538–545.

161. Ravindranath Y, Steuber CP, Krischer J, et al. High-dose cytarabine for intensification of early therapy of childhood acute myeloid leukemia: a Pediatric Oncology Group study. J Clin Oncol 1991;9(4):572–580.

162. Woods WG, Kobrinsky N, Buckley J, et al. Intensively timed induction therapy followed by autologous or allogeneic bone marrow transplantation for children with acute myeloid leukemia or myelodysplastic syndrome: a Childrens Cancer Group pilot study. J Clin Oncol 1993;11(8):1448–1457.

163. de Botton S, Coiteux V, Chevret S, et al. Outcome of childhood acute promyelocytic leukemia with all-trans-retinoic acid and chemotherapy. J Clin Oncol 2004;22(8):1404–1412.

164. Tallman MS, Rowlings PA, Milone G, et al. Effect of post-remission chemotherapy before human leukocyte antigen- identical sibling transplantation for acute myelogenous leukemia in first complete remission. Blood 2000;96(4):1254–1258.

165. Aplenc R, Alonzo TA, Gerbing BR, et al. Ethnicity and survival in childhood acute myeloid leukemia: a report from the Children's Oncology Group. Blood 2006;108(1):74–80.

166. Ravindranath Y, Yeager AM, Chang MN, et al. Autologous bone marrow transplantation vs intensive consolidation chemotherapy for acute myeloid leukemia in childhood. Pediatric Oncology Group. N Engl J Med 1996;334(22):1428–1434.

167. Chen AR, Alonzo TA, Woods WG, Arceci RJ. Current controversies: which patients with acute myeloid leukaemia should receive a bone marrow transplantation?—an American view. Br J Haematol 2002; 118(2):378–384.

168. Burnett AK, Wheatley K, Goldstone AH, et al. The value of allogeneic bone marrow transplant in patients with acute myeloid leukaemia at differing risk of relapse: results of the UK MRC AML 10 trial. Br J Haematol 2002;118(2):385–400.

169. Gibson BE, Webb D, Wheatley K. Does transplant in first CR have a role in pediatric AML? A review of the MRC10 and 12 trials. Blood 2000;96:522a.

170. Creutzig U, Reinhardt D. Current controversies: which patients with acute myeloid leukaemia should receive a bone marrow transplantation?—a European view. Br J Haematol 2002;118(2):365–377.

171. Cahn JY, Labopin M, Sierra J, et al. No impact of high-dose cytarabine on the outcome of patients transplanted for acute myeloblastic leukaemia in first remission. Acute Leukaemia Working Party of the European Group for Blood and Marrow Transplantation (EBMT). Br J Haematol 2000;110(2):308–314.

172. Mrozek K, Heinonen K, de la Chapelle A, Bloomfield CD. Clinical significance of cytogenetics in acute myeloid leukemia. Semin Oncol 1997;24(1):17–31.

173. Wheatley K, Burnett AK, Goldstone AH, et al. A simple, robust, validated and highly predictive index for the determination of risk-directed therapy in acute myeloid leukaemia derived from the MRC AML 10 trial.

United Kingdom Medical Research Council's Adult and Childhood Leukaemia Working Parties. Br J Haematol 1999;107(1):69–79.

174. Hasle H, Arico M, Basso G, et al. Myelodysplastic syndrome, juvenile myelomonocytic leukemia, and acute myeloid leukemia associated with complete or partial monosomy 7. European Working Group on MDS in Childhood (EWOG-MDS). Leukemia 1999;13(3):376–385.

175. Ravindranath Y, Chang M, Steuber CP, et al. Pediatric Oncology Group (POG) studies of acute myeloid leukemia (AML): a review of four consecutive childhood AML trials conducted between 1981 and 2000. Leukemia 2005;19(12):2101–2116.

176. Grimwade D, Walker H, Oliver F, et al. The importance of diagnostic cytogenetics on outcome in AML: analysis of 1,612 patients entered into the MRC AML 10 trial. The Medical Research Council Adult and Children's Leukaemia Working Parties. Blood 1998;92(7):2322–2333.

177. Smith FO, Alonzo TA, Gerbing RB, Woods WG, Arceci RJ. Long-term results of children with acute myeloid leukemia: a report of three consecutive Phase III trials by the Children's Cancer Group: CCG 251, CCG 213 and CCG 2891. Leukemia 2005;19(12):2054–2062.

178. Creutzig U, Zimmermann M, Ritter J, et al. Treatment strategies and long-term results in paediatric patients treated in four consecutive AML-BFM trials. Leukemia 2005;19(12):2030–2042.

179. Raimondi SC, Chang MN, Ravindranath Y, et al. Chromosomal abnormalities in 478 children with acute myeloid leukemia: clinical characteristics and treatment outcome in a cooperative pediatric oncology group study-POG 8821. Blood 1999;94(11):3707–3716.

180. Alonzo TA, Wells RJ, Woods WG, et al. Post-remission therapy for children with acute myeloid leukemia: the children's cancer group experience in the transplant era. Leukemia 2005;19(6):965–970.

181. Arceci RJ, Burnett A, Estey E, Hills R, Woods WG. Acute myelogenous leukemia in adolescents and young adults: Who should treat? Am Soc Clin Oncol 2006:533–542.

182. Kiyoi H, Naoe T, Nakano Y, et al. Prognostic implication of FLT3 and N-RAS gene mutations in acute myeloid leukemia. Blood 1999;93(9):3074–3080.

183. Meshinchi S, Woods WG, Stirewalt DL, et al. Prevalence and prognostic significance of FLT3 internal tandem duplication in pediatric acute myeloid leukemia. Blood 2001;97(1):89–94.

184. Kondo M, Horibe K, Takahashi, Y, et al. Prognostic value of internal tandem duplication of the FLT3 gene in childhood acute myelogenous leukemia. Med Pediatr Oncol 1999;33(6):525–529.

185. Thiede C, Steudel C, Mohr B, et al. Analysis of FLT3-activating mutations in 979 patients with acute myelogenous leukemia: association with FAB subtypes and identification of subgroups with poor prognosis. Blood 2002;99(12):4326–4335.

186. Kottaridis PD, Gale RE, Linch DC. Prognostic implications of the presence of FLT3 mutations in patients with acute myeloid leukemia. Leuk Lymphoma 2003;44(6):905–913.

187. Meshinchi S, Alonzo T, Gerbing R, Stirewalt D, Lange B, Radich J. Clinical significance of FLT3 internal tandem duplication in pediatric AML, a CCG 2961 study. Blood 2003;102:98a.

188. Zwaan CM, Meshinchi S, Radich JP, et al. FLT3 internal tandem duplication in 234 children with acute myeloid leukemia: prognostic significance and relation to cellular drug resistance. Blood 2003;102(7):2387–2394.

189. Meshinchi S, Stirewalt DL, Alonzo TA, et al. Activating mutations of RTK/ras signal transduction pathway in pediatric acute myeloid leukemia. Blood 2003;17:17.

190. Yamamoto Y, Kiyoi H, Nakano Y, et al. Activating mutation of D835 within the activation loop of FLT3 in human hematologic malignancies. Blood 2001;97(8):2434–2439.

191. Lacayo NJ, Meshinchi S, Kinnunen P, et al. Gene expression profiles at diagnosis in de novo childhood AML patients identify FLT3 mutations with good clinical outcomes. Blood 2004;104(9):2646–2654.

192. Meshinchi S, Arceci RJ, Sanders JE, et al. Role of allogeneic stem cell transplantation in FLT3/ITD-positive AML. Blood 2006;108(1):400–401.

193. Chou WC, Tang JL, Lin LI, et al. Nucleophosmin mutations in de novo acute myeloid leukemia: the age-dependent incidences and the stability during disease evolution. Cancer Res 2006;66(6):3310–3316.

194. Alcalay M, Tiacci E, Bergomas R, et al. Acute myeloid leukemia bearing cytoplasmic nucleophosmin (NPMc+ AML) shows a distinct gene expression profile characterized by up-regulation of genes involved in stem-cell maintenance. Blood 2005;106(3):899–902.

195. Grisendi S, Pandolfi PP. NPM mutations in acute myelogenous leukemia. N Engl J Med 2005;352(3):291–292.

196. Falini B, Mecucci C, Tiacci E, et al. Cytoplasmic nucleophosmin in acute myelogenous leukemia with a normal karyotype. N Engl J Med 2005;352(3):254–266.

197. Schnittger S, Schoch C, Kern W, et al. Nucleophosmin gene mutations are predictors of favorable progno-
     sis in acute myelogenous leukemia with a normal karyotype. Blood 2005;106(12):3733–3739.
198. Thiede C, Koch S, Creutzig E, et al. Prevalence and prognostic impact of NPM1 mutations in 1485 adult
     patients with acute myeloid leukemia (AML). Blood 2006;107(10):4011–4020.
199. Cazzaniga G, Dell'Oro MG, Mecucci C, et al. Nucleophosmin mutations in childhood acute myelogenous
     leukemia with normal karyotype. Blood 2005;106(4):1419–1422.
200. Shimada A, Taki T, Tabuchi K, et al. KIT mutations, and not FLT3 internal tandem duplication, are strongly
     associated with a poor prognosis in pediatric acute myeloid leukemia with t(8;21): a study of the Japanese
     Childhood AML Cooperative Study Group. Blood 2006;107(5):1806–1809.
201. Schnittger S, Kohl TM, Haferlach T, et al. KIT-D816 mutations in AML1-ETO-positive AML are associ-
     ated with impaired event-free and overall survival. Blood 2006;107(5):1791–1799.
202. Cairoli R, Beghini A, Grillo G, et al. Prognostic impact of c-KIT mutations in core binding factor
     leukemias: an Italian retrospective study. Blood 2006;107(9):3463–3468.
203. San Miguel J, Martinez A, Macedo A, et al. Immunophenotyping investigation of minimal residual disease
     is a useful approach for predicting relapse in acute myeloid leukemia patients. Blood 1997;90:2465.
204. Sievers EL, Lange BJ, Alonzo TA, et al. Immunophenotypic evidence of leukemia after induction therapy
     predicts relapse: results from a prospective Children's Cancer Group study of 252 patients with acute
     myeloid leukemia. Blood 2003;101(9):3398–3406.
205. Jaeger U, Kainz B.Monitoring minimal residual disease in AML: the right time for real time. Ann Hematol
     2003;82(3):139–147.
206. Nagler A, Condiotti R, Rabinowitz R, Schlesinger M, Nguyen M, Terstappen LW. Detection of minimal
     residual disease (MRD) after bone marrow transplantation (BMT) by multi-parameter flow cytometry
     (MPFC). Med Oncol 1999;16(3):177–187.
207. Lee S, Kim YJ, Eom KS, et al. The significance of minimal residual disease kinetics in adults with newly
     diagnosed PML-RARalpha-positive acute promyelocytic leukemia: results of a prospective trial.
     Haematologica 2006;91(5):671–674.
208. Lo-Coco F, Breccia M, Diverio D. The importance of molecular monitoring in acute promyelocytic
     leukaemia. Best Pract Res Clin Haematol 2003;16(3):503–520.
209. Grimwade D. The significance of minimal residual disease in patients with t(15;17). Best Pract Res Clin
     Haematol 2002;15(1):137–158.
210. Krejci O, van der Velden VH, Bader P, et al. Level of minimal residual disease prior to haematopoietic stem
     cell transplantation predicts prognosis in paediatric patients with acute lymphoblastic leukaemia: a report
     of the Pre-BMT MRD Study Group. Bone Marrow Transplant 2003;32(8):849–851.
211. Nemecek ER, Gooley TA, Woolfrey AE, Carpenter PA, Matthews DC, Sanders JE. Outcome of allogeneic
     bone marrow transplantation for children with advanced acute myeloid leukemia. Bone Marrow Transplant
     2004;34(9):799–806.
212. Sierra J, Storer B,Hansen JA, et al. Transplantation of marrow cells from unrelated donors for treatment of
     high-risk acute leukemia: the effect of leukemic burden, donor HLA-matching, and marrow cell dose.
     Blood 1997;89(11):4226–4235.
213. Robin M, Guardiola P, Dombret H, et al. Allogeneic bone marrow transplantation for acute myeloblastic
     leukaemia in remission: risk factors for long-term morbidity and mortality. Bone Marrow Transplant
     2003;31(10):877–887.
214. Laane E, Derolf AR, Bjorklund E, et al. The effect of allogeneic stem cell transplantation on outcome in
     younger acute myeloid leukemia patients with minimal residual disease detected by flow cytometry at the
     end of post-remission chemotherapy. Haematologica 2006;91(6):833–836.
215. Leung W, Hudson MM, Strickland DK, et al. Late effects of treatment in survivors of childhood acute
     myeloid leukemia. J Clin Oncol 2000;18(18):3273–3279.
216. Michel G, Socie G, Gebhard F, et al. Late effects of allogeneic bone marrow transplantation for children with
     acute myeloblastic leukemia in first complete remission: the impact of conditioning regimen without total-
     body irradiation—a report from the Societe Francaise de Greffe de Moelle. J Clin Oncol 1997;15(6):2238–2246.
217. Leahey AM, Teunissen H, Friedman DL, Moshang T, Lange BJ, Meadows AT. Late effects of chemother-
     apy compared to bone marrow transplantation in the treatment of pediatric acute myeloid leukemia and
     myelodysplasia. Med Pediatr Oncol 1999;32(3):163–169.
218. Parsons SK, Gelber S, Cole BF, et al. Quality-adjusted survival after treatment for acute myeloid leukemia
     in childhood: a Q-TWiST analysis of the Pediatric Oncology Group Study 8821. J Clin Oncol 1999;
     17(7):2144–2152.

219. Watson M, Wheatley K, Harrison GA, et al. Severe adverse impact on sexual functioning and fertility of bone marrow transplantation, either allogeneic or autologous, compared with consolidation chemotherapy alone: analysis of the MRC AML 10 trial. Cancer 1999;86(7):1231–1239.
220. Lipshultz SE, Rifai N, Dalton VM, et al. The effect of dexrazoxane on myocardial injury in doxorubicin-treated children with acute lymphoblastic leukemia. N Engl J Med 2004;351(2):145–153.
221. Estey EH. Treatment options for relapsed acute promyelocytic leukaemia. Best Pract Res Clin Haematol 2003;16(3):521–534.
222. Estey EH, Giles FJ, Beran M, et al. Experience with gemtuzumab ozogamycin ("mylotarg") and all-trans retinoic acid in untreated acute promyelocytic leukemia. Blood 2002;99(11):4222–4224.
223. Woolson RF, Lachenbruch PA. Rank analysis of covariance with right-censored data. Biometrics 1983; 39(3):727–733.
224. Ellenberg SS, Eisenberger MA. An efficient design for phase III studies of combination chemotherapies. Cancer Treat Rep 1985; 69(10):1147–1154.
225. Simon R, Thall PF, Ellenberg SS. New designs for the selection of treatments to be tested in randomized clinical trials. Stat Med 1994;13(5–7):417–429.
226. Herson J, Carter SK. Calibrated phase II clinical trials in oncology. Stat Med 1986;5(5):441–447.
227. Rubinstein LV, Korn EL, Freidlin B, Hunsberger S, Ivy SP, Smith MA. Design issues of randomized phase II trials and a proposal for phase II screening trials. J Clin Oncol 2005;23(28):7199–7206.
228. Estey EH. New designs for phase II trials: application to a trial of targeted therapies vs. chemotherapy in patients age > 60 with AML/high-risk MDS. Ann Hematol 2004;83 (suppl 1):S94–96.
229. Estey EH, Thall PF. New designs for phase 2 clinical trials. Blood 2003;102(2):442–448.

18 AML in Older Adults

Richard M. Stone

1. INTRODUCTION

Older adults with acute myeloid leukemia (AML) present a complex array of therapeutic dilemmas. As a result of host factors making chemotherapy less well tolerated, and disease factors making response to antineoplastic strategies less likely, difficult decisions abound. Therapeutic options, including aggressive chemotherapy, supportive care, or less intense therapy (e.g., clinical trials), have vastly different implications. The choice among these requires prolonged discussions with the patient and family members. Because of the poor results obtained in this age group, there is a need for the development of novel targeted, less toxic, and more effective therapies.

2. DIAGNOSIS AND CLASSIFICATION

The disease-related workup of an older adult with AML is similar to that in younger patients. Unexplained cytopenias, the presence of immature cells in the peripheral blood, or extramedullary deposits of myeloblasts should trigger a more precise delineation of the situation. A bone marrow examination should be performed with cells aspirated for morphological and cytochemical anaylsis, immunophenotype, and cytogenetics. Two classification systems are used. The older FAB system *(1)* is largely morphologically based and subcategorizes AML into eight subtypes: M0 through M7. The therapeutic approach to each is virtually identical except for M3 AML (acute promyelocytic leukemia [APML]). This entity, relatively unusual in older adults, is characterized by leukopenia, the presence of granule-laden malignant promyelocytes, and presentation with bleeding because of a disseminated intravascular coagulopathy *(2)*. Acute promyelocytic leukemia, confirmed by the finding of the characteristic t(15;17) chromosomal translocation and/or the associated APML-RARα fusion transcript, presenting at any age is treated with a combination of anthracycline-based chemotherapy and *all-trans*-retinoic acid *(3)*. The newer classification system, the so-called WHO scheme *(4)*,

From: *Contemporary Hematology: Acute Myelogenous Leukemia*
Edited by: J. E. Karp © Humana Press Inc., Totowa, NJ

emphasizes the importance of increasing cytogenetic and genetic understanding of acute leukemia. Moreover, this classification scheme denotes the presence of greater than 20% myeloblasts in the bone marrow as indicating AML, compared with the 30% requirement in the FAB classification system. Such a change is based in part on the finding that age and cytogenetics are much more important with regard to predicting response to chemotherapy than is the percentage of marrow blasts *(5)*.

3. PROGNOSIS

Although the white count and lactate dehydrogenase at presentation have some impact, the two most important prognostic characteristics for AML are the age of the patient and the chromosome findings at diagnosis *(6,7)*. Within the older age cohort, there is general agreement that patients 70–80 years of age fare more poorly than do those patients aged 55–70. Moreover, patients who present with AML in the ninth decade of life do extremely poorly. For younger adults there is a clear demarcation of prognosis based on chromosome findings at diagnosis *(7,8)*. About 15% of patients have chromosomal translocations that alter transcription factor biology, including inv16, t(8;21), and t(15;17), which are associated with a good prognosis if intensive chemotherapy is employed. Another 15% of patients have the type of chromosomal abnormalities typically seen in treatment-related AML or AML occurring after myelodysplastic syndrome (MDS), including loss of the long arm or all of chromosomes 5 or 7 or complex cytogenetic abnormalities. These patients have a dismal prognosis with chemotherapy. The other 70% of patients have so-called intermediate cytogenetics: normal, abnormalities at 11q23, trisomy 8, or other abnormalities. Recently, within the normal cytogenetic category, those with activating mutations in the FLT3 tyrosine kinase gene (occurring in about 30–40% of this cohort) have also been found to have an inferior prognosis *(9)*. These chromosomal patterns probably also have prognostic relevance for older adults *(6)*, but because of the generally overwhelmingly negative influence of patient age, the distinctions are less pronounced. Moreover, the increased incidence of adverse prognosis chromosomal abnormalities in older adults accounts in part for their inferior prognosis *(10)*. The percentage of older adults presenting with a so-called favorable chromosomal abnormality is much lower than the 15% value seen in the younger patients with this disease *(6)*.

The overall results with chemotherapy in older adults with AML are very discouraging. The likelihood of achieving remission is between 40 and 50% compared to 60–80% in younger adults with the same disease *(11)*. Those patients who achieve remission are much less likely to remain free of disease for long periods of time (disease-free survival is about 40–50% in younger adults who achieve remission compared with 10–20% in the older adults) *(11)*. The inability to achieve remission and/or to stay in remission yields a very disappointing cure rate of about 5–10% in this population.

The reasons for the inferior prognosis are a combination of host and disease factors. Clearly, older adults have a higher likelihood of comorbid diseases, decreased stem cell reserve, and an inability to excrete chemotherapy, which makes them much more susceptible to morbidity and mortality from sepsis *(12)*. Some of these issues can be subsumed into the performance status, which is an important prognostic factor at presentation; however, a more precise measure of fitness for treatment needs to be delineated. As already mentioned, the higher incidence of adverse chromosomal abnormalities suggests that AML in the older adult emanates from a more proximal stem cell in the hematopoietic hierarchy than that seen in the younger adults. Other data that support this notion include the increased likelihood of expression of molecules such as MDR1, which mediates drug resistance *(10)*. Moreover, there is a high incidence of presumed or proven antecedent hematological abnormalities in older adults that present with AML. Leith et al. have shown that older adults who have a prior history of MDS and have adverse chromosomes as well as high expression of the MDR1 gene product have a less than 15% likelihood of achieving remission with standard induction chemotherapy *(10)*.

4. TREATMENT

4.1. Standard Care

Treatment of patients with acute leukemia is divided into phases. The initial phase, or induction, is designed to eliminate all detectable evidence of leukemia in the blood, bone marrow, and extramedullary sites, thereby producing a remission. Remission induction represents the first step toward long-term disease control or potential cure. Induction chemotherapy generally involves a several-week period of aplasia, during which time the bone marrow is virtually devoid of recognizable hematopoietic elements, the blood counts are profoundly low, and patients are at risk for bleeding and opportunistic infections. As discussed above, older adults have a relatively high treatment-related mortality rate because of both disease and host-related factors. The second phase of antileukemic treatment is postremission therapy, designed to eliminate residual undetectable leukemic cells. In AML, postremission chemotherapy in younger adults can consist of either high-dose chemotherapy for several cycles, high-dose chemotherapy with myeloblative chemotherapy employing rescue by previously harvested autologous hematopoietic stem cells, or allogeneic stem cell transplantation. The likelihood of long-term disease control in patients with AML who achieve remission can range from as high as 80% in young patients whose blasts have chromosomal abnormalities associated with a good prognosis down to less than 10% in older patients and/or those whose blasts have chromosomal abnormalities associated with a poor prognosis.

If the decision is made to treat an older adult recently diagnosed with AML with induction chemotherapy, several days of an anthracycline such as daunorubicin or idarubicin and 7 days of continuous infusional cytarabine are usually administered. This so-called 3+7 regimen has remained the backbone of AML induction therapy for approx 30 years. It is difficult to conclude that one anthracycline or anthracycline-like agent has superiority over another. The most commonly used agent is probably daunorubicin at a dose of 45 mg/m^2 per day for 3 days. Although earlier reports suggested that idarubicin might produce better results *(13)*, more recent studies have not been able to demonstrate a superiority of either idarubicin or mitoxantrone compared with daunorubicin in this age cohort *(14,15)*. The dose of cytarabine used is 100–200 mg/m^2/day given by continuous intravenous infusion for 7 days. Attempts to intensify the cytarabine dose during induction have had mixed results in younger adults *(16,17)* and are probably not indicated for those over the age of 60. 6-Thioguanine is added to the induction regimen in AML for patients treated in the United Kingdom; moreover, the added benefit, particularly in older patients, is completely unclear *(18)*. The addition of etoposide to the anthracycline- and cytarabine-based regimen is feasible, particularly in younger adults, and may be associated with a disease-free survival (but not an overall survival) benefit, but there is no proof of its utility in this age group. Fludarabine does not appear to have a place in induction therapy of older adults *(19)*. It is also possible to intensify the daunorubicin dose apparently safely based on noncomparative results from a large trial performed by the CALGB *(20)*, but an ongoing trial performed by the Eastern Cooperative Oncology Group comparing 45 mg/m^2/day of daunorubicin for 3 days to 90 mg/m^2 for 3 days is being conducted only in adults under the age of 60.

Once an older adult with AML achieves remission and recovers from toxicity associated with induction therapy, the choice of postremission therapy is not straightforward. It does seem clear, however, that intensive postremission therapy is not indicated in this age cohort. CALGB 8525 was a landmark study *(11)* in which adults with AML of all ages were enrolled at diagnosis and given 3+7 induction; those who achieved remission were randomized to one of three doses of cytarabine in the postremission setting: (1) 100 mg/m^2 per day for 5 days by continuous iv infusion; (2) 400 mg/m^2 by continuous iv infusion for 5 days; or (3) 3 g/m^2 over 3 hours per dose q12h on days 1, 3, and 5 (total of six doses) (high-dose ara-C). Although younger adults randomized to the high-dose ara-C arm had a markedly superior disease-free and overall survival compared to patients randomized to one of the other of the lower-dose arms, there was absolutely no impact of dose in adults over the age of 60. Only about 14% of those patients who achieved remission had more than several years of disease control with any of the doses of cytarabine; moreover, it was very difficult to administer all four planned courses of high-dose ara-C to older adults. Attempts to intensify therapy with alternative regimens have also been unsuccessful. In CALGB 8923, adults 60 years of age or greater who achieved remission with standard induction chemotherapy were randomized to receive either four cycles of fairly low-dose ara-C (100 mg/m^2/day) or two cycles of a fairly intensive mitoxantrone/modified high-dose ara-C regimen *(21)*. Yet again, the overall outcome was poor and there was no difference based on postremission randomization. It should be noted that those few older adults that present with favorable chromosome AML prognosis (inversion of chromosome 16 or translocation 8;21) should be considered candidates for intensive postremission therapy based on the results suggesting a high likelihood of a long-term disease control with high-dose ara-C in patients with these cytogenetic abnormalities.

Should any postremission therapy be given to an older patient with AML? Based on studies done in the 1970s *(22)*, which randomized (mainly younger) patients in CR to either some chemotherapy or none, it is reasonable to administer some postremission therapy for an even small possibility of long-term disease-free survival. Exactly what the optimal regimen to be administered in the postremission setting is in this age cohort of patients with AML in remission is not clear; it seems reasonable to repeat the induction course or give modified high-dose ara-C for one or two cycles. An interesting study conducted by the HOVON-SAKK European Cooperative Group randomized older adults with AML in CR to either eight cycles of low-dose ara-C or observation after they received one cycle of repeat induction therapy. The results suggested that there was a disease-free but no overall survival benefit for patients randomized to the low-dose ara-C *(23)*.

Another special case pertains to the relatively few older adults who have APML. Because of the excellent results with *all-trans*-retinoic acid- and anthracycline-based therapy, older adults with APML should be treated with curative intent *(24)*. In most series, older age does represent a relatively adverse prognostic factor in APML, as does an elevated white count at diagnosis *(25,26)*. Moreover, the emphasis on anthracycline therapy in APML does merit scrutiny in older patients because of the potential effect on cardiac pump function. Nonetheless, good results have been obtained by treating older adults with *all-trans*-retinoic acid in combination with anthracycline-based chemotherapy followed by anthracycline and *all-trans*-retinoic acid postremission therapy. Whether or not it is worth adding maintenance *all-trans*-retinoic acid with oral metabolite therapy for a year as the currently suggested plan in younger adults *(27)* is unclear.

4.2. Hematopoietic Stem Cell Transplantation

Until recently, any form of stem cell transplantation was felt to be absolutely contraindicated in older adults with AML. The high-dose chemotherapy and or radiation therapy used in preparative regimens in both autologous and allogeneic myeloblative transplants is generally felt to be too toxic for patients in this age group, especially given potential hepatic and pulmonary compromise. Moreover, in the allogeneic setting, it is known that severe acute and chronic graft vs host disease is somewhat more likely in older adults. On the other hand, given the intrinsic nature of resistance disease that defines AML in older adults, it is just this cohort of patients who might potentially benefit from an intensive chemotherapy approach or certainly from the type of immunological approach present after some form of allogeneic stem cell infusion. Although still relatively unusual in this country, high-dose chemotherapy with autologous stem cell support is more commonly used in Europe as a postremission strategy in older adults with AML. Supportive results are derived from studies using high-dose chemotherapy with autologous peripheral blood stem cell rescue in patients with MDS, who, as mentioned before, have bone marrow findings similar to those of the typical patient with AML who is older. Manageable toxicity and good long-term disease outcomes have caused some European investigators to use this procedure for treatment of AML in first remission (28). Although autologous transplantation as consolidation after second remission has led to some long-term disease-free survivors in younger adults (29), the utility of such an approach in older adults who may have achieved a second remission is unclear.

Certainly the fastest growing segment of hematopoietic stem cell transplantation is in the area of nonmyeloblative or reduced intensity conditioning regimens for allogeneic transplants (30,31). Several recent studies have demonstrated the feasibility of this approach, which relies on graft vs leukemia as the major antineoplastic effect in older adults with a variety of conditions. Some of these studies have suggested that nonmyeloblative and myeloblative transplants are associated with similar long-term outcomes (31). However, the long-term efficacy of the nonmyeloblative allogeneic approach is not yet accurately known. There are even fewer data about the appropriateness of doing a nonmyeloblative matched unrelated donor transplant.

4.3. Treatment Decisions

Given the high morbidity and mortality costs of standard induction chemotherapy and postremission therapy in older adults with AML coupled with a relatively low chance for success, the appropriateness of such therapy is a reasonable question. However, based on available data it is very difficult to provide relevant information as to the consequences of either standard myelointensive approaches vs supportive or lower intensive strategies. Two European studies conducted in the 1980s attempted to address this question in a prospective fashion. Lowenberg et al. (32) randomized older AML patients to immediate intensive induction chemotherapy at diagnosis, or "watch and wait," until counts or clinical deterioration was noted, which would then prompt the use of induction chemotherapy. The watch-and-wait strategy was designed to test the idea of maximizing quality of life by withholding treatment while patients felt well. Those who were randomized to immediate chemotherapy experienced a slightly longer overall survival. However, the lack of an associated quality-of-life analysis and the relatively brief survival benefit with high upfront mortality diminished the enthusiasm with which such a recommendation can be adopted. Another trial conducted by French investigators compared standard chemotherapy to low doses of cytarabine (33). Again, those who received the more intensive chemotherapy experienced a higher CR rate and a slightly better long-term survival. However, there was a much higher upfront mortality in those who received intensive chemotherapy, and the survival benefit was brief without any comparison in terms of the quality-of-life costs. Therefore, while justification exists for use of early intensive chemotherapy in older adults with AML, there is still significant need to perform additional research. Sekeres et al. *(34)* conducted a study in which patients with high-grade MDS or AML were asked how they made the decision to choose either intensive chemotherapy or a less intensive/supportive approach. About half of the patients chose the standard approach; these patients seemed to be somewhat younger and have lower platelet counts. While documentation of an extensive discussion of treatment options was noted in the chart, patients felt that they were not presented with many treatment options and consistently overestimated their chances of cure with chemotherapy compared to the physician's opinion. The consequences of choosing induction chemotherapy included an immediate decrease in the quality of life, but after recovery from the acute side effects, patients were able to feel quite well, especially if remission was achieved.

4.4. The Use of Hematopoietic Growth Factors

The hematopoietic growth factors granulocyte-macrophage colony-stimulating factor (GM-CSF) and granulocyte colony-stimulating factor (G-CSF) are widely used after chemotherapy to lessen the duration and impact of neutropenia in solid tumor and lymphoma patients receiving myelointense chemotherapy. Their use in myeloid malignancies is less well developed and more controversial because of the initial concerns that G-CSF and GM-CSF would stimulate the receptors known to exist on the surface of leukemic cells and promote the growth of clonal genetic leukemia cells, thereby increasing the chance of disease resistance *(35)*. However, numerous randomized trials of induction chemotherapy with or without the use of hematopoietic growth factors have diminished the concerns about the leukemogenic potential of these agents. On the other hand, perhaps because of the profoundly myelosuppressive nature of leukemic induction chemotherapy and the inability of these agents to affect epithelial toxicity, their impact in managing the treatment-related complications of induction therapy in older adults with AML is limited *(36)*. Randomized trials with G-CSF in older adults with AML consistently show a reduction in the duration of neutropenia (about 5 days, and 2–3 days in the case of GM-CSF); however, except for one ECOG trial *(37)* there has been no beneficial effect on reducing infectious mortality or improving overall survival, which was the original hope. One trial with G-CSF as a supportive agent in older adults did show an improvement in the CR rate *(38)*, but this may have been due to the growth factor-induced alteration of bone marrow morphology because there was no lessening of infectious deaths nor improvement in overall survival. Although GM-CSF is approved as a supportive agent after induction therapy for older adults with AML, it is rarely used for that purpose. It does seem reasonable to administer G-CSF as a postremission chemotherapy based on clear-cut benefits in a trial conducted with this agent in younger adults with AML *(39)*.

4.5. New Treatment Approaches

Given the high toxicity cost and the relatively poor outcomes with standard chemotherapy-based approaches for the treatment of older adults with AML, new ideas are badly needed. One would hope that many such strategies will be derived from an increased understanding of the biology of these leukemias; however, patients with balanced translocations, the molecular genetics of which are relatively well understood, are rare in this age cohort. Nonetheless, two drugs have recently been approved for patients with AML, one of which was specifically designated for older adults. In a fashion similar to the reports from the Peoples Republic of China in the 1980s documenting responses using *all-trans*-retinoic acid in patients with advanced APML *(40)*, investigators from the same country used arsenic trioxide to produce similarly impressive results in patients with refractory and relapsed APML *(41)*. Complete remissions occurring via both an apoptic and differentiation-type mechanisms were also reported by American investigators *(42,43)*. Amazingly, even patients with advanced disease were able to experience profound reductions in tumor burden measured by quantitative polymerase chain reaction testing after treatment with arsenic trioxide. A major US intergroup trial recently completed accrual, which was dedicated to determining whether the use of arsenic trioxide in the early postremission setting might be beneficial. Arsenic trioxide, given intravenously daily over several weeks, is relatively well tolerated, although monitoring of electrolytes and QT interval is advisable because of reports of malignant ventricular arythimias.

The other new agent approved for treatment of older adults with AML is gemtuzumab ozogamicin (GO), a humanized monoclonal antibody–toxin conjugate *(44)*. In phase II testing of GO in relapsed AML patients, the CR rate was 30%, although half of these patients had imcomplete platelet recovery (CRp). CRp patients and those with traditional CRs appear to have the same national history. GO's place in the management of older adults with AML is still in development. The drug, although somewhat targeted, is still toxic in that profound myelosuppression, albeit generally without mucocytis, occurs. It should be given only by those experienced in its use. Second, reports of severe hepatic toxicity, even to the point of fatal venoocclusive disease, have been reported particularly in patients who receive this drug within a few months of allogeneic bone marrow transplantation *(45)*. Such severe hepatic toxicity has also been reported in patients receiving gemtuzumab alone or in combination with other therapeutic agents *(46)*. The role of GO as an agent to be used in the upfront treatment of older patients with AML has not conclusively been determined. A recent phase II study of GO in "non-chemotherapy eligible" patients aged greater than 60 with AML yielded a CR/CRp rate of 17% (33% in those aged 61–75) but was too toxic in more elderly patients *(47)*. Results from another phase II trial of GO as primary therapy (with interleukin [IL]-11) in older adults with AML suggested that the results were inferior to what would have been expected with chemotherapy *(48)*. Large cooperative groups are testing the value of adding GO to standard chemotherapy or using it late postremission to deal with minimal residual disease.

While a discussion of all agents in development for older adults with AML is beyond the scope of this chapter, one can subclassify approaches into those that could work as primary neoplastic agents on their own, those that are mainly developed to enhance therapeutic effect, and those that promote or require the assistance of the immune system. Agents that might have intrinsic activity against leukemia cells include novel chemotherapeutic drugs, inhibitors of the FLT3 tyrosine kinase, and farnesyltransferase inhibitors. Although no standard cytotoxic chemotherapeutic agents have been recently approved for use in AML, several agents are under development. The novel nucleoside analogs clofarabine *(49)* and troxicitabine *(50)* represent two such examples. Clofarabine has been approved for use in relapsed pediatric ALL.

Most activating mutations in the FLT3 tyrosine kinase gene involve a duplication of between 3 and more than 33 amino acids in the juxtamembrane region of the protein *(51)*. About 5% of those with AML have a point mutation in the activation loop. Either of these two acquired genetic abnormalities produce constitutive enzymatic activation and transforming activity as well as the ability to generate leukemias in murine models *(51)*. Just as imatinib mesylate is an effective agent in chronic myelogenous leukemia because of its ability to inhibit the abl kinase, it is hoped that one of more of the FLT3 small molecule tyrosine kinase inhibitors in development will prove to be similarly useful in AML, despite the recognition that florid leukemia probably requires and is dependent on more than one mutation. Several FLT3 inhibitors are currently in clinical trials; each has shown the ability to produce reductions in the peripheral blast count, but remissions are rare *(52,53)*. These drugs are now being evaluated in combination with chemotherapy.

The farnesyltransferase inhibitors inhibit a critical posttranslational modification of enzymes such as the ras family of proto-oncogenes, which are important agents in cell signaling. A phase I trial with one such farnesyltransferase inhibitor, tipifarnib, produced responses in patients with advanced leukemia *(54)*. A follow-up phase II trial in more than 200 patients with relapsed or refractory leukemia documented a response rate well under 10% *(55)*. However, renewed interest in tipifarnib as a potential agent for the treatment of older adults with AML is based on a trial in which older adults were given this single agent as their initial therapy. More than 100 patients who were either older than age 75 or between 65 and 75 years of age with a prior history of myelodysplasia were enrolled in this trial. The complete response rate was approx 15%, with an overall response rate of 25% *(56)*. Large studies are being conducted in Europe (randomized trial between best supportive care and tipifarnib in adults greater than 70 years with AML) and in North America (large phase II trial of two different doses and two different schedules [four arms] of tipifarnib) in older adults with newly diagnosed AML.

Agents that enhance the effect of chemotherapy and are not expected to have seen any activity on their own represent a more daunting developmental strategy. To prove efficacy, phase III trials comparing chemotherapy with or without the agent are required. The best example of this group is the so-called drug resistance modulators. One of the proposed reasons for the intrinsic level of disease resistance in older adults with AML is the relatively high expression of genes such as MDR1, which encodes the GP170 protein, capable of mediating efflux of a variety of naturally occurring chemotherapeutic substances. This efflux pump can be inhibited by the use of several types of agents including phenothiazines, cyclosporine, and the nonimmunosuppressive cyclosporine analog PSC-833. One study comparing chemotherapy with mitoxantrone, cytarabine, etoposide with or without PSC-833 failed to show a benefit with the agent in adults with relapsed AML *(57)*. Another study of induction chemotherapy with or without the same agent in older adults failed to be completed because of undue toxicity associated with the use of PSC-833, which increases the drug levels of etoposide and daunorubicin as a result of its effect on biliary metabolism *(20)*. However, a recent trial in relapsed AML did show a survival benefit when cyclosporin A was added to daunorubicin plus high-dose ara-C reinduction chemotherapy *(58)*. The Southwest Oncology Group is now conducting a trial in newly diagnosed older adults with AML randomized to chemotherapy with or without cyclosoprin A. The Eastern Oncology Cooperative Group is currently doing a clinical trial in which patients with previously untreated AML over the age of 60 receive either standard chemotherapy with or without the nonpharmacologically active drug resistance modulator zosuquidar.

Overexpression of genes that encode molecules preventing programmed cell death or apoptosis is associated with an increased level of chemotherapeutic resistance. In vitro studies have shown that downregulating such overexpression with agents such as oblimersen (an 18-mer anti-bcl-2 oliglonucleotide) can provide chemotherapy an increased ability to kill leukemia cells. An early-phase trial of oblimersen plus chemotherapy showed that it was feasible to administer these agents together to patients with AML *(59)*; the Cancer and Leukemia Group B is now conducting a large prospective randomized trial in which newly diagnosed older patients with AML receive either chemotherapy alone or chemotherapy plus an infusion of oblimersen (in both the induction and postremission settings). In vitro studies suggest that the protosome inhibitor bortezomib may potentiate the effects of chemotherapy in leukemia. Consequently, early-phase trials with chemotherapy and bortezomib in relapsed and older adults with AML are underway *(60)*. Documenting a benefit with this approach will probably require another large randomized prospective phase III trial.

4.6. Immunotherapeutic Approaches

Attempts to harness the patient's own immune system to assist in antileukemic therapy represent a longstanding developmental therapeutic approach. For example, in the 1970s the nonspecific immunostimulant bacille Calmette-Guérin (BCG) vaccine was tested in a randomized trial that failed to show a benefit *(61)*. More sophisticated means of using immunotherapy in AML have since been made available. Because of the presumed complex pathophysiology and intrinsic chemotherapeutic resistance that characterizes AML in the older population, it seemed appropriate to test these approaches in this patient cohort. The Cancer and Leukemia Group B conducted a large prospective phase III trial in older adults with AML in which patients received induction chemotherapy followed or not by the drug resistance modulator PSC-833 followed by two cycles of postremission therapy followed by a randomization to low-dose IL-2 or observation. The purpose of the low-dose IL-2 was to stimulate autologous T-cells and natural killer cells to potentially replicate the graft-vs-leukemia effect seen after allogeneic transplantation. Although prior studies of the use of low-dose IL-2 in patients receiving intensive antileukemia chemotherapy demonstrated feasibility, many patients dropped out before randomization or refused the 90-day course of IL-2, making the interpretation of this trial difficult *(20)*. Another method to enhance non-specific immunotherapy is represented by nonmyeloblative bone marrow transplantation, which is being used with increased frequency as a treatment strategy in older adults with AML, as discussed earlier in this chapter. The Southwest Oncology Group is now conducting an important trial in which older adults with AML who complete induction and postremission chemotherapy are "genetically" assigned to have a nonmyeloblative allogeneic transplant if they have a viable histocompatible sibling donor.

Making leukemic cells more visible to the immune system via a vaccine strategy is currently being tested by several investigators. Studies conducted by Dr. Moldrem at M.D. Anderson suggest that autologous antileukemic immunity can be generated by exposure to immuno-genic peptides. Others have shown that expression of cytokine genes, such as GM-CSF or IL-2, by leukemic cells can enhance presentation of presumptive leukemia antigens in murine systems *(62)*. Clinical studies in which leukemic cells are engineered to express GM-CSF or coculture with GM-CSF-expressing cells have been conducted *(63)*; however, phase III trials would be required to document clinical benefit.

5. CONCLUSION

AML in older adults remains a daunting therapeutic challenge. A high level of disease resistance and comorbid disease leads to a high degree of toxicity and low long-term efficacy with currently available chemotherapy-based strategies. Research is being done on ways to discuss the dilemma of chemotherapy treatment in older patients. Simultaneously, there are great efforts to devise less toxic and more effective therapies based on enhanced understanding of leukemic pathophysiology.

REFERENCES

1. Bennett J, Catovsky D, Daniel M, et al. Proposed revised criteria for the classification of acute myeloid leukemia: a report of the French-American-British cooperative group. Ann Int Med 1985;103:620.
2. Fenaux P, Chomienne C, Degos L. Acute promyelocytic leukemia: biology and treatment. Semin Oncol 1997;24:92–102.
3. Tallman MS, Nabhan C, Feusner JH, et al. Acute promyelocytic leukemia: evolving therapeutic strategies. Blood 2002;99:759–767.
4. Vardiman JW, Harris NL, Brunning RD. The World Health Organization (WHO) classification of the myeloid neoplasms. Blood 2002;100:2292–2302.
5. Estey E, Thall P, Beran M, et al. Effect of diagnosis (refractory anemia with excess blasts, refractory anemia with excess blasts in transformation, or acute myeloid leukemia [AML]) on outcome of AML-type chemotherapy. Blood 1997;90:2969–2977.
6. Grimwade D, Walker H, Harrison G, et al. The predictive value of hierarchical cytogenetic classification in older adults with acute myeloid leukemia (AML): analysis of 1065 patients entered into the United Kingdom Medical Research Council AML11 trial. Blood 2001;98:1312–1320.
7. Grimwade D, Walker H, Oliver F, et al. The importance of diagnostic cytogenetics on outcome in AML: analysis of 1,612 patients entered into the MRC AML 10 trial. The Medical Research Council Adult and Children's Leukaemia Working Parties. Blood 1998;92:2322–2333.
8. Byrd JC, Mrozek K, Dodge RK, et al. Pretreatment cytogenetic abnormalities are predictive of induction success, cumulative incidence of relapse, and overall survival in adult patients with de novo acute myeloid leukemia: results from Cancer and Leukemia Group B (CALGB 8461). Blood 2002;100:4325–4336.
9. Kottaridis PD, Gale RE, Linch DC. Prognostic implications of the presence of FLT3 mutations in patients with acute myeloid leukemia. Leuk Lymphoma 2003;44:905–913.
10. Leith CP, Kopecky KJ, Godwin J, et al. Acute myeloid leukemia in the elderly: assessment of multidrug resistance (MDR1) and cytogenetics distinguishes biologic subgroups with remarkably distinct responses to standard chemotherapy. A Southwest Oncology Group study. Blood 1997;89:3323–3329.
11. Mayer RJ, Davis RB, Schiffer CA, et al. Intensive postremission chemotherapy in adults with acute myeloid leukemia. Cancer and Leukemia Group B. N Engl J Med 1994;331:896–903.
12. Beghe C, Balducci L. Biological basis of cancer in the older person. Cancer Treat Res 2005;124:189–221.
13. Wiernik PH, Banks PL, Case DC, Jr., et al. Cytarabine plus idarubicin or daunorubicin as induction and consolidation therapy for previously untreated adult patients with acute myeloid leukemia. Blood 1992;79: 313–319.
14. Anderson JE, Kopecky KJ, Willman CL, et al. Outcome after induction chemotherapy for older patients with acute myeloid leukemia is not improved with mitoxantrone and etoposide compared to cytarabine and daunorubicin: a Southwest Oncology Group study. Blood 2002;100:3869–3876.
15. Rowe J, Neuberg D, Friedenberg W, et al. A Phase III study of three induction regimens and of priming with GM-CSF in older adults with acute myeloid leukemia: a trial by the Eastern Cooperative Oncology Group. Blood 2004;103:479–485.
16. Bishop JF, Matthews JP, Young GA, et al. Intensified induction chemotherapy with high dose cytarabine and etoposide for acute myeloid leukemia: a review and updated results of the Australian Leukemia Study Group. Leuk Lymphoma 1998;28:315–327.
17. Weick JK, Kopecky KJ, Appelbaum FR, et al. A randomized investigation of high-dose versus standard-dose cytosine arabinoside with daunorubicin in patients with previously untreated acute myeloid leukemia: a Southwest Oncology Group study. Blood 1996;88:2841–2851.
18. Hann IM, Stevens RF, Goldstone AH, et al. Randomized comparison of DAT versus ADE as induction chemotherapy in children and younger adults with acute myeloid leukemia. Results of the Medical Research Council's 10th AML trial (MRC AML10). Adult and Childhood Leukaemia Working Parties of the Medical Research Council. Blood 1997;89:2311–2318.
19. Ossenkoppele GJ, Graveland WJ, Sonneveld P, et al. The value of fludarabine in addition to ARA-C and G-CSF in the treatment of patients with high-risk myelodysplastic syndromes and AML in elderly patients. Blood 2004;103:2908–2913.

20. Baer MR, George SL, Dodge RK, et al. Phase 3 study of the multidrug resistance modulator PSC-833 in previously untreated patients 60 years of age and older with acute myeloid leukemia: Cancer and Leukemia Group B Study 9720. Blood 2002;100:1224–1232.

21. Stone R, Berg D, George S, et al. Post-remission therapy in older patients with de novo acute myeloid leukemia: a randomized trial comparing mitoxantrone and intermediate-dose cytarabine with standard-dose cytarabine. Blood 2001;98:548–553.

22. Bloomfield C. Postremission therapy in acute myeloid leukemia. J Clin Oncol 1985;3:1570–1572.

23. Lowenberg B, Suciu S, Archimbaud E, et al. Mitoxantrone versus daunorubicin in induction-consolidation chemotherapy—the value of low-dose cytarabine for maintenance of remission, and an assessment of prognostic factors in acute myeloid leukemia in the elderly: final report. European Organization for the Research and Treatment of Cancer and the Dutch-Belgian Hemato-Oncology Cooperative Hovon Group. J Clin Oncol 1998;16:872–881.

24. Jurcic J. Treating Acute Promyelocytic Leukemia in the Older Patient. The Am J Oncol Rev 2005;4: 344–349.

25. Sanz MA, Martin G, Gonzalez M, et al. Risk-adapted treatment of acute promyelocytic leukemia with all-trans-retinoic acid and anthracycline monochemotherapy: a multicenter study by the PETHEMA group. Blood 2004;103:1237–1243.

26. Sanz MA, Martin G, Rayon C, et al. A modified AIDA protocol with anthracycline-based consolidation results in high antileukemic efficacy and reduced toxicity in newly diagnosed PML/RARalpha-positive acute promyelocytic leukemia. PETHEMA group. Blood 1999;94:3015–3021.

27. Fenaux P, Chastang C, Chevret S, et al. A randomized comparison of all transretinoic acid (ATRA) followed by chemotherapy and ATRA plus chemotherapy and the role of maintenance therapy in newly diagnosed acute promyelocytic leukemia. The European APL Group. Blood 1999;94:1192–1200.

28. Gorin NC. Autologous stem cell transplantation in acute myelocytic leukemia. Blood 1998;92:1073–1090.

29. Yeager AM, Kaizer H, Santos GW, et al. Autologous bone marrow transplantation in patients with acute nonlymphocytic leukemia, using ex vivo marrow treatment with 4-hydroperoxycyclophosphamide. N Engl J Med 1986;315:141–147.

30. McSweeney PA, Niederwieser D, Shizuru JA, et al. Hematopoietic cell transplantation in older patients with hematologic malignancies: replacing high-dose cytotoxic therapy with graft-versus-tumor effects. Blood 2001;97:3390–3400.

31. Alyea EP, Kim HT, Ho V, et al. Comparative outcome of nonmyeloablative and myeloablative allogeneic hematopoietic cell transplantation for patients older than 50 years of age. Blood 2005;105:1810–1814.

32. Lowenberg B, Zittoun R, Kerkhofs H, et al. On the value of intensive remission-induction chemotherapy in elderly patients of 65+ years with acute myeloid leukemia: a randomized phase III study of the European Organization for Research and Treatment of Cancer Leukemia Group. J Clin Oncol 1989;7:1268–1274.

33. Tilly H, Castaigne S, Bordessoule D, et al. Low-dose cytarabine versus intensive chemotherapy in the treatment of acute nonlymphocytic leukemia in the elderly. J Clin Oncol 1990;8:272–279.

34. Sekeres MA, Stone RM, Zahrieh D, et al. Decision-making and quality of life in older adults with acute myeloid leukemia or advanced myelodysplastic syndrome. Leukemia 2004;18:809–816.

35. Vallenga E, Ostapovicz D, O'Rourke B, et al. Effects of recombinant K-3, GM-CSF on proliferation of leukemic clonogenic eeks in short term and long term cultures. Leukemia 1987;1:584–589.

36. Schiffer CA. Hematopoietic growth factors as adjuncts to the treatment of acute myeloid leukemia. Blood 1996;88:3675–3685.

37. Rowe JM, Andersen JW, Mazza JJ, et al. A randomized placebo-controlled phase III study of granulocyte-macrophage colony-stimulating factor in adult patients (>55 to 70 years of age) with acute myelogenous leukemia: a study of the Eastern Cooperative Oncology Group (E1490). Blood 1995;86:457–462.

38. Dombret H, Chastang C, Fenaux P, et al. A controlled study of recombinant human granulocyte colony-stimulating factor in elderly patients after treatment for acute myelogenous leukemia. AML Cooperative Study Group. N Engl J Med 1995;332:1678–1683.

39. Heil G, Hoelzer D, Sanz MA, et al. A randomized, double-blind, placebo-controlled, phase III study of filgrastim in remission induction and consolidation therapy for adults with de novo acute myeloid leukemia. The International Acute Myeloid Leukemia Study Group. Blood 1997;90:4710–4718.

40. Degos L, Dombret H, Chomienne C, et al. All-trans-retinoic acid as a differentiating agent in the treatment of acute promyelocytic leukemia. Blood 1995;85:2643–2653.

41. Shen ZX, Chen GQ, Ni JH, et al. Use of arsenic trioxide (As2O3) in the treatment of acute promyelocytic leukemia (APL): II. Clinical efficacy and pharmacokinetics in relapsed patients. Blood 1997;89:3354–3360.

42. Soignet SL, Frankel SR, Douer D, et al. United States multicenter study of arsenic trioxide in relapsed acute promyelocytic leukemia. J Clin Oncol 2001;19:3852–3860.

43. Soignet SL, Maslak P, Wang ZG, et al. Complete remission after treatment of acute promyelocytic leukemia with arsenic trioxide. N Engl J Med 1998;339:1341–1348.

44. Sievers EL. Efficacy and safety of gemtuzumab ozogamicin in patients with CD33-positive acute myeloid leukaemia in first relapse. Expert Opin Biol Ther 2001;1:893–901.

45. Wadleigh M, Richardson PG, Zahrieh D, et al. Prior gemtuzumab ozogamicin exposure significantly increases the risk of veno-occlusive disease in patients who undergo myeloablative allogeneic stem cell transplantation. Blood 2003;102:1578–1582.

46. Giles F, Estey E, O'Brien S. Gemtuzumab ozogamicin in the treatment of acute myeloid leukemia. Cancer 2003;98:2095–2104.

47. Amadori S, Suciu S, Stasi R, et al. Gemtuzumab ozogamicin (Mylotarg) as single-agent treatment for frail patients 61 years of age and older with acute myeloid leukemia:final results of AML-15B, a phase 2 study of the European Organization for Research and Treatment of Cancer and Gruppo Italiano Malattie Ematologiche dell'Adulto Leukemia Groups. Leukemia 2005;19:1768–1773.

48. Estey EH, Thall PF, Giles FJ, et al. Gemtuzumab ozogamicin with or without interleukin 11 in patients 65 years of age or older with untreated acute myeloid leukemia and high-risk myelodysplastic syndrome: comparison with idarubicin plus continuous-infusion, high-dose cytosine arabinoside. Blood 2002;99:4343–4349.

49. Kantarjian H, Gandhi V, Cortes J, et al. Phase 2 clinical and pharmacologic study of clofarabine in patients with refractory or relapsed acute leukemia. Blood 2003;102:2379–2386.

50. Giles FJ, Feldman EJ, Roboz GJ, et al. Phase II study of troxacitabine, a novel dioxolane nucleoside analog, in patients with untreated or imatinib mesylate-resistant chronic myelogenous leukemia in blastic phase. Leukemia Res 2003;27:1091–1096.

51. Gilliland DG, Griffin JD. The roles of FLT3 in hematopoiesis and leukemia. Blood 2002;100:1532–1542.

52. Smith BD, Levis M, Beran M, et al. Single-agent CEP-701, a novel FLT3 inhibitor, shows biologic and clinical activity in patients with relapsed or refractory acute myeloid leukemia. Blood 2004;103:3669–3676.

53. Stone RM, DeAngelo DJ, Klimek V, et al. Patients with acute myeloid leukemia and an activating mutation in FLT3 respond to a small-molecule FLT3 tyrosine kinase inhibitor, PKC412. Blood 2005;105:54–60.

54. Karp JE, Lancet JE, Kaufmann SH, et al. Clinical and biologic activity of the farnesyltransferase inhibitor R115777 in adults with refractory and relapsed acute leukemias: a phase 1 clinical-laboratory correlative trial. Blood 2001;97:3361–3369.

55. Harousseau JL, Reiffers J, Lowenberg J, et al. Zarnestra (R115777) in patients with relapsed and refractory acute myelogenous leukemia (AML): results of a multicenter Phase II study. Blood 2003;102:176a[614].

56. Lancet JE, Karp JE. Farnesyl transferase inhibitors in myeloid malignancies. Blood 2003;17:123–129.

57. Greenberg PL, Lee SJ, Advani R, et al. Mitoxantrone, etoposide, and cytarabine with or without valspodar in patients with relapsed or refractory acute myeloid leukemia and high-risk myelodysplastic syndrome: a phase III trial (E2995). J Clin Oncol 2004;22:1078–1086.

58. List AF, Kopecky KJ, Willman CL, et al. Benefit of cyclosporine modulation of drug resistance in patients with poor-risk acute myeloid leukemia: a Southwest Oncology Group study. Blood 2001;98:3212–3220.

59. Marcucci G, Byrd JC, Dai G, et al. Phase 1 and pharmacodynamic studies of G3139, a Bcl-2 antisense oligonucleotide, in combination with chemotherapy in refractory or relapsed acute leukemia. Blood 2003;101:425–432.

60. Attar EC, De Angelo DJ, Ballen KK, et al. Phase I Dose Escalating Trial of Bortezomid (Velcade) in Combination with Idarubicin and Cytarabine in Patients with Acute Myeloid Leukemia. Blood 2004;104:498 a[1799].

61. Omura GA, Vogler WR, Lefante J, et al. Treatment of acute myelogenous leukemia: influence of three induction regimens and maintenance with chemotherapy or BCG immunotherapy. Cancer 1982;49:1530–1536.

62. Dunussi-Joannopoulos K, Runyon K, Erickson J, et al. Vaccines with interleukin-12-transduced acute myeloid leukemia cells elicit very potent therapeutic and long-lasting protective immunity. Blood 1999;94: 4263–4273.

63. DeAngelo DJ. A Phase I study of vaccination with lethally irradiated, autologous myeloblasts engineered by adenoviral mediated gene transfer to secrete human granulocyte-macrophase colony stimulating factor. Blood 2001;98:463a.

19 Dameshek Smiles: Molecular Clues to the Chronic Myeloproliferative Disorders Unmasked

Jason Gotlib

CONTENTS

Summary

The classic chronic myeloproliferative disorders (MPDs) polycythemia vera (PV), essential thrombocythemia (ET), and idiopathic myelofibrosis (MF) have been historically grouped together because of their overlapping clinical phenotypes. The recent discovery of a single acquired point mutation (V617F) in the Janus kinase 2 (*JAK2*) gene in most patients with PV and about half of ET and MF patients provides a new starting point for exploring the genetic and biologic mechanisms of disease pathogenesis in these related disorders. This chapter highlights the different roads of discovery to the *JAK2* V617F mutation, both *in vitro* and *in vivo* experimental data relevant to the mutant JAK2 tyrosine kinase, and new questions raised by the discovery.

Key Words: *JAK2* V617F; polycythemia vera; essential thrombocythemia; idiopathic myelofibrosis; myeloproliferative disorder.

1. INTRODUCTION

In his prescient 1951 *Blood* editorial *(1)*, "Some Speculations on the Myeloproliferative Syndromes," Dr. William Dameshek eloquently elaborated on the overlapping clinical and histopathological features of the chronic myeloproliferative disorders:

"It is possible that these various conditions- 'myeloproliferative disorders'- are all somewhat variable manifestations of proliferative activity of the bone marrow cells, perhaps due

From: *Contemporary Hematology: Acute Myelogenous Leukemia*
Edited by: J. E. Karp © Humana Press Inc., Totowa, NJ

to a hitherto undiscovered stimulus. This may affect the marrow cells diffusely or irregularly with the result that various syndromes, either clear-cut, or transitional, result. Among them are the following: chronic granulocytic leukemia, polycythemia vera, idiopathic or "agnogenic"myeloid metaplasia of the spleen (and liver), thrombocythemia, megakaryocytic leukemia and erythroleukemia (Di Guglielmo's syndrome)." (1)

In a series of landmark research articles first appearing in March 2005, several groups identified a singular and novel mutation (V617F) in the Janus Kinase 2 (*JAK2*) tyrosine kinase gene in a substantial proportion of patients with polycythemia vera (PV), essential thrombocythemia (ET), and idiopathic myelofibrosis (MF) *(2–5)*. This recurrent somatic mutation results in constitutive activation of the JAK2 tyrosine kinase, and provides at least one biologic explanation for Dameshek's "undiscovered stimulus."

Perhaps influenced by Dameshek's editorial, polycthemia vera, essential thrombocythemia, and idiopathic myelofibrosis (agnogenic myeloid metaplasia with myelofibrosis, AMM) have been historically grouped together as the 'classic chronic myeloproliferative disorders.' Common themes which have emerged among these diseases include: (1) demonstration of clonal hematopoiesis in a proportion of cases and presumptive involvement of a multipotent hematopoietic progenitor *(6–10)*; (2) growth factor-independent colony formation *in vitro (11)*, and hypersensitivity of marrow/blood cells to hematopoietic growth factors; *(12–16)* (3) extramedullary hematopoiesis; (4) thrombotic and hemorrhagic diatheses; and (5) the potential for to evolution to myelofibrosis (e.g. PV and ET), and acute myelogenous leukemia.

PV patients can present with leukocytosis and/or thrombocythemia , and patients diagnosed with idiopathic MF may alternatively represent the "spent phase" of PV or ET (e.g. post-polycythemic or post-thrombocythemic myelofibrosis with metaplasia). This phenotypic mimicry, combined with a lack of distinct molecular markers, can lead to misdiagnosis of these disorders. However, the finding of an increased red blood cell mass distinguishes PV from all other chronic MPDs. Other diagnostic laboratory testing in PV is less useful (reviewed in *17*). For example, the serum erythropoietin level has a low sensitivity and negative predictive value. A clonal cytogenetic abnormality is found in <25% of PV patients *(17)*. Other clonality assays (see below) are available only on a research basis, and applicable only in informative women. Similarly, testing for endogenous erythroid colony formation (or other *in vitro* colony forming assays to assess growth factor hypersensitivity) is not widely available. Bone marrow morphology and CT measurement of spleen size can be normal or lack specificity for the diagnosis of PV *(17)*. Platelets from PV pts frequently show impaired expression of c-Mpl, the receptor for thrombopoietin *(17–19)*. Decreased expression of platelet c-Mpl can be used to distinguish PV from secondary erythrocytoses, but not from ET and MF which also show decreased expression of platelet Mpl *(17–22)*. Polycythemia rubra vera-1 (PRV-1) mRNA transcription is increased in circulating granulocytes in PV, but also in some pts with ET and MF, and therefore cannot be utilized as a unique marker for one particular MPD *(23)*.

2. CLONALITY ANALYSIS IN CHRONIC MPDs

X-chromosome linkage analysis of the glucose-6-phosphate dehydrogenase gene in the terminally differentiated cells (e.g. erythrocytes, granulocytes, and platelets) of females established the clonal origin of PV and ET. The implication of these early studies was that these chronic MPDs arose from a pluripotent hematopoietic progenitor *(6,8)*. Subsequently, polymerase chain reaction (PCR) of the X-linked phosphoglycerate kinase gene was used to demonstrate the heterogeneity of clonal involvement of different lineages (e.g. erythroid vs.

myeloid) in female PV patients *(9)*. Clonality can only be established in the minority of cases of PV, ET, and MF by clinically available tests such as conventional cytogenetics or fluorescent in-situ hybridization.

2.1. JAKs and STATs

The Jak kinases are non-receptor tyrosine kinases which consist of 4 family members in mammals: JAK1, JAK2, JAK3, and tyrosine kinase 2 (TYK2) *(24)*. The JAK-STAT (signal transducer and activation of transcription) pathway is a common signaling pathway utilized by numerous cytokines, growth factors, and interferons. Ligand binding results in receptor dimerization, and activation of JAK kinases that are constitutively associated with the receptor. These events lead to phosphorylation of tyrosine residues on the intracellular domains of the dimerized receptor, permitting docking of STAT proteins. Subsequent phosphorylation of STAT proteins by JAKs results in their dimerization, and translocation to the nucleus where gene transcription is activated *(25)*.

Starting from the carboxy terminus, JAKs consist of 7 distinct structural domains, JH1 -JH7, whch are recapitulated among the 4 JAKs *(26)*. The JAK homology 1 (JH1) is the kinase domain, and the JAK homology 2 (JH2) pseudokinase domain is juxtaposed to JH1. The JH2 domain lacks catalytic activity, but serves an important function as a negative regulator of kinase activity *(26)*. The amino terminus of JAKs contain a Band-4.1, ezrin, radixin, moesin (FERM) homology domain (JH6-JH7) which mediates binding to cytokine receptors, and also is a positive regulator of catalytic activity *(26)*.

JAK1, JAK2, and TYK2 have a broad cellular distribution, whereas JAK3 is primarily expressed in hematopoietic cells *(24)*. JAK-STAT signaling serves as a messenger system for diverse body processes including (1) fat metabolism through transmission of signals from leptin to JAK2; (2) body growth via growth hormone receptor association with JAK2; and (3) immune system function mediated by signaling from interferons and various interleukins to JAK1 and JAK3 *(26)*. Relevant to the discussion herein, JAK2 is critical for signaling by erythropoietin (EPO), thrombopoietin (TPO), and cytokines that utilize the interleukin-3 family of receptors (IL-3, IL-5, and GM-CSF) *(26)*.

2.2. Why Focus on JAK2?

Several observations foreshadowed the relevance of JAK2 to hematopoietic malignancy, particularly PV and autonomous erythropoiesis. First, the growth factors to which hematopoietic progenitors are hypersensitive in MPDs (EPO, SCF, GM-CSF, IL-3, TPO, and IGF-1), all employ JAK2 for signaling *(26,27)*. Second, mutation of the gene analogous to *JAK2* in *Drosophila*, termed *Hopscotch*, results in kinase activation and a leukemia-like phenotype *(28,29)*. Conversely, *JAK2* knockout mice exhibit embryonic lethality due to a failure of erythropoiesis *(30,31)*.

TEL-JAK2 [(t9;12)(p24;p13)] is a constitutive fusion tyrosine kinase that leads to both myeloid and lymphoid leukemias in a murine bone marrow transplant model *(32)*. TEL-induced oligomerization of TEL-JAK2 results in constitutive tyrosine kinase activity and transforms the murine hematopoietic cell line Ba/F3 to IL-3 independent growth *(32,33)*. TEL-JAK2 signaling is mediated through STAT1, STAT3, STAT5 *(34,35)*, and phosphatidylinositol 3′-kinase *(36)*. In addition, the TEL-JAK2 fusion activates the extracellular signal-regulated kinase (ERK), stress-activated protein/JUN kinase, and p38 signaling pathways *(37)*.

In 2005, the t(8;9)(p23;p24) translocation was identified by 3 groups as a recurrent molecular rearrangement which fuses the *PCM1* gene on 8p22 with the *JAK2* gene on 9p24

(38–40). *PCM1-JAK2* is found in a spectrum of hematologic malignancies including acute myelogenous leukemia, atypical (*BCR-ABL*-negative) chronic myelogenous leukemia, chronic eosinophilic leukemia, and pre-B cell acute lymphoblastic leukemia *(38–40)*. Recently, a *BCR-JAK2* fusion [(t(9;22)(p24;q11.2)] was identified in a patient with Philadelphia chromosome-negative CML.*(41)* The *BCR* breakpoint is identical to the p190 breakpoint observed in the majority of cases of *BCR-ABL*-positive ALL and in some patients with CML, and the JAK2 breakpoint was identical to the breakpoint found in the *TEL-JAK2* fusion found in T-ALL *(33)*. Constitutive activation of the chimeric tyrosine kinase results from fusion of the kinase (JH1) domain of *JAK2* to the coiled-coil (CC) oligimerization domain of *BCR (41)*.

3. DIFFERENT PATHS LEAD TO THE DISCOVERY OF THE *JAK2* V617F MUTATION

The discovery of the *JAK2* V617F mutation as a shared genetic derangement in PV, ET, and MF was reported almost simultaneously by 4 groups in the *Lancet (2)*, *Cancer Cell (3)*, *Nature (4)*, and *The New England Journal of Medicine (NEJM) (5)* in the Spring of 2005. The research team led by Kralovics and colleagues *(5)* had previously reported that approximately 30% of patients with PV exhibit loss of heterozygosity (LOH) on the short arm of chromosome 9 *(42)*. This group considered 9p LOH a stem cell defect that may harbor a mutation that contributes to the clonal expansion of hematopoietic cells in chronic MPDs. By employing a greater number of microsatellite markers, this group was able to home in on a minimal genomic region shared by all patients with 9p LOH, and sequencing revealed the *JAK2* mutation in affected patients.

James and colleagues' discovery of the *JAK2* mutation began with a functional approach *(4)*. This group had previously shown that inhibitors of several signaling molecules/pathways (e.g. JAK2, Src, and phosphatidylinositol-3-OH kinase) blocked endogenous erythroid colony (EEC) formation in PV patients *(43)*. Their focus on JAK2, and ultimately the sequencing of the *JAK2* V617F mutant, was driven by experiments showing that a small interfering RNA against JAK2 substantially reduced EEC formation from PV patient samples.

An emerging theme in the pathogenesis of myeloid malignancies, particularly chronic MPDs, is the constitutive activation of tyrosine kinases leading to abnormal cell growth. Examples include the *BCR-ABL* fusion gene, found in 95% of patients with chronic myeloid leukemia, the *D816V KIT* mutation in the majority of cases of systemic mastocytosis, *PDGFRA* or *PDGFRB* fusions in MDS/MPDs with or without eosinophilia, and the fibroblast growth factor receptor 1 (*FGFR1*) chimeric oncoproteins in the 8p11 stem cell myeloproliferative syndrome (reviewed in *44* and *45*). In patients with acute myelogenous leukemia, mutation of the *FLT-3* receptor tyrosine kinase gene (internal tandem duplication or D835 mutation) in 30–35% of patients is associated with a worse prognosis *(46)*. It was therefore a logical approach by two of the groups *(2,3)* to pursue a high throughput screening of the kinome, including some 85 tyrosine kinases, to identify putative mutations that could explain the pathogenesis of PV, ET, and IMF. Their large-scale tyrosine kinase sequencing effort successfully uncovered the *JAK2* V617F mutation.

3.1. The *JAK2* V617F Mutation

The *JAK2* mutation results from a guanine-to-thymine change encoding a valine-to-phenylalanine substitution at codon 617 (V617F) *(2–5)*. The V617F mutation occurs within the JH2 domain of JAK2, which is the pseudokinase, or autoinhibitory domain of the

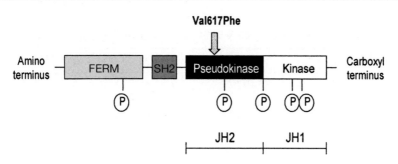

Fig. 1. Structural Schematic of the Jak2 Protein Showing the Position of the Val617Phe Mutation in the JH2 Pseudokinase Domain. FERM= 4.1 (f)-ezrin-radixin-moesin; SH2=SRC homology 2; JH1= Jak homology 1; JH2=Jak homology 2. P indicates an autophosphorylation site.

molecule (Figure 1). The JH2 domain negatively regulates the activity of the JH1 (kinase) domain (47,48). Molecular modeling of the JAK2 structure indicates the importance of the amino acid valine at position 617 for maintaining JH2-induced inhibition of the kinase domain in the inactive state; replacement by a phenylalanine residue is predicted to destabilize the inhibitory interaction, leading to constitutive JAK2 tyrosine kinase activity (49).

4. PREVALENCE OF THE *JAK2* V617F MUTATION IN CHRONIC MPDS AND OTHER HEMATOLOGIC MALIGNANCIES

Table 1 shows the prevalence of the *JAK2* V617F mutation in PV, ET, and MF among 8 studies (2–5,50–53). The cumulative frequency is 78% in PV, 41% in ET, and 50% in MF.

To date, the mutation has not been identified in secondary erythrocytoses, lymphoid malignancies such as chronic or acute lymphoid leukemias (51,54), and is rarely present in acute myelogenous leukemia, except for the French-American-British (FAB) subtype M7 (acute megakaryocytic leukemia) (52). In cases of AML in which the mutation is identified, such patients have usually had an antecedent history of PV, ET, or MF (52,54). In analyses of smaller cohorts of patients "atypical" myeloproliferative disorders (e.g. atypical/unclassified MPD, CMML, systemic mastocytosis, and idiopathic hyypereosinophilic syndrome, the *JAK2* V617F mutation is either not detected, or at a relatively low frequency compared to PV, ET, or MF (Table 2) (51,52,54–56). In three studies, a small proportion of MDS patients also exhibited the *JAK2* V617F mutation (52,54,55).

The *JAK2* V617F allele is not detected in normal individuals. In 12/313 (4%) of chronic MPD patients (11 PV, 1 MF), heterozygosity for the *V617F* allele was identified in buccal mucosal cells, indicating that germline transmission of the mutation is a rare event in patients with chronic MPDs (3). Seven of these 12 patients had PV, and DNA from their granulocytes showed a homozygous *JAK2 V617F* pattern, consistent with LOH at the 9p24 locus.

The *JAK2* V617F mutation is not detected in T-cells (2), and another study confirmed lack of involvement of both T-cells and B-cells in 3 patients homozygous for the mutation (56). However, in the CD34+ cell fraction, a mixed clonality pattern with wild-type *JAK2* was observed, with the mutant form predominating (57). These findings indicate that *JAK2* V617F is an acquired somatic mutation in the vast majority of patients, and that its phenotypic expression is limited to the myeloid lineage.

Table 1
Prevalence of the *JAK2* V617F Mutation in PV, ET, and MF

Study (ref.)	PV	ET	MF
Baxter et al. *(2)*	71/73 (97%)	29/51 (57%)	8/16 (50%)
Levine et al. *(3)*	121/164 (74%)	37/115 (32%)	16/46 (35%)
James et al. *(4)*	40/45 (89%)	9/21 (43%)	3/7 (43%)
Kralovics et al. *(5)*	83/128 (65%)	21/93 (23%)	13/23 (57%)
Zhao et al. *(50)*	20/24 (83%)	ND	ND
Jones et al. *(51)*	58/72 (81%)	24/59 (41%)	15/35 (43%)
Jelinek et al. *(52)*	25/29 (86%)	3/10 (30%)	18/19 (95%)
Antonioli et al. *(53)*	ND	74/130	ND
Totals	418/535 (78%)	197/479 (41%)	73/146 (50%)

PV, polycythemia vera; ET, essential thrombocythemia; MF, idiopathic myelofibrosis; ND = not determined.

5. EXPERIMENTAL EVIDENCE HIGHLIGHTING THE PATHOGENETIC RELEVANCE OF *JAK2* V617F TO CHRONIC MPDs

Prior studies have shown that erythroid and granulocyte-macrophage progenitor cells from polycythemia vera patients can grow in the absence of erythropoietin, as well as several other growth factors, including interleukin-3 and granulocyte-macrophage colony-stimulating factor *(12–15)*. In the initial study describing the *JAK2* V617F mutation, the mutation was detected from individual hematopoietic colonies derived from a patient with ET, incuding CFU-GM, BFU-E, and endogenous erythroid colonies (EEC) *(2)*. These results are consistent with the notion that the mutation arises in a pluripotent hematopoietic progenitor that gives rise to myeloid and erythroid lineages. There was a significantly higher frequency of the mutation in EPO-independent erythroid colonies (100%), versus CFU-GM and BFU-E *(2)*. As a corollary to this finding, only erythroid progenitors with the mutation could grow in the absence of exogenous EPO, whereas normal or mutant erythroid progenitors could grow in the presence of EPO *(2)*.

In another series of experiments, a small interfering RNA (SiRNA) that reduced JAK2 expression by 90% markedly reduced EEC formation, highlighting the dependence of endogenous erythroid colony growth on the JAK2 protein *(4)*. In addition, induction of apoptosis and dose-dependent inhibition of proliferation the HEL human erythroleukemia cell line (*JAK2* V617F homozygous-positive) was observed with a small molecule JAK2 inhibitor *(3)*. Such effects were not observed in the K562 cell line which expresses a constitutively activated BCR-ABL protein, but not mutant *JAK2 (3)*.

In *in vitro* experiments assessing the transforming potential of JAK2 on cell lines, expression of the mutant (but not wild type) JAK2 in the factor dependent cell line BaF3/EPO led to EPO hypersensitivity and growth factor-independent survival *(4)*. In addition, expression

Table 2
Prevalence of the *JAK2* V617F Mutation in Atypical MPDs, MDS, and Acute/Chronic Myeloid and Lymphoid Leukemias

Study (ref.)	Atypical CML/CMML	SM	HES	CNL	MDS	JMML	Ph+CML/ de novo AML[a]	B/T-cell ALL	CLL
Levine et al. (54)	9/116				2/48		1/219	0/176	0/45
Jelinek et al. (52)	10/68				1/68		0/127[b]	0/20	
Jones et al. (51)	30/152		2/134						
Steensma et al. (55)	3/119	2/8		1/6	5/101				
Tono et al. (56)						1/5			
Totals	52/455 (11.4%)	2/8 (25%)	2/134 (1.5%)	1/6 (17%)	8/217 (3.7%)	1/5 (20%)	1/346 (<1%)	0/196 (0%)	0/45 (0%)

CML, chronic myelogenous leukemia; CMML, chronic myelomonocytic leukemia; SM, systemic mastocytosis; HES, idiopathic hyperesosinophilic syndrome; CNL, chronic neutrophilic leukemia; MDS, myelodysplastic syndrome; JMML, juvenile myelomonocytic leukemia; Ph+, Philadelphia chromosome-positive; AML, acute myelogenous leukemia; ALL, acute lymphoblastic leukemia; CLL, chronic lymphocytic leukemia.

[a]M0–M6 AML.

[b]2/11 (18%) patients with megakaryocytic leukemia (M7) demonstrated the *JAK2 V617F* mutation (not shown).

of mutant JAK2 along with the EPO receptor in a Ba/F3 cell line led to EPO-independent STAT5 activation *(4)*.

The *in vivo* effects of the *JAK2* V617F mutation were tested in mice transplanted with bone marrow cells transduced with murine embryonic stem cell virus carrying mutant and wild-type *JAK2*, or empty vector *(4)*. Only introduction of the *JAK2* mutant led to erythrocytosis (hematocrit 60%) following their transplantation into lethally irradiated recipients. These *in vivo* results provide convincing evidence of the relevance of the *JAK2* mutation to the pathogenesis of human PV.

A series of experiments investigated the possible inhibitory effects of wild-type JAK2 on the cellular effects mediated by the mutant JAK2 protein *(4)*. Co-expression of wild-type JAK2 with the mutant protein restored EPO dependence in Ba/F3 cells. In addition, co-expression of wild-type and mutant JAK2 protein in 293T cells did not interfere with autophosphorylation of JAK2 V617F *(4)*. Therefore, wild-type JAK2 does not appear to directly down-regulate the activity of mutant JAK2; instead, it may compete for binding sites on receptors and interfere with the ability of mutant JAK2 to activate downstream signaling.

5.1. Heterozygosity vs Homozygosity for the JAK2 V617F Mutation

Homozygous *JAK2* V617F mutations occur in approximately 15–20% of MPD patients (25–30% of PV patients) *(2,3,5)*, and appear to result from loss of heterozygosity (LOH) from mitotic recombination, not from deletion of the normal *JAK2* allele at the 9p24 locus. In the study by Kralovics and colleagues *(5)*, 51/244 MPD patients exhibited 9p LOH. All 51 patients had the V617F mutation: 43/51 patients were homozygous and 8/51 were heterozygous. The remaining 193/244 MPD patients did not exhibit 9p LOH. Of these 193 patients, 66 were heterozygous, 127 were wild-type, and none were homozygous for the mutant allele. In one series *(2)*, DNA was available for analysis from 27 PV patients within a year of diagnosis, and seven (26%) were homozygous for the *JAK2 V617F* mutation. This was the same frequency of homozygosity observed within the entire PV cohort. These data indicate that patients with PV may exhibit homozygosity for the *JAK2* mutation in early in their course, and is not necessarily a feature of advanced or longstanding disease.

6. GENOTYPE-PHENOTYPE CORRELATIONS OF THE *JAK2* V617F MUTATION

Several studies have evaluated whether the *JAK2* V617F genotype translates into differences in clinical presentation. In one study *(2)*, no statistically significant differences in clinical or laboratory features at presentation were found in ET and MF patients with or without the *JAK2* V617F mutation. However, Levine et al found that several statistically significant differences were associated with mutation status *(3)*. For example, within their PV cohort, women were more likely than men to have a heterozygous or homozygous mutation. In a cohort of ET patients, age or sex was not related to *JAK2* mutation status *(53)*. However, in a multivariate analysis, the *JAK2* mutation was associated with a higher hemoglobin level in these ET patients. These individuals did not meet WHO criteria for PV.

Kralovics and colleagues found a statistically significant association between positivity for the *JAK2 V617F* mutation and 1) the rate of complications (fibrosis, thrombosis, and hemorrhage), 2) prior need for cytoreductive treatment, and 3) the increased age of patients *(5)*. Two studies confirmed that a longer duration of disease was associated with a homozygous mutation *(3,5)*. In one of these studies, this association was restricted to PV and ET patients

(89 vs. 61 months, p = .008), and not found in MF patients *(3)*. It is unknown whether the association between longer disease duration and homozygosity for the *JAK2* V617F mutation simply reflects the time required for two sequential genetic mutational events to occur: the first being acquisition of the *JAK2* mutation, and the second related to mitotic recombination at the 9p24 *JAK2* locus. However, the finding that the frequency of homozygous mutations in patients within year of diagnosis mirrors that of an entire PV cohort *(2)* would suggest otherwise, or that unknown additional factors may be relevant.

6.1. Biologic Correlates of the JAK2 **V617F** *Mutation*

Three biologic alterations which are characteristic of patients with chronic MPDs include the ablility to form endogenous erythroid colonies (EEC) in culture without exogenous erythropoietin, overexpression of PRV-1 mRNA in granulocytes, and decreased c-Mpl (thrompopoietin receptor) expression (see above). The *JAK2* V617F genotype was highly correlated with the ability to form EEC (64/65 patients, R =0.97), and PRV-1 overexpression (77/78 patients, R =0.98), both statistically significant (p < .0001) *(58)*. However, the association of EEC and PRV-1 overexpression was not found in ET patients *(53)*. In contrast, c-Mpl expression was not correlated with mutation status *(53,58)*, which is consistent with prior reports indicating no association between c-Mpl expression with either EEC formation or level of PRV-1 expression. In ET patients with EEC/PRV-1 overexpression, a higher incidence of clinical evolution to PV has been noted *(59)*. It is possible that that the "PV phenotype" that emerges in some ET patients reflects the presence of the *JAK2* V617F mutation, and that EEC formation and PRV-1 overexpression are co-segregating biologic markers.

RNA microarray analysis has been used to define altered gene expression patterns in PV patients vs. normal controls, and between PV patients with normal vs. mutant *JAK2*. Compared to patients without *JAK2* V617F, patients heterozygous or homozygous for the mutation exhibited upregulation of 13 genes, in addition to the *PRV1* and *NF-E2* (nuclear factor erythroid-derived 2) genes, whereas the gene *ANKRD15* was downregulated *(60)*. Changes in these gene expression patterns were also observed with activation of the JAK/STAT pathway in response to secondary neutrophilia or G-CSF treatment), suggesting that these gene signatures were more broadly related to activation of the JAK/STAT signaling axis *(60)*. RNA microarray and proteomic analyses are complementary approaches that may help further characterize the biologic changes and clinical phenotypes resulting from the *JAK2* mutation.

7. NEW "SPECULATIONS"

While the discovery of the *JAK2* V617F mutation provides at least a partial explanation for the longstanding enigma regarding the molecular pathogenesis of the classic chronic MPDs, the finding raises many new "speculations." For example, it is unknown how a single mutation leads to multiple clinical phenotypes. Although found in at least 80% of PV patients, the *V671F* mutation is also found in 40% and 50% of ET and MF patients, respectively, as well as in a low proportion of atypical MPD cases. Hypotheses that merit investigation include whether the mutation arises in different hematopoietic progenitors in these diseases, or becomes skewed toward a particular progenitor compartment over time. Another consideration is whether expression of mutant kinase activity is lineage dependent. For example, in *FIP1L1-PDGFRA* (F-P)–positive chronic eosinophilic leukemia (CEL), the gene for the F-P fusion tyrosine kinase can be detected in multiple lineages, including neutrophils, monocytes, and B- and T-lymphocytes, in addition to eosinophils; however, hypereosinophilia is the primary manifestation of disease and neutrophilia is uncommonly present *(45)*. In CEL, the cellular mechanisms which link constitutive F-P fusion tyrosine kinase activity with preferential eosinophil proliferation and/or decreased apoptosis in CEL are currently unknown. Similarly, the *JAK2* V617F mutation may require a particular cellular milieu and expression of cell-specific genes in order for a particular phenotype to become manifest. Although not yet demonstrated, accumulation of secondary mutations and/or individual genetic backgrounds may also modify the phenotypic expression of the mutation. Longitudinal analysis of larger cohorts of patients will be needed to confirm whether there is a gene dosage effect (e.g. heterozygosity vs homozygosity for *JAK2* V617F mutation) on clinical disease expression and aggressiveness. Additional studies will also be required to establish whether *JAK2* V617F-positive patients differ from similarly-treated patients with normal *JAK2* regarding the natural history of their disease (e.g. rates of thrombosis, hemorrhage, myelofibrosis, and evolution to AML).

8. FUTURE DIRECTIONS

Distinction of a chronic MPD vs. secondary (reactive) causes of erythrocytosis, thrombocytosis, and myelofibrosis can often be a diagnostic challenge. The *JAK2* V617F mutation is an unique clonal marker that now offers the potential for rapid and reliable diagnosis of PV and other myeloproliferative disorders. New diagnostic algorithms for PV (and other chronic MPDs) are being generated which incorporate *JAK2* mutation screening in conjunction with conventional clinical and laboratory assessments *(61)*. Since the *JAK2* mutation is found in approximately 80% of PV patients, it will likely become the supervening diagnostic screening modality in the patient presenting with an elevated hemoglobin, without obvious evidence of a secondary erythrocytosis or decreased plasma volume. For PV patients with an indeterminate (low-positive) or negative mutation screen for *JAK2* V617F, the Polycythemia Vera Study Group (PVSG) modified criteria *(62)* provide useful guidance for establishing the diagnosis of PV. The PVSG criteria may need to be re-evaluated in light of the discovery of the *JAK2* mutation. However, as the PVSG criteria allow for the diagnosis of PV based solely on the detection of a clonal marker, these criteria should be able to accommodate the new findings without the need for significant revision. With the molecular origins of an increasing number of chronic MPDs being revealed, a semi-molecular classification scheme of these disorders will likely emerge and should prove useful in this age of targeted therapeutics.

The genetic basis for *JAK2 V617F*-negative chronic MPDs, which currently comprises 10–20% of PV patients, and some 50% of MF and ET patients, is unknown. Future investigations are certain to focus on the mutational status and activity of negative regulators of JAK2 including SOCS-1,*(63)* SOCS-2,*(64)* SOCS-3,*(65)* SHP-1 *(66)*, and protein tyrosine phosphatase 1B *(67)*. (also reviewed in *25*). For example, bi-allelic disruption of the SOCS-1 gene in primary mediastinal B-cell lymphoma (PMBL) cell lines/patient samples leads to sustained JAK2 phosphorylation *(61)*. Impaired negative regulation of the JAK2 signaling axis may therefore be a primary pathogenetic event in PBML, and should be evaluated in the chronic MPDs.

Discovery of the JAK2 mutation is fostering investigations which focus on the downstream biological consequences of constitutive JAK2 activity. Using renal interstitial (NRK-49F) fibroblasts as a model of diabetic nephropathy and renal fibrosis, angiotensin II was found to induce

JAK2 activation and connective tissue growth factor (CTGF) expression *(68)*. Although not specifically studied in the context of MF, CTGF is implicated in various fibrotic disorders and induced in fibroblasts after activation with transforming growth factor-beta (TGF-β) *(69)*. In turn, TGF-β appears to play a pivotal role in the pathogenesis of MF. TGF-β produced by hematopoietic cells is pivotal for the development of myelofibrosis in mice with TPO overexpression *(70)*, and is a cytokine implicated in the ineffective hematopoiesis and osteosclerosis of MF *(71)*.

Akin to the development of imatinib as a selective BCR-ABL tyrosine kinase inhibitor in CML, targeted agents are now in development to block the constitutive tyrosine kinase activity of the *JAK2 V617F* mutant. However, since the JAK-STAT signaling pathway is utilized by many cytokines and is involved in ubiquitous body processes, especially immune cell function, the challenge for drug development will be to design a specific inhibitor of mutant JAK2 with an acceptable therapeutic index that preserves the activity of normal JAK2 and related family members.

REFERENCES

1. Dameshek W. Some speculations on the myeloproliferative syndromes. Blood 1951;6:372–375.
2. Baxter JE, Scott LM, Campbell PJ, et al. Acquired mutation of the tyrosine kinase JAK2 in human myeloproliferative disorders. Lancet 2005;365:1054–1061.
3. Levine RL, Wadleigh M, Cools J, et al. Activating mutation in the tyrosine kinase JAK2 in polycthemia vera, essential thrombocythemia, and myeloid metaplasia with myelofibrosis. Cancer Cell 2005;7:387–397.
4. James C, Ugo V, Le Couédic J-P, et al. A unique clonal JAK2 mutation leading to constitutive signalling causes polycythemia vera. Nature 2005;434:1144–1148.
5. Kralovics R, Passamonti F, Buser AS, et al. A gain-of-function of JAK2 in myeloproliferative disorders. New Engl J Med 2005;352:1779–1790.
6. Adamson JW, Fialkow PJ, Murphy S, Prchal JF, Steinmann L. Polycythemia vera: stem cell and probable clonal origin of the disease. New Engl J Med 1976;295:913–916.
7. Prchal JF, Adamson JW, Steinmann L, Fialkow PJ. Human erythroid colony formation in vitro: evidence for clonal origin. J Cell Physiol 1976;89:489–492.
8. Fialkow PJ, Faguet GB,Jacobson RJ, Vaidya K, Murphy S. Evidence that essential thrombocythemia is a clonal disorder with origin a multipotent stem cell. Blood 1981;518:916–919.
9. Gilliland DG, Blanchard KL, Levy J, Perrin S, Bunn HF. Clonality in myeloproliferative disorders: Analysis by means of the polymerase chain reaction. Proc Natl Acad Sci USA 1991;88:6848–6852.
10. Harrison CN, Gale RE, Machin SJ, Linch DC. A large proportion of patients with a diagnosis of essential thrombocythemia do not have a clonal disorder and may be at lower risk of thrombotic complications. Blood 1999;93:417–424.
11. Prchal JF, Axelrad AA. Letter: bone-marrow responses in polycythemia vera. New Engl J Med 1974;290:1382.
12. Zanjani ED, Lutton JD, Hoffman R, Wasserman LR. Erythroid colony formation by polycythemia vera bone marrow in vitro. Dependence on erythropoietin J Clin Invest 1977;59:841–848.
13. Dai CH, Krantz SB, Dessypris EN, Means RT Jr, Horn ST, Gilbert HS. Polycythemia vera, II: hypersensitivity of bone marrow erythroid, granulocyte-macrophage, and megakaryocyte-progenitor cells to interleukin-3 and granulocyte-macrophage colony-stimulating factor. Blood 1992;80:891–899.
14. Dai CH, Krantz SB, Koury ST, Kollar K. Polycythemia vera, IV: specific binding of stem cell factor to normal and polycthaemia vera highly purified erythroid progenitor cells. Br J Haematol 1994;88:497–505.
15. Correa PN, Eskinazi D, Axelrad AA, Circulating erythroid progenitors in polycythemia vera are hypersensitive to insulin-like growth factor-1 in vitro: studies in an improved serum-free medium. Blood 1994;83:99–112.
16. Axelrad AA, Eskinazi D, Correa PN, Amato D. Hypersensitivity of circulating progenitor cells to megakaryocyte growth and development factor (PEG-rHu MGDF) in essential thrombocythemia. Blood 2000;96:3310–3321.
17. Fruchtman S, Barosi G, Fung JJ, Guardiola P, et al. Clinical symposia report- myeloproliferative disorders: issues, controversies, and advances in treatment. Clin Adv Hematol Oncol. June 2004; 2–15.
18. Moliterno AR, Hankins WD, Spivak JL. Impaired expression of the thrombopoietin receptor by platelets from patients with polycythemia vera. N Engl J Med 1998;338:572–580.

19. Moliterno AR, Siebel KE, Sun AY, et al. A novel thrombopoietin signaling defect in polycythemia vera platelets. Stem Cells 1998;16:185–192.
20. Horikawa Y, Matsumura I, Hashimoto K, et al Markedly reduced expression of platelet c-mpl receptor in essential thrombocythemia. Blood 1997;90:4031–4038.
21. Li J, Xia Y, Kuter DJ. The platelet thrombopoietin receptor number and function are markedly reduced in patients with essential thrombocythemia. Br J Haematol 2000;111:943–953.
22. Harrison CN, Gale RE, Pezella F, et al. Platelet c-mpl expression is dysregulated in patients with essential thrombocythaemia but this is not of diagnostic value. Br J Haematol 1999;107:139–147.
23. Bock O, Serinsoz E, Neusch M, et al. The polycythaemia rubra vera-1 gene is constitutively expressed by bone marrow cells and does not discriminate polycythaemia vera from reactive and other chronic myelo-proliferative disorders. Br J Haematol 2003;123:472–474.
24. Aringer M, Cheng A, Nelson JW, et al. Janus Kinases and their role in growth and disease. Life Sciences 1999;64:2173–2186.
25. Shuai K, Liu B. Regulation of the Jak-Stat signaling in the immune system. Nature Rev 2003;3:900–911.
26. Yamaoka K, Saharinen P, Pesu M, Holt III VET, Silvennoinen O, Shea JO. The Janus kinases (Jaks). Genome Biol 2004;5:253–258.
27. Kaushansky K, et al. On the molecular origins of the chronic myeloproliferative disorders: it all makes sense. Blood 2005;105:4187–4190.
28. Hanratty WP, Dearolf CR. The *Drosophila* Tumorous-lethal hematopoietic oncogene is a dominant mutation in the *hopscotch* locus. Mol Gen Genet 1993;238:33–37.
29. Harrison DA, Binari R, Nahreini TS, Gilman M, Perrimon N. Activation of a Drosophila Janus kinase (JAK) causes hematopoietic neoplasia and developmental defects. EMBO J 1995;14:2857–2865.
30. Neubauer H, Cumano A, Muller M, Wu H, Huffstadt U, Pfeffer K. Jak2 deficiency defines an essential developmental checkpoint in definitive hematopoiesis. Cell. 1998;93:397–409.
31. Parganas E, Wang D, Stravopodis D, et al. Jak2 is essential for signaling through a variety of cytokine receptors. Cell 1998;93:385–395.
32. Schwaller J, Frantsve J, Aster J, et al. Transformation of hematopoietic cell lines to growth-factor independence and induction of a fatal myelo- and lymphoproliferative disease in mice by retrovirally transduced TEL/JAK2 fusion genes. EMBO J 1998;17:5321–5333.
33. Lacronique V, Boureaux A, Valle VD, et al. A TEL-JAK2 fusion protein with constitutive kinase activity in human leukemia. Science 1997;278:1309–1312.
34. Ho JM, Beattie BK, Squire JA, Frank DA, Barber DL. Fusion of the ets transcription factor TEL to Jak2 results in constitutive Jak-Stat signaling. Blood 1999;93:4354–4364.
35. Schwaller J, Parganas E, Wang D, et al. Stat5 is essential for the myelo- and lymphoproliferative disease induced by TEL/JAK2. Mol Cell 2000;6:693–704.
36. Nguyen MH, Ho JM, Beattie BK, Barber DL. TEL-JAK2 mediates constitutive activation of the phosphati-dylinositol 3′-kinase/protein kinase B signaling pathway. J Biol Chem 2001;276;32,704–32,713.
37. Ho JM, Nguyen MH, Dierov JK, et al. TEL-JAK2 constitutively activates the extracellular signal-regulated kinase (ERK), stress-activated protein/Jun kinase (SAPK/JNK), and p38 signaling pathways. Blood 2002; 100:1438–1448.
38. Reiter A, Walz C, Watmore A, et al. The t(8;9)(p22;p24) is a recurrent abnormality in chronic and acute leukemia that fuses PCM1 to JAK2. Cancer Res 2005;65:2662–2667.
39. Bousquet M, Quelen C, De Mas V, et al. The t(8;9)(p22;p24) translocation in atypical chronic myeloid leukaemia yields a new PCM1-JAK2 fusion gene. Oncogene. 2005 August 8; [Epub ahead of print].
40. Murati A, Gelsi-Boyer V, Adélaide J, et al. PCM1-JAK2 fusion in myeloproliferative disorders and acute erythroid leukemia with t(8;9) translocation. Leukemia 2005;19:1692–1696.
41. Griesinger F, Hennig H, Hillmer F, et al. A BCR-JAK2 fusion gene as the result of a t(9;22)(p24;q11.2) translocation in a patient with a clinically typical chronic myeloid leukemia. Genes Chromosomes Cancer 2005;44:329–333.
42. Kralovics R, Guan Y, Prchal JT. Acquired uniparental disomy of chromosome 9p is a frequent stem cell defect in polycythemia vera. Exp Hematol 2002;30:229–236.
43. Ugo V, Marzac C, Teyssandier I, et al. Multiple signaling pathways are involved in erythropoietin-independent differentiation of erythroid progenitors in polycythemia vera. Exp. Hematol 2004;32:179–187.
44. O'Brien S, Tefferi A, Valent P. Chronic myelogenous leukemia and myeloproliferative disease. Hematology (Am Soc Hematol Educ Program.) 2004;146–162.

45. Gotlib J. Molecular classification and pathogenesis of eosinophilic disorders: 2005 update. Acta Haematol 2005;114:7–25.
46. Gilliland DG, Griffin JD. Role of FLT3 in leukemia. Curr Opin Hematol 2002;9:274–281.
47. Saharinen P, Takaluoma K, Silvennoinen O. Regulation of the Jak2 tyrosine kinase by its pseudokinase domain. Mol Cell Biol 2000;20:3387–3395.
48. Saharinen P, Silvennoinen O. The pseudokinase domain is required for suppression of basal activity of Jak2 and Jak3 tyrosine kinases and for cytokine-inducible activation of signal transduction. J Biol Chem 2002; 277:47,954–47,963.
49. Lindauer K, Loerting T, Liedl KR, Kroemer RT. Prediction of the structure of human Janus kinase 2 (JAK2) comprising the two carboxy-terminal domains revceals a mechanism for autoregulation. Protein Eng 2001; 14:27–37.
50. Zhao R, Xing S, Li Z, et al. Identification of acquired JAK2 mutation in polycythemia vera. J Biol Chem 2005;280:22,788–22,792.
51. Jones AV, Kreil S, Zoi K, et al. Widespread occurrence of the JAK2 V617F mutation in chronic myeloproliferative disorders. Blood 2005;106:2162–2168.
52. Jelinek J, Oki Y, Gharibyan V, et al. JAK2 mutation 1849G>T is rare in acute leukemias but can be found in CMML, Philadelphia-chromosome negative CML and megakaryocytic leukemia. Blood 2005;106:3370–3373.
53. Antonioli E, Guglielmelli P, Pancrazzi A, et al. Clinical implications of the JAK2 V617F mutation in essential thrombocythemia. Leukemia 2005;19:1847–1849.
54. Levine RL, Loriaux M, Huntly BJP, et al. The JAK2V617F activating mutation occurs in chronic myelomonocytic leukemia and acute myeloid leukemia, but not in acute lymphoblastic leukemia or chronic lymphocytic leukemia. Blood 2005;106:3377–3379.
55. Steensma DP, Dewald GW, Lasho TL, et al. The JAK2 V617F activating tyrosine kinase mutation is an infrequent event in both "atypical" myeloproliferative disorders and myelodysplastic syndromes. Blood 2005;106:1207–1209.
56. Tono C, Xu G, Toki T, et al. JAK2 Val617Phe activating tyrosine kinase mutation in juvenile myelomonocytic leukemia. Leukemia 2005;19:1843–1844.
57. Lasho TL, Mesa R, Gilliland DG, Tefferi A. Mutation studies in CD3, CD19, and CD34 cell fractions in myeloproliferative disorders with homozygous JAK2 in granulocytes. Br J Haematol 2005;130:797–799.
58. Goerttler P, Steimle C, Marz E, et al. The Jak2V617F mutation, PRV-1 overexpression and EEC formation define a similar cohort of MPD patients. Blood 2005;106:2862–2864.
59. Griesshammer M, Klippel S, Strunck E, et al. PRV-1 mRNA expression discriminates two types of essential thrombocythemia. Ann Hematol 2004;83:364–370.
60. Kralovics R, Teo S-S, Buser AS, et al. Altered gene expression in myeloproliferative disorders correlates with activation of signaling by the V617F mutation of JAK2. Blood 2005;106:3374–3376.
61. Tefferi A, Gilliland DG. The JAK2V617F tyrosine kinase mutation in myeloproliferative disorders: status report and immediate implications for disease classification and diagnosis. Mayo Clin Proc. 2005;80:947–958.
62. Pearson TC, Messinezy M. The diagnostic criteria of polycythaemia rubra vera. Leuk Lymphoma 1996;22 (Suppl. 1):87–93.
63. Melzner I, Bucur AJ, Bruderlein S, et al. Biallelic mutation of SOCS-1 impairs JAK2 degradation and sustains phosphor-JAK2 action in the MedB-1 mediastinal lymphoma line. Blood 2005;105:2535–2542.
64. Leung KC, Doyle N, Ballesteros M, et al. Estrogen inhibits GH signaling by suppressing GH-induced JAK2 phosphorylation, an effect mediated by SOCS-2. Proc Natl Acad Sci USA 2003;100:1016–1021.
65. Ridderstrale M, Amstrup J, Hilton DJ, Billestrup N, Tornqvist H. SOCS-3 is involved in the downregulation of the acute insulin-like effects of growth hormon in rat adipocytes by inhibition of JAK2/IRS-1 signaling. Horm Metab Res 2003;35:169–177.
66. Jiao H, Berrada K, Yang W, Tabrizi M, Platanias LC, Yi T. Direct association with and dephosphorylation of Jak2 kinase by the SH2 domain-containing protein tyrosine phosphatase SHP-1. Mol Cell Biol 1996;16: 6985–6992.
67. Myers MP, Andersen JN, Cheng A, et al. TYK2 and JAK2 are substrates of protein-tyrosine phosphatase 1B. J Biol Chem 2001;276:47,771–47,774.
68. Lee CI, Guh JY, Chen HC, Hung WC, Yang YL, Chuang LY. Advanced glycation end-product-induced mitogenesis and collagen production are dependent on angiotensin II and connective tissue growth factor in NRK-49F cells.

69. Grotendorst. GR. Connective tissue growth factor: a mediator of TGF-beta action on fibroblasts. Cytokine Growth Factor Rev 1997;8:171–179.
70. Chagraoui H, Tulliez M, Smayra T, et al. Stimulation of osteoprotegerin production is responsible for osteosclerosis in mice overexpressing TPO. Blood 2003;101:2983–2989.
71. Tefferi A. Myelofibrosis with myeloid metaplasia. N Engl J Med 2000;342:1255–1265.

20 New Designs for Clinical Trials

Elihu Estey

CONTENTS

Summary

Designs for clinical trials have undergone little change in the past 30 years. Nonetheless, conventional designs have numerous inadequacies. Because it fails to use all available information accumulated during the trial and typically has an insufficient sample size, the 3+3 phase 1 design is often unlikely to select the correct dose implied in the 3+3 algorithm. The design fails to account for covariates, thus assuming, despite evidence to the contrary, that dose is the only determinant of toxicity. It does not monitor response, thus failing to recognize the phase 2 aspects of phase 1 trials and the phase 1 aspects of phase 2 trials; rather these features are often addressed in an *ad hoc* fashion. Phase 2 trials similarly ignore the realities of medical practice. Thus, although patients are interested in frequent data analyses, standard designs discourage these because of the connection between *p*-value and trial design and the desire to maintain a specified final *p*-value. In addition to being inadequately adaptive, phase 2 designs are frequently concerned with only a single outcome. Here we propose remedies for the shortcomings noted above. Such solutions are based on the Bayesian paradigm.

Key Words: 3+3 design; conventional two-stage designs; Bayesian methodology.

1. NEW DESIGNS FOR CLINICAL TRIALS

Over the past 10 years significant advances in basic biological sciences have regularly been translated into the management of patients with acute myeloid leukemia (AML). For example, the goal of therapy in acute promyelocytic leukemia (APL) is now molecular remission, bone marrows are now examined for internal tandem duplications in the Flt3 gene, and current clinical trials are investigating various new therapies posited to target molecular abnormalities thought critical for survival of AML, but not normal, blasts.

During these same years many papers describing new designs for clinical trials have appeared in the statistical literature. Nonetheless, and in contrast to the rapidity with which modern biological methods have found application in clinical medicine, the methods used to conduct clinical trials have remained fundamentally unchanged for 25 years at least. Specifically, a phase 1 trial using the 3+3 method is done to determine the dose of a new drug

From: *Contemporary Hematology: Acute Myelogenous Leukemia*
Edited by: J. E. Karp © Humana Press Inc., Totowa, NJ

to be administered in a subsequent phase 2 trial. The latter is typically a single-arm study that takes only one interim look at the data for purposes of deciding whether the new drug is so unlikely to be successful that the trial should be stopped before the planned number of patients is accrued. If, after the trial is completed, the results appear promising, a large randomized phase 3 study examines whether the standard or the new treatment is superior. Again, the number of interim analyses is kept low in order to maintain a 5% false-positive rate at the end of the study.

This chapter will review problems with current phase 1, 2, and 3 designs and propose alternatives that might be clinically useful, much as are modern molecular biological techniques. An underlying theme will be that the distinctions between phase 1 and 2, and between phase 2 and 3, are dysfunctional, serving the best interests of neither patients nor investigators. Accordingly, alternative designs will include those that combine aspects of phase 1 and 2, and phase 2 and phase 3.

2. PHASE 1 DESIGNS

2.1. The Conventional 3+3

In the standard 3+3 design, three patients are entered at a given dose. If none of these three has (severe) toxicity, the next three patients receive a higher dose, while if two or three have such toxicity, the next three patients are treated at a lower dose. Finally, if one of the first three patients has toxicity, another three are treated at the initial dose, with the dose subsequently escalated if one of these first six has toxicity, lowered if three or more have toxicity, and considered as appropriate if two of six have toxicity.

The 3+3 design is an algorithm that arrives at a dose without a specific objective criterion. However, because a toxicity rate of 3/6, but not 1/6, is considered excessive, we may infer that the phase 1 study aims to determine a dose where the probability of toxicity is between 17 and 50%, for example, about 25–35%. However, computer simulation of various plausible clinical scenarios indicates that the 3+3 design performs quite poorly in achieving this objective. Table 1 *(1)* shows an example, assuming a maximum sample size of 36 treated in 12 cohorts of 3 each. The first row in the table lists 6 doses, labeled 100 through 600. The second row illustrates a scenario where the true probability of toxicity at the 100 dose is very low, 0.01, with the probability of toxicity increasing with dose, until it becomes 0.76 at 600. (By "true" we mean what would be observed if an infinite number of patients had been treated.) Because the 300 dose produces a true toxicity rate of 0.26, we would like the design to select 300 as the appropriate dose for future patients. However, the third row of the table indicates that the 3+3 design will select this dose in only 41% of cases. The algorithm is as likely to select a dose (200) associated with a true probability of toxicity of only 0.09. The 3+3 also does poorly in the second scenario (Table 1, row 5), in which 100 is the appropriate dose, with higher doses producing true toxicity rates between 0.53 and 0.88. Here the 3+3 is as likely to terminate without selecting a dose as it is to select 100.

The 3+3 performs so poorly, and is thus said to have poor operating characteristics (OC), for two related reasons. First, it treats a relatively small number of patients: on average 16 in scenario 1, 13 in scenario 2, and 8 in scenario 3 (rows 4, 7, and 10 in Table 1). Second, it does not use all available information. In particular, the dose for the next cohort of three patients is determined only by the results in the previous cohort. Say two of the three patients in a given cohort had toxicity at a given dose. The 3+3 algorithm does not permit revisitation of that dose. However, it is intuitive that there would be more inclination to give the same dose

Table 1
Operating Characteristics of the 3+3 Design (4000 simulations per scenario)

Dose	100	200	300	400	500	600	No dose selected
True probability of toxicity	0.01	0.09	**0.26**[b]	0.47	0.64	0.76	—
Probability of selecting dose as appropriate	0.08	0.43	0.41	0.07	0	0	0
Number of patients treated at dose[a]	3.3	4.8	4.9	2.5	0.4		—
True probability of toxicity	**0.25**[b]	0.53	0.69	0.79	0.84	0.88	—
Probability of selecting dose as appropriate	0.47	0.05	0	0	0	0	0.48
Number of patients treated at dose[a]	5.4	2.6	0.3	0	0	0	—

[a] The number of patients treated is not an integer because of averaging over the 4000 simulations.
[b] The bolded doses are those most likely to produce the desired rate of toxicity (25–33%).
Adapted from ref. 1.

to the next cohort if the rate of toxicity at the four previous dose levels had been 0/3, 0/3, 0/3, and 0/3 than if there had been only two previous cohorts with toxicity rates of 1/6 and 1/6. Yet the 3+3 does not make this distinction, and its inability to use all the data contributes to its propensity to select doses that are below those desired as judged by the 3+3 algorithm, as in the first two scenarios in Table 1.

2.2. Bayesian Learning (2–4)

Given the above, it seems useful to employ phase 1 designs that use all the available data. Bayesian methods are valuable in this regard. The Bayesian paradigm is built around observed data and parameters, which we will denote by θ. Parameters are theoretical quantities that, while they are not observed, characterize important aspects of the drug being investigated. An example of a parameter is the probability of complete remission or the probabilities of toxicity at various doses. An important aspect of the Bayesian paradigm is that parameters are random quantities, with probability distributions describing one's uncertainty about them. The Bayesian paradigm begins with a prior distribution, $p(\theta)$, that characterizes one's uncertainty about θ before conducting a trial and observing the data. The next object is the likelihood, $L(\text{data} \mid \theta)$, which describes the probability of observing any specified data given any value of θ. Examples of likelihoods include the binomial distribution for binary events and the normal or "bell-shaped" curve for continuous variables. The basic idea of the Bayesian paradigm is to combine the observed data with the prior to arrive at a "posterior" distribution of θ, which describes one's uncertainty about θ after observing the data. Bayes' theorem arrives at the posterior by multiplying the prior by the likelihood of observing the data given the parameter: $p(\theta \mid \text{data}) \propto L(\text{data} \mid \theta) \times p(\theta)$.

Thus, the Bayesian paradigm bases inferences on the probabilities of parameters or hypotheses given data, whereas conventional "frequentist" (*p*-value based) methods do the reverse.

When making decisions or inferences based on accruing data, Bayes' theorem may be applied repeatedly, with the posterior at each stage becoming the prior for the next stage. The probability distributions in this sequence become increasingly informative about θ as the data accumulate. This process, known as "Bayesian learning," is especially useful in sequential data monitoring during a clinical trial. At each of many times, the current posterior probability distribution may be used to make a variety of decisions, including modifying doses (as in a phase 1 trial), dropping an inferior treatment arm, unbalancing a randomization in favor of a treatment or treatments that have relatively superior performance, or terminating the trial early because of either superiority of a treatment or futility.

The Bayesian approach is properly contrasted with the conventional, "frequentist" approach, which in particular uses p-values as a basis for inferring strength of evidence. While Bayesians view θ as a random quantity, frequentists assume that θ is fixed, but unknown. For a given frequentist test of hypothesis, the p-value is defined as the probability, under the null hypothesis, of observing a value of the test statistic as extreme, or more extreme, than that actually observed. Many scientists erroneously believe that the p-value is the probability that the null hypothesis is true given the observed data. In fact, this intuitively appealing quantity is a Bayesian posterior probability, not a p-value. Calculation of a p-value involves both observed and unobserved data, because the definition of the p-value includes any data that might have been observed under a predetermined experimental design. An obvious logical flaw is that a given data set could give rise to two or more different p-values, depending on which design was intended. For observational data, where there is no experimental design, the p-value of a given test may be a wide variety of different quantities, depending on what sort of assumptions one makes about how the data arose and the manner in which putative hypotheses are formulated.

Once a frequentist experimental design is specified, the investigator is permitted to look at the accruing data only if and when an interim test is specified by the design. If this constraint is violated, then the p-value must be adjusted upward to account for the fact that a false-positive decision might have been made. Indeed, many "group sequential" designs have been described to deal with the issue of interim analyses. Each design's statistical rules are constructed so that, accounting for the interim analyses, the overall false-positive probability (Type I error) will be maintained below a desired level, typically, $p = 0.05$. In practice, this is done by performing the interim tests at p-values much smaller than 0.05. However, the same overall p-value can lead to different decisions depending on the particular design employed. Regardless of the type of boundary however, the frequentist method punishes the investigator for looking at data. Consider a trial designed to have overall Type I error of 0.05. If the investigator looks at the data at any unplanned times and performs a test at each look, it is possible that all of the planned 0.05 Type I error has been spent before the trial is completed. Thus, when new data become available thereafter, the frequentist approach makes no allowance for using it along with the previous data! The same problem arises in a frequentist design for a trial in which the final planned test yields a p-value of 0.051, but additional data are subsequently obtained that strengthen the evidence in favor of a difference. The frequentist approach does not permit these subsequent data to be used, since they were not obtained as part of the planned experiment.

In contrast, Bayesian inference utilizes all of the available data, with inferences based on posterior probabilities computed from observed data. In particular, Bayesian inference does not involve unobserved data and is not affected by the experimental design, i.e., the data enter inferences only through the likelihood function. Consequently, not only can posterior

Table 2
Bayesian Logistic Regression Design in Practice

Cohort	Assigned dose	Patients with toxicity	Mean P(tox) at 100	Mean P(tox) at 200	Mean P(tox) at 300	Mean P(tox) at 400	Mean P(tox) at 500	Mean P(tox) at 600
Prior	—	—	0.06	**0.25**	0.47	0.64	0.75	0.82
1	200	0	0.03	0.11	**0.26**	0.41	0.52	0.61
2	300	1	0.04	0.12	**0.29**	0.47	0.60	0.68
3	300	0	0.03	0.08	**0.19**	0.35	0.48	0.57
4	300	0	0.02	0.06	0.15	**0.28**	0.41	0.51
5	400							

P(tox), mean probability of toxicity. A cohort of three patients is always treated at the dose closest to the target 0.25 (boldface).
Adapted from ref. *1*.

probabilities be used as an explicit measure of support for a hypothesis, but Bayesian inference makes more logical sense than frequentist inference.

2.3. Bayesian Logistic Regression

The Bayesian logistic regression (BLR) method for phase 1 assumes that the probability of toxicity increases with dose (as in Table 1) according to a logistic regression model. Such models allow one to combine information from patients treated at different dose levels, with this "borrowing strength" allowing more reliable prediction of the toxicity to be expected if a patient receives a given dose. In the BLR method, a prior on θ, the probabilities of toxicities over a range of doses must be determined (Table 2, row 2). Typically, the physician specifies a reasonable expectation of the probability of toxicity at 2 doses, e.g., 200 and 500 in Table 2. This information may then be used to derive the prior on θ. Table 2 illustrates how the incoming data alter these priors to generate posteriors. Patients are treated in cohorts of three, and the desired dose is one that produces a toxicity rate closest to 0.25. Thus, the first three patients receive dose 200. If none of these three has toxicity, the mean probabilities of toxicity change (Table 2, row 3). Because the 300 dose is now the one most likely associated with a probability rate of 0.25, the next cohort of three patients is treated at this dose. The trial proceeds accordingly, with each posterior serving as a new prior, until 36 patients (12 cohorts) have been treated, with the selected dose then being the one whose mean probability of toxicity is closest to the target 0.25. Note that with BLR a dose can be revisited, unlike with the 3+3.

The superiority of the BLR to the 3+3 can be appreciated by contrasting their OC. Table 3 does so, using the same clinical scenarios as Table 1. With both the 3+3 and the BLR, the simulations assume a cohort size of three and a maximum of 36 patients. In each scenario, the BLR is more likely than the 3+3 to select the dose producing a mean toxicity rate closest to 0.25; these "probabilities of correct selection" are 0.41 vs 0.72 in the first scenario and 0.47 vs 0.96 in the second scenario (Table 3, rows 3 and 6, respectively). Note that in both scenarios the 3+3 treats many fewer patients than the BLR. These and many other simulations indicate that the 3+3 simply does not treat enough patients to arrive at correct conclusions. Since the dose decided on in phase 1 usually is not subject to change thereafter, the poor OC of the 3+3 have significant implications for phase 2 and 3, as well as for phase 1, trials.

Table 3
**Operating Characteristics of 3+3 Contrasted With Those of Bayesian Logistic
Regression (BLR) (4000 simulations per scenario for each method)**

Dose	100	200	300	400	500	600	No dose selected
True probability of toxicity	0.01	0.09	0.26	0.47	0.64	0.76	—
Probability of selecting dose as approprite	0.08[a] 0[b]	0.43 0.21	**0.41**[c] **0.72**[c]	0.07 0.06	0 0	0 0	0 0
Number of patients treated at dose	3.3[a] 0.2[b]	4.8 11.3	4.9 20.5	2.5 3.7	0.4 0.4	0 0	— —
True probability of toxicity	0.25	0.53	0.69	0.79	0.84	0.88	—
Probability of selecting dose as appropriate	**0.47**[a,c] **0.96**[b,c]	0.05 0.04	0 0	0 0	0 0	0 0	0.48 0
Number of patients treated at dose	5.4[a] 27.9[b]	2.6 7.6	0.3 0.5	0 0	0 0	0 0	— —

[a] The values in this row are those with the 3+3.
[b] The values in this row are those with BLR.
[c] The boldface values are the probabilities of correct selection.
Adapted from ref. *1*.

Under the circumstances, it seems reasonable to replace the 3+3 with model-based dose-finding methods such as the BLR or the continuous reassessment method (CRM) *(5–7)*. Like the BLR, the CRM is a Bayesian dose-finding algorithm that, unlike the 3+3, is based on a parametric model and a fixed target for the probability of toxicity. In general, the BLR and CRM have similar OC under a variety of clinical scenarios, such as those illustrated in Tables 1 and 3.

2.4. Accounting for Covariates

With either the 3+3, BLR, or CRM, patients entered on a phase 1 trial are regarded as interchangeable. In particular, once it is known that they qualify for the study based on performance status < Zubrod 3 and serum bilirubin and creatinine levels <2, no account is made for covariates. Yet, is well known that in phase 2 trials in AML, results are profoundly influenced by covariates ("prognostic factors") such as age. It seems intuitive that the same might be true in phase 1 studies. For example, at any given dose, there might be more concern about a toxicity rate of 1/3 than a rate of 2/3 if all the former patients were <40 years of age and if all the latter patients were >75. Similarly, it may be incorrect to assume that, for example, the probability of toxicity following administration of a drug that is excreted by the liver is the same in a patient with a serum bilirubin of 0.6 and a patient with a bilirubin of 1.4, even though both of these values are "normal." Thus, examining the covariates that were independent predictors of "dose-limiting toxicity" in phase 1 or 2 trials of paclitaxel, estramustine, carboplatin, cisplatin, docetaxel, irinotecan + tomudex, and tipifarnib, Rogatko et al. *(8)* found that while dose was indeed such a covariate, so were performance status and weight loss (paclitaxel), performance status and alkaline phosphatase (estramustine), total bilirubin (carboplatin), alkaline phosphatase (cisplatin), alkaline phosphatase and bilirubin (docetaxel), alkaline phosphatase, cigarette smoking, and creatinine (irinotecan + tomudex), and alkaline phosphatase and albumin (tipifarnib). All patients had a performance status of 0 or 1 and had normal, or near-normal, liver and kidney function. These data suggest that rather than attempting to identify a single dose, phase 1 studies might focus on identifying a range of doses, with the specific dose recommended depending on a patient's covariates. Efforts to develop such designs are in progress. Suffice it to say that these designs will require more patients than are usually used in phase 1 trials. Given our aforementioned views that these trials currently enroll too few patients to sustain good OC even without accounting for covariates, it seems that it is generally desirable to increase the number of patients treated in phase 1.

2.5. Monitoring Response and Toxicity (9)

Phase 1 trials typically use toxicity, while ignoring response, as the basis for determining the dose to be given in a subsequent phase 2 study. A patient, however, participates in a phase 1 trial to achieve a response, not "no toxicity." If there were no hope of a given patient achieving a response in a particular phase 1 trial, the trial would be unethical. We thus consider it appropriate to monitor rates of both efficacy and toxicity as a function of dose in phase 1 trials. The following "phase 1–2" design uses both response and toxicity to do dose finding. The underlying Bayesian model assumes that three outcomes are possible: response, which can be any measure of efficacy, toxicity, or neither. Toxicity is defined to be so severe that, if it occurs, any measure of efficacy is either irrelevant or impossible, the latter case occurring when toxicity is fatal. The investigator must specify a minimum acceptable probability of response, $\theta_R{}^*$, and a maximum acceptable probability of toxicity, $\theta_T{}^*$. For each possible dose, d, we denote the probabilities (Prob) of response and toxicity by $\theta_R(d)$ and $\theta_T(\mathbf{d})$. The posteriors of $\theta_R(d)$ and $\theta_T(d)$ are updated after the response/toxicity data are obtained from each successive cohort, and the posterior probabilities $\mathrm{Prob}[\theta_R(d) < \theta_R{}^* \mid \mathrm{data}]$, i.e., that the dose is inefficacious, and $\mathrm{Prob}[\theta_T(d) > \theta_T{}^* \mid \mathrm{data}]$, i.e., that the dose is too toxic, are computed for each d. A dose is considered acceptable only if neither of these two probabilities is large, and if there are several acceptable doses, the dose with the highest response rate is assigned to the next cohort. If no doses are considered acceptable, the trial ends. As usual, as the data accumulate, a dose found to be acceptable at one point in the trial may later become unacceptable, and vice versa (Bayesian learning, Table 2).

As an example, consider a trial of a new drug to be given as first "salvage" therapy in patients with AML whose first remission was less than 1 year. Response is defined as complete remission (CR)—but could be defined as CR + CRp, etc.—and toxicity implies grade 3–4 toxicity. The investigator set $\theta_R{}^* = 0.125$ and, based on clinical experience, $\theta_T{}^* = 0.30$. Each of the four doses $d = 1, 2, 3,$ or 4 is considered unacceptable if $\mathrm{Prob}[\theta_R(d) < 0.125 \mid \mathrm{data}] > 0.90$ or $\mathrm{Prob}[\theta_T(d) > 0.30 \mid \mathrm{data}] > 0.95$. This says that a dose is unacceptable provided that, based on the incoming data, it is highly likely to produce either a response rate < 0.125 or a toxicity rate >0.30, with the criterion probabilities 0.9 and 0.95 defining the term "highly likely" for response and toxicity, respectively. Successive cohorts of three patients are treated, up to a maximum of 15 cohorts (45 patients), with the first cohort receiving the lowest dose. OC for the 3+3 and the phase 1–2 for each of three dose–outcome scenarios are summarized in Table 4. Under scenario 1, both response rate and toxicity increase with dose, and both doses 3 and 4 are acceptable (true probabilities response and toxicity >0.125 and <0.30 respectively). The phase 1–2 (correctly) selects one of these doses in 89% of simulations vs 35% for the 3+3. The second scenario is particularly interesting; here all the doses produce

Table 4
Contrasting Operating Characteristics of the Phase 1–2 and 3+3 Designs

Scenario	Doses	Dose 1	Dose 2	Dose 3	Dose 4	None	No. of treated P1–2 /3+3
1	True θ_R/θ_T	0.02/0.10	0.05/0.15	0.15/0.25[a]	0.20/ 0.30[a]	—	44/13
	% selected P1–2	0	0.02	0.36	0.53	0.09	
	% selected 3+3	0.13	0.27	0.26	0.09	0.26	
2	True θ_R/θ_T	0.01/0.05	0.02/0.10	0.05/0.15	0.02/0.25	—	29/14
	% selected P1–2	0	0	0	0.14	0.86	
	% selected 3+3	0.05	0.13	0.26	0.12	0.44	
3	True θ_R/θ_T	0.01/0.45	0.05/0.50	0.05/0.65	0.20/0.75	—	24/6
	% selected P1–2	0.02	0.04	0	0	0.94	
	% selected 3+3	0.33	0.07	0	0	0.60	

[a]Acceptable doses are shown in boldface.
Adapted from ref. 9.

acceptable toxicity, but none produce acceptable efficacy. Because it looks only at toxicity, the 3+3 (incorrectly) selects a dose for further study in 56% of simulations, while, because it looks at response and toxicity, the phase 1–2 does so in only 14% of simulations. In the third scenario, all doses are too toxic and hence unacceptable, but dose 4 does meet the response standard (12.5%). Nonetheless, it is never selected by the phase 1–2, showing that the design is safe. The probability of (correctly) selecting no dose in this scenario is again higher with the phase 1–2 than the 3+3. Note that in all scenarios the 3+3 treats fewer patients; however, as noted, the price for this is a considerably higher probability of incorrect conclusions about which dose(s) are appropriate for further study.

OC describe average behavior of a design. Another useful way to evaluate a dose-finding design's performance is to examine the doses that it chooses for the second cohort based on each the possible outcomes that may be seen with the first cohort. These are given in Table 5 for the phase 1–2 design, along with the corresponding decisions made by the commonly used 3+3 algorithm. There are four cases (boldface in Table 5) where the two designs disagree. In each of these cases, the decision made by the phase 1–2 method appears more rational, bearing in mind the targeted minimum response rate of 12.5% and upper toxicity bound of 30%. When two or three patients respond, the phase 1–2 design stays at the same dose, which makes sense because these are highly successful outcomes In contrast, the 3+3 algorithm only uses the fact that there are 0/3 toxicities, and it escalates the dose. When two patients have toxicity, the 3+3 rule uses only the fact that there are 2/3 toxicities and terminates the trial, whereas the phase 1–2 design treats another cohort at the same dose level, essentially because there is a reasonable hope of achieving the 12.5% response rate while controlling toxicity at 30%. For example, if two of three patients have toxicity, the probability is 19% that the toxicity rate is below the 30% upper accepted bound. Of course, as new data accumulate, these decisions are revisited.

The importance of simulation cannot be overemphasized. Thus, the OC determined from the simulations are the basis of the maximum sample size, cohort size, and criterion probabilities (0.9 and 0.95 in the above trial).

Table 5
Decisions for the Second Cohort Based on Outcome in First Cohort

Number with response	Number with toxicity	Number with neither response nor toxicity	Phase 1–2 decision for second cohort	3+3 decision for second cohort
0	3	0	Stop the trial	Stop the trial
3	0	0	**Stay at dose 1**	**Escalate to dose 2**
2	1	0	Stay at dose 1	Stay at dose 1
2	0	1	**Stay at dose 1**	**Escalate to dose 2**
0	2	1	**Stay at dose 1**	**Stop the trial**
1	2	0	**Stay at dose 1**	**Stop the trial**
1	1	1	Stay at dose 1	Stay at dose 1
0	1	2	Stay at dose 1	Stay at dose 1
1	0	2	Escalate to dose 2	Escalate to dose 2
0	0	3	Escalate to dose 2	Escalate to dose 2

Adapted from ref. *9.*

2.6. Summary

The current phase 1 → phase 2 paradigm could be profitably replaced by designs such as the combined phase 1–2 design described in the preceding paragraph. Larger sample sizes (e.g., 36–48) are required than in the usual phase 1, although by replacing the need for the usual phase 2, the phase 1–2 probably requires no more patients than entered currently when adding the numbers accrued in phase 2 to those accrued in phase 1. There is a savings in time in that there is no need to organize separate phase 1 and phase 2 trials. Certainly, as demonstrated by simulation studies, modern phase 1 designs, e.g., BLR, enable more accurate dose finding than the current 3+3.

3. PHASE 2 DESIGNS

3.1. The Conventional Method

Phase 2 trials often are viewed as a means to decide whether an experimental treatment, E, is sufficiently promising to warrant a phase 3 trial comparing E with a "standard" treatment or treatments, which we denote by S. In fact, all phase 2 trials inherently involve comparison of E to S. Patients in particular are not as interested in whether E is active—the typical concern of a phase 2 trial—as in whether E is more active than another drug. However, when the data on E and S arise from separate trials, as is conventionally the case, rather than from a single randomized trial, any E-vs-S treatment effect is hopelessly confounded with latent, between-trial effects. The existence of these effects can be illustrated by noting that results can differ far beyond what might be attributed to the "play of chance" when the same treatment is given in two separate trials; these differences persist after adjustment for prognostic covariates *(2).* In fact, trial effects may be much larger than any actual treatment effects. If trial effects are ignored, an erroneous decision to proceed (or not proceed) to phase 3 may be based on a confounded trial-treatment effect that is mistakenly assumed to be an actual treatment effect. It is logically inconsistent that the need to avoid confounding trial and treatment effects is addressing by randomizing in phase 3, yet it is often ignored in the evaluation of phase 2 data that determines whether the phase 3 trial will be conducted in the first place.

The Simon two-stage design is probably the most widely used design for phase 2 trials *(10)*.The design specifies a rate of no interest (p_0) and a rate of interest (p_1); these rates derive from historical data, again suggesting the comparative nature of phase 2 trials. Simon himself has criticized the standard two-stage design, noting that p_0 is itself a statistic with a variance, rather than a fixed value as assumed in the original Simon design *(11)*. This follows from the relatively small number of patients given the historical treatment. Ignoring this fact means that the actual false-positive (type 1 error) and false-negative (type 2 error) rates are considerably higher than the nominal ones usually noted in protocols. This can be addressed only by an increase in sample size. Another problem with two-stage designs is that they permit only one interim look at incoming results. However, patients would prefer more frequent looks, and, in fact, it is commonly known that physicians frequently examine the accumulating data, although, as described below, such looks affect the inferences drawn at the conclusion of the trial, but are frequently not mentioned in the relevant publications. As noted in the section on Bayesian learning, Bayesian methodology provides a way around this dilemma.

3.2. A Bayesian Selection Design (12)

An infrequently discussed issue is that of selecting which treatment(s) should be investigated in a large-scale trial when a number of candidate treatments are available but the number of patients is limited. Thus, the investigator must decide whether to study a relatively small number of treatments, each accruing a large number of patients, or, conversely, a larger number of treatments each accruing a smaller maximum sample size. Currently, the former method seems preferred. Ideally, the strength of preclinical findings and the absence of between-trial effects would support the current method. Recent history, however, suggests that an *a priori* rationale cannot replace clinical observation. For example, α-interferon undoubtedly lengthens survival in chronic phase chronic myelogenous leukemia, although a satisfactory explanation has remained unavailable for 20 years. Similarly, 2-chlorodeoxyadenosine's efficacy in hairy cell leukemia was discovered quite unexpectedly. The original impulse to investigate arsenic trioxide in APL owed more to Chinese medical culture than to an understanding of the pathogenetic role of the PML-RARα fusion gene. Without discounting the importance of "bench-to-bedside" research, these examples suggest the importance of empiricism in the discovery of effective therapies. It follows that an alternative to the current practice is to randomize smaller numbers of patients among a greater number of therapies.

The selection design described below provides a Bayesian framework for the latter approach. The design randomizes patients among several experimental treatments, say E_1, ..., E_k, with parameters θ_1,..., θ_k. Each θ_j is compared with the parameter θ_S of a standard treatment, S, using historical data on S, hence the prior on θ_S does not change, there being no S arm in the trial to update, whereas the distributions of θ_1, ...,θ_k are updated throughout the trial. As each patient outcome in each of the E_j arms becomes known, the prior for that arm is updated and the resultant posterior is compared to θ_S. For ethical reasons, the priors on each experimental treatment must be identical. A minimum improvement to be provided by each E_j compared to S may be specified. If it appears highly unlikely that the specified improvement will result for a given E_j, accrual on that arm closes. The maximum sample size per arm may be set so that the final posterior of each θ_j will have a given level of reliability, say a 95% credibility interval of a given width. At the conclusion of the trial, the E_j with the highest posterior mean or median is selected for subsequent large-scale investigation, provided it appears reasonably likely to give the desired improvement over S. Including an S arm is straightforward, the only technical difference being that the distribution of θ_S also is updated as data on S are obtained.

We applied this design to a trial in which patients with untreated AML and abnormal karyotypes were randomized among four treatments: liposomal daunorubicin + ara-C (LDA) +/– thalidomide (thal) and LD + topotecan (LDT) +/– thal. In AML patients with abnormal cytogenetics, the historical CR rate at MDACC was 291/591 (49%), leading us to use a β (291,300) prior for θ_S (Fig. 1A). Note that although this distribution is quite concentrated around its mean of 0.49, it quantifies uncertainty about θ_S. In contrast, a frequentist formulation would view θ_S as the fixed quantity 0.49. The prior for each θ_j was assumed to also have mean 0.49, but with a much greater dispersion, reflecting the lack of knowledge about these treatments (Fig. 1A). The targeted improvement was 0.15, and thus the targeted average CR rate was 0.49 + 0.15 = 0.64. Accrual into any of the four arms, E_j, was to be stopped if, after each cohort of five patients was evaluated, Prob[θ_S + 0.15 < θ_j | data] < 0.10. This means that the targeted improvement is very unlikely, with the cutoff probability of 0.10 quantifying the phrase "very unlikely." This produces the rule that a given arm would be dropped if the [no. of CRs]/[no. of patients evaluated] ≤ 1/5, 4/10, or 7/15. Otherwise, each arm would accrue 20 patients, with this number chosen to provide an 80% posterior probability interval for θ_j having a width of <0.25, assuming an observed mean CR rate of 0.64. If accrual to an arm were stopped, all subsequent patients, up to a total of 80, would be randomized among the remaining arms, again with evaluation after each cohort of five patients using stopping rules derived from the above expression.

The design parameters thus consisted of the targeted improvement (0.15), the per-arm sample size (20), and the stopping criterion probability (0.10). As always, computer simulation is done and the OC determined to be sure that these parameters are sensible. Table 6 illustrates the OC for the four-arm selection trial. First consider the OC for each arm (intra-arm OC; Table 6A). These include the sample size, which is random because an arm may terminate early, and the probability of early termination (PET). The values in this and similar tables are the means of 4000–10,000 simulated trials. In the scenario where the true CR rate is 39%, i.e., 10% lower than historical and hence very undesirable, the PET is 85% and the median sample size is only 10 (Table 6). Thus, the design is appropriately protective. Similarly, if the true CR rate equals the historical mean of 49%, the PET is also reasonably high, 59%. In contrast, if the true CR rate is the desired 64%, the PET is only 18%; equivalently, there is an 82% chance the arm will not be (incorrectly) terminated. Considering the interarm OC (Table 6B), if the true CR rate in three of the arms is the historical mean 49% but is the desired 64% in the fourth arm, the probability of (correctly) selecting the fourth arm for future study, equivalently the probability that the arm will accrue at least 20 patients and will have the highest observed CR rate, is 63%. If, in contrast, the true CR rate in all four arms is the historical 49%, the probability of (correctly) selecting none of the arms for further study is 32%, reflecting the small sample size, but this increases to 84% if all four arms have true CR rate 39%. If these OC are considered unacceptable, the design parameters may be altered, for example, by raising the criterion probability from 0.10 to 0.15. However, this sort of change decreases the false-positive rate but also increases the false-negative rate, and in general better values for both rates can be obtained only with larger sample sizes. Note that our nominally high false-negative rate of 37% must be compared with what would obtain in the absence of the design. If one of the four treatments were randomly selected for a single-arm trial, the effective false-negative rate is 75%, and it is larger if the single-arm trial is run with early stopping rules. It is important to note that our design has the goal of selecting the best treatment, among those not dropped because of lack of efficacy, compared to the standard, regardless of the degree of difference between the best and the second best experimental

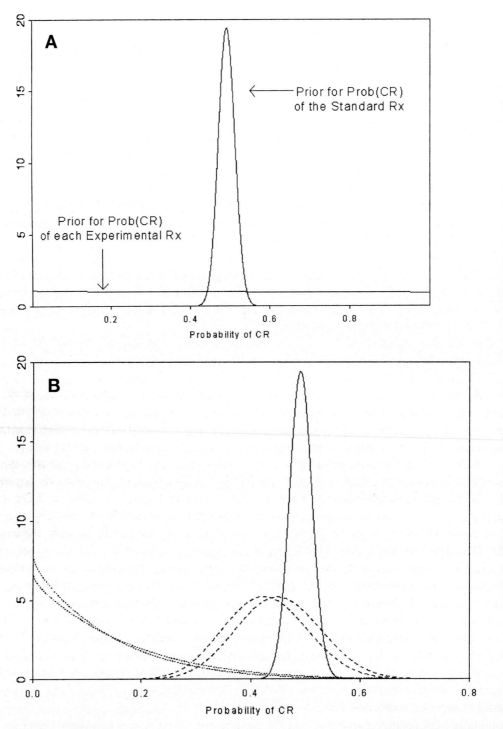

Fig. 1. **(A)** Prior probability distributions for the probability of complete remission (Prob(CR)) with standard treatment (S) and for each of the four experimental treatments (E).The mean of all distributions is 0.49, but the prior on S is informative given previous data in 591 patients, while the prior on each E is noninformative given the lack of data. **(B)** Posterior distributions for Prob(CR) with treatment arms LDT, LDT + thal, LDA, and LDA + thal after observing 0/6, 0/5, 18/40,and 17/40 CRs, respectively, compared with the prior Prob(CR) with S. The prior and posterior with S (solid line) are identical because no patients were

Table 6
Operating Characteristics (OC) of the Selection Design

A. Intra-arm OC

		Achieved sample size percentiles[b]		
True CR rate[a] (%)	Prob(early termination)	25th	50th	75th
39	0.85	5	10	15
49	0.59	10	15	20
64	0.18	20	20	20

B. Interarm OC

	Selection probabilities				
Clinical scenario	Arm 1	Arm 2	Arm 3	Arm 4	No arm
Arm 4 has true CR rate 64%, arms 1–3 have true CR rate 49%	0.09	0.09	0.09	0.63	0.10
All arms have true CR rate 49%	0.17	0.17	0.17	0.17	0.32
All arms have true CR rate 39%	0.04	0.04	0.04	0.04	0.84

[a]Mean historical CR (complete remission) rate = 49%.
[b]For example, with a true CR rate of 49%, in 25% of the 10,000 simulated trials, the sample size was 0–10, the median sample size was 15, and in another 25% of the trials the sample size was 20, the maximum.
Adapted from ref. 2.

treatment. This is very different from a design in which the goal is to decide whether the best treatment provides a specified degree of improvement over the others. Hypothesis-test-based designs have the latter goal, and the power of such a test is the probability that it correctly detects such an improvement. This type of goal requires a much larger sample size.

In the four-arm trial, accrual into the LDT and LDT + thal arms was stopped after the first six patients in LDT and the first five in LDT + thal failed to enter CR. Figure 1B depicts the resulting posterior probabilities. The figure shows that not only were LDT or LDT + thal unlikely to have the targeted 15% improvement over the historical CR rate, but they also were likely to be inferior to the LDA +/− thal arms. The remaining patients were randomized between the LDA and LDA + thal arms, which had observed CR rates of 18/40 and 19/40, respectively. The LDT arm had six rather than five patients, and the total sample size was 91 rather than 80, because of the 2-month time period required to evaluate each patient's CR.

The posterior probabilities that the two LDA arms are improvements are also small (Fig. 1B). Specifically, the posterior probability that LDA is on average 20% better than S is 0.001, and the posterior probability that it is 10% better is 0.039. The corresponding probabilities for LDA + thal are 0.0004 and 0.019. These probabilities, which have no frequentist (p-value-based) equivalent, led us to select none of the treatments for further study. These probabilities are much smaller than the designed cutoff of 0.10 because of the 2-month time lag between accrual and evaluation noted above.

---

given S in this trial. The curves for LDT and LDT + Th (dotted lines) remain relatively uninformative given the small sample sizes, but there is virtually no probability that the CR rates with these arms overlap the (higher) CR rates seen with S. The LDA and LDA + thal curves are more informative (dashed lines), and most of the probability density is to the left of the highest plausible CR rate produced by S. Thus, the posterior probability that LDA is 20% better than historical is 0.001, and the posterior probability that it is 10% better is 0.039. The corresponding probabilities for LDA + thal are 0.0004 and 0.019. (Adapted from ref. 2.)

An obvious advantage of the design was that it reduced exposure to LDT and LDT + thal. In contrast, suppose that a conventional Simon two-stage design (10) had been used within each of the four arms, for example to distinguish between response probabilities of 49% (the rate with S) and 64% (the desired 15% improvement) with Type I (false-positive) and Type II (false-negative) error rates of 10%. Using the "optimal" design, which minimizes average sample size when the response rate is "of no interest" (here 49%), 48 patients would have been treated in the first stage in each arm. Thus, 96 patients would have received LDT or LDT + thal, rather than 11. Because the LDA and LDA + thal arms would have gone on to the second stage, after which a total of 76 patients would have been treated in each of these arms, the overall sample size would have been 96 + 152 = 248, compared to the 91 treated here. Although the increase in sample size would have led to lower nominal false-positive and false-negative rates, the price would have been a less protective and much longer trial.

A difficulty with the randomized selection design is that it does not adaptively account for imbalances in prognostic covariates between patients on the different arms. Such an imbalance could occur as a result of the small sample sizes. This problem can be ameliorated by use of "dynamic allocation" when patients are randomized; for example, in the trial described above, we used such a scheme to achieve balance between arms with respect to cytogenetics, age, performance status, and presence of an antecedent hematological disorder. Finally, stopping after entry of a relatively small number of patients as in the LDT +/– thal arms could lead to failure to detect a small, perhaps biologically unique, subset of patients who might respond to a treatment, even though the average patient is highly unlikely to respond. It is unclear, however, whether any trial should proceed with such a goal in mind.

4. OTHER BAYESIAN DESIGNS

4.1. The Phase 2–3 Designs (13)

We have pointed out that using data from single-arm phase 2 trials to compare treatments introduces bias in the form of trial-treatment confounding. The need to avoid this problem in phase 3 makes it impossible to use any phase 2 data in the phase 3 comparisons. Even with randomization, however, decisions to move from phase 2 to phase 3 typically are based on early outcomes in phase 2, rather than survival or disease-free survival time. This requires the implicit assumption that the early outcome is to some extent associated with improved survival or disease-free survival. These problems motivated development of a new phase 2–3 design that randomizes between E and S throughout and makes repeated interim decisions during the trial based on both early response and survival time data. These decisions include (1) stopping the trial and concluding that E is associated with longer survival than S, (2) stopping the trial because of futility, i.e., concluding that E and S are associated with similar survival, (3) continuing the trial, or (4) expanding the phase 2 trial to incorporate other centers, at which point the "phase 3" trial begins. Accrual continues while the phase 3 trial is being organized, and the "seamless" nature of the phase 2–3 transition allows for the use of all phase 2 data in all phase 3 decisions.

4.2. Adaptive Randomization

Randomized trials are essential to minimize the confounding of treatment effects with the effects of latent, unobserved variables, when comparing a new therapy to a standard one However, randomization may be questioned on ethical grounds, especially when the standard treatment is suspected *a priori* to produce very poor results. Adaptive randomization (AR), which may be done using straightforward Bayesian criteria, satisfies both the scientific imperative of randomization to obtain unbiased comparisons and the desire to reduce the number of patients randomized to an ineffective therapy. In AR, the first group of patients is randomized with equal probability between two or more treatments. Thereafter, the AR algorithm uses the updated data from previous patients to favor the treatment that, in terms of the interim data, has on average superior outcomes. This design has been applied to a trial comparing troxacitabine + ara-C, troxacitabine + idarubicin, and idarubicin + ara-C for treatment of older patients with newly diagnosed AML *(14)*.

4.3. Multicourse Treatment Strategies (15)

A pervasive problem is that conventional phase 2 and phase 3 designs entirely ignore the possibility that administration of one therapy may affect outcome with a subsequent therapy. For example, because targeted therapies may affect multiple targets, a therapy directed at target X may also down/upregulate target Y, thereby influencing response to a future therapy aimed at Y. Debate often revolves around whether a less toxic, but potentially less curative therapy should be given a chance to fail before use of the more toxic and hence putatively more curative therapy. For example, should young patients with chronic myeologenous leukemia receive imatinib mesylate prior to allogeneic transplantation, or vice versa? Similarly, older patients with untreated AML might have a lower mortality rate if they receive a relatively nontoxic targeted therapy (A) first, and receive a cytotoxic therapy (B) only should A fail. However, the reverse B $\rightarrow$ A approach might be preferable if B's anti-AML effect is significantly greater than A's, outweighing any reduction in toxicity with the A $\rightarrow$ B strategy. In all of these cases, the issue is evaluation of a multicourse treatment strategy, rather than a particular treatment. Specifically, the question is which is the preferable sequence of treatments. Conventional statistical designs, however, regard each therapy as a distinct entity, and in particular they ignore the issue of the sequence in which two or more therapies are administered. As is the case with many current designs, this approach wastes information.

To address this problem we developed a design that incorporates historical data while accommodating multiple treatment courses, a trinary outcome in each course (CR, death, neither), and prognostic covariates. Based on a real-valued function of probabilities of CR and death, the methodology, within prognostic subgroups, drops inferior treatment strategies during the trial and selects the best two-course strategy at the end. We intend to apply this design to a trial in patients over age 59 with high-risk myelodysplastic syndrome. Patients are to be randomized among clofarabine + ara-C (CA), PKC412 (P) + low-dose ara-C (LDAC), tipifarnib (T) + LDAC, and low-dose decitabine(D). CA is considered a "high-intensity" option, while P-LDAC, T-LDAC, and D are considered "low-intensity." Patients not achieving at least major hematological improvement (International Working Group Criteria) after 3 months on CA are rerandomized among P-LDAC, T-LDAC, and D. Patients in whom the three low-intensity options are similarly unsuccessful receive CA. (This decision reflects reluctance to give patients two successive low-intensity therapies.) Thus, there are six strategies that can be analyzed: CA followed at failure by P-LDAC, T-LDAC, or D, and CA after failure of P-LDAC, T-LDAC, or D. Thus, we would be able to detect, for example, that CA is a better salvage therapy if preceded by P-LDAC than by T-LDAC.

5. CONCLUSION

There is an immense statistical literature on methods for the design and conduct of clinical trials. The conventional phase 1-2-3 paradigm remains the standard, with the great majority of trials classified as phase 1, phase 2, or phase 3. While the explanation for this practice

Table 7
Inadequacies of Conventional Designs Contrasted With Proposed Bayesian Alternatives

Trial type	Conventional	Bayesian
Phase 1	**3+3**	**Bayesian logistic regression, CRM**
	1) Ignores information from all cohorts except most recent	1) Uses information from all cohorts
	2) Treats too few patients	2) Generally treats more patients
	Result—dose selected less likely to produce specified amount of toxicity and hence less likely to be efficacious (assuming response between toxicity and response)	**Result**— more likely to select an effective dose
Phase 2	**Simon two-stage**	**Various Bayesian**
	1) Because p-values are tied to trial design, typically allows only one interim look so as to be able to preserve desired false-positive rate	Because they are not tied to design, Bayesian posterior probabilities are more flexible, in particular allowing more frequent monitoring, montoring of multiple outcomes, and derivation of predictive probabilities
	2) Rate of no interest derived from (relatively little) historical data is assumed to be a constant, rather than a statistic	
	Result—insufficiently adaptive; actual false-negative and false-positive rates often higher than nominal rates	**Result**—more adaptive; more relevant to realities of medical practice
Phase 1–2	—	Allows monitoring of both response and toxicity with typically 36–48 maximum sample size; thus is more efficient than typical sequence of phase 1 followed by phase 2

CRM, continuous reassessment method.

is unclear, it continues to have numerous undesirable effects. By ignoring the sort of multiplicities described here, standard methods often reduce clinical trial designs to abstractions that ignore many important aspects of the medical phenomena and waste potentially useful information. Consequently, important issues, such as how to select among various available treatments, the phase 2 aspect of phase 1 trials (and vice versa), the waste of phase 2 data in phase 3, the multi-course nature of therapeutics, etc., are not addressed. Questions that are addressed may be answered incorrectly, e.g., as consequences of using unreliable methods for dose finding in phase 1, basing comparisons on biased data from single-arm phase 2 trials, etc. In addition to their scientific flaws, conventional methodology often serves patients poorly. Patients are vitally interested in adaptive monitoring of response and toxicity, yet are entered into trials that are considerably less than fully adaptive. Our examples demonstrate that the Bayesian paradigm provides an ideal structure for accommodating the requisite complexity and more frequent data monitoring. Whether or not investigators adopt Bayesian methods, however, we are convinced that the inadequacy of current approaches should no longer be ignored (Table 7).

ACKNOWLEDGMENTS

The author has benefitted greatly from many discussions and collaborations with Dr. Don Berry and, especially, Dr. Peter Thall, both of the Department of Biostatistics and Applied Mathematics at the University of Texas M.D. Anderson Cancer Center.

REFERENCES

1. Thall P, Lee SJ. Practical model-based dose-finding in phase 1 clinical trials: methods based on toxicity. Int J Gynecol Cancer 2003;13:251–261.
2. Estey EH, Thall PF. New designs for phase 2 clinical trials. Blood 2003;102:442–448.
3. Berry DA. Statistical innovations in cancer research. In: Holland J et al., eds. Cancer Medicine, 6th ed. London: BC Decker, 2003;465–478.
4. Berger JO, Berry DA. Statistical analysis and the illusion of objectivity. Am Scientist 1988;76:159–165.
5. O'Quigley J, Pepe M, Fisher L. Continual reassessment method: a practical design for phase 1 clinical trials in cancer. Biometrics 1990;46:33–48
6. Piantadosi S, Fisher JD, Grossman S. Practical implementaion of a modified continual reassessment method for dose-finding trials. Cancer Chemother Pharmcol 1998;41:429–436.
7. Moller S. An extension of the continual reassessment method using a preliminary up-and-down design in a dose-finding study in cancer patints, in order to investigate a greater range of doses. Stat Med 1995;14:911–922.
8. Rogatko A, Babb JS, Wang H, Slifker MJ, Hudes GR. Patient characteristics compete with dose as predictors of acute treatment toxicity in early phase clinical trials. Clin Cancer Res 2004;10:4645–4651.
9. Thall P, Estey E, Sung H-G. A new statistical method for dose-finding based on efficacy and toxicity in early phase clinical trials. Invest New Drugs 1999;17:155–167.
10. Simon R. Optimal two-stage designs for phase II clinical trials. Controlled Clin Trials 1989;10:1–10.
11. Thall P, Simon R. Incorporating historical control data in planning phase 2 clinical trials. Stat Med 1990; 9:215–228.
12. Thall PF, Estey E. A Bayesian strategy for screening cancer treatments prior to Phase II clinical evaluation. Stat Med 1993;12:1197–1211.
13. Inoue LYT, Thall PF, Berry DA. Seamlessly expanding a randomized phase II trial to phase III. Biometrics 2002;58:823–831.
14. Giles FJ, Kantarjian HM, Cortes JE, et al. Adaptive randomized study of idarubicin and cytarabine versus troxacitabine and cytarabine versus troxacitabine and idarubicin in untreated patients 50 years or older with adverse karyotype acute myeloid leukemia. J Clin Oncol 2003;21:1722–1727.
15. Thall PF, Sung H-G, Estey EH. Selecting therapeutic strategies based on efficacy and death in multi-course clinical trials. J Am Statist Assoc 2002;97:29–39.

Index